Ashford

D0364162

WM 1886 H0601003 II

AMB

Sleep Disorders: A clinical textbook

The editors have made every effort to ensure the accuracy of drug dosage and other information contained in this book. However, this does not diminish the requirement to exercise clinical judgment, and the editors and publisher cannot accept responsibility for the use of the information in clinical practice.

The editors and publisher gratefully acknowledge the permission granted to reproduce the copyright material in this book. Every effort has been made to trace copyright holders and to obtain their permission for the use of copyright material. The publisher apologizes for any errors or omissions in this book and would be grateful if notified of any corrections that should be incorporated in future reprints or editions.

Sleep Disorders: A clinical textbook

edited by Antonio Ambrogetti, Michael Hensley and Leslie Olson

Ann

WM 168 H0601003

QUAY
BOOKS

A division of MA Healthcare Ltd

Quay Books Division, MA Healthcare Ltd, St Jude's Church, Dulwich Road, London SE24 0PB

British Library Cataloguing-in-Publication Data
A catalogue record is available for this book

© MA Healthcare Limited 2006
ISBN 1 85642 237 2

All rights reserved. No part of this publication may be reproduced, stored in a retrieval system or transmitted in any form or by any means, electronic, mechanical, photocopying, recording or otherwise, without prior permission from the publishers

Printed in Malta by Gutenberg Press Limted, Gudja Road, Tarxien PLA 19, Malta

Contents

List of contributors

Dr Antonio Ambrogetti MD, FRACP is Medical Consultant to Sleep Medicine, Charlestown, NSW and Visiting Medical Officer, Respiratory and Sleep Medicine at the John Hunter Hospital, Newcastle, Australia.

Dr Nicholas Antic MBBS, FRACP is Staff Specialist Respiratory Physician at the Adelaide Institute for Sleep Health, Repatriation General Hospital, Daw Park, South Australia.

Dr Liat Ayalon PhD is Fellow in the Department of Psychiatry, School of Medicine, University of California, San Diego, USA and at the Institute for Fatigue and Sleep Medicine, Sheba Medical Center, Ramat Gan, Israel.

Dr Delwyn Bartlett PhD is Research and Consultant Psychologist at the Woolcock Institute of Medical Research, Camperdown, NSW, Australia.

Dr Vincenza Castronovo PhD is a Psychologist at the Sleep Disorders Centre, IRCCS, H San Raffaele, Milano, Italy.

Dr Yaron Dagan MDDSC is Director of the Institute for Fatigue and Sleep Medicine, Sheba Medical Center, Ramat Gan, Israel.

Dr Huw Davies MB, BS, FRACP is Senior Consultant, Respiratory Medicine at the Repatriation General Hospital and Flinders Medical Centre, South Australia, Australia.

Dr Elizabeth Ellis MPhys, BHealth Law, PhD is Senior Lecturer at the Faculty of Health Sciences, University of Sydney, Sydney, Australia.

Professor Ron Grunstein MB, BS, PhD, FRACP is Head of the Sleep Research Group, Woolcock Institute of Medical Research, University of Sydney, Australia and Head of the Centre for Respiratory Faliure and Sleep Disorders, Royal Prince Alfred Hospital, Missenden Road, Camperdown, NSW, Australia.

Professor Michael Hensley MB, BS(Hons), PhD, FRACP, FAFHM is Dean of the Newcastle Medical School, The University of Newcastle, Newcastle and Director of the Newcastle Sleep Disorders Centre, John Hunter Hospital, Newcastle, Australia.

Dr David Hillman MB, BS, FRANZCA is Head of the Department of Pulmonary Physiology at the Sir Charles Gairdner Hospital, Verdun Street, Nedlands, Western Australia, Australia and Director of the WA Sleep Disorders Research Institute, Queen Elizabeth II Medical Centre, Nedlands, Western Australia, Australia.

Dr Lata Jayaram FRACP is Staff Specialist Respiratory Physician at the South Auckland Clinical School, Middlemore Hospital, Otahuhu, Auckland, New Zealand.

Associate Professor Doug McEvoy MBBS, MD, FRACP is Director of the Adelaide Institute for Sleep Health, Repatriation General Hospital, Daw Park, South Australia, Australia.

Dr Leslie Olson MB, BS, BSc(Med), Mlitt, PhD, FRACP is Senior Lecturer at the Faculty of Health, The University of Newcastle, Newcastle, Australia.

Amanda Piper PhD is Senior Physiotherapist at the Centre for Respiratory Failure and Sleep Disorders, Royal Prince Alfred Hospital, Camperdown, NSW, Australia and Research Fellow at the Woolcock Institute of Medical Research, Camperdown, Australia.

Dr Karen Waters FRACP, PhD is Director of the Paediatric Sleep Unit, The New Children's Hospital, Paramatta, NSW, Australia.

Introduction

Sleep medicine is a well-established science which has developed through the contributions of many health professionals, including among others, physiologists, psychologists, psychiatrists, neurologists and respiratory physicians. There are a great many journals and books which set out our current understanding of sleep and wakefulness from the perspective of physiology, psychology, neurology and respiratory medicine. We do not aim to add to their number.

This book is concerned with the clinical aspects of sleep disorders. It provides a description of the investigation of patients presenting with sleep complaints and their treatment in the event that a sleep disorder turns out to be the problem. The book is predominantly symptom-based, providing the easiest possible reference for health practitioners.

Each chapter is intended to be used independently and, therefore, a degree of repetition occurs throughout the book.

The first four chapters provide an introduction to basic science and its correlation with clinical practice. The second part of the book addresses the most common complaints reported by patients.

This textbook will be useful both to students of health science and to those practitioners who have no specialist training in sleep and wake disorders but who meet, on a daily basis, patients who might have sleep disorders. If we convince the reader of nothing else, we hope to convince him/her that this means that all healthcare practitioners form part of our primary audience — the only exceptions being those with specialist training in sleep disorders.

Antonio Ambrogetti
September 2005

Part I: The science behind sleep disorders

CHAPTER I

Neuroanatomy and pharmacology of sleep: clinical implications

Antonio Ambrogetti

A basic knowledge of the neuroanatomical structures of the sleep and wake function, its physiology and neurochemistry is important for clinicians to understand and identify presenting symptoms and to undertake rational treatment. This information enables the physician to explain: why emotions trigger cataplexy; why selective serotonin reuptake inhibitors (SSRIs) are useful in its treatment; why the sleep and wake function is deranged in some neurodegenerative diseases, such as Parkinson's disease or Alzheimer's dementia; and why warm feet help falling asleep.

This chapter contains a brief summary of the current understanding of the anatomical structures involved in sleep and wake regulation. Pictorial descriptions have been included where possible. It should be noted that the sleep and wake function is an integral part of the autonomic nervous system and is, therefore, intimately related to cardiorespiratory, neuroendocrine and metabolic control.

Introduction

Observation and interest in sleep, particularly dreams, can be traced back to the first documents of human history. However, initial observers were more interested in the 'soul' and 'mind', rather than sleep itself, which was taken for granted. The question of why we sleep is a recent one, and one that remains unanswered.

Sleep and wakefulness, as a distinct function within the medical science is only a recent definition compared with other systems, eg. cardiovascular, respiratory and renal. Understanding of these functions has benefited from recognizable anatomical structures, awareness of their physiology and connection between physio-anatomical abnormalities and clinical syndromes.

Sleep and wake function, similar to psychiatry, has suffered from the lack of easily identifiable macro-anatomy, and the mechanistic dualism of mind and body, whereby certain clinical syndromes, such as hysteria and insomnia, were labelled 'functional', meaning they were to do with the mind rather than the body.

Until the second half of the twentieth century, sleep was considered a passive phenomenon, with different theories about it being influenced by the prevailing ideas at the time (Thorpy,

2000). Although the central nervous system was considered a centre for sleep and wakefulness (consciousness), its function was seen as a passive conductive system (*Figure 1.1*) of external energy, usually light, conveyed through the eyes into the body and responsible for visual images and motor activity. Withdrawing the external input at night would lead to the winding down of the body and eventually to sleep.

The view of the brain and the nervous system as a passive relay started changing towards the end of the nineteenth century. The work of Camillo Golgi and Ramon Y Cajal showed it was not a network of connecting wires (syncytium), but rather a series of discrete, interconnecting cells with arborization, passing information from one cell to another via their axons and dendrites. About the same time, the ability to record electrical activity from the brain changed the idea of the brain being a passive organ to an active one capable of internally generating activity.

In the second half of the nineteenth century, a series of technical advances in neurophysiology, including electroencephalography (EEG) scalp recording, intracellular recording and electrical stimulation of the brain, provided the methodology needed to increase knowledge on sleep. The most important contribution, however, to understanding sleep organization came from the clinical observation of Constantine von Economo during the 'influenza' epidemic of 1917.

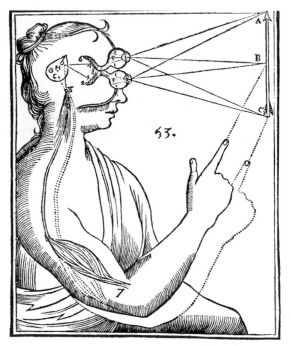

Figure 1.1: The energy (light) from the object reaches the pineal gland, considered the site of the soul by Rene Descartes, through the retina and the cerebral ventricles. The energy is then conveyed to the arm producing its movement. (Clarke and Dewhurst, 1996). Reprinted from 'Biologic Rhythms in Clinical and Laboratory Medicine', Y Touitou and E Haus, Figure 2, 1992 © Springer-Verlag.

Some of von Economo's patients manifested profound sleepiness, while others had severe insomnia. Following examination of the patient's brain, he concluded that lesions in the posterior area of the hypothalamus were associated with sleepiness and in the anterior hypothalamus with lack of sleep. Although the observation of lethargy associated with brainstem lesions had been previously reported (Hobson, 1995), von Economo concluded that these discrete 'areas' of the brain were actively involved in regulating wakefulness and sleep, moving away from a view of sleep as a passive phenomenon. It took a further 50 years for this view to be fully accepted.

Following von Economo's observations, a series of brain transection experiments, conducted by Frederick Bremer, were seen as evidence that sleep was a passive phenomenon due to withdrawal of proprioceptive and somatotropic sensory input (deafferentation theory). A transection in the upper brainstem (*Figure 1.2*) at the level of the superior colliculus (isolated forebrain) in the cat was associated with continuous sleep state, characterized by constricted pupils and, in a later experiment, by a slow EEG with spindling as seen during sleep (sleep spindles are EEG markers of stage 2 sleep onset).

This experiment seemed to confirm the idea that sleep resulted from withdrawal of sensory input. However, further experiments with section in the area between the spinal cord and the medulla (isolated brain), showed maintenance of sleep and wake cycling. Any doubts raised by these findings as to the soundness of the deafferentation theory of sleep were quelled by the explanation that sensory input from the cranial nerve was sufficient to maintain an awake state. This view was eventually disproved in the late 1940s.

Giuseppe Morruzzi and Horace Magoun demonstrated that electrical stimulation of a poorly localized group of neurons in the brainstem, which they called reticular formation (ascending reticular activating system) caused behavioral and EEG signs of arousal (*Figure 1.2*). It was also shown that selective lesions of the sensory input of the brainstem that did not damage the reticular formation, did not alter the sleep and wake pattern; but that selective lesions of the reticular activating system led to a prolonged sleep-like state (Lindsley *et al*, 1950; Lindsley *et al*, 1949).

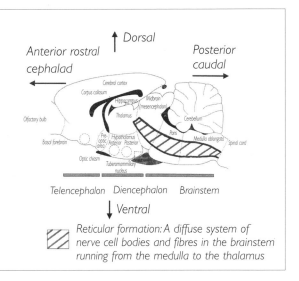

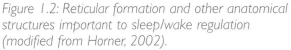

Figure 1.2: Reticular formation and other anatomical structures important to sleep/wake regulation (modified from Horner, 2002).

By the 1950s, wakefulness was shown to be an active process generated by the central nervous system, confirming the clinical observation and prediction of von Economo. Further, in the early 1940s, Walter Rudolf Hess showed that electrical stimulation of the thalamic area in cats induced an EEG pattern of sleep, confirming that sleep, like being awake, was an active function of the nervous system. It should be noted that damage of thalamic nuclei has been recently associated with the rare prion disease, fatal familial insomnia.

In 1953, rapid eye movement during sleep (Aserinski and Kleitman, 1953) was described, setting the scene for sleep as a dynamic circadian state, leading to the current definitions of wakefulness, slow-wave sleep, sleep (non-rapid-eye-movement [NREM] sleep) and paradoxical sleep (REM sleep).

During the twentieth century, other lines of research had emerged looking for *hypnotoxin* (sleep factors). These substances would accumulate in the body when awake, leading to sleep when a certain threshold was reached. The breaking down of these molecules during sleep would eventually lead to waking. This hypothesis made sense given that the process of falling asleep is somewhat gradual and slow (minutes) in keeping with a metabolic process, compared to the speed of neurons electrical transmission (milliseconds). In the early 1900s, research revealed that spinal fluid from sleep-deprived dogs, infused in the brain of a normal dog, induced sleep in the recipient. This observation led to the concept of *humoral* regulation of sleep and initiated a field of research in 'sleep factors' which is still ongoing (Hayaishi, 2000; Kimura *et al*, 2001).

Regulation of sleep and wakefulness should be seen in the context of autonomic nervous system function with interplay between cardiovascular and respiratory control, endocrine and metabolic homeostasis, immune system and circadian rhythm control. Taken within this context, it is hardly surprising that many molecules involved with immune and neuroendocrine regulation affect sleep and wakefulness (*Table 1.1*) (Dickstein and Moldofsky, 1999; Kimura *et al*, 2001; Kreuger and Karnovski, 1995; Steiger and Holsboer, 1997).

Table 1.1: Neuromodulators of sleep and wakefulness

Sleep-promoting molecules	Sleep-inhibiting molecules
• Interleukin-1 (IL-1)	• Interleukin-10 (IL-10)
• Tumour necrosis factor	• Corticotrophin releasing hormone (CRH)
• Prostaglandin D2	• Adrenocorticotropin hormone (ACTH)
• Growth hormone-releasing hormone (GHRH)	• Somatomedin
• Neuropeptide Y	• Thyrotropin-releasing hormone (TRH)
• Vasoactive intestinal peptide (VIP)	
• Delta sleep-inducing peptide (DSIP)	
• Uridine	

In modern neurophysiology, the search for sleep-related molecules centres on the study of neuro-transmitters, which mediate the activation and inhibition of the neuro pathways subserving sleep and wakefulness (see below). It is likely that many of these substances have modulatory effects on the sleep and wake function. Interleukin-1 (IL-1) seems to be a common sleep-promoting mediator for other molecules (Dickstein and Moldofsky, 1999). Substances such as growth hormone-releasing hormone (GHRH), neuropeptide Y, corticotropin-releasing hormone (CRH) and vasoactive intestinal peptide (VIP) also appear to be instrumental in the interaction between sleep and the neuroendocrine system.

Sleep and wake control

The mechanism of regulation of sleep and wake functions is located in the part of the brain which, from a phylogenetic point of view, derives from the primitive (reptilian) brain (*Figures 1.3* and *1.4*) and, to some degree, the paleomammalian/limbic system. The primitive brain contains the reticular formation and a group of more localized nuclei in the brainstem which regulates autonomic functions including, cardiorespiratory, endocrine, metabolic (including temperature control), as well as sleep and wakefulness.

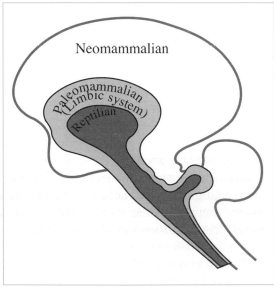

Figure 1.3: Phylogenetic zones of brain development (Salloway et al, 1997).

The limbic system is closely connected to the primitive brain and it is concerned with emotional response (mood, affect, and motivation). The neo-mammalian (neocortex) subserves higher functions and feeds back to the subcortical structures but has no primary function in sleep control.

Although wakefulness, slow-wave sleep and REM sleep constitute an integrated system, it is useful to consider them separately.

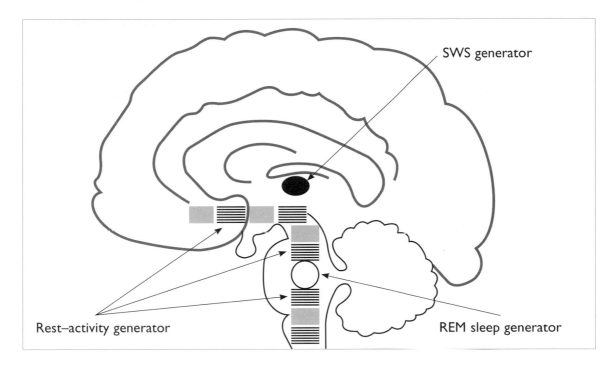

*Figure 1.4: Brainstem, hypothalamic and thalamic areas involved in sleep and wake regulation (reprinted from Sleep Medicine Reviews **5**(4) Lugaresi and Provini, 'Clinical Features and Pathophysiological Implications': 320. © 2001 with permission from Elsevier Science).*

The wake system

The state of being awake is actively driven by the interplay of aminergic neurons (norepinephrine/ noradrenaline, histamine, serotonin, dopamine neurons), cholinergic activity and the excitatory amino acid glutamate. These factors modulate the arousal system activity upward by increasing sensory input from the spinal cord, in particular auditory and pain input (Steriade, 1992). A recently described system, the orexin (hypocretin) system, which also interacts with the above neurons, appears to be an important modulator of alertness (*Table 1.2*).

Central to wake and sleep regulation is the activity of the thalamic reticular formation. This is essentially an extension of the reticular system of the brainstem around the thalamic nuclei. These cells contain the inhibitory neurotransmitter gamma-aminobutyric acid (GABA) and galanin — the GABA being the main inhibitory neurotransmitter in the brain. Activation of the thalamic reticular nuclei reduces stimulation input to the thalamus itself and the cortex, favoring sleep onset, including the appearance of spindles on the EEG (*Chapter 4, Figure 4.17*). This function has been described as a 'gate function'. When the neurons of the thalamic reticular nuclei are not active, the gate is open and cortical activation (wakefulness) is enhanced. When these neurons are active, the gate is closed and activation of the cortical structure is reduced, favoring sleep onset.

Table 1.2: Wake-promoting molecules	
Transmitter	**Predominant location**
• Norepinephrine (NE)	• Locus ceruleus
• Dopamine	• Midbrain
• Serotonin 5-HT	• Dorsal raphe nuclei
• Histamine (HA)	• Hypothalamus (posterolateral)
• Acetylcholine (ACh)	• Mesopontine areas and basal forebrain
• Glutamate	• Midbrain and thalamus
• Orexin (hypocretin)	• Hypothalamus (posterolateral)

The aminergic and cholinergic neurons promote the wake cycle in two ways:

- their input has an inhibitory action on the thalamic reticular nuclei: they open the gate (*Figure 1.5*)
- they have a direct activation effect on the cortex.

The aminergic neurons (*Figures 1.6, 1.7* and *1.10*) are active during the wake cycle and, when there is motor activity (serotonin), they reduce their firing during slow-wave sleep and cease activity during REM.

Histamine neurons are localized in the posterior hypothalamus (tuberomammillary area) and project rostrally to the preoptic area (Lin, 2000) and the cholinergic and aminergic neurons in the midbrain and pons (*Figure 1.8*).

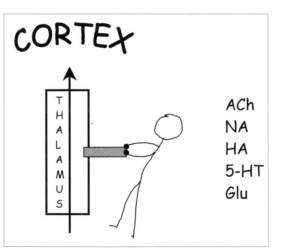

Figure 1.5: The thalamo-cortical gate is kept open by the depolarizing influence of acetylcholine (ACh), noradrenaline (NA), histamine (HA), serotonin (5-HT) and glutamate (Glu).

Animal studies suggest that histamine type 1 (H1) and 2 (H2) receptors facilitate cortical activation and, therefore, mediate the wake cycle. Histamine 3 (H3) receptors are autoreceptors and down-regulate their own activity. The sleep-promoting action of antihistamine medications is likely to be mediated by action on H1 receptors (and possibly H2).

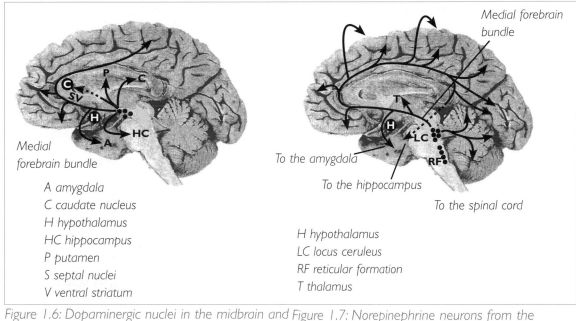

A amygdala
C caudate nucleus
H hypothalamus
HC hippocampus
P putamen
S septal nuclei
V ventral striatum

H hypothalamus
LC locus ceruleus
RF reticular formation
T thalamus

Figure 1.6: Dopaminergic nuclei in the midbrain and their connection to the thalamus and the ventral path to the basal forebrain. Reprinted from 'The Human Brain', 2nd edn, Nolte and Angevine. © (2000) reprinted with permission from Elsevier Science.

Figure 1.7: Norepinephrine neurons from the locus ceruleus and reticular formation, and their connections to the cortex (activating) directly through the ventral basal forebrain, and indirectly through the thalamus. Reprinted from 'The Human Brain', 2nd edn, Nolte and Angevine. © (2000) reprinted with permission from Elsevier Science.

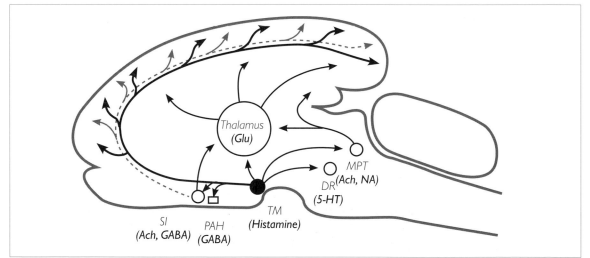

Figure 1.8: Histamine neurons and their connections: ACh, acetylcholine; DR, dorsal raphe nuclei; GABA gamma-aminobutyricacid; 5-HT 5-hydroxytryptamine (serotonin); MPT, mesopontine tegmentum; NE norepinephrine; PAH preoptic-anterior hypothalamus; SI substantia innominata; TM, tuberomammillary nuclei. Reprinted from Sleep Medicine Reviews, 4(5) Lin JS, 'Brain structures and mechanisms involved in the control of cortical activation and wakefulness, with emphasis on the posterior hypothalamus and histaminergic neurons: 471–503. © (2000) with permission from Elsevier Science.

Animal experiments suggest that antagonists of H3 receptors, which increase activity of histaminergic neurons by reducing autoinhibition, promote alertness. It is possible that H3 antagonists may be a third group of clinically useful alertness-enhancing compounds, apart from amphetamine and non-amphetamine (eg. modafinil) medication.

Acetylcholine has a more complex role, both in wakefulness and REM sleep. Cholinergic neurons are active both in wakefulness, promoting cortical activation through the thalamus and directly through the forebrain (*Figure 1.9*), and in REM sleep, through the cholinergic neurons in the pons (see below).

The serotonin and orexins (hypocretins) deserve examination, the latter because of their possible diagnostic role in hypersomnolence syndromes, and serotonin as the subject of extensive studies as well as its public profile.

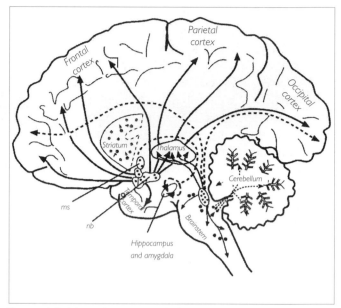

*Figure 1.9: Note that some cholinergic neurons from the pons relay in the thalamus, while others have direct connections with the cortex. Similarly, the cholinergic neurons from the basal forebrain connect with the thalamus, and directly with the cortex, including the limbic system. Reprinted from Trends in Neurosciences **22**, Perry et al, 'Acetylcholine in mind': 273–280. © 1999 with permission from Elsevier Science.*

Serotonin

The story of serotonin is complex but interesting, as it has been variously defined as a promising sleep-inducing substance and as a neurotransmitter involved, among other activities, in the wake cycle and motor behavior regulation (Jacobs and Fornal, 1999; Jouvet, 1999).

Serotonin was discovered by Vittorio Erspamer at the University of Pavia in the early 1930s in the enterocromaffin cells of the gastrointestinal tract, where it causes contraction of smooth muscle. He called the substance enteramine (Whitaker-Azmitia, 1999). The same substance was isolated in the late 1940s from a serum sample during research on hypertension and possible vasoconstrictors. The molecular structure was identified as 5-hydroxytryptamine (5-HT) and it was re-named 'serotonin'. Serotonin was recognized as a neurotransmitter in 1953 and since then it has been implicated in multiple functions, including sleep regulation, anxiety, sexual behavior, depression and psychotic illnesses.

Initially, a series of observations led to the serotonin theory of sleep. The injection of serotonin in the cerebral ventricle of animals and the administration of serotonin precursor (L-tryptophan) seemed to produce drowsiness and sleep (Ursin, 2002). Furthermore, selective destruction of the dorsal raphe nuclei, where serotonin neurons are principally located (*Figure 1.10*) caused insomnia. The degree of lack of sleep was proportional to the ablation produced.

Similarly, chemical inactivation of the serotonin system by p-chlorophenylalanine (PCPA) was followed by insomnia. At this time (early 1970s) serotonin appeared to be the long sought after sleep factor. However, the development of techniques to measure selectively individual cells showed that activity from the raphe nuclei cells was increased during wakefulness, reduced during slow-wave sleep and that there was no activity during REM. At the same time, stimulation of the same neurons produced wakefulness. Also, microinjection of serotonin in the brainstem area did not induce sleep. This evidence negated the idea of serotonin as the sleep neurotransmitter and terminated the serotonin theory of sleep, at least as initially formulated (Jouvet, 1999).

The observation that selective serotonin reuptake inhibitors (SSRIs), which presumably increase serotonin levels, are often associated with insomnia seems to confirm the more recent interpretation that serotonin is associated with the wake function. SSRIs are also strong REM suppressants, in keeping with current evidence of a serotonin role in REM sleep regulation (inhibitory).

The discovery of different 5-HT receptors, however, has revealed a rather complex interaction of serotonin with sleep and wake modulation

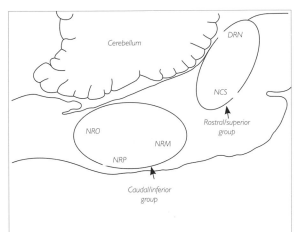

Figure 1.10: The raphe nuclei are a poorly localized group of neurons in the dorsal and mid-line zone of the medulla and pons. The rostral group has extensive and reciprocal innervation with thalamic nuclei and hypothalamic areas involved with wakefulness. They have important connections with cholinergic pontine nuclei in the regulation (suppression) of REM sleep. DRN, dorsal raphe nucleus; NCS, nucleus centralis superior; NRM, nucleus raphe magnus; NRO, nucleus raphe obscurus; NRP, nucleus raphe pallidus. Reprinted by permission of Elsevier Science from 'Activity of Serotonergic Neurones in Behaving Animals' by Jacobs and Fornal, Neuropsychopharmacology **21**: *9s–15s. © 1999 by American College of Neuropsychopharmacology.*

(*Figure 1.11*). For example, both 5-HT2 and 5-HT1A receptors seem to promote wakefulness. Some of the known antagonists to these receptors are associated with significant sedation. For example, nefazodone (Serzone™) and mirtazapine (Avanza™) are atypical antidepressants with sedative properties likely to be related to their antagonist effect on 5-HT2 receptors. Serotonin-containing neurons also have dense connections with suprachiasmatic nuclei, suggesting a probable integrative role between circadian rhythm and the sleep and wake cycle (Morin, 1999).

Hypocretins (orexins)

In 1998, the identification of two novel peptides isolated from the posterior hypothalamus was reported. They were called hypocretin because of the anatomical site from which they were isolated (*hypo*thalamus) and some homology with the peptide se*cretin* (Hungs and Mignot, 2001; Kilduff and Peyron, 2000; Samson and Resch, 2000).

In the same year, the same peptides were isolated by a different group of researchers who named them orexin A and B because the area of the hypothalamus from which the peptides were isolated is associated with regulation of feeding. Hypocretins and orexins were shown to be the same molecules. The orexin (hypocretin) A and B receptors were also cloned. Orexin-containing neurons are localized to the lateral hypothalamus but they connect extensively to other areas within the hypothalamus, the thalamus, the brainstem and the limbic system, with a stimulatory action.

From a sleep and wake point of view, hypocretin neurons have dense connections with the aminergic and cholinergic neurons in the locus coeruleus (norepinephrine), dorsal raphe

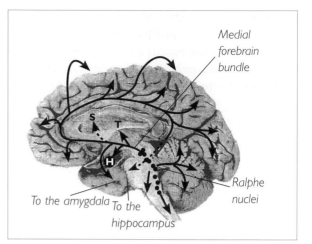

Figure 1.11: Serotoninergic neurons in the rostral and lower raphe nuclei, and their connections to the hypothalamus, basal forebrain/preoptic area. H, hypothalamus; S, septal nuclei; T, thalamus. Reprinted from 'The Human Brain', 2nd edn. Nolte J and Angevine J. © 2000 Mosby, Inc with permission from Elsevier Science.

nuclei (serotonin), tuberomammillary area (histamine) and pontine areas (cholinergic neurons). Not long after the hypocretins were described, a canine model of narcolepsy showed the genetic abnormality to be associated with dysfunction of the orexin 2 receptor, suggesting that orexin/hypocretin systems have a role in the pathogenesis of narcolepsy and possibly other hypersomnolence syndromes.

Animal studies have linked the alertness-promoting activity of modafinil (Modiadol™, Modavigil™, Provigil™) to the activation of the tuberomamillary histaminergic neurons and the orexin neurons. This might explain the alerting activity of modafinil as compared to amphetamines, which are thought to increase alertness by facilitating neural transmission of catecholamines (Scammell *et al*, 2000). Human studies suggest a potential diagnostic role in measuring hypocretin 1 in the cerebral spinal fluid (CSF and plasma) of patients with narcolepsy (Higuchi *et al*, 2002; Nishino *et al*, 2001).

Rapid-eye-movement sleep (REM sleep)

REM sleep is described as the behavioral state of sleep characterized by EEG activation (fast and low voltage), rapid eye movements and inhibition of muscle tone (*Figure 1.12*). Because the EEG in REM is similar to that in wakefulness, REM sleep is also referred to as paradoxical sleep (looks asleep but has an arousal EEG). REM sleep alternates with slow-wave sleep with an average periodicity of 90 minutes through the sleep episode.

During REM it is possible to identify tonic and phasic events as described in *Figure 1.13*.

Transection studies by the French researcher Michel Jouvet identified the pons reticular formation as the site of REM generation (lateral dorsal tegmentum and pedunculopontine tegmentum, LDT and PPT). Electrophysiological studies also showed that cholinergic neurons within the pontine reticular formation (the LDT and PPT) were actively discharging during REM sleep (REM-on neurons), and aminergic neurons decreased their activity during REM sleep (REM-off neurons).

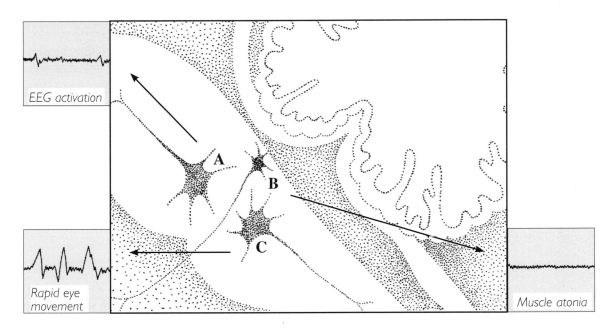

Figure 1.12: Sites of generation of REM sleep characteristic phenomena, EEG activation, rapid eye movements and muscle atonia (Hobson, 1988).

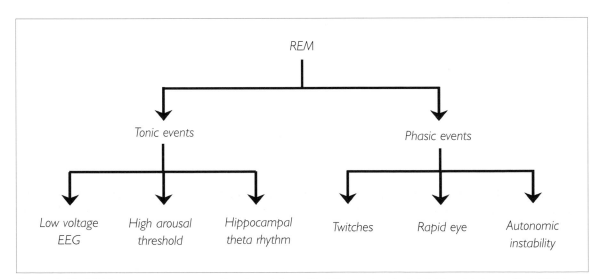

Figure 1.13: REM-generator neurons. Reprinted from 'The Dreaming Brain', J Allan Hobson. © 1988 by J Allan Hobson, MD. Printed by permission of Basic Books, a member of Perseus Books, LLC.

A reciprocal interaction between cholinergic and aminergic neurons has been proposed as the regulatory mechanism for REM (*Figure 1.14*). The REM-off neurons are silent during REM sleep and inhibit REM sleep when actively firing (during the wake cycle). These neurons are predominantly nor-adrenergic from the peri-locus ceruleus area, serotoninergic from the dorsal raphe nuclei and hystaminergic from the tuberomammillary area. In clinical depression, a decreased aminergic and serotoninergic drive would enhance cholinergic activity and result in decreased REM onset latency (see *Chapter 8*). It would also give a rationale for the antidepressant action of tricyclic antidepressant and selective serotonin reuptake inhibitors which restore serotonin and aminergic drive.

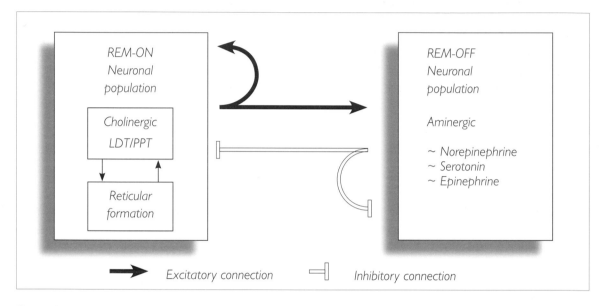

Figure 1.14: Reciprocal interaction between 'REM-ON' and 'REM-OFF' neurons. LDT, laterodorsal tegmental nuclei; PPT, pedunculopontine tegmental nuclei (Hishikawa and Shimizu, 1995).

The REM-on neurons are cholinergic, but are distinct from another group of cholinergic pontine neurons active during the wake cycle.

The series of events which leads to REM sleep is thought to involve a decrease in aminergic inhibitory action (decreased activity of noradrenergic and serotonergic REM-off neurons) which releases the activity of cholinergic REM-on neurons. What triggers the timing of this cascade of events and what terminates it is not yet clear. It is likely that GABA is a neurotransmitter involved in inhibition of aminergic activity (Mallich *et al*, 1999).

Connections within the pons and between the pons and the medulla are also responsible for the other phenomena of REM sleep, rapid eye movements and muscle atonia. Experimental ablation lesions around the locus ceruleus are associated with muscle atonia, suggesting the probable involvement of these areas on muscle tone control.

The malfunction of the REM sleep system is at the base of the common (although infrequently reported) REM behavior disorder. In this condition, the lack of muscle tone inhibition during REM sleep leads to patients acting out their dreams, sometimes with significant injury to themselves or bed partners.

Narcolepsy is a syndrome also associated with mal-regulation of the REM system, and study of narcolepsy has helped understanding of REM physiology. Animal studies suggest hypersensitivity and hyperactivity of the cholinergic and cholinoceptive system in narcolepsy. Microinjections of cholinergic agents in the pons produces cataplexy in the narcoleptic animal in much lower doses than in the control animal, in keeping with a hypersensitivity state.

Cataplexy can also be induced by injection in the basal forebrain which has direct connection with the limbic system. This finding could explain why cataplexy can be triggered by emotions, a possibility supported by animal studies. If this hypothesis is correct, hyperactivity of the cholinergic and cholinoceptive systems would also help explain the early REM sleep onset (Mignot and Nishimo, 1997).

The importance of pedunculopontine and forebrain structures in REM regulation is also highlighted by the sleep abnormalities seen in neurodegenerative disease such as Alzheimer's disease, Lewy body dementia and Parkinson's disease (*Chapter 8, Table 8.1*). In these conditions, there are episodes of visual hallucinations and REM behavior disorder as well as changes in quantity and timing of REM sleep. Similar syndromes are also seen following vascular damage to brainstem structures, eg. top of the basilar artery syndrome hallucinosis (Caplan, 1990)

Slow-wave sleep (non-REM sleep)

The terminology used to refer to slow-wave sleep can be somewhat confusing because slow-wave sleep is also used to refer to low-frequency high-amplitude EEG sleep stage (stages 3 and 4, 0.75-4Hz). Therefore, the term non-REM sleep is widely used although it is undesirable to refer to a process that is not involved in it. The term slow-wave sleep should be used instead.

Slow-wave sleep has an essential role in the homeostatic process of the sleep and wake cycle, being the state through which humans start sleep. Also, it seems that the perception of having slept depends to some extent on the length of continuous non-REM sleep prior to arousal (Sewitch, 1984).

Studies (McGinty and Szymusiek, 2001; Sherin *et al*, 1996) have shown that the anterior hypothalamic area is the site of sleep-promoting neurons. Different techniques have demonstrated that a population of neurons in the ventral lateral preoptic area (VLPO) and basal forebrain are active during sleep and dormant during the wake cycle (*Figure 1.15*). These findings confirm the clinical observation of von Economo when, seventy years ago, he hypothesized that the anterior hypothalamus was the site of sleep control.

Although the hypothalamic area is the site of activity for many sleep-promoting substances (*Table 1.1*), the inhibitory neurotransmitters,

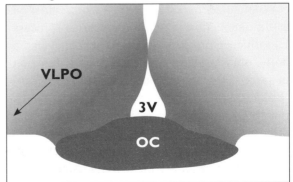

Figure 1.15: Coronal section at the level of the anterior hypothalamus showing the localized group of neurons in the ventrolateral preoptic area (VLPO) active during sleep. 3V, third ventricle; OC, optic chiasm. Reprinted with permission from Science **271**, Sherin et al 'Activation of ventrolateral preoptic neurons during sleep'. © 1996 American Association for the Advancement of Science.

GABA and galanin, and the neuromodulator adenosine are currently considered the major mediators of the process of sleep onset. Through the widespread connections of the VLPO neurons to the aminergic and cholinergic neurons of the brainstem, these inhibitory neurotransmitters facilitate sleep onset.

The preoptic area neurons also have connections with the suprachiasmatic nucleus and may be the mediators of circadian sleep and wake regulation. One indirect piece of evidence of circadian influence is the coupling of sleep and body temperature (Sewitch, 1984). Sleep onset is associated with a reduction in body temperature. Studies in animals show the presence of temperature-sensitive neurons in the anterior hypothalamus in a similar location to the sleep-promoting neurons. Some are sensitive to warmth; they are active during sleep and set in motion heat dissipation reflexes, such as skin vasodilatation. The peripheral vasodilatation decreases core body temperature and this is associated with sleep onset. These observations seem to give credit to the popular belief that having warm feet (using a hot water bottle) helps sleep onset (Krauchi *et al*, 1999; Pache *et al*, 2001).

Sleep and wake cycle regulation

Sleep and wake cycle regulation is the result of interaction between a variety of external and internal factors, with the retinohypothalamic tract and suprachiasmatic nuclei system functioning as integrative regulators between external influences (mainly the light and dark cycle) and internal homeostatic processes. From a clinical point of view, it is useful to conceptualize the sleep and wake regulation as the interaction between a circadian (process C) influence on sleep and wake tendency and a homeostatic component, mostly as a function of prior wakefulness (process S) (*Figure 1.16*) (Bobèly, 1982; Bobèly *et al*, 1998). Sleepiness, measured as arousal threshold increases, with prior periods of being awake with the maximum need to sleep in humans occurring after thirty hours of sleep deprivation (Dijk and Edgar, 1999). The increase in arousal threshold (eg. a higher intensity stimulus is required to wake the person from sleep) corresponds to an increase in delta power (0.75–40Hz) on the EEG, that is proportional to prior wakefulness and declines exponentially during sleep (*Figure 1.17*).

A homeostatic role of slow-wave sleep is also supported by the experimental evidence that, within a twenty-four-hour period, the amount of

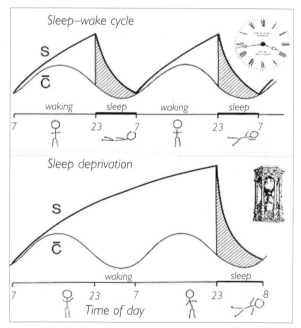

Figure 1.16: Two factor model. A component S during which the pressure for sleep increases as a function of prior wakefulness (possibly mediated by sleep factor). Process C, which influences sleep and wake propensity in accordance with light and dark cycle and other non-photic time givers (eg. meals, work, and social interaction). Note that sleep following sleep deprivation does not fully 'compensate' for prior lack of sleep (Borbèly, 1982).

slow-wave sleep is proportionally reduced if a nap has occurred prior to the main night's sleep episode (*Figure 1.18*).

The idea that with progressive wakefulness the body approaches a point where sleep onset is triggered is in keeping with the presence of a 'sleep factor(s)', which accumulates when the person is awake, eventually reaching a sleep threshold, and decreases during sleep.

Among the many possible sleep factors, adenosine is currently considered a strong candidate (Porkka-Heiskamen *et al*, 2002). Adenosine is an inhibitory neuromodulator shown to accumulate during wakefulness as a function of neuronal (and glial) metabolic activity as part of the adenosine–phosphate pathway (ATP, ADP and AMP). The inhibitory action of adenosine is mediated through adenosine receptors, receptor A1 being the most important one in the forebrain and mesopontine cholinergic areas. Animal experiments indicate that the adenosine level increases in the basal forebrain during sleep deprivation, and declines during sleep. Local injection in the forebrain and systemic administration of adenosine decreases wakefulness and increases sleep. In clinical practice, the adenosine receptor antagonists, caffeine and theophylline, reduce sleepiness and increase alertness.

Interacting with the above proposed homeostatic (process S) regulation is a circadian sleep and wake propensity controlled by the suprachiasmatic nuclei system (process C). The tendency to fall asleep (*Figure 1.19*) in individuals who are intensely sleep deprived (eg. kept awake overnight) varies during a 24-hour period (Lavie, 1996).

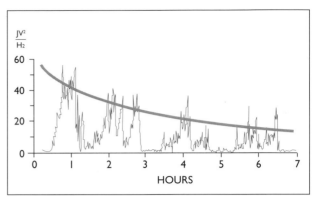

Figure 1.17: The amount of slow-wave sleep (measured as power density of the 0.75 to 4.5 Hz frequency EEG wave) declines exponentially through the sleep period (Borbèly, 1982).

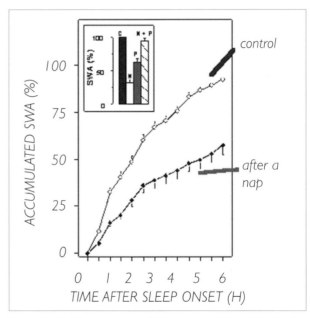

Figure 1.18: The amount of slow-wave sleep obtained during the main sleep episode is proportionally reduced by the amount obtained during a prior nap (Borbèly, 1982).

In another study by Lavie (1986), young volunteers were kept awake overnight and then put through a 24-hour schedule of 7 minutes sleeping followed by 13 minutes awake. The tendency to fall asleep was increased between 10.00PM and 4.00AM and in the afternoon (the 'siesta' period). However, sleepiness tendency was very low between 8.00AM and 9.00AM and, also, surprisingly very low between 8.00PM and 10.00PM despite the intense sleep deprivation. The author referred to the period refractory to sleep onset as 'forbidden zone', followed by a period when sleep was favored known as 'sleep gates'. The study also showed that although sleep gates varied between individuals, it was quite constant within a subject. The propensity to fall asleep had a rapid onset with an all-or-none pattern, rather than gradual and progressively increasing sleepiness.

The consistancy of the time when sleep is more likely to occur in each individual has some correspondence with clinical practice. Some patients say that they are unable to fall asleep if they have passed their preferred bedtime. Patients whose sleep gate is set past midnight present with a clinical syndrome of delayed sleep phase (see *Chapters 8* and *10*). It is an important clinical observation that a rise in melatonin precedes the sleep gate by approximately 1.5 hours (*Figure 1.20*), and that the timing of the sleep gate is correlated with melatonin secretion (Lavie and Luboshitzky, 1996). It is hypothesized that the melatonin action is mediated by the suprachiasmatic nuclei, which contain melatonin receptors.

The anatomical structures which drive circadian rhythm are the suprachiasmatic nuclei (SCN) (*Figure 1.21*). The suprachiasmatic nuclei are central to the temporal organization of the sleep and wake distribution through a 24-hour period. In a normal synchronized condition, sleep occurs within a time window of approximately 8 hours, and with wakefulness for the following 16 hours; a ratio of 1:2. Animal experiments have shown that once the suprachiasmatic nuclei are removed, the sleep and wake function loses its temporal organization. Evidence of lack of sleep and wake rhythmicity is also documented in humans, particularly following head trauma (even minor ones) or neurosurgical intervention (*Chapter 10*).

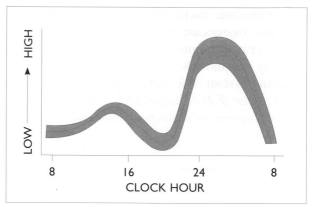

Figure 1.19: Note that at around 8.00PM the subjects had been grossly sleep deprived, yet sleep onset is difficult (forbidden zone). Sleep propensity increases quickly after 10.00PM. (the sleep gate opens). The two periods when sleep is more likely to occur are between midnight and 6.00AM and early afternoon. These are also the peak periods for motor vehicle accidents. Reprinted from Lavie, 'The Enchanted World of Sleep'. © 1996 Yale University Press.

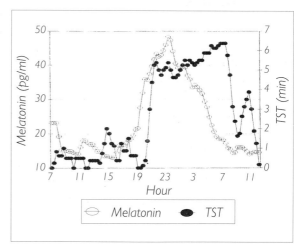

Figure 1.20: Melatonin surge occurs approximately 1.5 hours before the 'opening' of the sleep gate (Lavie and Luboshitzky, 1996).

The actual pathways and molecular mechanism of the SCN influence is not yet known, but the close proximity and connection of the sleep-active neurons of the VLPO (ventrolateral preoptic area) make this a likely pathway mediating the sleep gate (Dijk and Edgar, 1999).

The SCN also have reciprocal connections with wake-active aminergic neurons, and particularly the serotonergic neurons of the dorsal raphe nuclei (*Figure 1.22*). The relationship between the suprachiasmatic nuclei and the serotoninergic system is relevant given the recent evidence that serotonin agonists are able to cause phase shifts in the circadian rhythm (Dagan, 2002).

Other medications used in clinical practice (vitamin B12, metamphetamines, haloperidol and possibly estradiol (Refinetti, 2000) appear, at least in animals, to affect the rhythmicity of the circadian system. The mechanism of interaction is often not understood, but result from direct effect on the SCN or indirectly by interaction with melatonin levels (*Table 1.3*). Sleep deprivation does not appear to affect the melatonin rhythm.

Table 1.3: Drug effects on melatonin secretion in humans		
Increase	**Decrease**	**No effect**
• Chlorpromazine	• Alprenolol	• L-dopa
• Tranylcypromine	• Atenolol	• Dexamethasone
• Endorphin	• Metoprolol	• Flufenazine
• Fluvoxamine	• Propanolol	• Deprenyl
• Lithium	• Benzodiazepine	• Maprotiline
• Tetrahydrocannabinol	• Clonidine	

Among the substances that influence the circadian pacemaker, melatonin has an important role. Melatonin is produced not only by the pineal gland but also by the retina, and has a circadian rhythm that is not autonomous but depends on the suprachiasmatic nuclei. The production of melatonin is regulated by light exposure through the retina and the retinohypothalamic tract which feeds into the suprachiasmatic nuclei (*Figure 1.23*). It has been recently shown that receptors in the retina are separate and independent from the cones and rods, and are influenced by specific wavelengths (Brainard *et al*, 2001; Wehr, 1991). This new information should lead to a more selective use of light in the treatment of circadian sleep disorders, minimizing some of the risks associated with use of conventional light sources. Melatonin receptors are also present in the suprachiasmatic nuclei, suggesting that melatonin feeds back into the SCN.

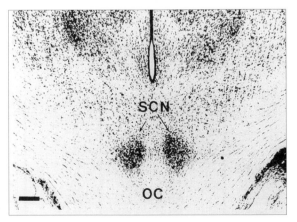

Figure 1.21: The suprachiasmatic nuclei (SCN) are situated just above, and on both sides of the optic chiasm (OC), and below the third ventricle (Moore, 1990).

In humans, both light and melatonin are able to phase shift sleep-and-wake timing and can be used in the management of circadian rhythm sleep disorders (*Chapter 10*).

Chapter summary

The states of wakefulness, slow-wave sleep and REM sleep are associated with recognized anatomical structures and neurochemistry (*Figure 1.24*) with close connection to the circadian pacemaker and other neurovegetative systems, in particular the neuroendocrine, cardiorespiratory and immune functions.

As *Figure 1.24* shows, there is a close similarity between wakefulness and REM sleep, except for the marked decrease in aminergic drive during REM sleep. Conversely, slow-wave sleep is characterized by decreased activity in both aminergic and cholinergic pathways with GABA, adenosine and perhaps other neurotransmitters being predominantly active. These three systems are subject to derangement leading to clinical syndromes that are of interest to sleep physicians.

As shown in *Figure 1.24*, it should be noted that increased sleepiness may not necessarily be the same as decreased wakefulness. Although there are methods that measure sleepiness tendencies, there are no reliable methods that measure the state of being awake. Decreased wakefulness is inferred by an increase in sleepiness, measured as short latency to sleep onset in a multiple sleep latency test or wakefulness maintenance test. Within the context of sleepiness and chronic fatigue states, there is a group of patients who may have derangement of their wakefulness/alertness regulation without necessarily being sleepy.

Finally, recent descriptions of the orexin/hypocretin system is adding to the understanding of sleep and wake regulation, possibly with diagnostic value and potential for further therapeutic advances.

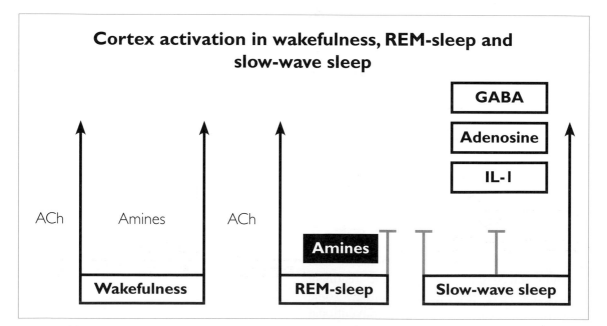

Figure 1.22: Schematic view of the interactions between the SCN and other sleep–wake related systems. ACh, acetylcholine; GABA, gamma-amino-butyric acid; IL-1, interleukin 1.

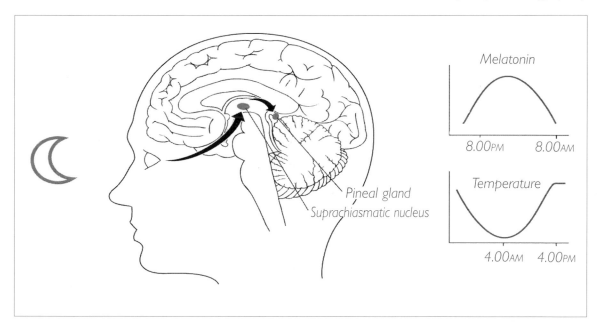

Figure 1.23: Melatonin circadian production is regulated by the SCN and influenced by light–dark cycle. With darkness melatonin level increases, while core body temperature reaches its nadir in the middle of the night.

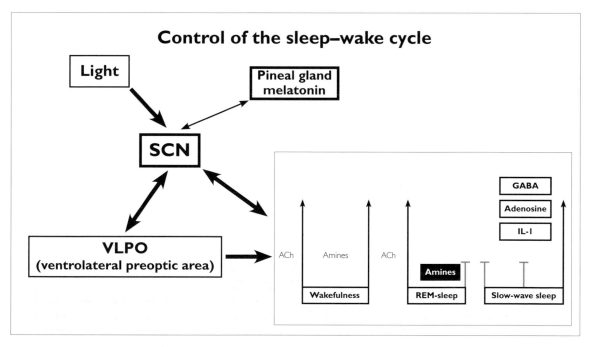

Figure 1.24: Major neurotransmitters in sleep–wake regulation. Note that acetylcholine (ACh) has a major role in wakefulness and REM sleep, and that a reduced adrenergic drive during wakefulness may allow REM-related symptoms to intrude during the day (hypnagogic hallucination, sleep paralysis and cataplexy).

References

Aserinski E, Kleitman N (1953) Regularly occurring periods of eye motility, and concomitant phenomena during sleep. *Science* **118**: 273–4

Borbèly A (1982) A two-process model of sleep regulation. *Hum Neurobiol* **1**: 195–204

Borbèly A, Tobler I, Acherman P, Geering B (1998) Bits of sleep. Explore the facts behind the mystery CD Version 1. Sleep Research Laboratory, University of Zurich

Brainard GC, Hanifin JP, Greeson JM, Byrne B, Glickman G, Gerner E, Rollag MD (2001) Action spectrum for melatonin regulation in humans: evidence for a novel circadian photoreceptor. *J Neuroscience* **21**(6): 6405–12

Caplan LR (1990) 'Top of the basilar' syndrome. *Neurology* **30**: 72–8

Clarke E, Dewhurst K (1996) *An Illustrated History of Brain Function. Imaging the Brain from Antiquity to Present.* 2nd edn. Norman Publishing, San Francisco

Dagan Y (2002) Circadian rhythm sleep disorders (CRSD). *Sleep Med Rev* **6**(1): 45–55

Dickstein JB, Moldofsky (H) (1999) Sleep, cytokines and immune function. *Sleep Med Rev* **3**(3): 219–28

Dijk DJ, Edgar DM (1999) Circadian and homeostatic control of wakefulness and sleep. In: Turek FW, Zee PC, eds. *Regulation of Sleep and Circadian Rhythms*. Marcel Dekker, New York

Hayaishi O (2000) Molecular mechanisms of sleep–wake regulation: a role of prostaglandin D2. *Phil Trans R Soc Lond* **355**: 275–80

Higuchi S, Usui A, Murasaki M, Matsushita S, Nishioka N, Yuoshino A *et al* (2002) Plasma orexin-A is lower in patients with narcolepsy. *Neurosci Lett* **318**(2): 61–4

Hishikawa Y, Shimizu T (1995) Physiology of REM sleep, cataplexy, and sleep paralysis negative motor phenomena. *Adv Neurology* **67**: 245–71

Hobson JA (1988) *The Dreaming Brain*. Basic Books, Philadelphia

Hobson JA (1995) *Sleep Scientific*. American Library, New York

Horner R (2002) University of Toronto. Available online: http://www.utoronto.ca/lsrnb/LectureNotes/sleepcoursenotes.html

Hungs M, Mignot E (2001) Hypocretin/orexin, sleep and narcolepsy. *BioEssays* **23**: 397–408

Jacobs BL, Fornal CA (1999) Activity of serotoninergic neurones in behaving animals. *Neuropsychopharmacology* **21**: 95–155

Jouvet M (1999) Sleep and serotonin: An unfinished story. *Neuropsychopharmacology* **21**(25): 245–75

Kilduff TS, Peyron C (2000) The hypocretins? Orexin lingand-receptor system: implication for sleep and sleep disorders. *Trends Neurosci* **23**(8): 359–65

Kimura T, Ho K, Yamamoto I (2001) Uridine receptor: Discovery and its involvement in sleep mechanism. *Sleep* **24**(3): 251–60

Krauchi K, Cajochen C, Werth E, Wirz-Justice A (1999) Warm feet promote the rapid onset of sleep. *Nature* **40**: 36–7

Krueger JM, Karnovski ML (1995) Sleep as a neuroimmune phenomenon: A brief historical perspective. *Adv Neuroimmunol* **5**: 5–12

Lavie P (1996) *The Enchanted World of Sleep*. Yale University Press, New Haven

Lavie P, Luboshitzky R (1996) Melatonin: possible role in human sleep and reproduction in sleep and sleep disorders; from molecules to behavior. In: Hayaishi O, Inoué S, eds. *Sleep and Sleep Disorders: From molecule to behaviour*. Academia Press, Tokyo

Lavie P (1986) Ultrashort sleep-waking schedule Part 3. 'Gates' and 'Forbidden Zones' for sleep. *Electroencephalography Clin Neurophysiol* **63**: 414–25

Lin JS (2000) Brain structures and mechanisms involved in the control of cortical activation and wakefulness, with emphasis on the posterior hypothalamus and histaminergic neurons. *Sleep Med Rev* **4**(5): 471–503

Lindsley DB, Bowden J, Magoun HW (1949) Effect upon EEG of acute injury to the brainstem activating systems. *Electroencephalography Clin Neurophysiol* **1**: 475–86

Lindsley DB, Schreiner LH, Knowles WB, Magoun HW (1950) Behavioural and EEG changes following chronic brainstem lesions in the cat. *Electroencephalography Clin Neurophysiol* **2**: 483–98

Lugaresi E, Provini F (2001) Agripnia excitata: clinical features and pathophysiological implications. *Sleep Med Rev* **5**(4): 313–22

Mallich NB, Kaur S, Jha KS, Seigel JM (1999) Possible role of GABA in the regulation of REM sleep with special reference to REM-OFF neurons in rapid eye movement sleep. In: Mallich BN, Inoue S, eds. *Rapid Eye Movement Sleep*. Marcel Dekker, New York

McGinty D, Szymusiek R (2001) Brain structures and mechanisms involved in the generation of NREM sleep: focus on the preoptic hypothalamus. *Sleep Med Rev* **5**(4): 323–42

Mignot E, Nishimo S (1997) Genetic and Pathophysiological Aspects of Narcolepsy. In: Hayaishi Q, Inoue S, eds. *Sleep and Sleep Disorders: From molecule to behaviour*. Academic Press, Tokyo

Moore R (1990) The circadian timing system and the organization of sleep-wake behavior. In: Thorpy M, ed. *Handbook of Sleep Disorders*. Marcel Dekker, New York

Morin L (1999) Serotonin and the regulation of mammalian circadian rhythmicity. *Ann Med* **31**: 12–33

Nishino S, Ripley B, Overeen S, Nevsimalova S, Lammers GJ, Vankova J *et al* (2001) Low cerebrospinal fluid, hypocretin (orexin) and altered energy homeostasis in human narcolepsy. *Ann Neurol* **50**: 381–8

Nolte J, Angevine Jr JB (2000) *The Human Brain in Photographs and Diagrams*. Mosby, St Louis

Pache M, Krauci K, Cajochen C, Wirz-Justice A, Dubler B, Flammer J, Kaiser HJ (2001) Cold feel and prolonged sleep onset latency in vasospastic syndrome. *Lancet* **358**: 125–6

Porkka-Heiskamen T, Alanko L, Kalinchuk A, Stemberg D (2002) Adenosine and sleep. *Sleep Med Rev* **6**(4): 321–32

Refinetti R (2000) *Circadian Physiology*. CRC Press, Washington

Salloway S, Malloy P, Cummings LJ (1997) *The Neuropsychiatry of Limbic and Subcortical Disorders*. American Psychiatric Press, Washington

Samson WK, Resch ZT (2000) The hypocretin/orexin story. *REM* **11**(7): 357–62

Scammell TE, Estabrooke IV, McCarthy MT, Chemilli RM, Yanagisawa M, Miller MS, Saper CB (2000) Hypothalamic arousal regions are activated during modafinil-induced wakefulness. *J Neurosci* **20**(22): 8620–8

Sewitch DN (1984) REM sleep continuity and the sense of having slept in normal sleepers. *Sleep* **7**(2): 147–54

Sherin JE, Shiromani PJ, McCorley RW, Saper CB (1996) Activation of ventrolateral preoptic neurons during sleep. *Science* **271**: 216–9

Steiger A, Holsboer F (1997) Neuropeptides and human sleep. *Sleep* **20**(11): 1038–52

Steriade M (1992) Basic mechanisms of sleep generation. *Neurology* **42**(6): 9–18

Thorpy M (2000) Historical perspective on sleep and man. In: Culebres A, ed. *Sleep Disorders and Neurological Diseases*. Marcel Dekker, New York

Ursin R (2002) Serotonin and sleep. *Sleep Med Rev* **6**(1): 57–69

Wehr TA (1991) The durations of human melatonin secretion and sleep respond to changes in day length (photoperiod). *J Clin Endocrinol Metab* **73**: 1276–80

Whitaker-Azmitia PM (1999) The discovery of serotonin and its role in neuroscience. *Neuropsychopharmacology* **21**(25): 2S–8S

CHAPTER 2

Chronobiology: an introduction

Antonio Ambrogetti

Introduction

Chronobiology (chronos=time, bios=life and logos=science) is the scientific discipline which studies time-dependent variation of functions in biological systems. Biological systems (Refinetti, 2000) encompass not only organisms (cells, organs, the entire body), but also groups of individuals (eg. seasonal mood changes in certain populations, reproductive patterns in certain animals). The time-dependent variations in body functions are usually referred to as biological rhythms, which are recurrent events within a biological system (*Figure 2.1*).

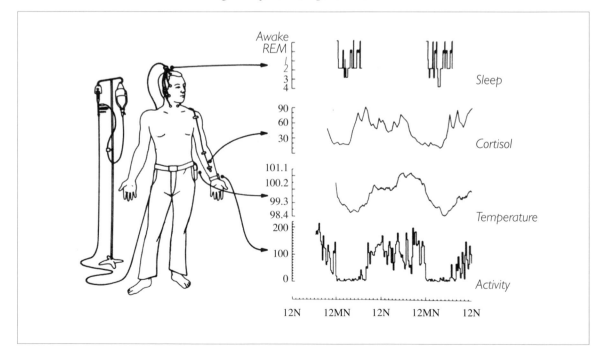

Figure 2.1: Body functions show a level of activity that varies in a predictable fashion (rhythm) over 24 hours (circadian) (Wehr and Goodwin, 1983). MN, midnight; N, noon.

Biological rhythms are characterized by self-sustaining, recurrent patterns, that can be described by a set of characteristics such as frequency, amplitude, peaks, troughs and phases (*Table 2.1*).

Table 2.1: Spectrum of biological rhythms

Category of rhythms	Period of rhythms	Term used to describe rhythms	Illustrative examples
Short periods	Seconds	High frequency oscillations	Electroencephalogram
Medium periods	30 min to 20 h	Ultradian	Sleep staging Pulsatile hormone secretion
	20 h to 28 h	Circadian	Most biologic functions
	28 h to 6 days	Infradian	Little studies thus far
Long periods	~ Week	Circaseptan	Work-related routine
	~ Month	Circamensual	Menstruation, fertility Neuroendocrine functions
	~ Year	Circannual	Many biochemical, endocrine, and physiological parameters

Reprinted from *American Journal of Hypertension*, **14**, Smolensky and Haus, © 2001 with permission from American Journal of Hypertension Ltd.

Central to chronobiology is the concept that time is relevant to both physiological and pathological processes. For example, blood pressure and body temperature vary depending on when during a 24-hour period measurements are made; asthma is usually more severe at 4.00AM than at 4.00PM. The presence of endogenous oscillators allows the synchronization and optimal timing of metabolic and physiological interdependent functions (Wirz-Justice, 1987). These ideas are often referred to as the biologic time structure of life form (Smolensky and D'Alonzo, 1993).

Chronobiology may appear to be at odds with the concept of homeostasis (Smolensky and D'Alonzo, 1993). Homeostasis refers to the idea that biological systems are organized to maintain a stable environment, which guarantees optimal and stable functions over time. Chronobiology, on the contrary, operates on the premise that function changes over time in a predictable and recurrent fashion and that 'rhythmicity is a fundamental property of living matter' (Reinberg, 2001).

Homeostasis and chronobiology, however, do not contradict each other if biological rhythms are seen as the upper and lower boundaries of a homeostatic system.

For a long time, the importance of the time of the day, and for period of the year, the manifestation of physiological and pathological processes was considered the result of external environmental factors, such as light and darkness cycles and variations in external temperature.

The first observation of an endogenous nature of biological rhythm (in-built in the organism) is credited to the French astronomer, Jean Jacques D'Ortous de Mairan (1729). He described how the leaves of Mimosa pudica change in position during the day (they open with light and fold at night-time). However, even when the plant was kept in constant darkness, the rhythm continued, pointing to an endogenous rhythm that was independent of the external influence of the light and dark cycle (*Figure 2.2*).

The observation that light and dark affect plants' rhythms was extended by Linnaeus who created a 'flower clock' (*Figure 2.3*).

However, it was another 100 years before the relevance of endogenous rhythms were conceptualized as relevant to physiological and pathological processes by Julien Joseph Virey in 1814 (Reinberg *et al*, 2001). Virey made the distinction between endogenous rhythm and environmental influences, and entraining by the 24-hour light and dark cycle. He stressed the importance of time of the day in the occurrence of gout and asthma and for drug administration. Virey's ideas were ignored for another 150 years until the 1950s when chronobiology became the subject of systematic research, creating the foundation for a body of knowledge relevant to many areas of biological science, including medicine and specifically the sleep and wake function.

Circadian rhythms

Many rhythms with different periods have been described as involving physiological and neurobehavioral functions. However, rhythms with a periodicity of 24 hours are particularly important to clinicians and health practitioners.

In the late 1950s, the German born researcher, Franz Halberg, coined the term circadian to refer to biological rhythms of approximately 24-hour duration (Halberg *et al*, 1959). Circadian (circa=about, diem=a day) rhythm is fundamental to many body functions and is important for adapting biological systems

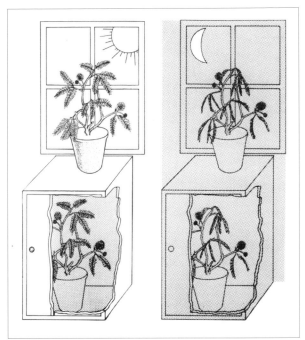

Figure 2.2: The opening and closing of the plant leaves persists even when the plant is maintained in constant darkness, indicating a rhythm independent of the light and darkness cycle (Moore-Ede, 1982).

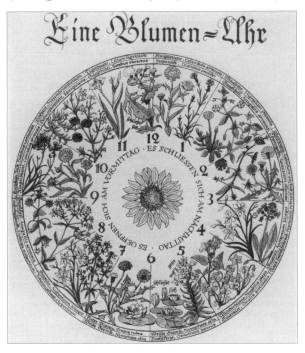

Figure 2.3: Linnaeus' flower clock, 1751 (Moore-Ede et al, 1982), see text.

to the environmental changes (light and dark cycle) associated with the earth's rotation (Pittendrigh, 1960). Circadian rhythm is ultimately essential to promote survival and reproduction (Moore, 1997).

The question as to whether the rhythms are 'approximately' 24 hours, rather than 'exactly' 24 hours is not completely clarified, but it is suggested that entrainment to 24 hours relative to light–darkness fluctuation is more difficult in animals whose natural clock is closer to 24 hours (Moore-Ede *et al*, 1982). Therefore, it seems that a rhythm which is approximately 24 hours may provide more flexibility for adjustment to the natural environment.

Circadian rhythms can be defined by the following characteristics (Johnson *et al*, 2003).

Free-running period

When circadian rhythms (eg. activity–rest cycles) are studied in animals and humans in stable conditions, isolated from environmental cues, they show a stable (free-running) rhythm, slightly longer or shorter than 24 hours. Most free-running rhythms persist for a long time, showing a precise timing.

Temperature compensation

As the underlying molecular mechanism of action of the internal clock is likely to be based on metabolic enzymatic processes, changes in internal temperature could affect the period of the clock. An increase in temperature would shorten the clock, and a decrease in temperature would lengthen it. This would be undesirable, particularly for organisms that do not thermoregulate and, to a lesser extent, even for homeothermic mammals. The exact mechanism of temperature compensation (maintaining a stable period despite fluctuation in temperature) is not fully understood (Johnson *et al*, 2003).

Entrainment

Entrainment is the process by which an internal rhythm (function), which is free-running with a period of approximately 24 hours, is 'carried along' so that its period conforms exactly to the 24-hour period of the environment (Johnson *et al*, 2003).

Although the terms entrainment and synchronization are often used synonymously, a distinction is made between the two. In entrainment the biological rhythm is entrained to a period, which is, on average, equal to the one of the entraining agent (Zeitgeber) and with a stable phase relationship between the two. Synchronization implies that the wave form of the entrained and entraining rhythms coincide.

Because organisms in real-life situations are subjected to many environmental factors, identification of which entraining agents are relevant to a particular biological rhythm is difficult, unless the following set of established criteria are demonstrated:

❖ *Absence of other time cues.* The rhythm being studied needs to be demonstrated to be free-running before the potential Zeitgeber is applied, and should be free-running with the same period after the Zeitgeber is removed.

❖ *Period control.* The rhythm studied should adjust its rhythm to be equal to the period of the Zeitgeber.

❖ *Stable phase relationship.* There should be a stable and reproducible relationship between the rhythm being entrained and the entraining agent.

❖ *Phase control.* Once the influence of the Zeitgeber is terminated, the biological rhythm being studied should resume its free-running period with a phase determined by the Zeitgeber cycle.

Recognition of these properties is important to differentiate environmental factors which act as Zeitgebers from other stimuli, which may affect the expression of a function without necessarily affecting the underlying biological clock. For example, the rest-activity rhythm could be affected by significant temperature changes where the animals studied may be more active during cold periods to keep warm and, therefore, give the impression of entrainment to the external temperature. However, when such temperature conditions are removed, the rest and activity cycle will resume with a phase dependent on the prior free-running period, rather than the period of the temperature cycle. This apparent entrainment without actually affecting the rhythm clock is referred to as 'masking' (Johnson *et al*, 2003; Minors and Waterhouse 1989; Wever, 1979).

The capacity of synchronizing with the light and dark cycle is mediated by an endogenous clock situated in the suprachiasmatic nuclei (SCN), a group of neurons (*Chapter 1*) which process light information from the retinohypothalamic tract, melatonin secretion and hypothalamic and brainstem arousal and sleep system (*Figure 2.4*). The circadian timing system (CTS) is composed of the neural structures which regulate the circadian rhythm by:

❖ Providing pacemaker activity.
❖ Entraining the body to environmental stimuli (light being the fundamental one).

The SCN receive direct input from the retina through a pathway (the retinohypothalamic tract), which is independent of the visual pathways, the main neurotransmitter being glutamate. The main neurotransmitter in the SCN is GABA, suggesting a predominantly inhibitory activity. Within the SCN, there are two groups of cells: the first (core) is connected to the retinohypothalamic tract, and the second (shell) with other brainstem structures. It is likely that the SCN provides the pacemaker synchronization for behavioral and physiological circadian rhythms through these output connections (*Figures 2.5* and *2.6*) (Moore, 1996).

The biological clock needs to be flexible enough to adjust (synchronize) to the relative length of the daylight/night period, which changes across seasons, and is also affected by artificial light exposure. This level of flexibility is restricted to a 'range of entrainment' (Zee and Turek, 1999) of between twenty to twenty-eight hours. Rhythms shorter than twenty hours are referred to as ultradian and those above twenty-eight hours as infradian. For example, the rhythmicity of REM sleep (average of ninety minutes) is an example of ultradian rhythm (*Figure 2.7*), and the menstrual period is an infradian rhythm.

Animal studies provide insight in the cellular/molecular mechanisms which underlie the biological clock regulation (Refinetti, 2000). A schematic representation is shown in *Figure 2.8* from a study of fruit flies (*Drosophila melanogaster*).

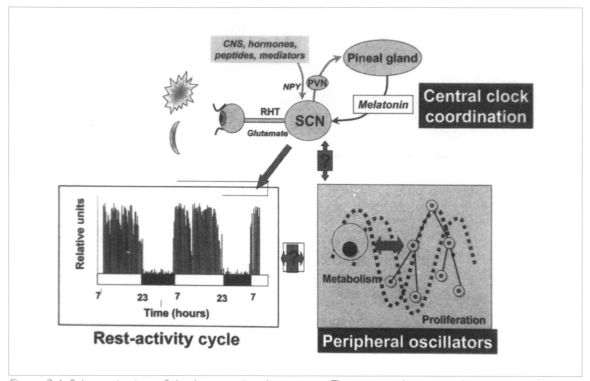

Figure 2.4: Schematic view of the human circadian system. The mammalian suprachiasmatic nucleus (SCN) is a biological clock located at the floor of the hypothalamus. It displays an approximate 24-hour cycle through the expression of several genes and biochemical functions. Its period (cycle duration) is calibrated by the alternation of light (directly) and darkness (through melatonin secretion by the pineal gland). The SCN generates the rest–activity cycle (left) and coordinates many circadian rhythms in the body, and possibly those that modulate cellular metabolism and proliferation (right). NPY-neuropeptide; PVN-paraventricular nucleus; RHT-retinohypothalamic tract.

The gene *per* (for period) localized in the X chromosome, is responsible for the synthesis of the protein PER which accumulates in the cytoplasm and generates a negative feedback loop to the transcription of the messenger RNA. In the fruit fly, different alleles of the *per* gene have been identified which code for different rhythm lengths (Refinetti, 2000). A second gene called *tim* (for timeless) was also identified in the fruit fly on chromosome 2. The *tim* gene codes for TIM protein, which physically interacts with the PER protein in the cytoplasm. TIM and PER binding modulates the re-entry of the PER protein in the nucleus. *tim* production appears to be affected by light. The exposure to light, for example, would increase the degradation of TIM and, therefore, increase the negative feedback on the per gene transcription mechanism which would shorten the cycle.

Further studies (Refinetti, 2000) have identified other genes *clock* and *cyc* whose protein CLOCK and CYC provide a positive feedback for the transcription of both *per* and *tim* genes, providing further flexibility and adaptation capability to the internal clock. Analogous genes have been found in mammals.

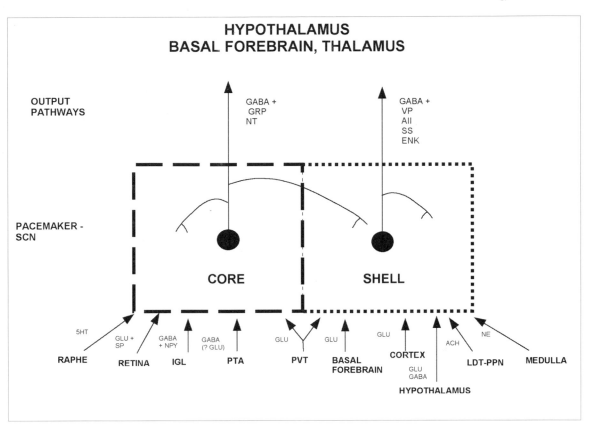

Figure 2.5: Schematic view of the suprachiasmatic nuclei (SCN) structure, input and output connections (modified from Moore, 1997). The SCN is organized in two areas, a core which receives input predominantly from optic pathways from the retina (directly) and from the intergeniculate leaflet (IGL) indirectly. The shell area receives input mostly from non-photic pathways (hypothalamus, basal forebrain). The main neurotransmitters are gama-aminobutyric acid (GABA) which is inhibitory, glutamate (GLU) which is excitatory, and serotonin (5-HT),and norepinephrine (NE). A variety of neuropeptides are often co-localized with the neurotransmitters in the SCN and its connecting pathways: substance P (SP), vasopressin (VP), vasoactive intestinal polypeptide (VIP), somatostatin (SS), angiotensin II (AII), enkephalin (ENK), gastrin-releasing peptide (GRP), neuropeptide Y (NPY), neurotensin (NT).

Circadian rhythms in humans

Studies of human subjects (and other mammals) during 'constant routine' have shown that, in the majority of cases, the circadian clock has a spontaneous period (length) usually slightly longer than 24 hours (*Figure 2.9*) (Wever, 1979). During a constant routine, many environmental factors which, in usual conditions, help to entrain the internal clock to the 24-hour cycle are kept constant to reduce their effects on the underlying endogenous rhythm. Light, food consumption, motor activity, social interaction and mental activity are kept constant to minimize the effect on the variable to be studied, such as temperature and sleep and wake pattern. Core body temperature and a melatonin 24-hour profile are often used as markers of the circadian rhythm.

The actual length (period) of the human circadian pacemaker is still the subject of debate. Initial studies conducted in underground bunkers suggested an average period of 24.5 hours, which is similar to that found in totally blind people who are free-running (the inability to perceive light makes them unable to entrain their rhythm to the 24-hour day cycle) (Sack and Lewy, 2001). Studies conducted using the 'forced desynchrony' protocol suggested a circadian period closer to 24 hours (ie. 24.2) (Dijk and Czeisler, 1995). During a forced desynchrony protocol, the entraining effect of the sleep and wake pattern is eliminated by enforcing a twenty-eight-hour day (nine hours and twenty minutes of darkness), which is beyond the entraining range. Under these conditions, the circadian rhythm is estimated using the profile of core body temperature and melatonin.

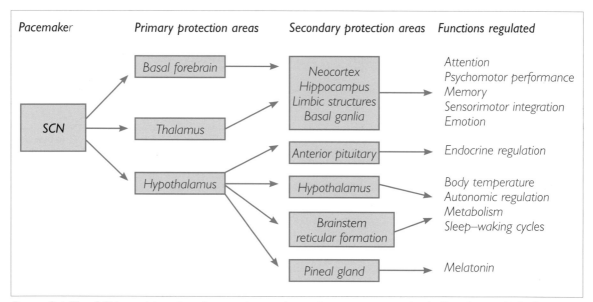

*Figure 2.6: The SCN provides circadian pacing and entrainment to many body functions, which then in turn feed back onto the SCN (Moore, 1996). Reprinted with permission from the Annual Review of Medicine, **48.** © 1997 by Annual Reviews www.annualreviews.org.*

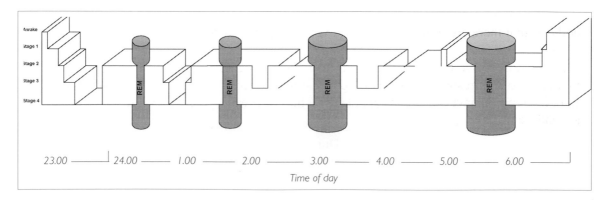

Figure 2.7: REM sleep recurs on average every 90 minutes.

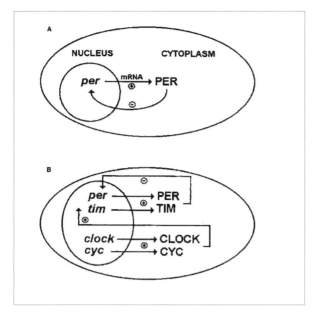

Figure 2.8: See text for explanation. From 'Circadian Physiology' by A Refinetti (2000), reproduced by kind permission of CRC Press.

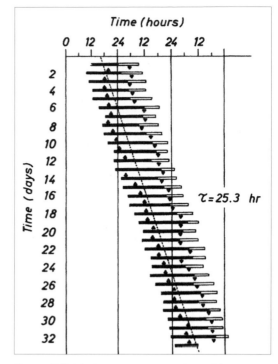

Figure 2.9: Under constant routine without environmental time cues, rest and activity and core body temperature have rhythm longer than 24 hours. Dark bar activity, clear bar rest, dots body temperature trough and peak. From 'The Circadian System of Man. Results of Experiments under Temporal Isolation' by Rutger A Wever, reproduced by kind permission of Springer-Verlag. © 1998–2001 Springer-Verlag.

The variable effect of exogenous factors on endogenous rhythm is referred to as 'masking effect'. Masking is the influence of one variable (internal or external) on another (Minors and Waterhouse, 1989; Wever, 1979;). Because motor activity is known to affect body temperature, the temperature rhythm (and other rhythms) may appear synchronous with the rest and activity cycle (*Figure 2.10*).

Experiments conducted in subjects kept in temporal isolation and constant routine (without time cues) for more than two weeks (Dijk and Edgar, 1999), indicated that rest and activity rhythm and body temperature rhythm would cycle with different periods (internal de-synchronization) (*Figure 2.11*), giving credit to the hypothesis that there are multiple 'clocks', even though the SCN seems to function as a 'master clock' (*Figure 2.4*).

However, the issue of whether one clock drives all circadian rhythms or there are multiple oscillators is still unresolved. Studies in totally blind subjects suggest that sleep propensity and melatonin free-run have the same circadian rhythm suggesting the same circadian pacemaker (Sack and Lewy, 2001).

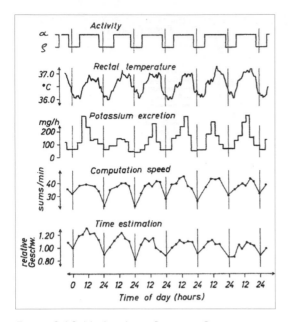

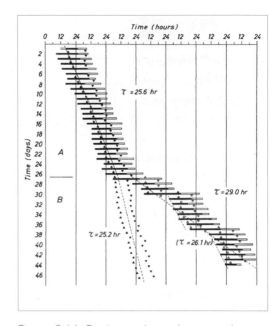

Figure 2.10: Under the influence of a strict 24-hour routine, both physiological and psychological functions show a synchronized 24-hour rhythm. From 'The Circadian System of Man. Results of Experiments under Temporal Isolation' by Rutger A Wever, reproduced by kind permission of Springer-Verlag. © 1998–2001 Springer-Verlag.

Figure 2.11: During prolonged temporal isolation, temperature continues cycling with a ~ 25-hour rhythm, while activity and rest can vary widely. From 'The Circadian System of Man. Results of Experiments under Temporal Isolation' by Rutger A Wever, reproduced by kind permission of Springer-Verlag. © 1998–2001 Springer-Verlag.

Clinical implications of chronobiology

Circadian rhythms are relevant to health practitioners from both a diagnostic and therapeutic point of view. Particular conditions and symptoms are more likely to occur at certain times of the day (*Figure 2.12* and *Table 2.2*).

For example, blood pressure shows a typical circadian pattern with lower values (dipping) at night-time (*Figure 2.13*). When a group of hypertensive subjects experienced 24 hours' monitoring as compared to sporadic blood pressure reading, the criteria for hypertension were not met in a sizeable group of them (Neutel and Smith, 1997).

Given the 24-hour profile of blood pressure, the time of the day the measurements are made, the time of administration of antihypertensive medication and their profile of action (half-life, blood concentration) becomes critical. As blood pressure is higher in the morning, some slow release anti-hypertensive formulations may be more effective given at night than at other times of the day (Smolensky and Haus, 2001; Smith, 2001).

Table 2.2: Circadian rhythms: impact on the diagnosis of medical conditions

Allergy: Cutaneous reactions to intradermal antigen tests 2- to 3-fold greater in evening than in morning.

COPD: Airway patency best in the afternoon and poorest overnight. Morning best time to assess severity of asthma and differentiate between fixed and reversible airway disease.

Glaucoma: Intraocular pressure highest during sleep and lowest in afternoon. Early morning eye exams best for assessing at-risk patients; false-negative diagnosis more at a risk in the afternoon.

Circadian rhythm sleep disorders: Sleep phase delay syndrome (abnormally retarded sleep onset and offset times) and non-24-hour sleep–wake syndrome (period of the sleep–wake cycle considerably different from 24-hour), best diagnosed by wrist actigraphy.

Diabetes: Results of glucose tolerance test different in the morning than in the afternoon, different times of the menstrual cycle, and different seasons of the year.

Laboratory chemistry: Plasma cortisol, melatonin, testosterone, and certain other hormone concentrations differ radically over the 24 hours as do certain other commonly assessed blood constituents and parameters in hematology, such as the number of circulating granulocytes, lymphocytes, and their subtypes.

Blood pressure assessment: SBP and DBP decline in sleep by 10% to 20% from daytime level. In uncomplicated essential hypertension, the pattern is similar, but the BP amplitude and/or 24-hour mean are abnormally elevated. In secondary hypertension, SBP and DBP may be normal or near normal in the day but abnormally high in sleep.

BP = blood pressure; COPD = chronic obstructive pulmonary disease; DBP = diastolic blood pressure; SBP = systolic blood pressure

Reprinted from *American Journal of Hypertension* **14**(9), Smolensky MH and Haus E, 'Circadian rhythms and clinical medicine with applications to hypertension': © 2001 with permission from the American Journal of Hypertension Ltd.

The application of chronobiology concepts to therapy is referred to as chronotherapeutics. Chronotherapeutics uses the information on the time-dependency of medication action (chronopharmacology). The time of the day the medication is administered affects its absorption, distribution and elimination rate (chronokinetics). Toxicity of medication is also time dependent (chronotoxicology). This is potentially relevant in cancer chemotherapy. Following the administration of a lethal dose of an anticancer drug, the survival of rodents varies two- to eight-fold depending on the time of the day the medication is administered (circadian chronotolerance) (Levi, 2002). This is clinically important as a chemotherapeutic agent can be given at the time of the day when toxicity is minimal (*Figure 2.14*), allowing a higher dose to be administered with potentially better anticancer effect.

The combination of rhythms in absorption, receptor numbers, and metabolic transformation results in differences in beneficial and undesirable side-effects of treatment (chronesthesy). For example, given the increase in gastric acid secretion at night-time, administration of H2 inhibitors (eg. cimetidine, ranitidine, famotidine) is usually recommended in the evening. However, the net effect on the gastric pH varies even when the medication plasma level is maintained stable by constant infusion, presumably due to circadian variation in the number and/or responsiveness of gastric receptors, an example of chronoesthesy (Lemmer, 1996).

Another clinically relevant example of chronoesthesy is the circadian variation in the anti-coagulant effect of heparin at constant infusion (*Figure 2.15*) with maximum activity at around 4.00AM (Decousus *et al*, 1985). Other practical examples of chronotherapeutics are described in *Table 2.3*.

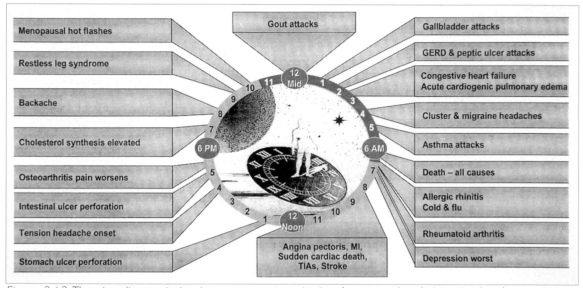

Figure 2.12: The circadian variation in symptoms severity is relevant to the clinician in the diagnostic process. GERD, gastroesophaeal reflux disease; MI, myocardial infarction; TIA< transient ischaemic attacks. Reprinted from American Journal of Hypertension 14(9), Smolensky MH and Haus E, 'Circadian rhythms and clinical medicine with applications to hypertension': 280s–290s. © 2001 with permission from the American Journal of Hypertension Ltd.

Circadian regulation of sleep

With the exception of infants (*Chapter 10*), sleep in humans is monophasic, consisting of a single, prolonged sleep episode in the 24 hours, with an average sleep to wake ratio of 1:2 (eight hours sleep and sixteen hours awake). As previously discussed, the subjective sleep/activity rhythm is synchronized to the 24-hour cycle by external cues (Zeitgebers, time-givers). Although light is considered the major time-giver, directly through the suprachiasmatic nuclei and indirectly through the melatonin, non-photic time cues are also important (meals, work routines, exercise, social interactions).

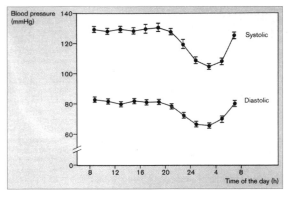

Figure 2.13: *Both systolic and diastolic pressures follow a circadian pattern with 'dipping' at night. This pattern is sometimes lost in some patients with chronic hypertension, especially in cases secondary to renal or endocrine pathology (Neutel and Smith, 1997; Lemmer, 1996).*

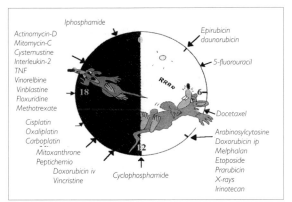

Figure 2.14: *The toxicity of chemotherapeutic drugs varies with the time of administration through the 24 hours, a feature that can be used to maximize efficacy and minimize side-effects (Levi, 2002).*

Sleep and wakefulness regulation results from the balance between the homeostatic process driven by prior wakefulness and a circadian drive (*Figure 2.16*). Animal and human studies suggest that:

1. The homeostatic drive to sleep tendency is increased by prior wakefulness. Sleep pressure becomes intense after thirty hours of continuous wakefulness (*Figure 2.17*) (Agnew and Webb, 1971; Dijk and Edgar, 1999).

2. Sleep structure, as described by conventional sleep stages, is the net result of sleep-wake function and circadian rhythm (*Figure 2.18*). REM sleep propensity, for example, increases as the sleep episode progresses (sleep–wake dependence) but is also more likely to correspond with core body temperature troughs (circadian system dependence). Slow-wave sleep, on the contrary, is more likely to occur at the beginning of the sleep episode and decline as sleep progresses (Dijk and Czeisler, 1995).

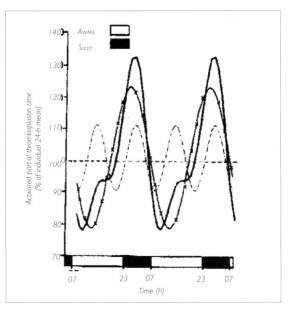

Figure 2.15: *The anticoagulant effect (activated partial thromboplastin time [APTT]) during constant infusion of heparin shows a circadian and an ultradian (shorter than 24 hours) variation. From The British Medical Journal 1985,* **290**, *341–344, with permission from the BMJ Publishing Group.*

3. The circadian endogenous clock provides a drive which promotes wakefulness even in the presence of sleep deprivation, opposing the homeostatic process (*Figure 2.19*).

4. The interaction between the sleep propensity driven by prior wakefulness and circadian influence results in peak alertness around 8AM–9.00AM and just before the main sleep

episode, around 8.00PM–9.00PM. These times of the day correspond to the 'forbidden zones' and 'sleep gates' described in *Chapter 1*.

5. Sleep tendency has a bimodal distribution in the 24-hour period, with a major peak corresponding to the core body temperature trough (between midnight and 6.00AM) and a second peak close to body temperature maximum, around 3.00PM (*Figure 2.20*). This afternoon period of increased sleep propensity corresponds to the 'siesta' of some cultures. It is also the time of the day when motor vehicle accidents are more likely to occur and is the 'midday dip' of many performance measures (Strogatz *et al*, 1987).

6. The timing of the sleep and wake cycle is complex and varies with age (Dijk and Duffy, 1999) but sleep propensity increases as core body temperature decreases, reaching a maximum approximately two hours prior to spontaneous awakening. The time between the core body temperature nadir and spontaneous awakening, however, is variable between individuals and tends to decrease with age (*Figure 2.21*) (Dijk and Duffy, 1999). This is a possible reason for the tendency in the elderly to wake earlier than they did at a younger age. The decreased ability to maintain sleep is associated with a decrease in slow-wave sleep and sleep spindles, as measured by reduction of EEG power density in the delta (1–4 Hz) and beta (12–15 Hz) frequencies.

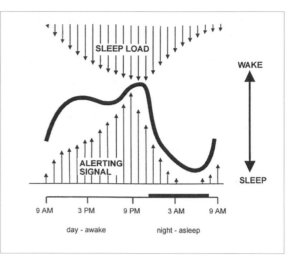

Figure 2.16: Opposing homeostatic and circadian drives determine wake and sleep maintenance. Note that in the second part of the sleep episode (dark bar), the sleep pressure decreases rapidly but sleep is maintained by a low circadian drive to wakefulness (Dijk and Edgar, 1999).

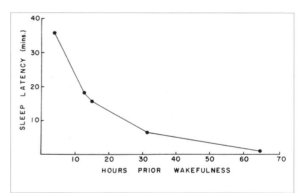

*Figure 2.17: The longer prior wakefulness the faster the latency to sleep. From Psychonomic Science 1971 **24**(6) Agnew Jr HW, Wilse B and Webb 'Sleep latencies in human subjects: Age, prior wakefulness, and reliability'.*

Abnormalities of the sleep and wake circadian rhythm leads to recognized sleep disorder syndromes (circadian rhythm sleep disorders, *Chapter 10*). These conditions are successfully treated by using entraining agents (chronobiotics), such as light and melatonin (Dawson and Armstrong, 1996).

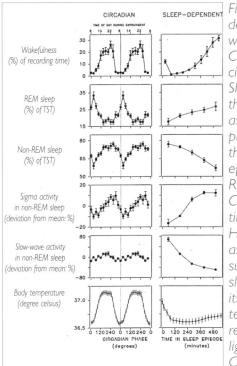

Figure 2.18: Separation of circadian (left) and sleep-dependent components (right) of different aspects of wakefulness, sleep parameters and body temperature. Circadian waveforms were deduced by assigning the data to circadian bins irrespective of time since start of sleep episode. Sleep-dependent changes were deduced by determining the time elapsed since the start of sleep episodes and assigning the data to 112 min bins, irrespective of circadian phase. Circadian waveform data are double plotted at the midpoints of the bins. Wakefulness in scheduled sleep episodes expressed as a percentage of total sleep time. B, REM sleep expressed as a percentage of total sleep time. C, non-REM sleep expressed as a percentage of total sleep time. D, sigma activity (ie. sleep spindle activity: 12.75–15.0 Hz) in non-REM sleep. Data were for each subject expressed as a deviation from its mean value and then averaged over subjects. E, Slow-wave activity (0.75-4.5 Hx) in non-REM sleep. Data were for each subject expressed as a deviation of its mean value and then averaged over subjects. F, core body temperature. The first point in the sleep-dependent graph represents the average value during the last 30 min before lights out. From The Journal of Neuroscience 15(5), Dijk and Czeisler. © 1995 by the Society of Neuroscience.

The effect of light on the sleep–wake rhythm

Light is the strongest environmental agent that synchronizes the internal clock to the 24-hour period. Sleep and wake respond to light exposure according to a phase response curve (PRC), which is fairly uniform for most organisms (*Figure 2.22*).

The light PRC describes the differential sensitivity of the endogenous circadian pacemaker to light exposure (Hoban *et al*, 1989; Minors *et al*, 1991).

The effect of light on the direction of phase shift depends on the time of the day, intensity and duration of exposure. Exposure to light during the day usually has no phase shifting properties. When exposure occurs in the evening it tends to phase delay with increasing effects through the night. However, after core body temperature nadir, light exposure tends to have the opposite effects with phase advance. A typical application is the use of light in the morning to phase advanced patients with delayed sleep phase syndrome.

Initially it was thought that high intensity light (>2500 lux) was necessary to exert an entraining effect, however, it is now accepted that low intensity (eg. 180 lux) has the potential to cause phase shifts (Boivin *et al*, 1994, Boivin *et al*, 1996; Czeisler *et al*, 1986; Czeisler, 1995; Dawson *et al*, 1993; Hoban *et al*, 1989). This is of practical importance because this low intensity is within the range of ordinary room light.

Table 2.3: Chronotherapies currently in clinical use

- Once-daily and alternate-day morning corticosteroid dosing minimizes risk of adrenal suppression and other side-effects.

- Bedtime corticosteroid dosing controls excessive hormone secretion in congenital adrenal hyperplasia.

- Asymmetrical morning high and late-afternoon low-dose corticosteroid substitution chronotherapy for Addison's disease best corrects fatigue and abnormal circadian time structure.

- Evening ingestion of certain HMG-CoA reductase antagonist medications optimizes their cholesterol-lowering effect.

- Nitroglycerin transdermal patch medication worn during the 24-hour period when angina risk is greatest., and removed in time to avoid sensitization to medication.

- Evening H2-receptor antagonist ingestion best controls nocturnal peptic ulcer and gastroesophageal reflux disease.

- Evening NSAID treatment optimizes attenuation of morning symptoms of rheumatoid arthritis; midday and/or afternoon NSAID treatment best for osteoarthritis that is typically worse in evening.

- Bedtime ADH analogue dosing helps alleviate nocturnal bedwetting in children and nocturia in adults.

- Bedtime (but not morning) aspirin dosing best prevent pregnancy-induced hypertension and pre-eclampsia.

- Evening theophylline chronotherapy (Uniphyl), producing highest drug concentration in sleep, optimizes control of nocturnal asthma and COPD.

- Evening verapamil chronotherapy (Verelan PM™ and Covera-HS™) achieves more complete 24-hour BP control than once-a-day conventional constant-release medications.

- Timed melatonin and bright-light chronotherapies enhance speed of adjustment to alteration of sleep–wake routine, after rapid transmeridian displacement by airplane or rotation between day and night shifts.

- Timed bright-light chronotherapy is effective for seasonal affective disorder (SAD), premenstrual dysphoric disorder (PMDD), and circadian rhythm sleep disorders (advanced and delayed sleep phase syndromes and non-24-hour sleep–wake cycle disorder).

- Luteal phase (commencing 6–14 days before menses) therapy of premenstrual dysphoric disorder (PMDD) using alprazolam, clomipramine, citalopram, fluoxetine or sertraline.

- Infusion of cancer medications in synchrony with circadian rhythms minimizes drug-induced toxicity, enabling more aggressive treatment.

Reprinted from *American Journal of Hypertension* **14**, Smolensky MH *et al*, © 2001 with permission from American Journal of Hypertension Ltd.

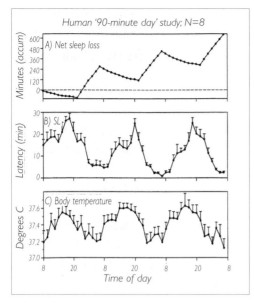

Figure 2.19: *The tendency to fall asleep (sleep latency, middle panel) maintains a circadian rhythm, in synchrony with body temperature (bottom panel) even in the presence of progressive sleep deprivation (homeostatic drive, top panel) (Dijk and Edgar, 1999).*

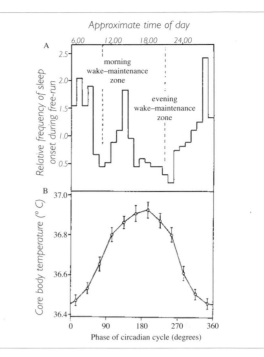

Figure 2.20: *Note the two peaks of sleep tendency, one corresponding to body temperature trough (~ 4.00AM) and one close to temperature peak (~ 3.00PM) (Dijk and Duffy, 1999).*

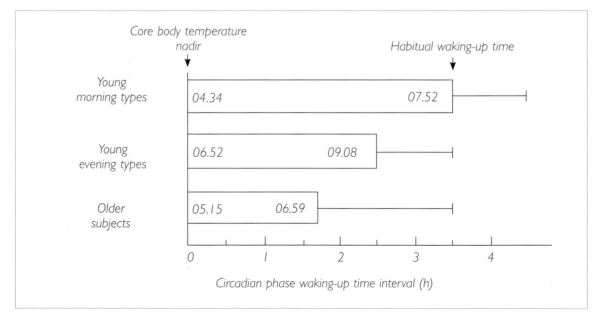

Figure 2.21: *The relation between core body temperature and spontaneous awakening changes with age (Dijk and Duffy, 1999), see text.*

In some patients with delayed sleep phase syndrome, even the light from a television set or a computer may be a contributing factor to delayed sleep onset, which presents clinically as difficulty initiating sleep (insomnia) and/or daytime sleepiness due to insufficient sleep time.

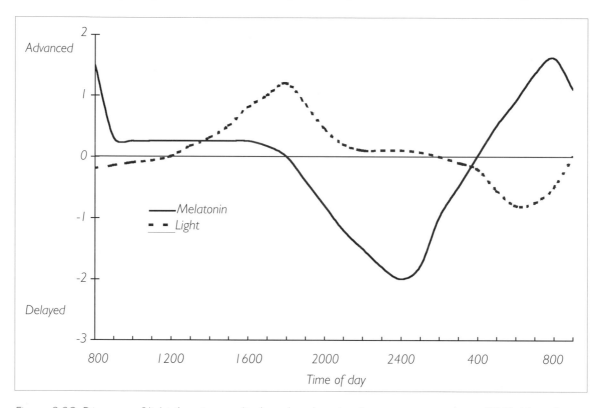

Figure 2.22: Diagram of light (continuous line) and melatonin phase response curves (PRC). Note the reciprocal characteristics of these two chronobiotic agents. Administered in the evening, melatonin tends to phase advance, while light phase delays, and vice versa in the morning (based on Arendt, 1997).

The use of light in practice

Given its phase-shifting properties, light is used in the management of different conditions (*Table 2.4*) (Eastman, 1992; Eastman and Martin, 1999; Campbell *et al*, 1993; Campbell, 1995; Czeisler, 1990).

It must be emphasized that the use of light is only part of a more comprehensive programme including regular sleep and wake time and other measures of sleep hygiene. Light can be delivered by using natural sources, light boxes, light visors or dawn simulators.

Table 2.4: Uses of light in clinical practice

- Delayed sleep phase syndrome.
- Advanced sleep phase syndrome.
- Management of shift work.
- Sleep maintenance insomnia.
- Seasonal affective disorder.

Exposure to daylight is ideal as it delivers high light intensity (approximately 10000 lux). Having breakfast on the verandah or walking in the morning for 20–30 minutes is ideal when possible.

In winter, the use of artificial light sources such as light boxes, either by direct exposure or reflected to the wall, can deliver up to 2500 lux or more depending on the distance from the light source. In practice, the use of light boxes is somewhat cumbersome and compliance is low. Light visors are more practical but deliver low intensity light (200–400 lux). The use of spectacles that deliver selected light frequency in the blue-green part of the spectrum (430–480 nm) is experimental but potentially useful if shown to be effective (Wright and Lack, 2001; NSVV Committee on Light and Health, 2003). Dawn simulators are a small device which can be used with different light sources and allow the bedroom to be lit progressively at a predetermined time in the morning. It should be noted that exposure to light is potentially hazardous (*Table 8.6, Chapter 8*).

Melatonin

Although light is probably the most effective agent in manipulating sleep and wake timing, it is not particularly practical. Melatonin is gaining acceptance as a potentially useful entraining drug (chronobiotic) (Geoffriau *et al*, 1998). Melatonin is synthesized by the pineal gland and other organs (eg. retina and gut) from tryptophan (*Figure 2.23*). It is metabolized by the liver and has a short half life. The plasma level depends on melatonin secretion as there is no known melatonin storage.

Regulation of melatonin secretion depends on neural input to the pinealocytes with the adrenergic receptors being the predominant ones. In fact, beta-blockers such as atenolol and propranolol can reduce melatonin secretion (*Table 1.3, Chapter 1*).

The role of melatonin in the regulation of the sleep–wake cycle remains controversial. Specifically, its role may include a direct effect on sleep (hypnotic effect), and an effect on the circadian oscillator (Dijk and Cajochen, 1997). Administration of melatonin to normal volunteers during the day when the level of endogenous melatonin is low and the circadian sleep tendency is minimal, results in a dose-dependent reduction in sleep-onset latency.

A phase-reponse curve (PRC) for melatonin is proposed (*Figure 2.22*) which is approximately 12 hours out of phase with the light PRC (Lewy *et al*, 1998). Light has a dose-dependent inhibitory effect on melatonin, with green light being the most active and red light ineffective. Melatonin in the evening has an advance phase-shifting effect (opposite to a light pulse) and is useful in the management of delayed sleep phase syndrome. A high concentration of melatonin receptors are present in the suprachiasmatic nuclei, suggesting that melatonin modulates its phase shifting by feedback action on the SCN.

By the same token, the coupling of onset of melatonin secretion and sleep onset points towards an important role for melatonin in sleep–wake regulation. Abnormal melatonin secretion, either low amplitude (as in the elderly, *Chapter 8*), or abnormal timing (eg. delayed sleep phase syndrome) can disrupt sleep and wake physiology (*Figure 2.24*) (Oren *et al*, 1995).

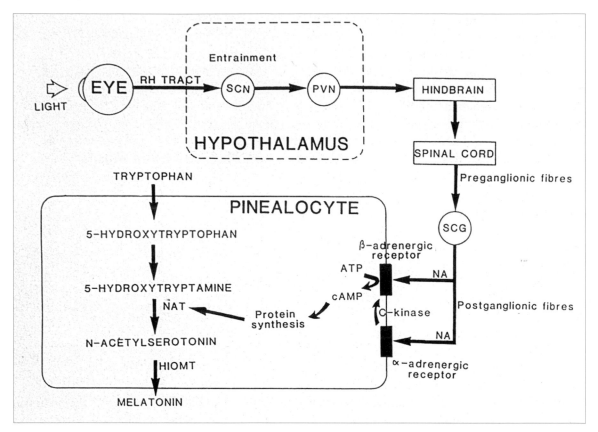

Figure 2.23: The modulation of melatonin production is influenced by adrenergic control through post-ganglionic innervation via the superior cervical ganglion (SCG). ATP, adenosine triphosphate; CAMP, cyclic-adenosine monophosphate; HIOMT, hydroxyindole-O-methyltransferase; NAT, N-acetyltransferase; PVN, paraventricular nucleus; RH, retinohypothalamic tract; SCG, superior cervical ganglion; SCN, suprachiasmatic nucleus. (From Touitou and Haus, 1994).

The secretion of melatonin is similar in men and women and decreases in amplitude with aging (Zhao *et al*, 2002). There is some evidence that melatonin can improve sleep quality in the elderly by consolidating sleep (Dijk and Cajochan, 1997). In the elderly who have difficulty maintaining sleep, the use of slow-release formulation of melatonin to keep its level elevated in the second part of the night, may be helpful. Other clinical applications of melatonin are discussed in *Chapters 6* and *11*.

The language of chronobiology

Chronobiology has led to the development of a new terminology, which allows researchers to describe rhythmic events. Trigonometric functions are used to describe in mathematical terms the recurrent nature of rhythmic functions (*Figure 2.25*).

The use of trigonometric function allows the identification of specific parameters that are helpful in defining a rhythm (*Figure 2.26*). The period τ (pronounced 'tau') represents a complete cycle of a rhythmic event. The amplitude (a) describes half of the distance between the lowest value and the peak value of the function (not of the data set). The peak value is referred to as acrophase and the lower value of the cycle as bathyphase.

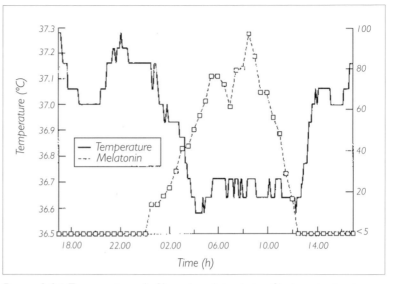

An average value for the rhythm is a more difficult parameter to obtain. Researchers use rhythm-adjusted means (*Figure 2.26*). In real experiments the data

*Figure 2.24: Temperature (left) and melatonin profile in a patient with delayed sleep-phase syndrome. Note how the trough in body temperature and the peak of melatonin are still coupled but delayed at 6–10.00AM compared to the usual 3–4.00AM. From Neurology in Practice 1995 **58**: 379, Oren et al, 1995. Reproduced with permission from BMJ Publishing Group.*

points are often unequally sampled and their mean is likely to either overestimate or underestimate the real mean value. To overcome this problem, a MESOR (midline estimating statistic of rhythm) is used instead. The MESOR represents the midway value between the highest and the lowest points of the function fitted to the data (Touitou and Haus, 1994).

The location in time of the rhythm, particularly when comparison is made between different functions, is described by the rhythm phase (φ). The phase of a rhythm is determined by a reference point chosen by the researcher (eg. wake time for the sleep and wake circadian rhythm or onset of motor activity). This allows identifying circadian time (CT) as opposed to usual clock time. If, for example, 7.00AM is the onset of daylight and it is taken as circadian time 0 (CT 0), then 8.00PM (20 hours) is referred to as CT 13. The relation between circadian rhythms can be described as 'phase angle difference'. For example, if the onset of melatonin secretion at dusk occurs at circadian time 13 (CT 13, or 20 hours), and onset of sleep is at CT 15 (21 hours), the 'phase angle difference' between the two rhythms is 2 hours.

A rhythm phase is relevant in the practical case of entrainment. As discussed above, an endogenous rhythm may tend to be slightly longer than 24 hours. If, for example, the internal clock in free-running condition is 23 hours, it would be out of phase with the 24-hour night and dark cycle. If one were to label the period of the endogenous 23-hour rhythm as a τ, and the 24-hour light and dark rhythm as T, then the difference in phase would be $\Delta\varphi = \tau$-T (Refinetti, 2000). The difference in phase would then be -1 hour. In this case, the endogenous clock is too fast and, therefore, needs to be 'delayed' 1 hour a day to adjust (entrain) to the 24-hour light and dark cycle.

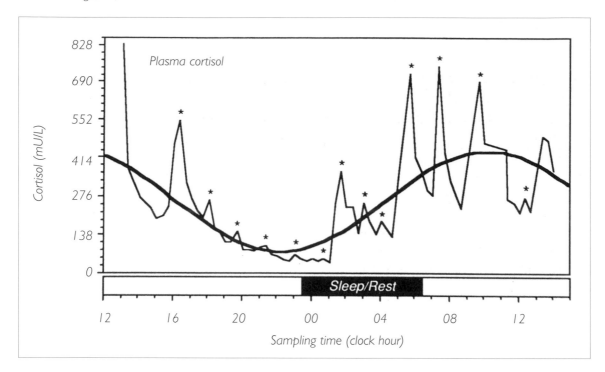

Figure 2.25: Fitting a sinusoid curve (sine or cosine) to the data estimates of a rhythm provides a useful way of describing a rhythm. From 'Biological Rhythms in Clinical and Laboratory Medicine', Touitou Y and Haus E, p. 8 , Figure 2, 1994. © 1994 Springer-Verlag.

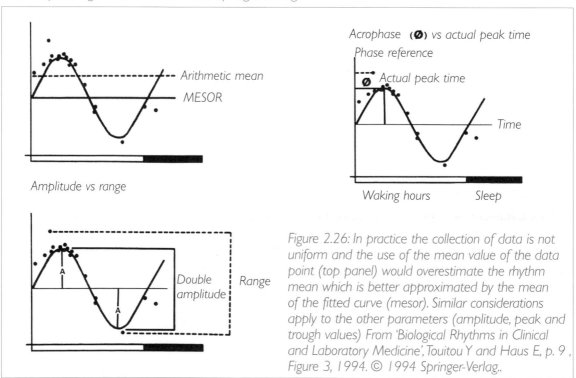

Figure 2.26: In practice the collection of data is not uniform and the use of the mean value of the data point (top panel) would overestimate the rhythm mean which is better approximated by the mean of the fitted curve (mesor). Similar considerations apply to the other parameters (amplitude, peak and trough values) From 'Biological Rhythms in Clinical and Laboratory Medicine', Touitou Y and Haus E, p. 9 , Figure 3, 1994. © 1994 Springer-Verlag..

References

Agnew HW Jr , Webb WB, Wilse B (1971) Sleep latencies in human subjects: Age, prior wakefulness, and reliability. *Psychon Sci* **24**(6): 253–4

Arendt J (1997) The pineal gland, circadian rhythms and photoperiodism. In: Redfern PH, Lemmer B, eds. *Physiology and Pharmacology of Biological Rhythms*. Springer, Berlin, Heidelberg, New York

Boivin DB, Duffy JF, Kronauer RE, Czeisler CA (1994) Sensitivity of the human circadian pacemaker to moderately bright light. *J Biological Rhythms* **9**(3–4): 315–31

Boivin DB, Duffy JF, Kronauer RE, Czeisler CA (1996) Dose-response relationships for resetting of human circadian clock by light. *Nature* **379**: 540–2

Campbell SS (1995) Effects of timed bright-light exposure on shift-work adaptation in middle-aged subjects. *Sleep* **18**(6): 408–16

Campbell SS, Dawson D, Anderson MW (1993) Alleviation of sleep maintenance insomnia with timed exposure to bright light. *JAGS* **41**(8): 829–36

Czeisler CA (1995) The effect of light on the human circadian pacemaker. Circadian clocks and their adjustment. Wiley, Chichester (Ciba Foundation Symposium 183): 254–302

Czeisler CA, Allan JS, Strogatz SH, Ronda JM, Sanchez R, Rios D *et al* (1986) Bright light resets the human circadian pacemaker independent of the timing of the sleep-wake cycle. *Science* **233**: 667–71

Czeisler CA, Johnson MP, Duffy JF, Brown EN, Ronda JM, Kronauer RE (1990) Exposure to bright light and darkness to treat physiologic maladaptation to night work. *N Engl J Med* **322**: 1253–9

Dawson D, Armstrong SM (1996) Chronobiotics — drugs that shift rhythms. *Pharmacol Ther* **69**(1): 15–36

Dawson D, Lack L, Morris M (1993) Phase resetting of the human circadian pacemaker with use of a single pulse of bright light. *Chronobiol Int* **10**(2): 94–102

Decousus H, Croze M, Levi F, Jaubert J, Perpoint B, Reinberg A, Queneau P (1985) Circadian changes in anticoagulant effect of heparin infused at a constant rate. *Br Med J* **290**: 341–4

Dijk DJ, Cajochen C (1997) Melatonin and the circadian regulation of sleep initiation, consolidation, structure, and sleep EEG. *J Biological Rhythms* **6**: 627–35

Dijk D, Czeisler CA (1995) Contribution of the circadian pacemaker and the sleep homeostat to sleep propensity, sleep structure, electroencephalographic slow waves, and sleep spindle activity in humans. *J Neuroscience* **15**(5): 3526–38

Dijk D, Duffy JF (1999) Circadian regulation of human sleep and age-related changes in its timing, consolidation and EEG characteristics. *Ann Med* **31**: 130–40

Dijk D, Edgar DM (1999) Circadian and homeostatic control of wakefulness and sleep. In: Turek FW, Zee PC, eds. *Regulation of Sleep and Circadian Rhythms*. Marcel Dekker Inc, New York

Eastman CI (1992) High-intensity light for circadian adaptation to a 12-h shift of the sleep schedule. *Am J Physiol* **263**: R428–R436

Eastman CI, Martin SK (1999) How to use light and dark to produce circadian adaptation to night shift work. *Ann Med* **31**: 87–98

Elliott WJ (2001) Cyclic and circadian variations in cardiovascular events. *Am J Hypertens* **14**: 2915–55

Geoffriau M, Brun J, Chazot G, Claustrat B (1998) The physiology and pharmacology of melatonin in humans. *Horm Res* **49**: 136–41

Halbert F, Haloberg E, Barnum CP, Bittner JJ (1959) Physiologic 24-hour periodicity in human beings and mice, the lighting regimen and daily routine. In: Withrow RB, ed. *Photoperiodism and Related Phenomena in Plants and Animals*. AAAS, Washington

Hoban TM, Sack RL, Lewy AJ, Miller S, Singer CM (1989) Entrainment of a free-running human with bright light. *Chronobiol Int* **6**: 347–53

Johnson CH, Jeffrey A, Elliott, Foster R (2003) Entrainment of circadian programs. *Chronobiol Int* **20**(5): 41–74

Lemmer B (1996) The clinical relevance of chronopharmacology in therapeutics. *Pharmacological Res* **33**(2): 107–15

Levi F (2002) From circadian rhythms to cancer chronotherapeutics. *Chronobiol Int* 19(1): 1–19

Lewy AJ, Ahmed S, Latham Jackson JM, Sack RL (1992) Melatonin shifts human circadian rhythms according to a phase-response curve. *Chronobiol Int* **9**(5): 380–92

Lewy AJ, Bauer VK, Ahmed S, Thomas KH, Cutler NL, Singer CM *et al* (1998) The human phase response curve (PRC) to melatonin is about 12 hours out of phase with the PRC to light. *Chronobiol Int* **15**(1): 71–83

Minors DS, Waterhouse JM (1989) Masking in humans: the problem and some attempts to solve it. *Chronobiol Int* **1**: 29–53

Minors DS, Waterhouse JM, Wirz-Justice A (1991) A human phase-response curve to light. *Neurosci Lett* **133**: 36–40

Moore RY (1996) Circadian rhythms: basic neurobiology and clinical applications. *Annu Rev Med* **48**: 253–66

Moore RY (1997) Chemical neuroanatomy of the mammalian circadian system. In: Redfern PH, Lemmer B, eds. *Physiology and Pharmacology of Biological Rhythms*. Springer, Berlin: chap 4

Moore-Ede MC, Sulzman FM, Fuller CA (1982) *The Clocks that Time Us*. Harvard University Press, Cambridge

Neutel JM, Smith DHG (1997) The circadian pattern of blood pressure: cardiovascular risk and therapeutic opportunities. *Curr Opin Nephrol Hypertens* **6**: 250–6

NSVV Committee on Light and Health (2003) *Light and Health in the Workplace*. Nederlandse Stichting Voor Verlichtingskunde, Arnhem, Netherlands

Oren DA, Turner EH, Wehr TA (1995) Abnormal circadian rhythms of plasma melatonin and body temperature in the delayed sleep phase syndrome. *J Neurol Neurosurg Psych* **58**: 379–85

Pittendrigh CS (1960) Circadian rhythms and the circadian organizaiton of living systems. *Cold Spring Harbor Symp Quant Biol* **25**: 159–82

Refinetti R (2000) *Circadian Physiology*. CRC Press, Boca Raton

Reinberg A (2001) *Chronobiology: Concepts and Definitions*. Mediterranean Society for Chronobiology, 11th Graduate Course in Chronobiology, Antalya ,Turkey

Reinberg A, Lewy H, Smolensky M (2001) The birth of chronobiology: Julien Joseph Virey 1814. *Chronobiol Int* **18**(2): 173–86

Sack LR, Lewy AJ (2001) Circadian rhythm sleep disorders: lessons from the blind. *Sleep Med Rev* **5**: 189–206

Smith DHG (2001) Pharmacology of cardiovascular chronotherapeutic agents. *Am J Hypertens* **14**: 296S–301S

Smolensky MH (1996) Chronobiology and chronotherapeutics. applications to cardiovascular medicine. *AJH* **9**: 11S–21S

Smolensky MH, D'Alonzo GE (1993) Medical chronobiology: concepts and applications. *Am Rev Respir Dis* **147**: S2–S19

Smolensky MH, Haus E (2001) Circadian rhythms and clinical medicine with applications to hypertension. *Am J Hypertens* **14**: 280S–290S

Strogatz SH, Kronauer RE, Czeisler CA (1987) Circadian pacemaker interferes with sleep onset at specific times each day: role in insomnia. *Am J Physiol* **253**: R172–R178

Touitou Y, Haus E (1994) *Biological Rhythms in Clinical and Laboratory Medicine*. Springer-Verlag, New York

Wever RA (1979) *The Circadian System of Man. Results of Experiements Under Temporal Isolation*. Springer-Verlag, New York

Wirz-Justice (1987) A circadian rhythms in mammalian neurotransmitter receptors. *Prog Neurobiol* **29**: 219–59

Wright HR, Lack LC (2001) Effect of light wavelength on suppression and phase delay of the melatonin rhythm. *Chronobiol Int* **18**(5): 801–8

Zee PC, Turek FW (1999) *Introduction to sleep and circadian rhythm in regulation of sleep and circadian rhythms*. Editors Turek FW, Zee PC. Marcel Dekker Inc, New York

Zhao ZY, Xie Y, Fu YR, Bogdan A, Touitou Y (2002) The circadian rhythm of melatonin: a cross-sectional study of Chinese subjects 30–110 years of age. *Chronobiol Int* **19**(6): 1171–82

Appendix (chronobiology glossary)

The following glossary is a brief description of the most common terms used in chronobiology research. (Reproduced with permission of The American Association of Medical Chronobiology and Chronotherapeutics.)

Acrophase:
Measure of timing of a rhythm in relation to a defined reference time point selected by the investigator (eg. local midnight for circadian rhythms). Used for data which can be described by the fitting of a mathematical model, eg. a cosine curve, and represents the crest time of the cosine curve best fitting to the data. May be expressed in (negative) degrees as the lag from the acrophase reference ($360° = 1$ period) or in calendar time units (eg. hours and minutes for circadian rhythms, days or months for infradian rhythms).

Amplitude (A):
The measure of one half of the extent of the rhythmic change estimated by the mathematical model (eg. cosine curve) best fitting to the data (eg. the difference between the maximum and the rhythm-adjusted mean (MESOR) of the best fitting curve).

Autorhythmometry:
Self-measurement of biologic rhythms by the subject examined.

Bathyphase:
The time of the lowest point of a mathematical model (eg. cosine curve) fitted to a time series and describing a rhythm. If a sine or a cosine curve is fitted, the bathyphase will differ $180°$ from the acrophase, measured in relation to a defined reference time point selected by the investigator (eg. local midnight for circadian rhythms). May be expressed in degrees as the lag from the phase reference ($360° = 1$ period) or in calendar time units (eg. hours and minutes for circadian rhythms, days or months for infradian rhythm).

Biologic time structure:
The sum of nonrandom time-dependent biologic changes, including growth, development, and aging, and a spectrum of rhythms with different frequencies.

Biologic clocks:
Self-sustained oscillators which generate biologic rhythms in absence of external periodic input (eg. at the gene level in individual cells).

Biologic rhythm:
A regularly recurring (periodic) component in a series of measurements of a biologic variable obtained as a function of time.

Chronergy:
Represents the rhythmic change of the response of the organism to a drug (its total effect) according to its chronokinetics and its chronesthesy.

Chronesthesy:
Rhythmic (thus predictable-in-time) changes in the susceptibility or sensitivity of a target biosystem (cell or organism) to an agent. May be caused by temporal changes in receptors of target cells or organs, membrane permeability, etc.

Chronobiology:
The science of investigating and objectively quantifying phenomena and mechanisms of the biologic time structure, including the rhythmic

manifestations of life. Term derived from chronos (time), bios (life), and logos (science).

Chronobiotic:	An agent capable of influencing biologic rhythm parameters (eg. the phase setting).
Chronodesm:	Time-qualified reference intervals. Reference intervals constructed along the time scale by Gaussian or non-Gaussian methods. Include time-qualified prediction and tolerance intervals.
Chronogram:	Display of data as a function of time.
Chronopathology:	Changes in an individual's biologic time structure preceding, coincident or following functional disorders or organic disease and/or time-dependent manifestation of disease.
Chronopharmaco-dynamics:	Temporal variations in the mode of action of a drug.
Chronopharmaco-kinetics	The study of the temporal changes in absorption, distribution, metabolism, and elimination of a drug. Describes the influence of the time of administration of a drug on the mathematical parameters which describe these processes in terms of absorption rate, peak drug concentration (Cmax), time-to-peak drug concentration (Emax), area under the concentration time curve (AUC), half-life ($t^{1}/_{2}$), etc.
Chronotherapy:	Use of treatment timed according to the stages in the sensitivity-resistance cycles of target (or nontarget) tissues and organs (or of the organism as a whole) to enhance the desired pharmacologic effect and/or reduce undesirable side effects of drugs or other therapeutic agents.
Chronotolerance:	Time-dependent tolerance of an organism to environmental stimuli and xenobiotics.
Chronotoxicology:	Time-dependent variation in toxicity.
Circadian:	About 24 hours. The term describes rhythms with an about 24-h (>20 to <28 h) cycle length whether they are synchronized with a 24-h periodic surrounding or not.
Circadiseptan:	A rhythm with a period of about 14 (± 3) days.
Circannual:	A rhythm with a period of about 1 year (± 2 months), synchronized with or desynchronized from the calendar year.
Circaseptan:	A rhythm with a period of about 7 (± 3) days, which may or may not be synchronized with the calendar week.
Circatrigintan:	A rhythm with a period of about 30 (± 5) days. Includes, in mature women during the time of ovarian activity, the menstrual cycle. The term is preferred to the term 'menstrual' because rhythms of this frequency are found in premenarchal girls, postmenopausal women and in men.

Circavigintan: A rhythm with a period of about 20 (± 3 days).

Clinospectrometry: Resolving of a spectrum of rhythms and trends (cline) by (computer-implemented) time series collection and analysis. With rhythms quantified as algorithmically formulated phenomena validated in inferential statistical terms.

Cosinor procedure: A mathematical–statistical method of describing a rhythm by determining by least squares technique the cosine curve best fitting to the data and exploring the presence of a rhythm by examining the null hypothesis for amplitude in an F-test. If a rhythm can be described by this procedure the cosinor yields a rhythm-adjusted mean (MESOR), an amplitude as measure of the extent of the rhythm, and an acrophase as indication of its timing with variance estimates for each.

Cosinor: Single cosinor — a cosinor procedure applicable to single biologic time series. Population mean cosinor — the cosinor procedure applicable to parameter estimates from three or more biologic time series for assessing the rhythm characteristics of a population. The parameter estimates are based on the means of estimates obtained from individuals in the samples.

Daily: Occurring every day.

Dampened oscillation: Oscillation decreasing (dampened) in amplitude due to inevitable loss of energy.

Desynchronization: State of two or more previously synchronized rhythmic variables that have ceased to exhibit the same frequency and/or the same acrophase relationships and show different than usual and/or changing time relations.

Diurnal: Day related (in contrast to nocturnal), eg. diurnal (vs nocturnal) activity pattern.

Endogenous rhythm: Presumably genetically fixed biologic rhythm, persisting in an environment without outside time cues.

Entrainment: Coupling of two rhythms of the same frequency to one of them (the entraining agent or synchronizer) determining the phase of the other. Coupling of endogenous rhythms to environmental oscillator of the same frequency and/or determination of the phase of biologic rhythms by an internal pacemaker.

Episodic variation: Apparently irregular (nonrhythmic) variation of a biologic variable, eg. episodic secretion of certain hormones (used by some as synonymous with 'pulsatile').

External desynchronization: Desynchronization of a biologic rhythm from an environmental cycle.

Feedsideward coordination: Interaction of several rhythms (multifrequency coordination). Involves rhythmic and predictable sequences of effects depending upon the phase of each of the rhythms involved. 'Feedsideward' may manifest itself as rhythmic alteration of stimulation, no effect or inhibition by an action of a rhythmic entity upon two other interacting entities.

Free-running:	Continuance of an endogenous bioperiodicity at least slightly but consistently different from any known environmental schedule, ie. from its usual synchronizer or usual pacemaker rhythm.
Frequency (f):	The number of cycles occurring per time unit; f is the reciprocal of the period (t).
Frequency ranges:	Groups of frequencies (or periods) frequently encountered in biologic rhythms. (Circadian frequency range: rhythm with periods of about 1 day, ie. by definition > 20 to < 28 h).)
Infradian rhythm:	Rhythm with a period longer (by definition > 28 h) than the circadian range; the term includes circaseptan, circatrigintan, circannual, and other rhythms of lower frequency.
Internal desynchronization:	State in which two or more previously synchronized variables within the same organism have ceased to exhibit the same frequency and/or the same acrophase relationships and show different from usual and/or changing time relations.
Jet lag:	Desynchronization and its clinical effect after rapid movement over several time zones (after transmeridian flights).
Lighting regimen:	The light–dark cycle (LD), or constant light (LL), or constant dark (DD) conditions used for chronobiologic studies.
Longitudinal sampling:	Study of the same subject or of a group of subjects over numerous cycles.
Longitudinal study:	Study of the same individual over a prolonged time span (eg. aging).
Marker rhythm:	Rhythm of use in monitoring an organism's biologic timing and/or the timing of a related rhythm showing a fixed time relation to the rhythm used as 'marker'. Can be used where appropriate for decision-making in applied or basic physiologic or pharmacologic work, eg. for time of sampling, timing of therapy, or for assessing therapeutic response (without any implication of causal relations between the rhythmic process and its marker). See also Reference Rhythm.
Masking of a rhythm:	Alteration of the usual shape and/or parameters of a rhythm due to random or nonrandom environmental stimuli, persisting for the duration of the stimulus only (without persistent alteration of endogenous rhythm components), eg. change in body temperature after a hot bath.
MESOR:	Midline Estimating Statistic of Rhythm. The value midway between the highest and the lowest values of the (cosine) function best fitting to the data. The 'M' is equal to the arithmetic mean only for equidistant data covering an integral number of cycles.
Pacemaker:	A functional entity capable of self-sustaining oscillations which synchronize other rhythms (eg. the suprachiasmatic nucleus in man).
Peak:	The highest point in a series of measurements obtained as a function of time.

Period (τ):   Duration of one complete cycle in a rhythmic variation.

Phase: The value of a rhythmic biological variable at a certain time. Each instantaneous state of an oscillation represents a phase.

Phase advance: Involves the earlier occurrence of a rhythm's phase, usually the acrophase (denoted by a plus sign).

Phase delay: Involves the later occurrence of a rhythm's (acro) phase (denoted by a minus sign).

Phase drift: During free running of an endogenous rhythm with a period slightly but consistently different from its usual environmental synchronizer, the rhythm's acrophase will occur during every synchronizer cycle at a different time (eg. clock hour in the case of circadian rhythms) in relation to the phase reference.

Phase reference: Time point chosen by the investigator as reference for the estimation of the timing of a rhythm (eg. local midnight for circadian rhythms).

Phase response curve: Graphical plot indicating how the amount and the duration of a phase shift, induced by a single stimulus, depend upon the rhythm's stage at which the stimulus is applied.

Phase shift: Single relatively abrupt or gradual change in the timing of a rhythm (completed within a finite time span) and described by the difference between the initial and final (acro) phase.

Photoperiod: In a light–dark regimen the duration of the light span (eg. in light–dark = LD 12:12 h, the photoperiod L = 12 h).

Plexogram: Display of original data covering spans longer than the period of a rhythm investigated along an abscissa of a single period (irrespective of time order of data collection).

Pulsatile variation: Variation of a biologic function with an irregular period higher than circadian of which a regular recurrence (rhythm) cannot be documented. May be the result of circadian-ultradian interactions or of other rhythmic and/or nonrhythmic mechanisms (used by some as synonymous with 'episodic').

Reference rhythm: A rhythm in one variable used as a time reference for other rhythms, events, or actions (see also Marker rhythms).

Rhythm: A regularly recurring and thus, to a certain degree, predictable (periodic) component of a (biologic) time series, demonstrated by inferential statistical means.

Scotoperiod: In a light-dark regimen the duration of the dark span (eg. light-dark = LD 12:12 h, the scotoperiod D = 12 h).

Seasonal variation: Change in a biologic system brought about by seasonal changes of temperature, lightspan, etc, and not observed in the absence of such changes.

Self-sustained oscillation: System that can make use of a constant source of energy (to counteract energy losses) and is able to continue to oscillate without outside energy input.

Shift work: Transient or permanent change in work schedule in relation to the social surroundings (eg. 3 x 8-h work shifts).

Suprachiasmatic nucleus: Group of hypothalamic neurons situated above the optic chiasm exhibiting an endogenous circadian oscillation acting as circadian pacemaker, receiving external phase information via the retina.

Synchronization: State of a system when two or more variables exhibit periodicity with the same frequency and specifiable acrophase and phase relation.

Synchronizer: Environmental periodicity determining the temporal placement of a biologic rhythm along an appropriate time scale. Synonyms: entraining agent, time-giver, Zeitgeber.

Synchronizing agent: See Synchronizer.

Time-giver: See Synchronizer.

Time series: A series of measurements obtained as a function of time.

Transmeridian flight: Movement over time zones (see Jet lag).

Transverse sampling: Sampling of a group of subjects over one cycle of a rhythm.

Transverse study: Comparison of two groups differing by a parameter (eg. age, sex) studied at one time (eg. over one cycle).

Trough: The lowest point in a series of measurements obtained as a function of time.

Ultradian rhythm: Biologic rhythm with a period shorter than circadian (less than 20 hours).

Zeitgeber: See Synchronizer. It has to be understood that the 'Zeitgeber' does not 'give time' (does not induce a rhythm) but determines its arrangement in time (synchronizes).

CHAPTER 3

Sleep history and investigations

Leslie Olson

Sleep histories

Most medical illness affects sleep in some way and, in many cases, the link between disease and symptoms is disturbed sleep. Sleep histories are simple to take and relatively easy to interpret.

Caution is required in interpreting sleep histories for two reasons. The first is that patients only have a limited knowledge of their sleep. Sleep causes retrograde amnesia for the 10 minutes or so before sleep onset, and arousals from most stages of sleep are followed by a period of confusion and disorientation. Therefore, accounts of the time of sleep onset and the frequency of arousals are highly subjective. A bed partner's objectivity may also be unreliable although description of abnormal nocturnal behavior can be useful. Patients can, however, provide information that is diagnostically helpful, such as the time that the events occur in abnormal behaviors (sleep-walking typically occurs before 1.00AM and REM-sleep-related phenomena typically occur after 2.00AM).

The second reason for caution in interpreting sleep histories is that changes in sleep patterns are most important when they are sustained over a long period, but the unreliability of sleep histories is magnified when one asks about sleep over months or years.

A further point about sleep histories is that, unlike the symptoms of most medical illnesses, most complaints of sleep disorders are sensations that normal people experience. Fatigue or sleepiness in the daytime or interrupted night-time sleep are not abnormal sensations in the sense that exertional chest pain is abnormal. A clear distinction needs to be made between a history appropriate for a patient with a primary complaint related to sleep, and a screening history for patients with other disorders.

Attention needs to be given to aspects of the history that are most reliable, and structured instruments should be used to assess symptoms. The questions that offer the greatest reliability are those that address specific consequences of nocturnal events. For example, asking a patient 'Do you snore badly?' is not helpful, but asking 'Does your bed partner move out of the bedroom because of your snoring?' is. Asking 'Are you tired and sleepy in the daytime?' is not helpful, but asking 'Do you actually fall asleep in the daytime at work?' is.

Sleep histories can have good sensitivity but it is uncommon for a history alone to offer good specificity. In patients with coexisting illnesses, the specificity of history is generally poor and most patients require a formal sleep study to make an accurate diagnosis. The only exception to this generalization is severe obstructive sleep apnea in patients who are otherwise healthy.

Structured sleep interview

It is useful to obtain an overview of the patient's sleep and wake pattern. A systematic inquiry using a structured interview is practical and helpful, particularly for practitioners who confront sleep problems intermittently or are approaching sleep and wake disorders for the first time. An example of a structured interview is shown in *Appendix A, pp 81–83* at the end of this chapter.

History of bedtime and night-time versus daytime function

A detailed history of daytime activity is essential. Ask about the nature of the occupation, commuting time, hours of work and issues such as overtime and work done at home which are often not volunteered. Activities apart from work should also be discussed, in particular, physical activity and the time of day it is carried out. Strenuous activity too close to bedtime (within 1–2 hours) may be detrimental to sleep onset in some individuals. Questions about when the last holiday (3–4 weeks) was taken can help uncover whether the patient is overworking, which is often associated with sleep deprivation.

Weekdays versus weekends

All patients should be asked about sleep patterns on both week days and weekends. It is common for someone who rises at 5.30AM on weekdays to 'sleep in' until 8.30AM or 9.00AM at the weekend, a pattern which may suggest chronic sleep deprivation. Recreational activity on Friday and Saturday nights may reveal behavior which can result in insufficient time to sleep.

Recreational substances

Specific questions should be asked about the use of nicotine, caffeine, alcohol, amphetamine and cannabis, in terms of current and/or past use.

Concurrent medical conditions and medications

Many medical conditions can affect sleep quality, notably gastroesophageal reflux, asthma, angina, heart failure, diabetes and prostatism. Similarly, a detailed list of current medications may reveal drugs known to affect sleep quality and continuity (eg. beta-blockers, theophylline, cortisone, ACE inhibitors).

Current stresses and psychiatric symptoms

The clinician should try to uncover underlying stresses in the patient's life, and/or personality traits or psychiatric symptoms which may be relevant. For this purpose, self-reported questionnaires, such as the depression, anxiety and stress scale (DASS) and the patient health questionnaire can be useful screening tools (*Appendix B, pp 83–84* and *Appendix C, pp 85–89*).

Specific aspects of the sleep history

Snoring and apnea

The principal symptoms of obstructive sleep apnea (OSA) are snoring, apnea reported by bed partners, and daytime sleepiness or fatigue. Snoring exhibited by OSA patients is loud and constant and can nearly always be identified by asking about disruptive snoring ('Do you snore every night or almost every night?' and, 'Does your snoring disturb the sleep of others?'). Significant symptoms of sleep apnea include frequent episodes of apnea or hypopnea with sleep fragmentation (20 to 30 per hour), which are maintained for most hours, virtually every night, for years. For this reason, regular bed partners will have observed the apnea. Asking 'Have you ever been told that you stop breathing while you are asleep?' usually reveals this. In middle-aged male patients with a regular bed partner, these three questions have good sensitivity, and answers of 'No' to all three make sleep apnea relatively unlikely. Snoring, however, is common (about 50% of middle-aged males snore regularly) and apnea during sleep is not always abnormal, so the specificity of these questions is poor.

Patients with regular disruptive snoring and reported apnea are very common, and conducting formal sleep studies on all such patients is impractical. Specificity may be increased by refining history taking, but when the identification of sleep disorders is a clinical priority, a formal sleep study should be conducted. While clinical priorities will vary, in developed medical systems a sleep study is always needed for a patient with disruptive snoring, witnessed apnea and a degree of daytime sleepiness that impairs quality of life or safety.

Although patients are only aware of a small number of their apneas and arousals, waking during the night is an important symptom of sleep apnea. Most patients with sleep apnea wake twice or more each night, and patients who rarely wake at night are very unlikely to have sleep apnea. A few patients will report waking with a clear-cut feeling of upper airway obstruction. This symptom is only common with severe sleep apnea, but is worth asking because it has relatively high specificity. Care is needed to distinguish choking arousals due to sleep apnea from gastro-esophageal reflux. In obstructive sleep apnea, the sensation is brief, usually 1 to 2 seconds, just the time to be fully awake. In gastroesophageal reflux the choking is prolonged, 20–30minutes, and associated with coughing. Apnea termination may be associated with large scale body movements and restlessness. Waking with the bed-clothes disarrayed is common in sleep apnea but this symptom is neither sensitive nor specific.

Sleep apnea headache

Headache is commonly thought to be a symptom of sleep apnea but, in fact, this is uncommon. The characteristic headache of sleep apnea is due to hypercapnia during sleep and occurs only with severe sleep apnea. This headache is described as dull and generalized, but its most important feature is that it clears rapidly — within 15 or 20 minutes — after waking. Because of this rapid clearing, patients rarely complain of this headache as a primary problem and never without other symptoms of sleep apnea. Headaches that last all day, even if consistently present on waking, are infrequently due to sleep apnea.

Bed partner's histories

If the bed partner can be interviewed, both the history of snoring and apnea can be refined, particularly in relation to apnea. Obstructive apneas need to be distinguished from central apneas or breathing pauses, which are more likely to be normal. Obstructive apneas occur during periods of loud snoring, and interrupt snoring abruptly. The first breath when breathing returns is still partially obstructed and is, therefore, often particularly loud and gurgling.

Bed partners often describe obstructive apneas graphically and just as often may provide a clear description of short breathing pauses following progressively softer snores. Cheyne–Stokes breathing in older patients with cardiac failure or cerebrovascular disease can also be quite precisely described by attentive bed partners.

Daytime sleepiness

The presence of daytime sleepiness usually makes sleep apnea worth investigating. For many patients there is no reason to be concerned about sleep apnea in the absence of daytime sleepiness. Where this is not the case, for instance with chronic lung disease and neuromuscular disorders, only formal sleep studies can provide the information that is needed. When taking a history for daytime sleepiness, it is important to find out when the patient falls asleep, not how sleepy they feel. Many patients with insomnia, for example, say that they are tired all the time, and always on the point of falling asleep — but never actually do. Patients with significant daytime sleepiness do fall asleep. To determine the severity of daytime sleepiness it is necessary to find out the circumstances in which it occurs.

It is helpful to develop a series of questions to rate sleepiness. For example, a response about mild sleepiness can be assessed by asking 'Do you fall asleep watching your favorite television programmes?' More marked sleepiness can be detected by asking 'Can you watch television at all without falling asleep?'. It is often helpful to ask about specific programmes, such as important football matches, as patients will reliably remember if they have missed the second half. Patients with marked sleepiness may say that they do not fall asleep watching television, however, they adopt methods to stay awake, such as sitting on a kitchen stool to watch television programmes they are anxious to see. A partner's account is often revealing, and may suggest greater sleepiness.

Other common situations worth asking about are car driving and public/social occasions. If asked, 'Can you drive for two hours without a stop?' nearly all non-sleepy adults answer 'Yes', and answering 'No' implies moderate sleepiness. Asking 'Do you fall asleep if you are in a group of people but not actively involved in conversation?' and 'Can you stay awake if you are in a concert or theatre?' detects moderate sleepiness. Asking 'Do you fall asleep in conversations with one other person?' and 'Have you fallen asleep eating a meal?' detects severe sleepiness.

The Epworth sleepiness scale (ESS) (*Appendix D, p. 90*) uses a series of similar questions. For practitioners who only occasionally see patients with sleep disorders, or who wish to screen patients with medical illnesses for sleep disorders, it is probably the best way to standardize questions for assessing sleepiness (Johns, 1991; 1992; 1994). However, the questions of the ESS have a significant degree of social specificity and practitioners in communities other than the Anglo-Celtic community for which the ESS was developed might need to develop their own variant for optimal performance. The ESS asks patients to imagine their chances of falling asleep if they have not experienced the situations described and patients with depression commonly have misleadingly high scores. It should be kept in mind that personality and psychological traits also influence responses to the ESS (Olson *et al*, 1998). The ESS assesses sleepiness tendency over the preceding week. Other scales such as the Stanford sleepiness scale (SSS) (*Appendix E, p. 90*), and the Karolinska sleepiness scale (KSS) (*Appendix F, p. 91*) assess sleepiness at the time the questionnaire is completed. The SSS and KSS are more useful as research than clinical tools, and the ESS remains the most suitable questionnaire in the clinical setting.

Sleepiness questionnaires should not be used to exclude sleepiness, as the correlation between subjective measure (questionnaire) and objective (multiple sleep latency test) measure of sleepiness is very low (Benbadis *et al*, 1999; Chervin, 2000).

Sleepiness is often difficult to distinguish from fatigue and lack of energy. Fatigue due to sleep disorders is consistently associated with sleepiness. This is revealed by questions about episodes of inappropriate sleep and the severity of fatigue. The frequency and inappropriateness of sleep episodes increase simultaneously. Fatigue, without episodes of inappropriate sleep, is rarely due to sleep disorders. Younger, employed patients are more likely to complain of morning fatigue than sleepiness. Women are generally less likely to report inappropriate sleep and more likely to complain of fatigue and weariness, and inability to achieve tasks and goals (Ambrogetti, *et al*, 1991) (*Figure 3.1*). This pattern of complaint often suggests anxiety or depression. The difficulty in identifying sleep apnea in females as the cause is increased because men are less likely to complain about their partner's snoring or observe apnea.

Inadequate or unrefreshing sleep

Two broad groups of patients fall under this heading:

- those with a primary complaint of daytime sleepiness who admit to unrefreshing sleep
- those whose primary complaint is unrefreshing sleep — 'I just can't get a good night's sleep'.

Care is required in the second group because their complaint may be a result of their daytime problems and not a true description of unrefreshing sleep at all. As in the case of insomnia, daytime situational sleepiness must be distinguished from fatigue.

A further critical point is whether the patient wakes unrefreshed — whether wake-up time is the worst part of the day — or wakes feeling reasonable and then goes down-hill. Patients who complain of waking tired in the mornings despite adequate sleep duration are likely to have a sleep disorder. Conversely, a patient who regularly wakes bright and refreshed is unlikely to have sleep apnea, even if they become sleepy later on in the day — though they may have narcolepsy. As noted above, a key problem is to separate fatigue from sleepiness: a patient who complains of unrefreshing sleep but has no abnormal daytime sleepiness probably does not have a sleep disorder.

Another problem is distinguishing disrupted or fragmented sleep from inadequate sleep duration. Ask about sleep duration in great detail — day-by-day and week-by-week. Bedtime, lights out time, and what fills the period between bedtime and lights out, the subjective time to fall asleep, the timing and duration of all awakenings of which the patient is aware, the final wake up time and the time of getting out of bed should be recorded both for week days and weekends and holidays. (Patients whose chronic daytime sleepiness is substantially improved when they have a holiday when they sleep longer just need more holidays — but caution is required: weekend catch-up sleep is not usually sufficient to make up for chronic sleep deprivation, so patients do not often report a marked beneficial effect of prolonged weekend sleep.) If there are arousals from sleep it is important to ask if the patient has difficulty going back to sleep afterwards (patients with OSA rarely do). Sleep timing over the years is also important as sleep phase disorders (*Chapter 10*) are life-long, although the unreliability of memory and the impact of work and social constraints may make this history difficult to interpret.

The most important clauses of inadequate sleep leading to medical consultation for daytime sleepiness are voluntary sleep restriction by adolescents, and involuntary sleep loss of shift workers.

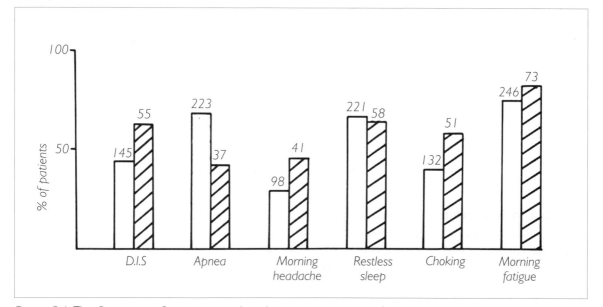

Figure 3.1: The frequency of symptoms other than excessive somnolence in men and women with snoring but without obstructive sleep apnea (OSA). DIS = difficulty initiating sleep. Figures above each bar represent absolute numbers of patients, out of 91 women and 327 men. Hatched columns represent women.

Shift work

Shift workers sleep less than non-shift workers. Night shift, in particular, is associated with sleep durations of between 5 and 6 hours per 24 hours and often less. If a patient does shift work, it is important to elicit the shifts that they do and the roster pattern. The common options are 7-day rotating shifts (ie, 7-day [8.00AM–4.00PM] shifts, 7-afternoon [4.00PM–12.00PM], and 7-night [12PM–8.00AM]) shifts and rapid or 'European' rotation (often with 12-hour shifts, two-day shifts [8.00AM–8.00PM] then 2 night shifts [8.00PM–8.00AM]). Find out where in this cycle days off are situated and how many of these there are. The direction of rotation is also important (ie. 'forward rotation' = day–afternoon–night–day off or 'backward rotation' = night–afternoon–day–day off). Forward rotation causes less sleepiness but some workers prefer backward rotation because the first shift being a night shift provides them with an extra day off at the end of the rotation.

The duration of shift working is perhaps the most important information of all, because long-term tolerance of shift work is a reliable indicator of either short sleep need or delayed sleep phase. Night shift workers usually only have short sleeps (5 to 6 hours), so anyone who has done night shifts regularly for a few years probably only needs this amount of sleep to function well. The exceptions are patients with delayed sleep phase (people with sleep onset after midnight), who characteristically tolerate shift work well because they sleep well in the daytime. The importance of these factors is that in later life when the person has retired, the short sleep need or the delayed sleep phase become a burden and the cause of insomnia.

Another influence on tolerance of shift-work is age. A shift pattern that a 25-year-old can tolerate will become progressively harder to tolerate with age, and there are few regular shift workers aged over 50. An individual who has tolerated shift work for years may present when 50 with insidious onset of fatigue and sleepiness, and since snoring is common in this age group, an erroneous diagnosis of OSA is easy to make.

Night shifts are not the only issue. Starting daytime work early or rising early to commute long distances are common causes of daytime sleepiness in individuals with some degree of delayed sleep phase (inability to fall asleep until late at night). Even minor and otherwise unimportant degrees of delayed sleep phase can lead to restricted sleep when long travel times, commonplace in modern cities, are needed before work. It may take 2 or 3 years for sleepiness to lead a patient to seek medical help, and the role of the patient's hours of work or commuting may not be obvious.

For adolescents, late nights are the usual problem. It is customary to treat 17- and 18-year-olds as adults, but in the area of sleep needs they are not. Most adolescents need more sleep than adults but social pressures and the desire to adopt adult behavior mean that they may not obtain even as much sleep as most adults. The situation is exacerbated when sleep is irregular and when social activities eliminate the opportunity to use weekends for catch-up sleep. The net result is that sleepiness is common in normal adolescents and may become extreme.

One difficulty with history-taking in these cases — shift workers, commuters and adolescents — is that the day-to-day variability of hours of sleep is difficult for patients to remember and hard for practitioners to represent in a clinical history. Bedtimes are especially problematic: most people cannot remember what time they went to sleep last night, let alone a week ago.

Many patients present because they have had an accident at work or while driving, or because their work performance is considered poor and there is a possibility that the incident is linked to a sleep problem. Sleep physicians see many adults for whom superannuation payouts, compensation, social security benefits or claims against employers for wrongful dismissal hang on factors related to sleep, and the relative importance of shift work and lifestyle.

In many countries, adolescents undergo final school assessments that determine access to tertiary education. A threat of inadequate performance in this assessment causes anxiety and may lead to exaggeration in the history. The situation is compounded because narcolepsy commonly begins in late adolescence and is the major differential diagnosis. Treating narcolepsy usually produces a gratifying improvement in work or school performance and there may be strong pressure to make this diagnosis. However, even quite extreme sleepiness in adolescents can be transient and a definite diagnosis of narcolepsy should not be made without strong evidence, usually clear-cut cataplexy.

In older patients, medical illnesses are a common cause of unrefreshing sleep and complaints of fatigue. There are three issues to contend with:

- identifying coexisting sleep disorders that affect the underlying illness
- identifying coexisting sleep disorders that account for symptoms that might otherwise be attributed to the underlying illness
- identifying important effects on sleep of the underlying illness.

For all practical purposes, the first two points come down to identifying sleep apnea. However, because snoring and observed apnea are common, sleep apnea is often seen as the explanation for disturbed and unrefreshing sleep in these patients. In most cases, only formal investigation can exclude it. Another difficulty is that in illnesses, such as chronic obstructive airway disease (COAD), even slight degrees of upper airway obstruction can be important in the genesis of nocturnal hypoventilation, so that non-disruptive or intermittent snoring is clinically relevant. For this reason, formal sleep studies are indispensable.

Many illnesses affect sleep and lead to complaints of unrefreshing sleep. In most cases these effects are straightforward: nocturia in prostatism, renal failure and uncontrolled diabetes mellitus or arousal due to pain in arthritis. A few illnesses have effects on sleep which are important either because therapy is, or is imagined to be, beneficial. The most important of these are cardiac failure and cerebrovascular disease, both discussed elsewhere.

In a number of common disorders, poor sleep is a characteristic feature and the cause is less straightforward. Poor sleep is common early in Parkinson's disease and is often exacerbated later on by therapy with levodopa. Poor nocturnal sleep and daytime sleepiness are common in dementia, although whether this is part of the disease or a result of lack of exercise and lack of stimulation in the daytime, leading to daytime napping and poor night-time sleep, is unclear.

Disturbed sleep is commonly due to alcohol and caffeine intake. In taking a history of alcohol and caffeine intake it is important to record not only the quantity consumed but also the timing. Caffeine has a long half-life (9–12 hours). Caffeine consumed at lunch time may still result in effective blood levels in the early hours of the morning. The onset of caffeine's effect is relatively slow, so caffeine taken in the evening does not cause sleep-onset insomnia but early morning waking. Alcohol reduces sleep latency during the intoxication phase but as the level falls, wakefulness appears, so those who fall asleep with significant blood levels are likely to have sleep disruption.

Insomnia

The distinction between inadequate and unrefreshing sleep and insomnia is, to some degree, artificial. The first question to ask any patient with insomnia is 'Why do you perceive your difficulties with sleep to be a problem?'. Since many patients first seek medical help for insomnia after many years of poor sleep, it is important to ask what has changed to lead them to seek help. A surprisingly large number of patients with insomnia find it difficult to answer these questions, and many others make it clear that the problem is really either depression or life-changes that have nothing to do with sleep.

The first aim of history-taking in patients with insomnia is to identify symptomatic insomnia, most commonly due to sleep apnea, pain, or drugs such as caffeine. This is usually straightforward, although a confident diagnosis may require a formal sleep study.

The second stage is to identify patterns that suggest that the patient has a short sleep need or a sleep phase shift ('disorder'). In the case of short sleep need, the clues are a prolonged history of asymptomatic short sleep, often with the first complaint coinciding with retirement. As noted above, a history of prolonged night shift work or working two jobs without daytime sleepiness are common backgrounds for short sleep need. With phase shifts, a history of good sleep when on afternoon or night shift is helpful in suggesting delayed sleep phase. It is critical to establish the patient's level of daytime alertness. A patient who only ever sleeps 5 hours, but performs normally in the daytime and wakes alert and refreshed, probably only needs 5 hours' sleep.

The pattern of insomnia is helpful in identifying phase shift and short sleep need. Patients with delayed sleep phase usually describe an inability to fall asleep until a consistent but late hour, and then normal sleep terminated by the alarm, and, when they are able to sleep on their preferred schedule (at weekends, for example), they sleep well. However, many patients with delayed sleep phase may not have the opportunity to sleep on an optimal schedule because of family commitments. Care needs to be taken not to discard the hypothesis of delayed sleep phase because sleep is no better at weekends or on holidays. Patients may have tried to sleep later with no benefit, but it may take some weeks of sleep on an optimal schedule to make the impact of schedule change clear: the impact of one or two nights is not helpful. Sleep patterns on prolonged holidays (3–4 weeks), if the patient allows himself to go to sleep and get up without restriction, may be helpful.

Because of chronic sleep deprivation, patients with delayed sleep phase often fall asleep quite early, particularly if they consume alcohol with their evening meal. They then awake 1 or 2 hours later and are unable to go back to sleep — particularly if they also have caffeine with their evening meal. This is a common and non-specific pattern of poor sleep and the diagnosis of delayed sleep phase can then be difficult to make.

Other clues to the presence of delayed sleep phase may be obtained from the patient's work habits. Persons with delayed sleep phase often fill the first hour or two of work time with low level or routine activity, and in the afternoon their output increases. Work problems most often afflict those whose schedule and productivity are fixed by others.

Advanced sleep phase is infrequently a cause of complaint. These patients rarely have chronic sleep deprivation because no one prevents them going to bed at 8.00PM or 9.00PM. They wake up at 4.00AM or 5.00AM feeling fine, and cannot go back to sleep.

Another important aspect is the timing of arousals. Normal, end-of-cycle arousals occur every 90–120 minutes, and most patients with insomnia and frequent arousals describe waking with this periodicity (ie. they go to sleep at 11.00PM, then wake at 12.30AM, 2.00AM and 3.30AM). Subjective arousals with a much shorter cycle should prompt consideration of an organic cause, such as pain or obstructive sleep apnea (objective arousals, recorded on polysomnography, are a different matter). The patient's report of the duration of these arousals is of little use, partly because of the false impression that they are awake for much of the night, especially between 2.00AM and 4.00AM. The pattern of arousal once or twice between sleep onset and 2.00AM, and then a period of wakefulness or light and unsatisfying sleep until 4.00AM or 4.30AM, followed by sound sleep truncated by an alarm, is common and non-specific.

Restless leg syndrome and periodic limb movement disorder

Most patients with restless leg syndrome (RLS) and periodic limb movement disorder (PLMD) report the movements straightforwardly and the diagnosis is not normally difficult. The complaints may be of insomnia, usually at sleep onset, or of leg discomfort before going to bed, or the disruption of the bed partner's sleep.

If the primary complainant is the bed partner, the history is of repetitive movement for which most use the word 'kicking' (rather than 'twitching'). The movements are consistently described as kick-like, of large amplitude, usually affecting the legs but at times the upper limbs, and occur a few times a minute (rather than a few times a second). Apart from this consistency of the movements, most movement disorders including Parkinson's disease and Huntington's chorea, are characterized by the disappearance of movements during sleep. The differential diagnosis is of other sleep disorders that cause large-scale body movements, such as sleep apnea, rather than the disorders that cause abnormal movements during wakefulness.

If the complaint is insomnia, the key element of the history is the co-existence of leg movements and the compulsion to move the legs. Movement (usually getting up and walking around) immediately eliminates the urge to move the legs, but this relief lasts only as long as the movement. The symptoms occur in the evening and the time of onset becomes slowly earlier as the patient ages. Symptoms are never present in the morning alone and disappear at some point during the night. Symptoms may appear in the arms but always occur in the legs first, usually for some years. Most patients have only sleep onset insomnia and it is uncommon for the movements to disrupt sleep but, occasionally, patients have difficulty going back to sleep after spontaneous arousals during the night.

The only additional features of history to be sought are those of renal failure and iron deficiency, both associated with RLS and PLMD. Many patients will have been given a benzodiazepine and a positive response is an additional helpful pointer to the diagnosis of PLMD.

Abnormal nocturnal behavior

Common sleep-related nocturnal behaviors such as sleep-walking and REM-sleep behavior disorder (RBD) cause dramatic events that are remembered and, therefore, usually lead to the detailed and often characteristic histories. The detail of the history usually depends on the testimony of a bed partner. In patients who sleep alone, it is hard to rule out epilepsy and psychiatric illness. Occasionally, patients with RBD whose behavior involves violent, sexually charged dreams are deeply offended by the 'desires' apparently exposed. They see this as a moral rather than medical issue and conceal the events or the dreams associated with them.

Other important elements are the timing of the behavior and whether, if they are awoken during the events, they are lucid or confused. Sleep-walking occurs in deep slow-wave sleep, usually in the first half of the night, while REM-sleep behavior disorder is more likely in the second half of the night. A person woken from deep slow-wave sleep will be confused and disorientated, while someone woken from REM sleep knows at once where they are and that they have been asleep. The same applies to patients woken from sleep-walking; they may continue elements of the abnormal behavior even when awake and may take up to 30 seconds to return to normal alertness. Sleep-walking rarely starts in adult life and nearly all adult sleep-walkers report sleep-walking in childhood. REM-sleep behavior disorder, in contrast, is uncommon in the young and usually afflicts men over 50 years.

One difficult task in relation to these disorders is to rule out epilepsy, psychiatric illness and drug-induced or factitious abnormal behavior as alternative diagnoses, particularly when the question of 'crime while asleep' arises. This task is made more difficult because even several consecutive sleep studies often do not contain a convincing example of the behavior under complaint. The history is critical and the key is a detailed account of what happens during such behavior. Sleep-walking occurs when the cortex is asleep but subcortical motor pathways are awake; therefore, sleep-walking can involve coordinated behavior but not purposeful or adaptive behavior. RBD is normally confined to the bedroom, and violence is directed indiscriminately at the bed partner and at inanimate objects in the bedroom.

Patients who are severely sleep-deprived may, during perfectly normal wakefulness, carry out complex activities, then go back to sleep immediately and, because of the amnesic effects of sleep, wake in the morning with no memory of their nocturnal activities (sleep drunkenness). In these cases, because the cortex is awake the behavior can be complex and adaptive. However, the degree of sleep deprivation required to produce this phenomenon makes the cause obvious.

Sleep investigations

Polysomnography (12 or more channels)

Polysomnography is a collection of physiological signals — ECG, pulse oximetry, and so on — recorded all at once and stored for later analysis (*Figure 3.2*) (American Sleep Disorders Association [ASDA], 1997a,b; Douglas *et al*, 1992; Portier *et al*, 2000). The conventional ensemble of recorded parameters has never been validated properly as a clinical tool and exists in its present form more because of the need to define the procedure of 'polysomnography' for reimbursement purposes, than because it is clinically optimal. The concept of a single procedure called 'polysomnography' that will provide definitive diagnostic information on any sleep disorder is misleading.

Polysomnography should be thought of as measurements of aspects of physiology that answer clinically important questions: Did the patient sleep? Did they stop breathing? Did they do it a lot, and why? Aspects of physiology which are easy to measure and may be relevant to sleep disorders are: scalp EEG, skin surface EMG of external eye muscles, the postural muscles of the neck and jaw and of the tibialis anterior (the main muscle involved in PLMD), qualitative motion of the rib-cage and abdomen to define paradoxical motion and, therefore, upper airway obstruction and arterial

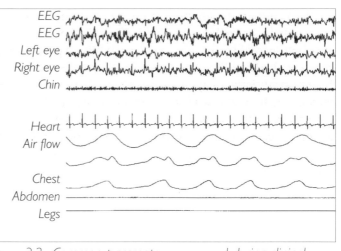

Figure 3.2: Common parameters measured during clinical polysomnography. Note that air flow, chest and abdomen activities are in synchrony.

oxygen saturation by pulse oximetry. Transcutaneous measurement of tissue PCO_2 is not part of routine sleep study set up in adults, but now common in infants and young children. Esophageal pressure — as a measure of pleural pressure and respiratory effort — and diaphragm EMG are tricky to measure but within the reach of good laboratories. The movement of air in and out of the mouth and nose is easy to record but hard to quantify, and accurate and precise measurement of tidal volume is not feasible for clinical purposes.

The scalp EEG, skin surface EMG of external eye muscles and postural EMG are used to 'stage' sleep. The system of 'stages' of sleep most widely used was defined by Rechtschaffen and Kales (1968) on the basis of studies in normal subjects (*Figure 3.3*). The criteria used for staging are skin surface electrical potentials (via EEG) over the cranial vault which reflect predominantly cortical activity. The recordings are divided into 'epochs', usually either 20 or 30 seconds long, and each epoch is assigned the stage that occupies a majority of the epoch. This system has a number of shortcomings, the principal one being that patches of EEG lasting less than 10–15 seconds or so are ignored unless they occur repetitively and frequently enough to take up more than half of an epoch. Conversely, very frequent but very short episodes of arousal from sleep can cause the recording to be classified as stage wake. Finally, although the stages do have some physiological significance (for example, the intensity of an external stimulus required to cause arousal increases steadily from stage 1 to stage 4), they are morphologically and not physiologically defined and the classification is arbitrary.

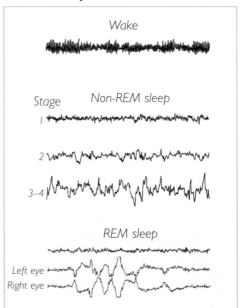

Figure 3.3: Sleep stages are scored according to a set of criteria (Rechtschaffen and Kales, 1968).

In terms of clinical polysomnography, sleep staging provides information about the amount and depth of sleep. For all sleep disorders, other than obstructive sleep apnea, this is indispensable. It is only occasionally important, however, in patients suspected of sleep apnea. It is common for patients sleeping in a laboratory to have little or no REM sleep, and a few have no sleep at all. Sleep apnea is nearly always most marked in REM sleep and a false conclusion of mild sleep apnea can be reached if the clinician does not know that the patient had no REM sleep in the laboratory. Although it is uncommon for apnea to be entirely absent in other stages, the index of events calculated over a whole night will be low if no REM sleep occurs, and may be below the diagnostic cut-off. For this reason, some patients with sleep apnea will be missed if sleep stages are not recorded.

Sleep staging is important in sleep apnea for patients with motor neurone disease (MND) and with muscular dystrophies. These patients usually have poor sleep, often, with little, or no REM sleep. When they enter REM they experience severe oxygen desaturation and wake up, resulting in severe sleep fragmentation and loss of REM sleep. When the pressure to sleep and enter sustained REM sleep eventually becomes overwhelming, gross desaturation occurs. At first this is only intermittent, but if sleep stages are not recorded the absence of REM sleep will not be recognized and a false conclusion that breathing is adequate during sleep may be drawn.

The most difficult and controversial aspect of sleep staging is the identification of arousals (ASDA, 1992; Kingshott *et al*, 1998; Magalang UJ *et al*, 1996; Mathur and Douglas, 1995). This task is critical because it is frequent arousal ('sleep fragmentation') that accounts for daytime sleepiness in many sleep disorders. In patients with snoring due to upper airway obstruction, the increased respiratory effort can cause arousal without any reduction in breathing (the so-called 'upper airway resistance syndrome'). Detecting and quantifying arousal is essential if patients with daytime symptoms due to upper airway obstruction during sleep are to be managed appropriately.

Technically, detecting arousals is relatively easy: there is a burst of high frequency EEG activity, often with a sharp rise in EMG activity and sometimes with body movement. The difficulty arises with defining the minimum duration and intensity that counts as an arousal so that arousal frequency can be quantified. A number of definition systems have been developed, and the different definitions can result in widely differing arousal counts. It is important to know which one a laboratory uses before trying to interpret its results. The recent trend has been for definitions to include shorter and less intense events, so that arousal counts are higher. However, there is still a significant subjective element in arousal counting, and accuracy depends heavily on the experience and care of the laboratory technicians.

In patients with insomnia, sleep staging is useful to answer two questions. Many patients who complain of getting little or no sleep turn out to sleep quite well in the laboratory (so-called 'subjective insomnia' or 'sleep-state misperception'). Sleep staging in patients suspected of delayed sleep phase can, if the patient sleeps well, demonstrate that sleep begins late, but sleep structure is otherwise normal.

The pulse oximeter measures arterial oxygen saturation. The output is usually represented as a continuous line, although this is slightly misleading because the machine actually makes a series of separate measurements, in most cases, a few times a minute. Oximeter output may not accurately follow the shape of rapid changes in oxygen saturation, although this is rarely important. The oximeter measures saturation far less accurately at very low levels. Here false readings may occur, such as the many patients with severe sleep apnea who are said by pulse oximeter to have arterial saturation of 40% or less for long periods.

In laboratory polysomnography, the oximeter's role is to define the severity and frequency of arterial desaturation. This sounds like a core function, especially in relation to sleep apnea. However, unless the patient has COAD and the question is whether a given level of oxygen supplementation is adequate, the contribution of oximetry is limited. The symptoms of sleep apnea are not due to hypoxia and oxygen desaturation is not necessary for a diagnosis of sleep apnea, nor is any particular level of desaturation a reason to treat sleep apnea.

The detection of breathing also represents a significant problem, and the deficiencies of current methods are a major weakness of current sleep monitoring technology (AASM Task Force, 1999; Berry *et al*, 1984; Gottlieb *et al*, 1999; Strohl and Redline, 1996; Manser *et al*, 2002; Moser *et al*, 1994; Redline *et al*, 2000). It is easy to detect complete cessation of breathing — apnea — and any of several methods are adequate and will give reliable apnea counts. However, in sleep apnea, episodes of apnea are less frequent than hypopnea: reduced tidal volumes due to upper airway obstruction. There are a number of methods capable of measuring tidal volume accurately when the airway is sealed — by an airtight mask or a mouthpiece and nose-clip or a cuffed endotracheal tube. Although research studies with airtight masks have been done, sleep is inevitably disrupted and, for clinical purposes, less disruptive methods of estimating breathing are used. All of these are unsatisfactory and unreliable. It is conventional to define hypopnea as a 50% fall in the breathing signal, but this is an arbitrary value. For practical purposes, the identification of hypopnea is subjective and, although each laboratory should achieve internal consistency, the hypopnea counts of different laboratories may not be comparable.

The final element in conventional polysomnography is a method for demonstrating paradoxical rib-cage and abdominal motion. Normally, the rib-cage and abdominal dimensions both increase on inspiration. When respiratory efforts are made but the airway is obstructed there is 'paradoxical' rib-cage and abdominal motion: one gets bigger while the other gets smaller. The classification of apnea as central, obstructive or mixed was once thought to be important, and although this distinction no longer seems important, the measurements are still made. It is easy to measure rib-cage and abdominal activity semiquantitatively, and thus to determine reliably whether there is paradoxical motion and no airflow, indicating obstructive apnea, or no motion and no airflow, indicating central apnea (*Figure 3.4a, b, c*).

An alternative means of making the distinction between central and obstructive apnea is to measure esophageal (ie. pleural) pressure with a balloon catheter placed in the esophagus, to see whether respiratory efforts are present or absent in the absence of air flow. This is not worthwhile for clinical purposes, but it allows an accurate estimate of both the size of the increased effort and the pattern of the response, and this is sometimes important for research purposes. Diaphragmatic EMG is difficult to do non-invasively, and even for research purposes adds little to esophageal pressure.

The above discussion suggests two important points. The first is that what is measured during a patient's sleep study should be determined by the questions raised by their particular presentation. The second key point is that the methods currently used for a number of key physiological parameters are seriously inadequate. Counts of hypopneas and of arousals are the least consistent aspects of a sleep recording — both between different scorers, when the same scorer looks twice at the same record, and between human and computer scorers. The fact that these are the most important aspects of the study when sleep apnea is at issue is an important reason why polysomnography is a doubtful 'gold standard' for the diagnosis of sleep apnea.

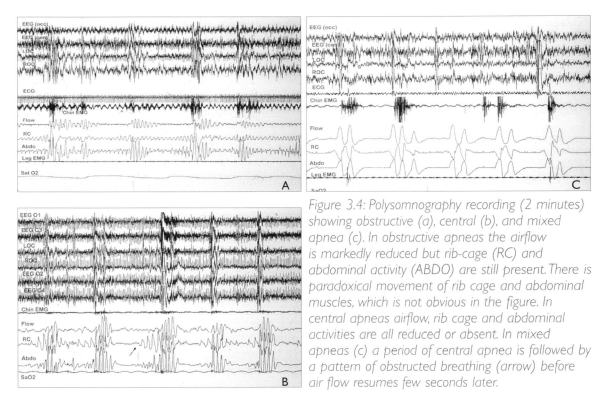

Figure 3.4: Polysomnography recording (2 minutes) showing obstructive (a), central (b), and mixed apnea (c). In obstructive apneas the airflow is markedly reduced but rib-cage (RC) and abdominal activity (ABDO) are still present. There is paradoxical movement of rib cage and abdominal muscles, which is not obvious in the figure. In central apneas airflow, rib cage and abdominal activities are all reduced or absent. In mixed apneas (c) a period of central apnea is followed by a pattern of obstructed breathing (arrow) before air flow resumes few seconds later.

Limited and portable sleep study systems (4–6 channels)

Laboratory polysomnography is expensive in terms of equipment, laboratory space and technical staff. Setting up a polysomnography laboratory requires a substantial amount of clinical and technical expertise. To reduce the costs and allow a wider range of institutions and clinicians to provide some clinical sleep services, systems have been developed that eliminate some of the trickier aspects of polysomnography. The systems that result are compact and readily portable, so that studies can be conducted either in a laboratory or in a patient's home (Chesson *et al*, 2003; Portier *et al*, 2000). Setting up and connecting the patient is regulated and simplified, and analysis is highly automated so that studies require minimal or no technical supervision for recording and do not have to be manually scored.

In general, the physiological measures that are provided by these systems are oxygenation, ECG, some measure of respiration and a measure of rib-cage and abdominal paradox. EEG and EMG, although theoretically easy to do, require a significant amount of skill to set up, and a high standard of recording is hard to maintain without a skilled technician continuously present, so they are omitted unless the system is intended for supervised use in a sleep laboratory.

The choice of parameters indicates that, for practical purposes, these systems are directed at the diagnosis of obstructive sleep apnea. Their performance in this task is good in patients with clear-cut sleep apnea, but poor in patients with borderline disease. However, patients with borderline disease probably do not benefit symptomatically from treatment of sleep apnea, so limited sleep study systems are normally quite acceptable. In more complex situations, the absence of the capacity to stage sleep is a problem. In situations where a sleep study is wanted to exclude sleep apnea in patients with a low pre-test probability, of whom the great majority of cases will be of mild or borderline sleep apnea, limited and portable monitoring is unlikely to be adequate.

Minimal sleep monitoring systems (1–2 channels)

Sleep apnea is only usually worth treating when there are daytime symptoms. Certainty is needed that there are nocturnal apneas due to upper airway obstruction. The presence of disruptive snoring points directly to upper airway obstruction and all that is needed is a means to detect apnea. The severity of apnea is not, in itself, an indication for treatment (although the likelihood that a patient has symptoms is related to severity), so the components of polysomnography dedicated to quantifying severity are, for most purposes, superfluous.

Minimal monitoring only requires pulse oximetry (*Figure 3.5*), although some investigators have added snoring detection. Pulse oximetry may initially appear to be a poor choice, since apneas and hypopneas can occur with little oxygen desaturation and sleep fragmentation can occur with none. However, patients with sleep apnea and daytime symptoms rarely have no oxygen desaturation at all during sleep. Monitoring is not intended to detect apneas, but simply to identify patients with the disease sleep apnea and, as such, oximetry can be an effective screening tool (Gyulay *et al*, 1993; Olson *et al*, 1999).

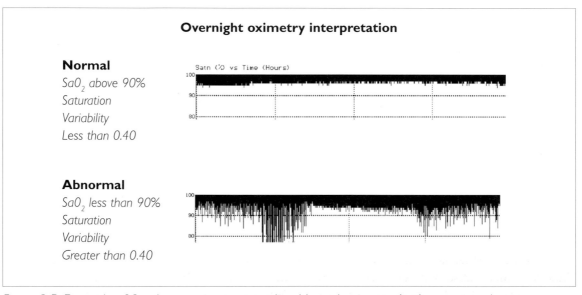

Figure 3.5: Example of four hours oximetry recording. Normal oximetry (top), unequivocal severe obstructive sleep apnea (bottom).

There are three ways to analyze the pattern of the oximeter tracing to diagnose sleep apnea. The first two are easily computerized and interpretation rules can be set out so that inexperienced practitioners can use these methods as screening tools. Desaturation events can be counted: usually a 4% fall below baseline is taken as the definition of an 'event' and oxygen desaturation index (ODI–ODI4 if 4% desaturation events are counted) is calculated. In this case an oxygen desaturation index (ODI) of less than 10 or so is a reasonable normal value. This procedure has reasonable sensitivity and specificity, but is inferior to other methods because it remains wedded to the idea that event detection rather than diagnosis is the aim of monitoring.

Better performance is obtained by looking for variability of the saturation recording, without regard to individual dips of arbitrary size. Oximeter output is not continuous, but rather a discrete measurement made every 12 seconds or so. The difference between each value and the next is calculated and divided by the number of readings minus 1. This is the saturation variability index, and values over 0.4 have sensitivity over 90%, but specificity of only about 60%; higher values have progressively greater specificity. Finally, the oximeter output can be printed out so that the whole night is represented by about 20 cm of paper or video screen. With experience, it is possible to make an educated guess at which patients have sleep apnea just by looking at the pattern of the tracing, particularly if a careful history has been taken as well.

The pulse oximeter is cheap and so small hospitals and individual practitioners can buy one, and, because it is robust and reliable, an efficient service is easy to organize. Patients are not intimidated by it and can easily be taught to use it unsupervised. The implication of the relatively low specificity of simple overnight oximetry is that a substantial number of patients have to be referred for more complex sleep studies, but in patient groups with low pre-test probabilities (eg. young people with high blood pressure or healthy snorers with no daytime symptoms) oximetry is an efficient first step.

Split-night sleep studies

Split study refers to a plysomnography protocol to perform a diagnostic recording in the first part of the night, followed by the application of nasal continuous positive airway pressure (CPAP) treatment in the second half, in patients being investigated for obstructive sleep apnea. This protocol is aimed at reducing the cost associated with performing a diagnostic study one night and a titration study a second night, when an appropriate pressure to abolish snoring and apnea is determined (*Chapter 5*). In the right clinical contest, and provided strict criteria are met, split studies help in maximizing health resources utilization (Elshaug *et al*, 2005; Rodway and Sanders, 2003).

The multiple sleep latency test

The multiple sleep latency test (MSLT) is the most validated objective measure of daytime sleepiness (American Sleep Disorders Association, 1992; Carskadon and Dement, 1982; Mitler *et al*, 1982; Reynolds *et al*, 1982; Richardson *et al*, 1978). The MSLT consists of four to five twenty-minute naps every 2 hours during the day, usually at 10.00AM, 12 midday, 2.00PM and 4.00PM and, possibly, a fifth one at 6.00PM. The patient is monitored with EEG and submental EMG and is requested to lie quietly in a bed and try to sleep. The patient is requested not to sleep between naps and to avoid stimulant substances such as coffee or engaging in stimulatory activity.

An overnight polysomnography the night before the MSLT should be part of the protocol, and a sleep diary for a week before the investigation is also a useful measure to help interpret the results.

The protocol varies slightly depending on the clinical question. If the clinician is interested in quantifying sleepiness tendency, the nap is terminated soon after sleep onset. The mean sleep latency is calculated as the average of the four or five nap attempts. If the clinical question is to corroborate a diagnosis of narcolepsy, the nap is terminated either soon after the first episode of early onset REM or 15 minutes after sleep onset. In the right clinical context, a short sleep latency (eg. <5 minutes) with two naps with early-onset REM would be considered supportive of the diagnosis. When narcolepsy is a consideration, usually five nap attempts are implemented unless two early-onset REMs have occurred in the previous four naps (Aldrich *et al*, 1997; Carskadon *et al*, 1981).

The MSLT has both test–re-test reliability as well as inter-rater reliability (Benbadis *et al*, 1995; Zwyghuizen-Doorenbos *et al*, 1988). Sleep onset is determined by the occurrence of the first epoch of any sleep, including REM sleep. However, different criteria have been applied at times, including the need for three epochs (30 seconds) of stage 1 as well as the occurrence of stage 2 before sleep onset is scored. Different criteria would result in a different estimate of mean sleep latency (Benbadis *et al*, 1996). Current recommendations indicate that sleep onset should be scored with the occurrence of any epoch of sleep including the first epoch of stage 1.

A mean sleep latency above 10 minutes in adults is considered normal. There is, however, a large standard deviation (10.4 ± 4.3 minutes in the four naps protocol, and 11.6 ± 5.2 in the five naps protocol), which results in significant overlap between patients with complaint of sleepiness and 'normal' controls (symptom-free subjects) (Littner *et al*, 2005). There are, in fact, individuals with normal levels of alertness and no complaints of daytime sleepiness who can fall asleep quickly, within less than 8 minutes. This ability to fall asleep easily, referred to as 'sleepability' (Harrison *et al*, 1996) may be a genetically determined characteristic. Therefore, the MSLT needs to be interpreted within the context of the clinical presentation, because a short-sleep latency does not indicate in itself a decreased level of alertness. Values below 5 minutes are within the pathological range of sleepiness and between 5 and 10 minutes is increased sleepiness tendency. Although the MSLT is highly standardized, individual factors, such as motivation and circadian rhythm, can influence test results (Harrison *et al*, 1996; Clodoré *et al*, 1986). The environment as well as the set-up can, in some individuals, be intimidating enough to prevent sleep onset.

One technical limitation of scoring sleep onset is that current criteria do not account for microsleeps that may occur during the recording period. It is important that brief episodes of EEG consistent with light sleep (eg. below 15 seconds in a 30-second epoch) should be reported, even though they will not be scored as sleep onset which requires more than 50% of an epoch showing EEG consistent with sleep.

Indications for MSLT include: the diagnosis of narcolepsy and of idiopathic somnolence; to assess objectively sleepiness in patients who complain of being unable to stay awake; to document reduction in sleepiness following treatment of other sleep disorders, in particular, in the case of medicolegal implications (eg a truck driver with severe sleep apnea being treated with nasal CPAP (see *Chapter 13*). The MSLT may also be part of the investigation of a patient complaining of insomnia when daytime sleepiness is an important component of the symptoms.

Maintenance of wakefulness test (MWT)

The MWT assesses the ability of the patient to remain awake, whereas the MSLT measures tendency to fall asleep. Technically, the MWT is similar to the MSLT. The test consists of four, 40-minute periods separated by 2-hour intervals where the patient is monitored by EEG, electromyogram and electroculogram and is sitting comfortably with their back and head supported by pillows. Only a dim light is allowed and the patient is requested to remain awake for 40 minutes (Doghramji *et al*, 1997; Mitler *et al*, 1982). A shorter version lasting 20 minutes is also being proposed (Mitler *et al*, 1998). The test is terminated soon after sleep onset according to sleep onset criteria similar to the MSLT.

In subjects with no complaint of sleepiness, the mean sleep latency in a MTW using 40 minutes is 35.2 ± 7.9 minutes. When a 20-minute trial is undertaken, the mean sleep latency is 18.7 ± 2.6 minutes (Doghramji *et al*, 1997). Comparison of MSLT and MWT shows low correlation suggesting that the two tests measure different aspects of sleepiness/alertness (Sangal *et al*, 1992).

OSLER test (Oxford sleepiness refractory test)

The Osler test is an indirect measure of alertness. It is similar in principle to the MWT, but does not require EEG monitoring. The subject is asked to remain awake in a sound proof and darkened room for four periods of 40 minutes through the day, and to press a digital button in response to a light generated by a diode for 1 second every 3 seconds. The action of the button and the light events are automatically recorded by the instrument and analyzed by a computer programme. Failure to respond to seven consecutive lights is taken as sleep onset. A mean sleep latency is then generated out of the four attempts (Bennett *et al*, 1997). The Osler test seems to compare well with the MWT in discriminating between normal subjects, obstructive sleep apnea patients and sleep-deprived patients (Bennett *et al*, 1997; Priest *et al*, 2001). Further analyses of the characteristics of the Osler test are under investigation. It may be possible, for example, to identify microsleep (sleep lasting less than 3 seconds) (Priest *et al*, 2001), and to reduce the number of tests to three or even one (Mazza *et al*, 2002). The Osler test could be used to assess response to treatment when sleepiness is a major symptom. It would not be useful in situations where detection of sleepiness associated with a REM sleep abnormality is diagnostically important (eg. narcoleptic syndromes).

Actigraphy

Reduction in motor activity is one of the features of a sleeping person. This characteristic has been used as one of the initial research tools to study sleep. At the beginning of the last century, actigraphy recorded motor activity during sleep using an electromagnet attached to the bed spring. The signal generated by the electromagnet translated movement into a running paper trace.

More sophisticated technology is now used, such as piezo-electric movement detectors miniaturized in watch-like instruments. The data is stored in digital format for up to 4 weeks, depending on the memory of the instrument and, on the sampling frequency, which can be from half a second up to one-minute intervals (*Figure 3.6*). The complexity of the actigraphy varies from logging movement changes to collecting data on light exposure, as well as the possibility of event marking.

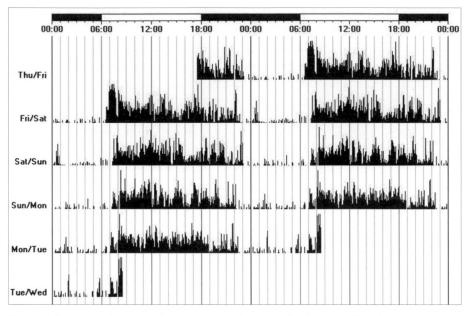

Figure 3.6: Actigraphy trace. Note that resting time (reduction of activity starts around 11.00PM, and get-up time (resumption of activity) around 6.30–7.00AM, in a very regular pattern.

Recommendation for the use of actigraphy in the evaluation of sleep disorder has been published for both research and clinical settings (American Sleep Disorders Association, 1995; Sadeh *et al*, 1995; Sadeh and Acebo, 2002). Actigraphy is particularly useful in circadian rhythm sleep disorders (*Chapter 10*).

A variety of algorithms, usually instrument-specific, have been developed to try to derive useful sleep parameters from activity and rest rhythms. Total sleep time is usually well correlated with polysomnographic measurement. However, extrapolation of sleep stages is not accurate enough. In particular, actigraphy cannot be used as a substitute for polysomnography.

Validity of actigraphy varies depending on the population studied. Although accuracy is high in normal individuals, it is decreased in patients with insomnia. More specifically, periods where patients may be lying quietly in bed may be mistaken for sleep. This is particularly relevant in patients with insomnia. Conversely, patients with movement disorder during sleep may show activity in keeping with wakefulness when the patient is actually asleep. Actigraphy has been used in all age groups from infants to the elderly, including patients with dementia and Parkinson's disease because it is easy to use and minimally intrusive.

References

AASM Task Force (1999) Sleep-related breathing disorders in adults: recommendations for syndrome definition and measurement techniques in clinical research. *Sleep* **22**(5): 667–89

Åkerstedt T, Gillberg M (1990) Subjective and objective sleepiness in the active individual *Intern J Neurosci* **52**: 29–37

Aldrich MS, Chervin RD, Malow BA (1997) Value of the multiple sleep latency test (MSLT) for the diagnosis of narcolepsy. *Sleep* **20**(8): 620–9

Ambrogetti A, Olson LG, Saunders NA (1991) Differences in the symptoms of men and women with obstructive sleep apnea. *Aust NZ J Med* **21**(6): 863–7

American Sleep Disorders Association Report (1986) Guidelines for the multiple sleep latency test (MSLT): A standard measure of sleepiness. *Sleep* **9**(4): 519–24

American Sleep Disorders Association Report (1992) The clinical use of the multiple sleep latency test. *Sleep* **15**(3): 268–76

American Sleep Disorders Association and Sleep Research Society (1992) EEG arousals: scoring rules and examples. *Sleep* **15**(2): 173–84

American Sleep Disorders Association Report (1995) Practice parameters for the use of actigraphy in the clinical assessment of sleep disorders. *Sleep* **18**(4): 285–7

American Sleep Disorders Association and Sleep Research Society (1997) Practice parameters for the indications for polysomnography and related procedures. *Sleep* **20**(6): 406–22

Benbadis SR, Mascha E, Perry MC, Wolgamuth BR, Smolley LA, Dinner DS (1999) Association between the Epworth sleepiness scale and the multiple sleep latency test in a clinical population. *Ann Intern Med* **130**: 289–92

Benbadis SR, Perry MC, Wolgamuth BR, Bendelson WB, Dinner DS (1996) The multiple sleep latency test: Comparison of sleep onset criteria. *Sleep* **19**(8): 632–6

Benbadis SR, Perry M, Wolgamuth BR, Turnbull J, Mendelson WB (1995) Daytime sleepiness. Mean versus median for the multiple sleep latency test. *Sleep* **18**(5): 342–5

Benbadis SR, Qu Y, Perry MC, Dinner DS, Warnes H (1995) Interrater reliability of the multiple sleep latency test. *Electroencephalogr Clin Neurophysiol* **95**: 302–4

Bennett LS, Stradling JR, Davies RJO (1997) A behavioural test to assess daytime sleepiness in obstructive sleep apnea. *J Sleep Res* **6**: 142–5

Berry D, Webb W, Block A (1984) Sleep apnea syndrome. A critical review of the apnea index as a diagnostic criterion. *Chest* **86**(4): 529–31

Bishop C, Rosenthal L, Helmus T, Roehrs T, Roth T (1996) The frequency of multiple sleep onset REM periods among subjects with no excessive daytime sleepiness. *Sleep* **19**(9): 727–30

Carskadon MA, Dement WC (1982) The multiple sleep latency test: What does it measure? *Sleep* **5**: S67–S72

Carskadon MA, Harvey K, Dement WC (1981) Multiple sleep latency tests during the development of narcolepsy. *West J Med* **135**: 414–17

Chervin RD (2000) The multiple sleep latency test and Epworth sleepiness scale in the assessment of daytime sleepiness. *J Sleep Res* **9**(4): 399–401

Chesson AL, Berry RB, Pack A (2003) Practice parameters for the use of portable monitoring devices in the investigation of suspected obstructive sleep apnoea in adults. *Sleep* **26**(7): 907–13

Clodoré M, Foret J, Benoit O (1986) Diurnal variation in subjective and objective measures of sleepiness: The effects of sleep reduction and circadian type. *Chronobiol Int* **3**(4): 255–63

Doghramji D, Mitler MM, Sangal RB, Shapiro C, Taylor S, Walsleben J *et al* (1997) A normative study of the maintenance of wakefulness test (MWT). *Electroencephalogr Clin Neurophysiol* **103**: 554–62

Douglas NJ, Thomas S, Mohammed AJ (1992) Clinical value of polysomnography. *Lancet* **339**: 347–50

Elshaug AG, Moss JR, Southcott AM (2005) Implementation of a split-night protocol to improve efficiency in assessment and treatment of obstructive sleep apnoea. *Internal Med J* **35**: 251–4

Gottlieb DJ, Whitney CW, Bonekat WH, Iber C, James GD, Lebowitz M *et al* (1999) Relation of sleepiness to respiratory disturbance index: the Sleep Heart Health Study. *Am J Resp Crit Care Med* **159**(2): 502–7

Gyulay S, Olson LG, Hensley MJ, King MT, Murree Allen K, Saunders NA (1993) A comparison of clinical assessment and home oximetry in the diagnosis of obstructive sleep apnea. *Am Rev Respir Dis* **147**: 50–3

Harnich MJ, Chard SR, Orr WC (1996) Relationships between measures of objective and subjective sleepiness. *Sleep Res*: 492

Harrison Y, Bright V, Horne JA (1996) Can normal subjects be motivated to fall asleep faster? *Physiol Behav* **60**(2): 681–4

Hoddes E, Zarcone V, Smythe H, Phillips R, Dement WC (1973) Quantification of sleepiness: A new approach. *Psychophysiology* **10**(4): 431–6

Johns MW (1991) A new method for measuring daytime sleepiness: The Epworth sleepiness scale. *Sleep* **14**(6): 540–5

Johns MW (1992) Reliability and factor analysis of the Epworth sleepiness scale. *Sleep* **15**(4): 376–81

Johns MW (1994) Sleepiness in different situations measured by the Epworth sleepiness scale. *Sleep* **17**(8): 703–10

Kingshott RN, Engleman HM, Deary IJ, Douglas NJ (1998) Does arousal frequency predict daytime function? *Eur Respir J* **12**: 1264–70

Littner MR, Kushida C, Wise M, Davila DG, Morgenthaler T, Lee-Chiong T *et al* (2005) Standards of Practice Committee of the American Academy of Sleep Medicine. Practice parameters for clinical use of the multiple sleep latency test and the maintenance of wakefulness test. *Sleep* **28**(1): 113–21

Magalang UK, Kelemen GS, Seeds KM, Schwab RJ (1996) The incidence and reproducibility of sleep arousals in normal subjects. *Sleep Res*: 511

Manser RL, Rochford P, Naughton MT, Pierce RJ, Sasse A, Teichtahl H *et al* (2002) Measurement variability in sleep disorderes medicine: the Victorian experience. *Internal Med J* **32**: 386–93

Mathur R, Douglas NJ (1995) Frequency of EEG arousals from nocturnal sleep in normal subjects. *Sleep* **18**(5): 330–3

Mazza S, Pepin JL, Deschaux C, Naegele B, Levy P (2002) Analysis of error profiles occurring during the OSLER test: a senstive mean of detecting fluctuations in vigilance in patients with obstructive sleep apnea syndrome. *Am J Resp Crit Care Med* **166**(4): 474–8

Mitler MM, Gujavarty KS, Browman CP (1982) Maintenance of wakefulness test: A polysomnographic technique for evaluation treatment efficacy in patients with excessive somnolence. *Electroencephalogr Clin Neurophysiol* **53**: 658–61

Mitler MM, Gujavarty KS, Sampson MG, Browman CP (1982) Multiple daytime nap approaches to evaluating the sleep patient. *Sleep* **5**: S119–S127

Mitler MM, Walsleben J, Sangal B, Hirshkowitz M (1998) Sleep latency on the maintenance of wakefulness test (MWT) for 530 patients with narcolepsy while free of psychoactive drugs. *Electroencephalogr Clin Neurophysiol* **107**: 33–8

Moser NJ, Phillips BA, Berry DTR, Harbison L (1994) What is hypopnoea, anyway? *Chest* **105**: 426–8

Olson LG, Ambrogetti A, Gyulay SG (1999) Prediction of sleep-disordered breathing by unattended overnight oximetry. *J Sleep Res* **8**(1): 51–5

Olson LG, Cole MF, Ambrogetti A (1998) Correlations among Epworth sleepiness scale scores, multiple sleep latency tests and psychological symptoms. *J Sleep Res* **7**: 248–53

Portier F, Portmann A, Czernichow P, Vascaut L, Devin E, Benhamou D *et al* (2000) Evaluation of home versus laboratory polysomnography in the diagnosis of sleep apnea syndrome. *Am J Respir Crit Care Med* 162: 814–8

Priest B, Brichard C, Aubert G, Liistro G, Rodenstein DO (2001) Microsleep during a simplified maintenance of wakefulness test. A validation study of OSLER test. *Am J Resp Crit Care Med* **163**(7): 1619–25

Rechtschaffen A, Kales A, eds (1968) *Manual of Standardized Terminology: Techniques and Scoring System for Sleep Stages of Human Subjects*. Calif, Los Angeles

Redline S, Kapur V, Sanders H, Stuart F *et al* (2000) Effects of varying approaches for identifying respiratory disturbances on sleep apnea assessment. *Am J Respir Crit Care Med* **161**: 369–74

Reynolds III CF, Coble PA, Kupfer DJ, Holzer BC (1982) Application of the multiple sleep latency test in disorders of excessive sleepiness. *Electroencephalogr Clin Neurophysiol* **53**: 443–52

Richardson GS, Carskadon MA, Flagg W, Van Den Hoed J, Dement WC, Mitler MM (1978) Excessive daytime sleepiness in man: multiple sleep latency measurement in narcoleptic and control subjects. *Electroencephalogr Clin Neurophysiol* **45**: 621–7

Rodway GW, Sanders MH (2003) The efficacy of split-night studies. *Sleep Med Rev* **7**(5): 391–401

Sadeh A, Acebo C (2002) The role of actigraphy in sleep medicine. *Sleep Med Rev* **6**(2): 113–24

Sadeh A, Hauri PJ, Kripke DF, Lavie P (1995) The role of actigraphy in the evaluation of sleep disorders. *Sleep* **18**(4): 288–302

Sangal RB, Sangal JM, Belisle C (1997) MWT and ESS measure different abilities in 41 patients with snoring and daytime sleepiness. *Sleep Res* **101**(4): 493

Sangal RB, Thomas L, Mitler MM (1992) Maintenance of wakefulness test and multiple sleep latency test. Measurement of different abilities in patients with sleep disorders. *Chest* **101**: 898–902

Strohl KP, Redline S (1996) Recognition of obstructive sleep apnea. *Am J Resp Crit Care Med* **154**: 279–89

Zwyghuizen-Doorenbos A, Roehrs T, Schaefer M, Roth T (1988) Test–retest reliability of the MSLT. *Sleep* **11**(6): 562–5

Appendix A: History-taking for initial consultation

Trigger for this consultation

What actually precipitated the individual to seek treatment? Describe briefly.
Who made the appointment for this consultation (may be important in terms of later compliance with treatment)?

Background

How did the individual sleep as a child and teenager?
How was this sleep difficulty perceived by other family members?
Is there any other family member who has difficulties with sleep including sleep apnea/parasomnias, etc?
Who was it and for how long did this family member experience difficulties, or is it still continuing?

Cognitions about sleep

How does the individual think about his/her sleep?
How much sleep does the individual think that he/she should achieve to feel good the next day?
What are the consequences to the individual when he/she does not sleep?
How does he/she describe himself/herself in relation to sleep?

Present sleep/wake pattern	lark or owl?
Pre-bed activities	timing of food, alcohol, exercise, relaxation time
Actual bedtime	
Initiation	sleep latency
Medication	what taken, when and how often
Length of sleep before first wake	_____
Number of wakes	_____
Length of sleep after first wake	_____
Final waking time	_____
Final getting up time	_____
Naps	when? where?
Differences in sleep patterns on weekends	_____
Differences in sleep patterns on holiday	_____

Primary sleep syndromes

Symptoms of obstructive sleep apnea.
History of snoring — does the individual wake with a dry mouth, headache, a start, or choking sensation?
Reports of witnessed apneas — a bed partner to confirm this.

Central apnea? In the elderly it is possible to miss symptoms of central apneas with sleep maintenance insomnia.

Restless legs syndrome — increasing and often unbearable creepy-crawly sensation, only relief is to move. What is it like for the individual to try to sit still in the movies at a play or concert?

Periodic limb movements — reports of kicking bed partner and/or messy bed in the morning.

Other movement disorders — REM behavior disorder predominantly in middle-aged men.

Parasomnias — history of sleep-walking/talking as a child. When did this behavior stop or has it continued? Frequency and time of night?

Bruxism — reports from dentist, has a dental splint/mouthguard been recommended?

Narcolepsy

Hypnagogic hallucinations — intense visual or auditory experiences when the patient is about to fall asleep (drowsy but still awake) or when the person is waking up from sleep (hypnopompic hallucinations). The individual may need to get up to determine whether the dream is real or not — more likely to occur with sleep deprivation or increased anxiety levels.

Sleep paralysis — sensation of not being able to move on waking or while drifting off to sleep. The person is able to breathe and move his eyes but nothing else. Sleep paralysis is usually frightening, at least the first few episodes. Not to be confused with the feeling of being so tired that the patient does not feel like getting up.

Cataplexy — during moments of intense excitement, anger, laughter, sex, loss of muscle control particularly in legs and face. Can literally 'fall in a heap'.

Automatic behavior — the person can perform certain complex activity without full awareness, eg. driving without full awareness. Automatic behavior occurs at some stage to everybody, but is very frequent in narcoleptic syndromes.

Social and environmental factors

Caffeine containing products (coffee, tea, cola drinks, 'energy drinks', chocolate) — amount and frequency.

Smoking or history of smoking — when stopped smoking?

Alcohol — how much per day? Type of alcohol and changes in intake between week days, weekends and holidays. Is alcohol used as a means of inducing sleep? Any history of binge drinking?

Recreational drugs (cannabis, speed, benzodiazepines)

Exercise — type of exercise, how often and for how long? Differing patterns — weekends vs weekdays. Exercising too close to bed time (<2 hours) may interfere with sleep onset in some individuals.

Other medications — over and above hypnotic medications. Antihypertensive medications, beta-blockers — timing of these medications important information in relation to initiation difficulties.

Ask about herbal and over-the-counter medication, such as valerian and antihistamines.

Ask about social drug use especially marijuana, cocaine, ecstasy, etc and codeine derivatives.

Occupation — full-time or part-time work; is work enjoyable? Stress factors? Shift worker? Possible retirement? Financial concerns?

Personal relationships — single or with partner; supportive, conflictive or no comment/feedback.

Children — number of children, gender, age where living now and overall relationship with children.

'Time out' — what does the individual do for himself/herself to relax/unwind? Sport, reading, hobbies, etc.

Living environment — house, flat, noisy neighbors, traffic noise, neighbors as shift workers.

Bedroom environment — amount of light and heat in the bedroom, comfort of the bed and whether the bed partner snores.

Other factors

Relevant medical history:

Any medical condition that may impact on sleep/wake patterns.

Include questions relating to asthma, bronchitis, emphysema, hypertension, cardiac family history, and renal history.

Pain-related conditions: osteo- and rheumatoid arthritis.

Migraines/headaches.

Psychiatric history (especially depression and postnatal depression, generalized anxiety disorders and panic disorders). Include questions about family members.

Post-traumatic stress disorder — ask about dreams/nightmares.

Menopause or perimenopausal symptoms.

Surgical history:

Any surgical procedures — also include motor vehicle accidents/bike accidents.

If hospitalized — how long for and what was the impact of that time in hospital on sleep?

Any complications?

From: Delwyn Bartlett, PhD Royal Prince Alfred Hospital

Appendix B: Depression, anxiety and stress scale (DASS)

Name: Date:

Please read each statement and circle a number 0, 1, 2 or 3 which indicates how much the statement applied to you over the past week. There are no right or wrong answers. Do not spend too much time on any statement.

The rating scale is as follows:

0   Did not apply to me at all
1   Applied to me to some degree, or some of the time
2   Applied to me to a considerable degree, or a good part of time
3   Applied to me very much, or most of the time

1.	I found myself getting upset by quite trivial things	0	1	2	3
2.	I was aware of dryness of my mouth	0	1	2	3
3.	I couldn't seem to experience any positive feeling at all	0	1	2	3
4.	I experienced breathing difficulty (eg, excessively rapid breathing, breathlessness in the absence of physical exertion)	0	1	2	3
5.	I just couldn't seem to get going	0	1	2	3
6.	I tended to over-react to situations	0	1	2	3
7.	I had a feeling of shakiness (eg. legs going to give way)	0	1	2	3
8.	I found it difficult to relax	0	1	2	3
9.	I found myself in situations that made me so anxious I was most relieved when they ended	0	1	2	3
10.	I felt that I had nothing to look forward to	0	1	2	3
11.	I found myself getting upset rather easily	0	1	2	3
12.	I felt that I was using a lot of nervous energy	0	1	2	3
13.	I felt sad and depressed	0	1	2	3
14.	I found myself getting impatient when I was delayed in any way (eg. lifts, traffic lights, being kept waiting)	0	1	2	3
15.	I had a feeling of faintness	0	1	2	3
16.	I felt that I had lost interest in just about everything	0	1	2	3
17.	I felt I wasn't worth much as a person	0	1	2	3
18.	I felt that I was rather touchy	0	1	2	3
19.	I perspired noticeably (eg. hands sweaty) in the absence of high temperatures or physical exertion	0	1	2	3
20.	I felt scared without any good reason	0	1	2	3
21.	I felt that life wasn't worthwhile	0	1	2	3

Please turn the page

Reminder of rating scale:

0   Did not apply to me at all
1   Applied to me to some degree, or some of the time
2   Applied to me to a considerable degree, or a good part of time
3   Applied to me very much, or most of the time

22. I found it hard to wind down	0	1	2	3
23. I had difficulty in swallowing	0	1	2	3
24. I couldn't seem to get any enjoyment out of the things I did	0	1	2	3
25. I was aware of the action of my heart in the absence of physical exertion (eg, sense of heart rate increase, heart missing a beat)	0	1	2	3
26. I felt down-hearted and blue	0	1	2	3
27. I found that I was very irritable	0	1	2	3
28. I felt I was close to panic	0	1	2	3
29. I found it hard to calm down after something upset me	0	1	2	3
30. I feared that I would be 'thrown' by some trivial but unfamiliar task	0	1	2	3
31. I was unable to become enthusiastic about anything	0	1	2	3
32. I found it difficult to tolerate interruptions to what I was doing	0	1	2	3
33. I was in a state of nervous tension	0	1	2	3
34. I felt I was pretty worthless	0	1	2	3
35. I was intolerant of anything that kept me from getting on with what I was doing	0	1	2	3
36. I felt terrified	0	1	2	3
37. I could see nothing in the future to be hopeful about	0	1	2	3
38. I felt that life was meaningless	0	1	2	3
39. I found myself getting agitated	0	1	2	3
40. I was worried about situations in which I might panic and make a fool of myself	0	1	2	3
41. I experienced trembling (eg. in the hands)	0	1	2	3
42. I found it difficult to work up the initiative to do things	0	1	2	3

Appendix C: Patient health questionnaire

The brief form of PRIME-MD® Patient Health Questionnaire is a useful self-reported screening test for depression and anxiety, developed by Dr Robert L Spitzer, Professor of Psychiatry at Columbia University. Some more detailed and expanded questionnaires are also available, from the author (contact Dr Robert L Spitzer at rls8@columbia.edu).

Research Quick Guide to Patient Health Questionnaire (PHQ) and Brief PHQ

Purpose. The Patient Health Questionnaire (PHQ) is designed to facilitate the recognition and diagnosis of the most common mental disorders in primary care patients: somatoform, depressive, anxiety, eating and alcohol disorders. The Brief PHQ only covers depressive disorders and panic disorder. Both instruments include questions about functional impairment, recent psychosocial stressors, and for women, questions about menstruation, pregnancy and childbirth. For patients with depressive symptoms a Total Depression Score can be calculated and repeated over time to monitor change.

Who should take the PHQ or Brief PHQ. Ideally, either questionnaire should be used with all new patients, all patients who have not completed the questionnaire in the last year, and all patients suspected of having a mental disorder.

Making a diagnosis. Since the questionnaire relies on patient self-report, definitive diagnoses must be verified by the clinician, taking into account how well the patient understood the questions in the questionnaire, as well as other relevant information from the patient, his or her family or other sources. In addition, the diagnoses of major depressive disorder (rather than syndrome) and other depressive disorder requires ruling out normal bereavement (mild symptoms, duration less than 2 months), a history of a manic episode (bipolar disorder) and a physical disorder, medication or other drug as the biological cause of the depressive symptoms. Similarly, the diagnoses of panic disorder and other anxiety disorders require ruling out a physical disorder, medication or other drug as the biological cause of the anxiety symptoms.

Interpreting the PHQ or BPHQ. At the bottom of pages that begin with 'FOR OFFICE CODING' (in small type) are criteria for judgments about diagnoses assessed on that page. The names of the categories are abbreviated, eg. major depressive syndrome is maj dep syn.

Additional clinical considerations. After making a provisional diagnosis with the PHQ or Brief PHQ, there are additional clinical considerations that may affect decisions about management and treatment.

Have current symptoms been triggered by psychosocial stressor(s)?
What is the duration of the current disturbance and has the patient received any treatment for it?
To what extent are the patient's symptoms impairing his or her usual work and activities?
Is there a history of similar episodes, and were they treated?
Is there a family history of similar conditions?

Customizing the PHQ or brief PHQ by omitting pages

Option	Questionnaire ingredients	No of pages	Coverage
A	PHQ	4	Mental disorders (somatoform, mood, anxiety, eating, alcohol) Functional impairment Stressors Menstruation, pregnancy, childbirth
B	First 3 pages of the PHQ	3	Mental disorders Functional impairment
C	Brief PHQ	2	Depressive disorders and panic disorder Functional impairment Stressors Menstruation
D	First page of Brief PHQ	I	Depressive disorders and panic disorder

Example of diagnosing major depressive disorder and calculating total depression score

Patient: A 43-year-old woman looks sad and complains of fatigue over the past month.

2. Over the last <u>2 weeks</u>, how often have you been bothered by any of the following	Not at all	Several days	More than half the days	Nearly every day
a Little interest or pleasure in doing things?.	☐	☐	☐	☒
b Feeling down, depressed, or hopeless?	☐	☒	☐	☐
c Trouble falling or staying asleep, or sleeping too much?	☐	☐	☒	☐
d Feeling tired or having little energy?	☐	☐	☐	☒
e Poor appetite or overeating?	☐	☒	☐	☐
f Feeling bad about yourself — or that you are a failure or have let yourself or your family down?	☐	☐	☒	☐
g Trouble concentrating on things, such as reading the newspaper or watching television?	☐	☐	☐	☒
h Moving or speaking so slowly that other people could have noticed? Or the opposite — being so fidgety or restless that you have been moving around a lot more than usual?	☒	☐	☐	☐
i Thoughts that you would be better off dead or of hurting yourself in some way?	☐	☒	☐	☐

FOR OFFICE CODING: Maj Dep Syn if #2a or b and five or more of #2a–2i are at least "More than half the days" (count #2i if present at all). Other Dep Syn if #2a or b and two, three, or four of #2a–2i are at least "More than half the days" (count #2i if present at all).

Major depressive disorder diagnosis. The criteria for major depressive syndrome are met since the patient checked #2a 'Nearly every day' and five of items #2a to 2i were checked 'More than half the days' or 'Nearly every day'. Note that #2i, suicidal ideation, is counted whenever it is present.

In this case, the diagnosis of major depressive disorder (not syndrome) was made since questioning by the physician indicated no history of a manic episode; no evidence that a physical disorder, medication, or other drug caused the depression; and no indication that the depressive symptoms were normal bereavement. Questioning about the suicidal ideation indicated no significant suicidal potential.

Total depression score. This is calculated by assigning scores of 0, 1, 2, and 3, to the response categories of 'Not at all,' 'Several days,' 'More than half the days,' and 'Nearly every day,' respectively. The total depression score is the sum of the scores for the nine items, and ranges from 0 to 27. In the above case, the score is 16 (3 items scored 1; 2 items scored 2; and 3 items scored 3).

In a study of 3000 primary care patients, the mean total depression score was 5.0. The standard deviation was 5.8. The mean score for patients with major depressive disorder (N=290) was 18.6; for patients with any mood disorder (N=473) the mean score was 15.1.

Developed by Drs Robert L Spitzer, Janet BW Williams, Kurt Kroenke and colleagues, with an educational grant from Pfizer Inc. For research information, contact Dr Spitzer at rls8@columbia.edu. The names PRIME-MD® and PRIME-MD TODAY® are trademarks of Pfizer Inc.

Brief patient health questionnaire

This questionnaire is an important part of providing you with the best health care possible. Your answers will help in understanding problems that you may have.

Name_____ Age_____ Sex: 0 Female 0 Male Today's date_____

1. Over the last <u>2 weeks</u>, how often have you been bothered by any of the following	Not at all	Several days	More than half the days	Nearly every day
a Little interest or pleasure in doing things	☐	☐	☐	☐
b Feeling down, depressed, or hopeless	☐	☐	☐	☐
c Trouble falling or staying asleep, or sleeping too much	☐	☐	☐	☐
d Feeling tired or having little energy	☐	☐	☐	☐
e Poor appetite or overeating	☐	☐	☐	☐
f Feeling bad about yourself — or that you are a failure or have let yourself or your family down	☐	☐	☐	☐
g Trouble concentrating on things, such as reading the newspaper or watching television	☐	☐	☐	☐

h	Moving or speaking so slowly that other people could have noticed? Or the opposite — being so fidgety or restless that you have been moving around a lot more than usual	☐	☐	☐	☐
i	Thoughts that you would be better off dead or of hurting yourself in some way	☐	☐	☐	☐

2.	Questions about anxiety	No	Yes
a	In the <u>last 4 weeks</u>, have you had an anxiety attack: suddenly feeling fear or panic? If you checked 'NO', go to question #3.	☐	☐
b	Has this ever happened before?	☐	☐
c	Do some of these attacks come suddenly out of the blue, that is, in situations where you don't expect to be nervous or uncomfortable?	☐	☐
d	Do these attacks bother you a lot or are you worried about having another attack?	☐	☐
e	During your last bad anxiety attack, did you have symptoms like shortness of breath, sweating, your heart racing or pounding, dizziness or faintness, tingling or numbness, or nausea or upset stomach?	☐	☐

3. If you checked off any problems on this questionnaire so far, how difficult have these problems made it for you to do your work, take care of things at home, or get along with other people?

Not difficult at all	Somewhat difficult	Very difficult	Extremely difficult
☐	☐	☐	☐

FOR OFFICE CODING: Maj Dep Syn if answers to #1a or b and five or more of #1a–1i are at least 'More than half the days' (count #1i if present at all). Other Dep Syn if #1a or b and two, three, or four of #1a–1i are at least 'More than half the days' (count #1i if present at all).
Pan Syn if all of #2a–2e are 'YES.'

1.	In the <u>last 4 weeks</u>, how much have you been bothered by any of the following problems?	Not bothered	Bothered a little	Bothered a lot
a	Worrying about your health	☐	☐	☐
b	Your weight or how you look	☐	☐	☐
c	Little or no sexual desire or pleasure during sex	☐	☐	☐
d	Difficulties with husband/wife, partner/lover or boyfriend/girlfriend	☐	☐	☐
e	The stress of taking care of children, parents, or other family members	☐	☐	☐
f	Stress at work outside of the home or at school	☐	☐	☐

g	Financial problems or worries	☐	☐	☐
h	Having no one to turn to when you have a problem	☐	☐	☐
i	Something bad that happened recently	☐	☐	☐
j	Thinking or dreaming about something terrible that happened to you in the past like your house being destroyed, a severe accident, being hit or assaulted, or being forced to commit a sexual act	☐	☐	☐

		No	Yes
5.	**In the <u>last year</u>, have you been hit, slapped, kicked or otherwise physically hurt by someone, or has anyone forced you to have an unwanted sexual act?**	☐	☐
6	**What is the most stressful thing in your life right now?**		
7.	**Are you taking any medicine for anxiety, depression or stress?**	No ☐	Yes ☐
8.	**FOR WOMEN ONLY: Questions about menstruation, pregnancy and childbirth.**		
	a. Which best describes your menstrual periods?		

Periods are unchanged	No periods because pregnant or recently gave birth	Periods have become irregular or changed in frequency, duration or amount	No periods for at least a year
☐	☐	☐	☐

		No (or does not apply)	Yes
b	During the week before your period starts, do you have a serious problem with your mood – like depression, anxiety, irritability, anger or mood swings?	☐	☐
c	If YES: Do these problems go away by the end of your period?	☐	☐
d	Have you given birth within the last six months?	☐	☐
e	Have you had a miscarriage within the last six months?	☐	☐
f	Are you having difficulty getting pregnant?	☐	☐

Adapted from the PRIME-MD® Patient Health Questionnaire © 1999, Pfizer Inc. For research information, contact Dr Robert L Spitzer at rls8@columbia.edu.

Appendix D: Epworth sleepiness scale

How likely are you to doze off or fall asleep in the following situations, in contrast to feeling just tired? This refers to your usual way of life in recent times. Even if you have not done some of these things recently try to work out how they would have affected you. Use the following scale to choose the most appropriate number for each situation.

0	**1**	**2**	**3**
Never doze	**Slight chance of dozing**	**Moderate chance of dozing**	**High chance of dozing**

How likely are you to doze off or fall asleep   (please circle your answer)

1.	While sitting and reading?	0	1	2	3
2.	While watching TV?	0	1	2	3
3.	While sitting inactive in a public place (eg. theatre, meeting)?	0	1	2	3
4.	While a passenger in a car for an hour without a break?	0	1	2	3
5.	While lying down to rest in the afternoon when circumstances permit?	0	1	2	3
6.	While sitting and talking to someone?	0	1	2	3
7.	While sitting quietly after lunch without alcohol?	0	1	2	3
8.	While in a car stopped for a few minutes in traffic?	0	1	2	3
			ESS score		/ 24

The higher the score the more the propensity to fall asleep. Values above 10 are suggestive of increased sleepiness tendency. The score is particularly useful to assess treatment response in the same patient over time.

Appendix E: Stanford sleepiness scale

1. Feeling active and vital; wide awake.
2. Functioning at high level; but not at peak.
3. Relaxed; awake; not at full alertness; responsive.
4. A little foggy; not at peak; let down.
5. Fogginess; beginning to lose interest in remaining awake; slowed down.
6. Sleepiness; prefer to be lying down; fighting sleep; woozy.
7. Almost in reverie; sleep onset soon; lost struggle to remain awake.
(X. Asleep).

From Hoddes *et al*, 1973.

Appendix F: Karolinska Scale

1	2	3	4	5	6	7	8	9
Extremely alert		Alert		Neither alert nor sleepy		Sleepy — no difficulty staying awake		Extremely sleepy — fighting sleep

From Åkerstedt and Gillberg (1990) Subjective and objective sleepiness in the active individual. *Intern J Neurosci* **52**: 29–37.

CHAPTER 4

Basic concepts of polysomnography

Vincenza Castronovo

Introduction

Polysomnography, derived from the Greek roots 'poly' meaning many, 'somno' meaning sleep and 'graphy' meaning to write, refers to multiple parameters recorded from subjects while they sleep.

The term polysomnography (PSG) was proposed by Holland, Dement and Raynal in 1974 to describe the recording of multiple, simultaneous physiological parameters. It refers to an overnight test fundamental for the evaluation and diagnosis of sleep disorders. The electrophysiological measures for assessing sleep involve the monitoring of cortical brain waves, eye movements and muscle activity.

PSG is a complex procedure that should be performed by specifically trained personnel.

The first part of this chapter covers the main aspects of PSG and provides a step-by-step approach to traditional in-laboratory PSG recording techniques. The second part refers to basic principles of conventional criteria for sleep-stage scoring, as well as microstructural aspects (in particular cyclic alternating pattern, CAP).

Part one: Polysomnography

Polysomnography is essential for diagnosing and evaluating sleep disorders, such as sleep-disordered breathing and parasomnias (abnormal behaviors or movements during sleep) (American Sleep Disorders Association, 2005a).

Equipment — the polysomnograph

A polysomnograph is a machine that converts the body's bio-electrical signals to a graphical representation which can help determine what happens during sleep. The main component is a series of amplifiers. There is a combination of alternating current (AC) channels and direct current (DC) channels. Typically, at least twelve to sixteen channels are used for standard recordings. The data from the amplifiers are written onto a moving chart, or stored into a computer which converts analog signals to digital ones. These digital signals are then stored by the computer for subsequent analysis.

Different activities, such as brain waves (EEG), eye movements (EOG), muscle activity (EMG), heart rate (ECG), blood oxygen levels (SaO$_2$) and respiration are usually monitored. Each of these activities is represented by graphical tracings on a polysomnogram. The tracings continue through the night as a patient sleeps. The input bioelectric signals recorded are generally very small, ranging from one microvolt to one millivolt. For this reason, these signals are amplified and filtered to preserve the frequency band of interest.

In terms of frequency, the signals may be very slow, from 0.001 to 0.01 Hertz (Hz) (ie. respiration) or very fast, from 1000 to 2000 Hz (ie. muscle activity). In practice, the most relevant range is from 0.3 to 20 Hz. Therefore, polysomnography requires proper amplification and filtering to ensure that an appropriate window for recording specific frequencies is established and filters do not eliminate important data. It is essential that technicians, regardless of the system used, have adequate knowledge of the impact of the correct use of filters on the data collected during PSG.

Calibration

Calibration is an important technical procedure that ensures adequate functioning of amplifiers and appropriate settings for recording the specific parameters of interest (*Figure 4.1*). All filter and sensitivity settings (*Table 4.1*) should be clearly documented in each channel recorded.

Epoch view

The epoch length is the amount of time that appears on each page of the recording. The process of sleep stage scoring and analysis of abnormalities is done by an epoch-by-epoch review of the data.

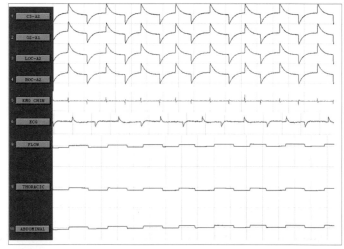

Figure 4.1: *Calibration showing the different amplifiers' settings for the different physiological signals recorded during polysomnography.*

The most common epoch view for traditional polysomnography is 10 mm/second, providing a 30-second epoch. Another widely accepted paper speed is 15 mm/second, which gives a 20-second epoch length. A paper speed of 30 mm/second should be used when recording patients with suspected sleep-related seizure activity. This speed enhances the ability to visualize EEG data, specifically the spike activity associated with epileptic discharges.

Table 4.1: Most common amplifier settings for polysomnography				
	Sensitivity (μVolt/cm)	**Low frequency filter (HZ)**	**Time constant**	**High frequency filter (Hz)**
EEG	50	0.3	0.5	30
EOG	50	0.3	0.5	30
EMG	50 (adjust as necessary)	10	0.05	>90
ECG	1 millivolt/cm (adjust as necessary)	1	0.5	15
Respiration	50 (adjust as necessary)	0.15	1–2	15

Electrode application

The patient should arrive at the sleep laboratory one to two hours before the start of the sleep study, to allow time to attach the electrodes for electrophysiological monitoring and fill out the required forms. In some cases a physical examination will also be conducted during this time.

The technician places small sensors called electrodes on the patient's scalp, face, chin, chest and legs. The process is not painful and takes only about 30 minutes. During this process, the patient is informed about the procedure and given the opportunity to ask questions. A common question is: 'Do you really expect me to sleep in all this?' Surprisingly, most people have little difficulty going to sleep wearing all the wires and sensors. After the

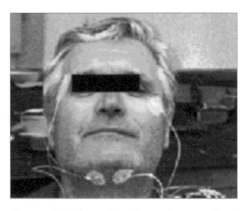

Figure 4.2: Man with electrodes attached for all-night polysomnographic evaluation.

patient is 'wired-up' they are given some time to relax before the test begins. The test usually starts around the time the patient normally goes to bed. The polysomnograph will reveal when drowsiness ends and sleep begins. *Figure 4.2* shows a man prepared for a typical recording.

Close to the recording room there is an instrumentation room for the polysomnograph and other equipment. Sleep laboratories employ closed-circuit television cameras and microphones to maintain visual and two-way audio communications between the patients in the sleep room and the technician in the instrumentation room. A videotape recorder or digital video is used to record the patient's movements and sounds during sleep. Additionally, a 'split screen' technique to simultaneously record tracings of the polysomnograph and movements during sleep is frequently

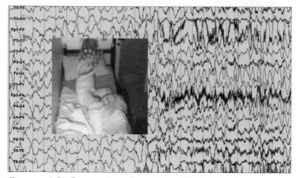

Figure 4.3: Example of a video-EEG simultaneous recording: tracings of PSG and movements from the video are recorded and stored together for further analysis.

used, especially for those patients where video-recording is fundamental for the differential diagnosis (*Figure 4.3*).

Determining sleep

The objective definition of wakefulness, slow-wave sleep, non-REM sleep and REM sleep is based on the patterns of brain waves (the electroencephalogram, EEG) eye movements (the electrooculogram, EOG) and muscle activity (the electromyogram, EMG).

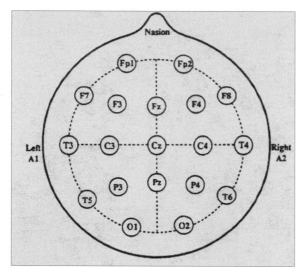

Figure 4.4: Diagram showing sites for the complete 10–20 system electrode placement.

Electroencephalography

Brain-wave activity from the central area and from the occipital area determines EEG attributes of the sleep state. Standard electrode derivations are C3/A2 or C4/A1 and O1/A2 or O2/A1. In many situations there may be a need for additional electrodes, in particular when it is necessary to evaluate or rule out EEG abnormalities. In these cases, more EEG electrodes are used according to the 10–20 system of the International Federation (Jasper, 1958) that defines the exact location of EEG electrodes (*Figure 4.4*).

The EEG electrodes, gold or silver–silver chloride cup electrodes filled with conductive paste, are generally attached to the scalp using small patches of gauze soaked in collodion and dried with compressed air to ensure long-term placement (at least 8 hours). Other methods using only electrode paste are acceptable and sometimes necessary in certain conditions (eg. children in intensive care units). The standard manual recommends referential recording of EEG leads, either C3 or C4 and O1 or O2, referenced to an indifferent auricularly placed electrode on the contralateral mastoid or ear lobe (C3/A2 or C4/A1 and O1/A2 or O2/A1) (*Figure 4.5*). The main reason for these EEG placements to distinguish sleep stages is because the elements characteristics of stage 2 non-REM, such as vertex sharp waves, K complexes and spindles, are mostly evident in the central area. Also, high-voltage slow waves, characteristic of stage 3–4 non-REM sleep, are maximally seen in frontal regions and yet show on central derivations. Alpha rhythm, typical of an awake person with eyes closed, by contrast is maximal over the occipital regions.

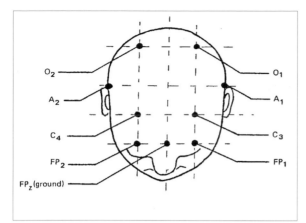

Figure 4.5: Illustration of the placement of EEG electrodes (O1, O2, C3, C4) as well as the placement of reference electrodes (A1 and A2). FPz is the ground.

Electro-oculography

Eye-movement monitoring (electro-oculogram, EOG), is based on recording the potential difference between the back of the eye and the front of the eye (cornea–retinal potential difference in the eye). The retina is electronegative with respect to the cornea and this generates voltage potentials when the eye moves between two well-positioned electrodes. The EOG electrodes are placed slightly lateral to the outer canthus of each eye: 1 cm above the outer canthus of the right eye (ROC) and 1 cm below the outer canthus of the left eye (LOC) or vice versa. The standard manual recommends referential recording of two EOG leads referred to the same auricular reference (ROC-A1 and LOC-A1) (*Figures 4.6, 4.7, 4.8*). With this placement of electrodes it is possible to detect vertical as well as horizontal eye movements.

There are two reasons for recording eye movement activity during sleep. The first is to record rapid eye movements, typical of REM sleep, and the second is for assessing the onset of sleep that is accompanied by slow-rolling eye movements (SEMs). Although these slow eye movements are not essential to sleep staging, they often provide useful information.

Gold cup electrodes, or silver–silver chloride electrodes, are applied to the surface of the skin with an adhesive tape. This method avoids the risk of collodion contacting the patient's eyes.

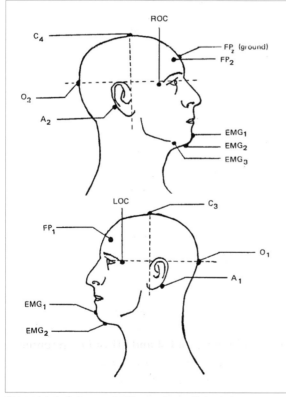

Figure 4.6: Schematic illustration of the placement of all electrodes necessary to determine sleep stages. Additional electrodes almost always include ECG, leg movements and a variety of respiratory parameters. EMG, electromyogram; LOC< left ocular canthus; ROC, right ocular canthus.

Electromyography

In a standard PSG the recording from muscles beneath the chin (mentalis and submentalis muscles) is used as a criterion for staging REM sleep. Most EMG recordings during sleep require taping electrodes to the skin over the muscle group of interest. Usually three electrodes, attached with adhesive tape, are placed beneath the chin overlying the mentalis and submentalis muscles, to allow for an alternative electrode in case a problem develops in one (*Figures 4.8, 4.9, 4.10*). The EMG is recorded bipolarly; any combination of the three placements can be used.

The EMG recordings from other muscle groups are sometimes used to assess certain sleep disorders (eg. periodic limb movement of the anterior tibialis muscle).

Electrocardiography

The ECG electrodes (gold or silver cup applied with tape or adhesive disposable electrodes) are applied to the surface of the skin. One is usually placed just beneath the right clavicle and the other one on the left side at the level of the seventh rib. The ECG is always monitored to assess autonomic function and to rule out possible abnormalities during sleep.

Additional parameters are monitored during sleep according to a specific protocol for the evaluation of specific sleep disorders. Respiration during sleep is one of the most commonly monitored parameters.

Respiration

Sleep studies are used to detect, characterize and determine the possible causes and degree of severity of apneas, hypoventilation and oxygen desaturation during sleep, and to evaluate possible relationships between sleep-disordered breathing, oxygen desaturation, and disrupted sleep.

During the night, ventilatory effort and airflow during sleep are monitored using a variety of methods.

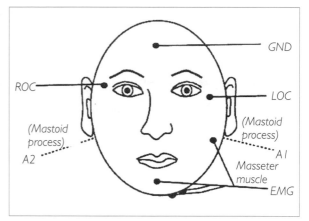

Figure 4.7: Complete diagram of the placement of EOG electrodes (ROC and LOC) and EMG electrodes (recording activity from mental, submental and masseter muscles). GND, ground electrode.

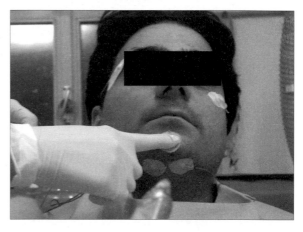

Figure 4.8: Application of EMG electrodes.

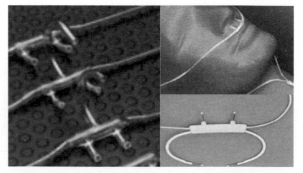

Figure 4.9: Thermistor used to record air flow at the nose and mouth.

Those mostly used include:

- air flow at nose and mouth: oronasal thermistors or flow sensors (nasal cannula) (*Figure 4.9*)
- efforts: movements of the chest and abdomen for assessing ventilatory activity are detected by strain gauges or piezo-electric sensors fastened around the chest and abdomen. These sensors respond to changes in expansion which occur with effort to breathe (*Figure 4.10*). Another technique (rarely used today because it is invasive) uses a small pressure transducing system to monitor changes in intrathoracic pressure by means of a balloon (pressure transducer) introduced into the thorax through the nose and down the esophagus
- EMG of intercostal muscles: electrodes placed on the skin over the intercostal muscle (between the ribs) detect movement with respiratory effort. This technique is particularly useful in differentiating obstructive from central apnea
- snoring: a miniaturized microphone placed over the substernal notch is used to record breathing sounds (*Figure 4.11*).

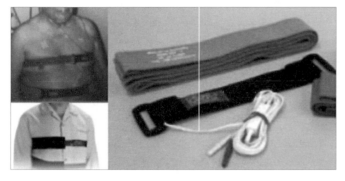

Figure 4.10: Piezo-electric belts applied at the thorax and abdomen used for recording respiration (thoracic and abdominal efforts).

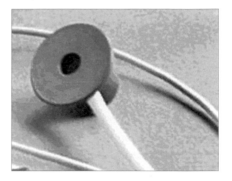

Figure 4.11: Microphone used to detect snoring sounds.

Measurement of oxygen saturation

Oxygen levels in the arterial blood are measured by means of an oximeter (*Figure 4.12*). The oximeter is a device that measures the percentage of hemoglobin in arterial blood in the form of oxyhemoglobin (percentage of arterial oxygen saturation). The device uses a probe (*Figure 4.13*) placed on the ear or finger to pass a light beam through living tissue. The instrument then compares the amount of light absorbed, with absorption by tissue, with known levels of oxygen saturation. The quantity of light absorbed indicates oxygen saturation.

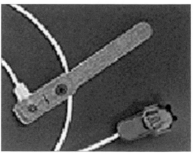

Figure 4.13: Flexible oximeter finger probe used to record SaO$_2$.

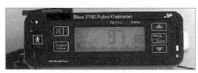

Figure 4.12: Oximeter used to detect oxygen saturation.

Physiologic calibrations

Before recording, electrodes should be visually inspected to assess their correct placement. An impedance check should always be obtained and documented (<5000 Ω).

Physiologic calibration is performed before the beginning of the recording. This calibration allows for documentation of proper functioning of the electrodes (EEG, EOG, EMG chin, respiration, EMG legs), and other monitoring devices and provides baseline data for review and comparison when scoring the PSG. The specific instructions given to the patient are:

- keep eyes open and then closed for 20–30 seconds (for EEG)
- look to left and right, up and down and blink the eyes (for EOG) (*Figure 4.14*)
- grit teeth, clench jaw, or smile (for EMG chin)
- inhale and exhale and hold breath for 10 seconds (for respiration)
- flex right and left foot (for EMG legs).

After physiologic calibrations are completed, the technician determines if any adjustment to electrodes or other monitoring devices is needed before the PSG begins. If a poor signal is noted during the physiologic calibrations, it is imperative that every effort is made to correct the problem as the condition is likely to get worse through the remaining portions of the recording.

When a satisfactory calibration procedure is done and all other aspects of patient and equipment preparation are completed, lights are turned out in the patient's room and the patient is told to assume a comfortable sleeping position and try to fall asleep. The lights-out time should be clearly noted.

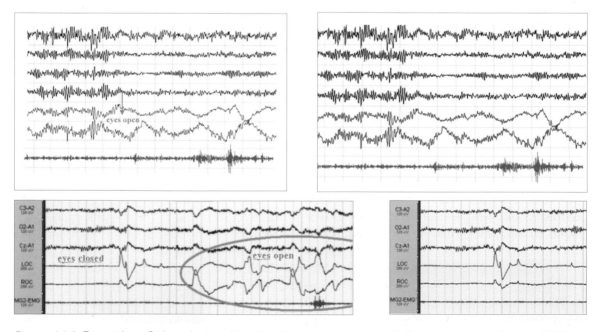

Figure 4.14: Examples of physiologic calibration showing eyes closed (left part: alpha rhythm on EEG channels) and eyes open (right part: rapid EOG movements).

Documentation

For an 'optimal' PSG complete documentation is essential. This includes patient identification (patient's full name and medical record number), date of recording and a full description of the study (including information on the channels recorded).

Specific parameters recorded on each channel should be clearly noted, as well as a full description of sensitivity, filters, and calibration settings for each channel. The time of the beginning and the end of the recording must be noted, as well as specific events that occur during the night.

The technician is also responsible for providing a clinical description of unusual events. For example, if a patient experiences an epileptic seizure during the study, the clinical manifestations of the seizure must be detailed — deviation of eyes or head to one side or the other, movement of extremities, vocalization, presence of incontinence, duration of seizure, and post-ictal status. Similar information should be reported on any clinical event observed in the laboratory, such as motor activity (eg. sleep-walking, sleep-talking). Physical complaints reported by the patient should also be reported.

Ending the study

Clinical circumstances and laboratory protocol dictate whether the patient is woken at a specific time or is allowed to awaken spontaneously. After waking, to end the study, the patient should be asked to perform the physiologic calibration movements to ensure that the electrodes and other monitoring devices are still functioning properly.

A subjective evaluation by the patient is made. The patient is asked to estimate how long it took to fall asleep, the amount of time spent asleep and if there were any disruptions during the sleep period. Patients should report on the quality of sleep and on the level of alertness experienced on awakening.

Conclusion

PSG is a complex, labor-intensive procedure. It requires specialized technical skills and knowledge of normal sleep and sleep disorders. Technicians need to be experts with sleep laboratory equipment, competent in dealing with medically ill patients, and capable of dealing with emergencies that may arise in the sleep laboratory during the night.

This field is faced with many challenges, not only in terms of developing standards of practice and procedures, but also in keeping up with ongoing developments of technology.

Throughout its evolution, PSG has proven to be both a fundamental tool for enhancing the understanding of sleep and its disorders and an essential diagnostic procedure.

Part two: Classification of human sleep

In 1953, Aserinski and Kleitman demonstrated the occurrence of periods of sleep characterized by conjugate rapid eye movements with an activated EEG pattern consisting of low amplitude waves and increased rates of heartbeat and respiration that led to the description of REM sleep. Dement and Kleitman, in 1957, observed that REM sleep appeared to recur in a cyclical fashion throughout the night, interspersed by periods of non-REM sleep. Sleep is not a unitary process. REM sleep, non-REM sleep and wakfulness have come to be thought of as the three states of consciousness. In 1968, the classification of Rechtschaffen and Kales differentiated REM from slow-wave sleep (non-REM sleep), which is divided into four stages, and provides the most widely accepted guidelines for staging human sleep.

It is useful to clarify some general concepts (referring primarily to the EEG) before going into the sleep stage scoring procedure. For EEG, frequency (Hz, Hertz) is the number of cycles (each cycle is the complete series of potential changes before the series repeats) per second. The common EEG frequency bands used for sleep scoring are:

- alpha (8–12 cycles per second, cps)
- beta (>12 cps)
- delta (<4 cps)
- theta (4–7 cps).

Another parameter is the amplitude that measures the wave from trough to peak.

When a sleep recording is scored, a sleep stage is assigned to each epoch (most commonly the epoch length is 30 seconds). A score that most appropriately characterizes the predominant pattern occurring during that interval is assigned to each epoch. The criteria detailed below are specifically for adults, although they have also been used to characterize sleep in children and adolescents. A separate set of criteria are necessary in newborns and older infants.

Stages of sleep are by convention divided into 'quiet' (non-REM) sleep, which consists of stages 1, 2, 3 and 4, and paradoxical (REM) sleep. The distribution of sleep stages follows a typical pattern. From wakefulness, subjects go through a short period of stage 1 into stages 2, 3, and 4 (slow-wave sleep, SWS) successively, which is interrupted approximately every 90 minutes by a period of REM sleep (*Figure 4.15*). The REM episodes tend to last from a few minutes to between 20 and 30 minutes or more in the early morning hours.

In normal young or middle-aged adults, approximately one quarter of time asleep is spent in REM sleep. Stages III and IV (SWS) seem to occur in the first part of the night and the amount of sleep in these sleep stages decreases with age.

The following parameters are essential when analyzing the sleep profile:

- total sleep time (TST): actual time spent asleep
- time in bed (TIB): time spent in bed
- sleep efficiency (SE):ratio between TST and TIB
- sleep latency (SL): amount of time required to fall asleep
- wakefulness after sleep onset (WASO): amount of time awake after initial sleep onset

- non-REM sleep stages (S1, S2, S3, S4) and REM sleep percentages
- REM latency (REM-L): latency to the first appearance of stage REM sleep.

After the study is completed, a sleep specialist needs to review and interpret the PSG to establish a diagnosis, taking into consideration the clinical history, and provide treatment recommendations if evidence of a sleep disorder is found.

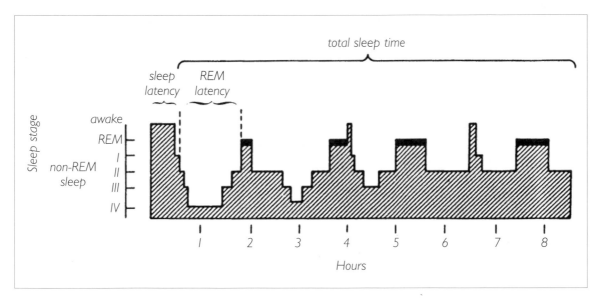

Figure 4.15: Graph defined as a 'Hypnogram' showing the sequence of sleep stages in a young, normal adult.

Sleep stage scoring

The patterns of EEG, EOG and EMG activity define REM and non-REM states as well as the different stages of non-REM sleep. Categorizing human polysomnographic recordings into these behavioral states is called 'sleep scoring'. The manual of Rechtschaffen and Kales provides the most widely accepted criteria for sleep scoring.

The different EEG patterns are illustrated all together in *Figure 4.16*. Alpha bands predominate the EEG during relaxed wakefulness with eyes closed, and have a frequency of 8–12 Hz. They are most prominent over the occipital cortex. Non-REM stage 1 is a transitional phase between wakefulness and sleep. The EEG is characterized by a relatively low voltage, mixed frequency activity of 2–7 Hz.

Stage 2 is defined by the presence of transient sleep spindles and K complexes (*Figure 4.17*). A sleep spindle consists of EEG activity of 12–14 Hz lasting from 0.5 seconds to 1.5 seconds. A K complex is an EEG waveform of about 0.5 seconds' duration, with a well-delineated negative component immediately followed by positive deflection.

The occurrence of delta waves in the EEG defines stages 3 and 4. A delta wave has an amplitude greater than 75 microvolts (measured peak to trough) (*Figure 4.18*). The frequency is

1–2 Hz. Stage 3 has from 20% to 50% delta waves in the EEG, while stage 4 has greater than 50% delta activity. Stages 3 and 4 are often collectively referred to as slow-wave sleep or delta sleep. However, notice that in some literature, stages 1, 2, 3 and 4 (non-REM sleep), are also referred to as slow-wave sleep, which can create confusion (*Chapter 1*). The EEG pattern during REM sleep is similar to that of stage 1, with the exception that 'saw-tooth' waves are frequently present (*Figure 4.19*).

The dramatic change in the EOG and the EMG further delineates REM from non-REM states. Although slow eye movements occur during stage 1 at sleep onset, eye-movement activity is negligible during stages 2, 3, and 4. REM sleep, in contrast, is characterized by rapid, conjugated eye movements. The frequency of rapid eye movements is sometimes quantified for various purposes as REM-density, usually expressed as the percentage of REM sleep occupied by phasic events.

EMG levels of stages 1, 2, 3 and 4 are typically lower than those of wakefulness, but tonic EMG is at its lowest level during REM sleep. This suppression of the EMG reflects an inhibitory influence on motor activity during REM sleep (*Chapter 1, Figure 1.14*).

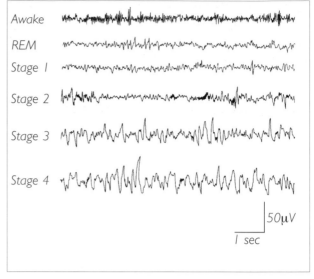

Figure 4.16: Different EEG patterns typical of the different states of consciousness (wake, non-REM and REM sleep).

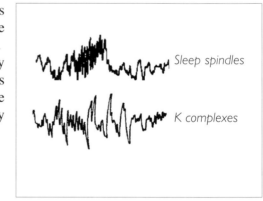

Figure 4.17: Sleep spindles and K complex characteristics of stage 2 non-REM.

EEG power spectral patterns

It is possible to analyze the ongoing EEG with techniques other than sleep stage scoring criteria. Computer programmes can quantify the amount of EEG activity attributable to certain sleep-specific frequencies, such as delta frequency and sleep-spindle frequency. This approach involves computers programmed to apply analysis of variance statistical techniques that quantify the EEG power in selected frequency bands (*Figure 4.20*).

The greater the power, the deeper the sleep, or the greater the tendency to sleep. One of the most

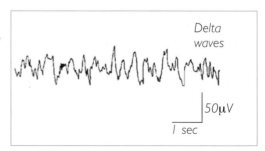

Figure 4.18: Delta waves, characteristics of stage 3 and 4 non-REM.

reproducible findings with this type of measurement is that slow-wave sleep increases after sleep deprivation, or sleep restriction, and decreases after sleep extension.

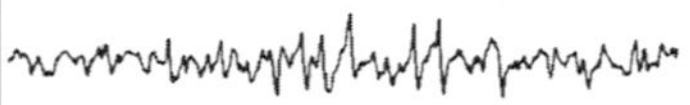

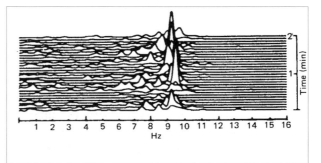

Figure 4.19: Saw-tooth waves, characteristics of REM sleep.

Saw-tooth waves

Multiple sleep latency test (MSLT)

MSLT is a measure of sleep tendency in terms of how quickly a person falls asleep (sleep latency). Carskadon and Dement (1975) demonstrated that sleep latency could measure physiological sleep tendency at any time of the day or night.

The MSLT procedure involves a person spending a standard night in the laboratory and then being offered 20-minute opportunities to nap at 2-hour intervals throughout the next day. The person is not allowed to sleep betweeen naps and caffeinated beverages are not permitted (American Association of Sleep Disorders, 2005b). The person is asked to try to sleep at each nap session. This procedure includes polysomnographic monitoring, so it is possible to determine the exact moment of sleep onset. Since sleep tendency fluctuates, multiple nap sessions are used. With this technique, excessively sleepy people fall asleep significantly more rapidly than controls or people who are not excessively sleepy.

The sleep stages

The determination of the sleep stage is based on the combined information from the EEG, EOG and EMG (*Table 4.2*). The final assessment is based on the dominant sleep stage in each epoch. The most widely accepted criteria for defining the stages are those of Rechtschaffen and Kales. In summary, sleep stages may be defined as follows.

Wakefulness

During relaxed wakefulness, with the eyes closed, the EEG shows rhythmic alpha activity waves (8–13 cycles per second) maximally seen with occipital derivations (D_1–D_2) but also occurring in the central one (vertex (C_3–C_4). This pattern attenuates with attention tasks and when eyes are open (EEG is characterized by low voltage mixed frequency). EOG show rapid eye movement and eye blinks (when open) and few or no eyes movements (when closed).

Figure 4.20: Power spectral analysis of the EEG. Horizontal axis represents frequency (in Hz) and vertical axis contains successive time samples of consecutive EEG activity over a 2-minute period. Most of the power in this diagragm is between 8 HZ and10 Hz.

Involuntary, slow, rolling eye movements (with eyes closed) often characterize the EOG in the epochs preceding stage 1 non-REM. Muscle tone is generally high and voluntary movements produce phasic increases of EMG amplitude (*Figure 4.21*).

Table 4.2: Summary of sleep scoring criteria

Stage	EEG	EOG	EMG
Wakefulness	Eyes closed: alpha, prominent in occipital derivations that attenuates with attention. Eyes open: low voltage mixed frequency	Voluntary control; blinks, REMs, SEMs if drowsy	Tonic activity, relatively high, voluntary movement
N-REM Stage I	Low voltage mixed frequency. Theta activity, vertex sharp waves	SEMs	Tonic activity, slight decrease from wakefulness
Stage 2	Relatively low voltage mixed frequency in the background. Sleep spindles and K complexes	Occasionally SEMs near to sleep onset	Tonic activity, low level
Stages 3–4	20–50% delta waves >50% delta waves	Picks up EEG	Tonic activity, low level
REM	Relatively low voltage mixed frequency, saw-tooth waves, theta activity	Phasic REMs	Tonic suppression, phasic twitches
Movement time	Obscured	Obscured	Very high activity

SEM, slow eye movement

Non-REM Sleep

The four non-REM sleep stages are distinguished principally by changes in the EEG pattern.

Stage I

Alpha activity is greatly decreased (less than 50% of the record). There is a low-amplitude, mixed-frequency activity (3–7 cycles per second). Vertex sharp wave bursts are common. Bursts of relatively high voltage, synchronous, theta activity (4 Hz–8 Hz) are common during the onset of stage 1 sleep in children and young adolescents. The slow eye movements (SEMs) precede the EEG transition to stage 1 sleep from wakefulness. Muscle tone is maintained during all non-REM sleep stages with a gradual decrease of the signal amplitude possibly occurring in the wake-to-sleep transition. As the subject progresses toward stage 2, the slower activity predominates (*Figure 4.22*).

Stage 2

The EEG background is a pattern of relatively low-voltage, mixed frequency activity. This stage is characterized and distinguished from stage 1 by the appearance of two specific types of intermittent EEG events, the spindles and the K complexes. Spindles are brief bursts of rhythmic, 12–14 cycles per second waves, lasting from 0.5 to 1.5 seconds. The frequency of appearance is about three to eight spindles per minute in normal adults (in older people sleep spindles tend to loose their classic morphology and have a lower frequency, lower amplitude and shorter duration). Some drugs, such as benzodiazepines, tend to increase the density of sleep spindles (De Gennaro and Ferrara, 2003).

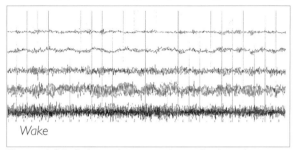

Figure 4.21: Polygraphic recording of relaxed wakefulness in a normal young adult with eyes closed (traces are the following: two EOGs, two EEGs and one EMG).

K complexes, the other EEG waveforms characteristic of stage 2 sleep, are composed of a high-amplitude, negative wave (upward deflection) followed by a positive component. The duration should not exceed 0.5 seconds. K complexes are maximal over the vertex and sometimes spindle activity may override the K complex. The typical density in young normal adults is about one to three per minute, although there is considerable individual variability. It should be noted that, in addition to its spontaneous appearance during stage 2 sleep, the K complex can occur at other times during sleep in response to auditory stimuli. K complexes can be visible also on EOG channels. In stage 2, the EMG is tonically active (*Figure 4.23*) (Colrain, 2005).

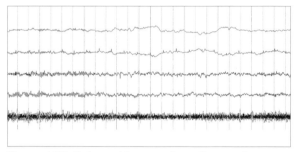

Figure 4.22: Polygraphic recording of stage 1 non-REM; slow rolling eye movements and attenuation of alpha rhythm mark the onset of stage 1 non-REM.

Stages 3 and 4

These stages are characterized by the appearance of high-voltage slow-wave activity (delta waves) of an amplitude peak to peak of at least 75 microvolts, and a frequency between 0.5 and

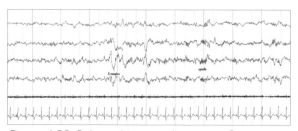
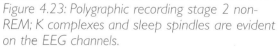

Figure 4.23: Polygraphic recording stage 2 non-REM; K complexes and sleep spindles are evident on the EEG channels.

3 cycles per second. Collectively, these stages are often referred to as slow-wave sleep or delta sleep. When delta activity is between 20 and 50% of the epoch, stage 3 is scored (*Figure 4.24*). In stage 4, delta activity makes up more than 50% of the epoch (*Figure 4.25*). Sleep spindles and K complexes may or may not be present during stages 3 or 4. Eye movements do not occur. On EOG, high-voltage, slow-wave activity is seen. EMG is tonically active although the tracing may occasionally achieve very low levels.

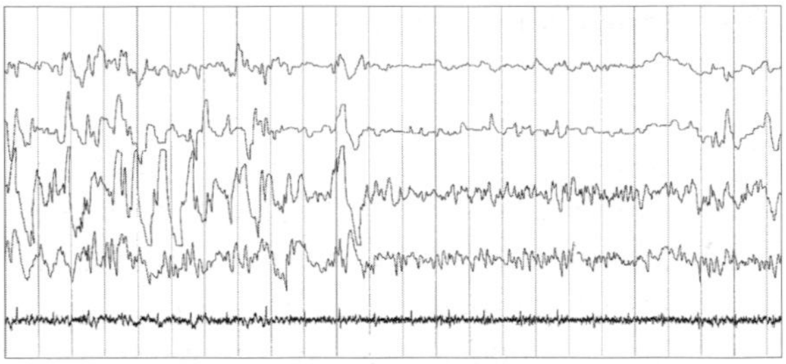

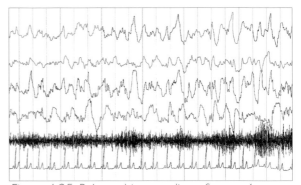

Figure 4.24: Polygraphic recording of stage 3 non-REM; high-voltage slow activity (delta waves) in 20-50% of the scoring epoch (as shown in this figure).

REM sleep

The staging of REM sleep is based on the recognition of the presence of three specific findings, 'desynchronized' EEG, bursts of rapid eye movements, and suppression of EMG activity. The EEG activity returns to a mixed frequency pattern similar to stage 1. A specific EEG pattern of 'saw-tooth' waves is fairly common and achieves the highest amplitude at the vertex with a frequency in the theta range (4–8 Hz) (*Figure 4.19*). The EOG shows bursts of rapid eye movement with the density varying, depending on the time of the night (earlier REM episodes contain fewer rapid eye movements than later episodes) (*Figure 4.26*, top two channels). The EMG drops to very low amplitude, indicating the decrease in tone of the submentalis muscles (*Figure 4.26*, bottom trace).

Figure 4.25: Polygraphic recording of stage 4 non-REM; predominance of delta waves in the EEG (also seen on the EOG channels).

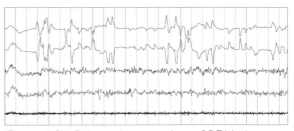

Movement time

Figure 4.26: Polygraphic recording of REM sleep; rapid eye movements are evident on the EOG channels; EMG tone is decreased; EEG channels show low-voltage mixed-frequency pattern.

Gross postural readjustments are fairly common during sleep. When movements arise from sleep or immediately preceding sleep (drowsy state), and obscure EEG activity for at least half of the scoring epoch, that epoch is defined as 'movement time' (*Figure 4.27*).

Transient arousal

EEG arousals are usually defined as alpha rhythm intrusions, lasting 2 seconds or longer but not associated with any stage or state change in the epoch scoring. These brief arousals are sometimes associated with body movements or respiration events. A task force of the American Sleep Disorders Association (ASDA) has defined a set of scoring rules for coding EEG arousals during sleep (*Figure 4.28*).

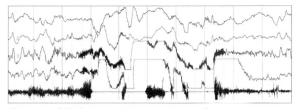

Figure 4.27: Polygraphic recording of movement time; amplifiers blocking excessive muscle activity and obscurity of the EEG are shown.

The REM–non-REM cycle

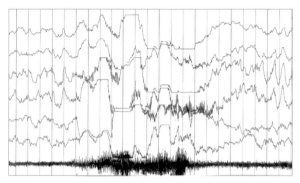

Figure 4.28: Arousal between 3 and 15 seconds in total duration with an EEG shift to faster frequency with maintained sleep.

As mentioned earlier, the sleep stages do not occur at random, but rather appear in cyclic fashion. In general, a normal young adult goes from waking into a period of non-REM sleep lasting 70–90 minutes prior to the first REM period. In an ideal situation, the sequence of stages is: waking, stage 1, stage 2, stage 3, stage 4, stage 3, stage 2 and REM. The first REM period is followed by a repetition of the non-REM stages (stage 2, stage 3, stage 4, stage 3, stage 2) and then another REM episode occurs. The interval from the beginning of one REM period to the beginning of the next is defined as the sleep cycle. The duration of the REM-to-REM cycle is generally thought to be about 90 minutes, but may vary from 70 to 120 minutes. However, the mean duration of sleep cycles may change during the night with different patterns in different age groups (Feinberg, 1974).

Excluding the first cycle of the night, subsequent cycles show progressively decreasing amounts of slow-wave sleep. The amount of slow-wave sleep in the first cycle is age dependent, decreasing with progressing age (*Figure 4.29*). With the exception of the elderly, the REM episode in the first cycle is shorter than those in subsequent cycles, during which it gets progressively longer. In general (with the exception of the elderly) slow-wave sleep is greatest early in the night and decreases as the night advances. REM sleep occurs in relatively small amounts early at night and increases as the night advances.

Sleep stages and age

Total sleep time and total nightly amounts of individual sleep stages are age dependent (Feinberg and Carlson, 1968; Roffwarg *et al*, 1966). In general, total sleep time is greatest in infancy, decreases in childhood, and remains relatively stable from the young adult years until old age, where it declines. In contrast, the number of awakenings during the night may increase with age in a linear fashion (*Figure 4.30*).

The percentage of REM sleep is highest in infancy and childhood, drops and then levels off in adulthood to decline in old age. Slow-wave sleep is highest in infancy and then changes in a hyperbolic curve that decreases with age (*Figure 4.31*). Typical values for the whole night in a young adult might be as follows: 50% stage 2, 25% REM, 10% stage 3, 10% stage 4, and 5% stage 1.

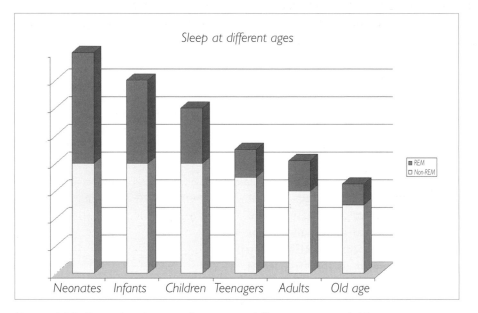

Figure 4.29: Sleep distribution of stages at different ages: in children, in young adults and in the elderly.

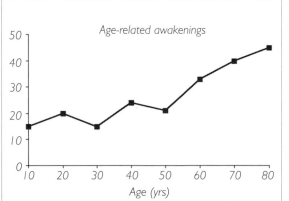

Figure 4.30: Graph of number of awakenings during the nocturnal sleep at different ages.

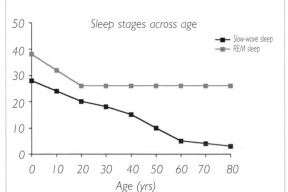

Figure 4.31: Graph of percentage of SWS and REM sleep at different ages.

Effects of temporal variables on sleep

Sleep is influenced by a variety of temporal variables other than age and time asleep which have been already mentioned. The length of wakefulness prior to sleep is directly related to the total amount of delta sleep and inversely related to the time required to fall asleep (the sleep latency). While it is not unexpected that the longer a person has been awake, the more quickly he falls asleep, it is perhaps surprising that the sleep latency is strongly influenced by the time of day at which sleep occurs, the so-called circadian effect. It is easier to fall asleep at midnight than at 4.00PM, even when the length of prior wakefulness is held constant.

Difficulties in falling asleep and staying asleep are well known to transoceanic jet travellers and shift workers. In contrast to delta sleep, REM sleep is influenced much more by the time of the day than by the length of prior wakefulness. REM sleep occurs more frequently during the morning hours than during the afternoon and evening hours. This effect is relatively independent of the length of wakefulness prior to going to sleep and to the amount of prior sleep. Naps in the morning have been shown to have more REM sleep than naps in the afternoon. On the other hand, naps in the afternoon have more slow-wave sleep than naps in the morning, because of the increased period of wakefulness since arising in the morning. Furthermore, following an afternoon nap, slow-wave sleep is reduced during nocturnal sleep for similar reasons.

In summary, temporal variables such as age, length of time asleep, length of wakefulness prior to the sleep period, and time of day at which sleep occurs, are important determinants of sleep characteristics. The underlying physiological and biochemical mechanisms for these temporal effects are mostly unknown.

Physiological variables related to the sleep stages

In addition to the physiological changes that largely define REM sleep, such as decreased muscle tone, a variety of metabolic and autonomic nervous system changes occur. During REM sleep there is increased cerebral blood flow, increased brain temperature and increased oxygen consumption. Erections may occur in males during REM sleep.

Part three: Sleep microstructure — arousal and cycling alternating pattern

The sleeping brain disposes of multiple arousal solutions that allow adaptive adjustments of the ongoing state to internal and external inputs. Transient EEG phenomena, lasting less than the scoring epoch, defined as 'phasic events', have been described within sleep recordings, allowing identification of what is known as the microstructure of sleep. EEG patterns, as arousals, have immediate repercussions on the continuity and depth of sleep.

According to the ASDA criteria, EEG arousals are sudden frequency shifts towards faster rhythms (mostly alpha and beta) that briefly interrupt the continuity of sleep stage background (*Figures 4.32* and *4.33*). For this reason, arousals are considered as major markers of sleep fragmentation and are responsible for producing functional daytime impairment. Even if arousals have been investigated in condition of sleep disturbances (eg. periodic limb movements, sleep breathing disorders, insomnia) the literature indicates that arousals are spontaneous manifestations of sleep even in the absence of sleep disturbance. In normal subjects, the mean duration of arousals remains unmodified across the life span (average length of about 15 seconds), but the increase in number with age is considered as the physiological basis of sleep fragility in the elderly.

The scoring of arousals relies on transient EEG changes mostly characterized by patterns of wakefulness. In contrast, the abrupt appearance of slow-wave activities as K complexes and delta bursts have been, until recently, neglected. These cortical events have been demonstrated to be associated with activation of neurovegetative functions (heart rate, blood pressure).

Transient, synchronized EEG patterns (K complexes and delta bursts) whether or not associated with an arousal, can be endowed with activating properties. The attribute of activation is not limited to conventional arousals but is extended to a number of complex EEG features (intermittent alpha rhythm, vertex sharp waves, bursts of K complexes, K-alpha complexes, delta bursts, arousals). These different activation patterns do not have the same activating power. The different EEG features clearly indicate a hierarchical spectrum of increasing strength from the weaker, high-amplitude delta burst, to the stronger, low-voltage alpha rhythm. Most activation complexes appear during non-REM sleep with a spontaneous occurrence every 20–40 seconds. Rhythms are defined as cyclic alternating pattern (CAP) in relation to their repetitive emergence.

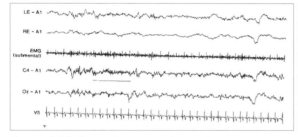

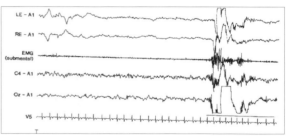

Figure 4.32: Arousal in stage 2 non-REM sleep (the EEG frequency change in this epoch is scored as an arousal despite the absence of an EMG amplitude increase).

Figure 4.33: Arousal in REM sleep (the EEG frequency change in this epoch is scored as an arousal as there is both an EMG amplitude increase and an EEG change greater than 3 second duration).

From K complexes to cyclic alternating pattern (CAP)

The K complex is considered to be an elementary expression of arousal during sleep. It is a spontaneous marker of non-REM sleep (especially of stage 2), but may also be triggered by sensory stimulation. The K complex densities (number of K complexes per minute of sleep) have overnight fluctuations according to their distribution within the sleep cycle. Peaks in densities (when the K complexes can be clustered in sequences) are often observed in connection with stage transitions. However, natural non-REM sleep is marked by other oscillations below 1 Hz. These very slow oscillations refer to the cyclic alternating pattern (CAP), a physiological correlate of non-REM sleep associated with changes in vigilance, muscle tone and autonomic activities.

Both arousals and CAP variables are scored independently of the standardized rules (Rechtschaffen and KalesK). The coding system of arousals is based on event-counting as a measure of sleep fragmentation. In contrast, CAP reflects a condition of unstable sleep. For this reason, arousal count and CAP scoring are considered distinct systems for the microstructural exploration of sleep. Arousal index increases linearly with age, while CAP rate values follow a U-shaped outline across the life span. Arousal quantification and CAP analysis have occupied a leading role in the investigation of sleep instability and fragmentation, respectively.

Cyclic alternating pattern (CAP)

The cyclic alternating pattern (CAP) can be considered the EEG marker of arousal instability during sleep. From the limits of conventional sleep parameters (macrostructure), further investigation of sleep microstructure is done by paying particular attention to K complexes and other arousal-related phasic events of non-REM sleep.

CAP is a spontaneous, periodic EEG activity of non-REM sleep and is characterized by sequences of transient EEG events, distinct from the background activity that recur at up to 1-minute intervals (*Figure 4.34*).

CAP occurs in all non-REM stages, both under normal and pathological conditions, whenever the level of arousal is unstable. Independently of the specific EEG features, CAP translates to a sustained oscillatory condition between a greater arousal level (phase A) and a lesser arousal level (phase

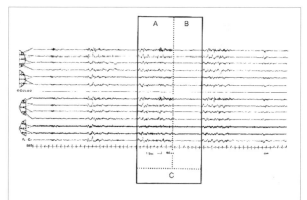

Figure 4.34: Example of cyclic alternating pattern, CAP in stage 2 non-REM. The box shows the CAP cycle (C) composed of a phase A (A) and the following phase B (B). There is a bipolar EEG derivation montage: from the top 6 channels these are, Fp2-F4, F4-C4, C4-P4, P4-O2, F8-T4, T4-T6; OCULOG (ROC-LOC); bottom 7 channels Fp1-F3, F3-C3, C3-P3, P3-O1, F3-T3, T3-T5, Fz-Cz; EKG (electrocardiogram).

B). Arousal instability during CAP is associated with a concomitant activation of the polygraphic parameters (EEG, cardiorespiratory rate, muscle tone) during phase A and with their attenuation during phase B. In non-REM sleep, the A phases are formed by the EEG arousal-related phasic events peculiar to the single stages, and the B phases, by the intervals of background theta–delta activity (see below). The absence of CAP within the sleep EEG coincides with a condition of sustained arousal stability, which is defined as non-CAP.

CAP rate

The CAP time is the temporal sum of all CAP sequences. CAP time can be calculated throughout total non-REM sleep and within the single non-REM stages. The percentage ratio of CAP time to total sleep time is referred to as CAP rate. CAP rate can be measured in non-REM sleep (percentage ratio of total CAP time to total non-REM sleep time), and in the single non-REM stages (percentage ratio of CAP time in a given stage to the total duration of that stage throughout sleep). In human sleep, CAP rate is an index of arousal instability that shows a U-shaped evolution (*Figure 4.35*) along the life span (teenagers mean 43.4%; young adults 31.9%; middle aged: 37.5%; elderly 55.3%). The values of

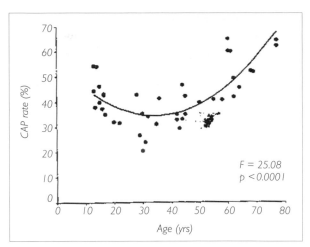

Figure 4.35: Distribution of CAP rate across the life-span.

CAP rate correlate with the subjective appreciation of sleep quality (the higher the CAP rate, the poorer sleep quality). As a marker of arousal instability, CAP rate is increased by perturbing conditions and decreased by hypnotic medication.

Phase A subtypes

Variations during CAP involve different degrees of muscle tone, heart rate and respiratory activity that increase during phase A and decrease during phase B. On the basis of the information derived from EEG activities, muscle tone and neurovegetative responses, a three-stage hierarchy of arousal strength has been identified:

1. Subtypes A1 (*Figure 4.36*): predominance of slow, high voltage EEG patterns (intermittent alpha rhythm in stage 1; sequences of K complexes or delta bursts in the other non-REM stages) associated with weak modifications of muscle tone and cardiorespiratory rate. The A1 subtypes show a decline from adolescence (71%) to young adulthood (61%), a plateau between young adulthood and middle age (62%), and then a drop from adulthood to senescence (47%).

2. Subtypes A2 (*Figure 4.37*): balanced mixture of slow and rapid EEG features (K complexes with alpha and beta activities, K-alpha, arousals with slow wave synchronization) linked with a moderate increase of muscle tone and

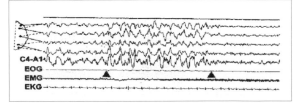

Figure 4.36: Delta burst in slow-wave sleep typical of A1 subtype. Top 4 channels are bipolar parasagittal derivation of the right side, C4-A1, EOG, EMG, EKG. A1 subtype.

vegetative alterations. The A2 subtypes
increase from adolescence (20%) to young
adulthood (28%), remain quite stable
throughout mature adulthood (27%), and
then rise during senescence (35%).

3. Subtypes A3 (*Figure 4.38*): prevalence
   of rapid low-amplitude EEG rhythms
   (transient activation phases or arousals)
   coupled with marked increase of muscle
   tone and cardiorespiratory rate. The
   A3 subtypes increase slightly from
   adolescence (9%) to young (11%) and
   mature (11%) adulthood, and then rise
   during senescence (18%).

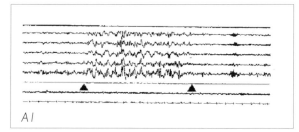

Figure 4.37: A2 subtype.

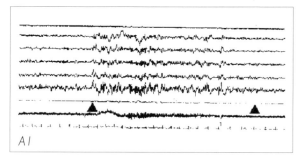

Figure 4.38: A3 subtype.

Scoring rules for CAP and non-CAP

CAP is organized in sequences of two or more CAP cycles (*Figure 4.39*). A CAP cycle consists of
a phase A and a phase B, each lasting between 2 and 60 seconds. All CAP sequences begin with
a phase A and end with a phase B.

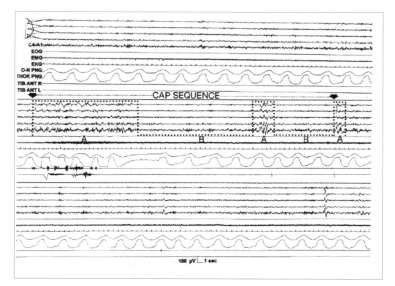

Figure 4.39: Consecutive recording of non-CAP (top), CAP (middle) and non-CAP (bottom). The middle part shows the minimal requirements for the definition of a CAP sequence (at least 3 phase A in succession).

In non-REM sleep, the phase A patterns are composed of single or clustered arousal-related phasic
events peculiar to the single sleep stages:

* intermittent alpha rhythms (EEG synchronization) (*Figure 4.40*) and sequences of vertex
  sharp waves (EEG synchronization), in stage 1

- sequences of two or more K complexes alone (EEG synchronization) (*Figure 4.41*) or followed by alpha-like components (EEG desynchronization) and beta rhythms (EEG de-synchronization), in stage 2
- delta bursts (EEG synchronization) which exceed by at least a third the amplitude of the background activity, in stages 3 and 4
- transient activation phases (EEG desynchronization), in all non-REM stages and EEG arousals (EEG de-synchronization), in all the stages
- CAP sequences commonly precede the transition from non-REM to REM sleep and end just before REM sleep onset. During REM sleep, which is characterized by the lack of EEG synchronization, CAP does not occur.

As CAP is a global EEG phenomenon involving extensive cortical areas, bipolar longitudinal montages warrant the most clear detection of CAP (Fp1/F3, F3/C3, C3/P3, P3/O1 or the other side). Monopolar EEG derivations (C3/A2 or C4/A1 and O1/A2 or O2/A1), eye movements channels and submentalis EMG that are used for the conventional sleep staging and arousal scoring are also essential for scoring CAP. The identification of CAP should be preceded by the definition of sleep stages according to Rechtschaffen and Kales conventional criteria.

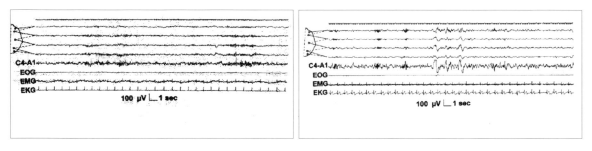

Figure 4.40: Intermittent alpha rhythm in stage 1 non-REM.

Figure 4.41: K complex sequences associated with spindles in stage 2 non-REM.

References and further reading

American Sleep Disorders Association (1997) *The International Classification of Sleep Disorders, Diagnostic and Coding Manual.* ASDA, Rochester

American Association of Sleep Medicine (2005a) Practice parameters for the indications for polysomnography and related procedures: An update for 2005. *Sleep* **28**(4): 499–521

American Association of Sleep Medicine (2005b) Practice parameters for clinical use of the multiple sleep latency test and the maintenance of wakefulness test. *Sleep* **28**(1): 113–21

American Electroencephalographic Society (1994) Guideline fifteen: guidelines for polygraphic assessment of sleep-related disorders (polysomnography). *J Clin Neurophysiol* **11**(1): 116–24

American Sleep Disorders Association (ASDA) (1992) EEG arousals: scoring rules and examples. A preliminary report from the Sleep Disorders Atlas Task Force of the American Sleep Disorders Association. *Sleep* **15**: 174–84

American Sleep Disorders Association, Standards Practice Committee (1995) Practice parameters for the use of polysomnography in the evaluation of insomnia. *Sleep* **18**: 55

American Sleep Disorders Association (1997) Practice parameters for the indications for polysomnography and related procedures. *Sleep* **20**: 406

American Thoracic Society Medical Section of the American Lung Association (1989) Indications and standards for cardiopulmonary sleep studies. *Am Rev Respir Dis* **139**(2) 559–68

Aserinski E, Kleitman N (1953) Regularly occurring periods of eye motility, and concomitant phenomena during sleep. *Science* **118**: 273–4

Bloch KE (1997) Polysomnography: a systematic review. *Technol Health Care* **5**(4): 285–305

Bornstein SK (1982) Respiratory monitoring during sleep: polysomnography. In: Guilleminault C, ed. *Sleeping and Waking Disorders: Indications and Techniques.* Addison-Wesley, Menlo Park. CA: 183–210

Boselli M, Parrino L, Smerieri A, Terzano MO (1998) Effect of age on EEG arousals in normal sleep. *Sleep* **21**: 351–7

Broughton RJ (1987) Polysomnography: principles and applications in sleep and arousal disorders. In: Niederrneyer E, Lopes da Silva F, eds. *Electroencephalography: Basic Principles, Clinical Applications and Related Fields.* 2nd edn. Urban & Schwatzenberg, Baltimore: 687

Butkov N (1996) *Atlas of Clinical Polysomnography.* Synapse Media, Medford, OR

Carskadon MA (1982) Basics for polygraphic monitoring of sleep. In: Guilleminault C, ed. *Sleeping and Waking Disorders: Indications and Techniques.* Addison-Wesley, Menlo Park CA: 1–16

Carskadon MA (1994) Measuring daytime sleepiness. In: Kryger MH, Roth T, Dement WC, eds. *Principles and Practice of Sleep Medicine.* 2nd edn. Saunders, Philadelphia: 961

Carskadon MA, Dement WC (1975) Sleep studies on a 90-minute day. *Electroencephalography Clin Neurophysiol* **39**(2): 145–55

Carskadon MA, Rechtschaffen A (1989) Monitoring and staging human sleep. In: MH Kryger, T Roth, WC Dement, eds. *Principles and Practice of Sleep Medicine.* WB Saunders, Philadelphia: 665–8

Chesson AL Jr, Ferber RA, Fry JM *et al* (1997) The indications for polysomnography and related procedures. *Sleep* **20**(6): 423–87

Coleman RM, Pollack C, Weitzman ED (1980) Periodic movements in sleep (nocturnal myoclonus): relation to sleep-wake disorders. *Ann Neurol* **8**: 4–16

Colrain IM (2005) The K complexes: a 7-year decade history. *Sleep* **28**(2): 255–73

Cooper R, Osselton W, Sbaw JC (1974) *EEG Technology.* 2nd edn. Butterworths, London

Cross O (1992) Technical tips: patient specific electrode application techniques. *Am J EEG Technol* **32**: 86

Davies RO, Bennett LS, Stradling SR (1997) What is an arousal and how should it be quantified? *Sleep Med Rev* **1**: 87–95

De Gennaro L, Ferrara M (2003) Sleep spindles: an overview. *Sleep Med Rev* **7**(5): 423–40

Dement WC (1978) *Sleep Apnea Syndromes*. Alan Liss, New York: 357

Dement WC, Kleitman N (1957) Cyclic variations of EEG during sleep and their relation to eye movements, body motility and dreaming. *Electroencephalogr Clin Neurophysiol* **9**: 673

Dement WC, Rechtschaffen A (1968) Narcolepsy: Polygraphic aspects, experimental and theoretical considerations. In: Gastaut H, Lugaresi E, Berti Ceroni G, eds. *The Abnormalities of Sleep in Man*. Aulo Gaggi Editore, Bologna: 147

Dement WC, Zarcone V, Guilleminault C *et al* (1973) Diagnostic sleep recording in narcoleptics and hypersomniacs. *Electroencephalogr Clin Neurophysiol* **35**: 220

Dietrich B (1997) Polysomnography in drug development. *J Clin Pharmacol* **37**(sSuppl 1): 70S–78S

Feinberg I (1974) Changes in sleep cycle patterns with age. *J Psychiatric Res* **10**(3–4): 283–306

Feinberg I, Carlson VR (1968) Sleep variables as a function of age in man. *Arch Gen Psychiatry* **18**(2): 239–50

Ferini-Strambi L, Bianchi A, Zucconi M, Oldani A, Castronovo V, Smirne S (2000) The impact of cyclic alternating pattern on heart rate variability during sleep in healthy young adults. *Clin Neurophysiol* **111**: 99–101

Guilleminault C (1982) *Sleeping and Waking Disorders: Indications and Technique*. Addison-Wesley, Menlo Park, California: 435

Guilleminault C, Stoohs R (1995) Arousal, increased respiratory efforts, blood pressure and obstructive sleep apnea. *J Sleep Res* **4**(suppl. 1): 117–24

Halasz P (1998) Hierarchy of micro-arousals and the microstructure of sleep. *Neurophysiol Clin* **28**: 461–75

Halasz P, Kundra O, Rajna P, Pal I, Vargha M (1979) Microarousals during nocturnal sleep. *Acta Physiol Acad Sci Hung* **54**(1): 1–12

Holland JV, Dement WC, Raynal DM (1974) Polysomnography: A response to a need for improved communication. Presented at the l4th Annual Meeting of the Association for the Psychophysiological Study of Sleep. Jackson Hole, WY

Jasper HH (1958) The ten–twenty electrode system of the International Federation. *Electroencephalogr Clin Neurophysiol* **10**: 371–5

Keenan SA (1992) Polysomnograpby: technical aspects in adolescents and adults. *J Clin Neurophysiol* **9**: 21–31

Keenan SA (1994) Polysomnographic techniques: an overview. In: Chokroverty S, ed. *Sleep Disorders Medicine: Basic Science, Technical Considerations, and Clinical Aspects*. Butterworth-Heinemann, Boston: 149–69

Martin RJ, Block AJ, Cohn MA (1985) Indications and standards for cardiopulmonary sleep studies. *Sleep* **8**(4): 371–9

Mathur R, Douglas NJ (1995) Frequency of EEG arousals from nocturnal sleep in normal subjects. *Sleep* **18**: 330–3

McGregor P, Weitzman ED, Pollack CR (1978) Polysomnognaphic recording techniques used for diagnosis of sleep disorders in a sleep disorders center. *Am J EEG Technol* **18**: 107

Nicolas A (1997) Microstructure du sommeil: physiologie. In: Benoit O, Goldenberg F, eds. *Exploration du Sommeil et de la Vigilance Chez l'Adulte*. Editions Médicales Internationales, Cachan: 173–201

Orr WC, Bollinger C, Stahl M (1982) Measurement of gastroesophageal reflux during sleep by esophageal pH monitoring. In: Guilleminault C, ed. *Sleeping and Waking Disorders: Indications and Techniques*. Addison-Wesley, Menlo Park, CA: 331

Parrino L, Boselli M, Spaggiari MC, Smerieri A, Terzano MO (1998) Cyclic alternating pattern (CAP) in normal sleep: polysomnographic parameters in different age groups. *Electroencephalogr Clin Neurophysiol* **107**: 439–50

Rechtschaffen A, Kales A (1968) *A Manual of Standardized Terminology, Techniques and Scoring System for Sleep Stages of Human Subjects*. Brain Information Service/Brain Research Institute, University of California, Los Angeles

Reite M, Buysse D, Reynolds C. Mendelson W (1995) The use of polysomnography in the evaluation of insomnia. An American Sleep Disorders Association review. *Sleep* **18**: 58

Roffwarg HP, Muzio JN, Dement WC (1966) Ontogenic development of the human sleep-dream cycle. *Science* **152**: 604–19

Rosa AC, Parrino L, Terzano MO (1999) Automatic detection of cyclic alternating pattern (CAP) sequences in sleep: preliminary results. *Electroencephlogr Clin Neurophysiol* **110**: 585–92

Schieber SP, Muzet A, Ferriere PJR (1997) Les phases d'activation transitoire spontanées au cours du sommeil chez l'homme. *Arch Sci Physio* **1**(25): 443–65

Smith JR (1990) Transferring EEG polysomnography technology to the home environment. In: Miles LE, Broughton RI, eds. *Medical Monitoring in the Home and Work Environment*. Raven Press, New York: 217–29

Tachibana N, Sugita Y, Terashima K, Teshima Y, Shimizu T, Hishikawa Y (1994) Scoring REM density. *Neurology* **44**: 987–8

Terzano MG, Mancia D, Salati MR, Costani O, Decembrino A, Parrino L (1985) The cyclic alternating pattern as a physiologic component of normal NREM sleep. *Sleep* **8**: 137–45

Terzano MG, Parrino L (1991) Functional relationship between micro- and macrostructure of sleep. In: Terzano MO, Halasz P, Declerck AC, eds. *Phasic Events and Dynamic Organization of Sleep*. Raven Press, New York: 101–19

Terzano MG, Parrino L (2000) Origin and significance of the cyclic alter-nating pattern (CAP). *Sleep Med Rev* **4**: 101–23

Terzano MG, Parrino L, Boselli M, Smerieri A, Spaggiari MC (2000) CAP components and EEG synchronization in the first three sleep cycles. *Clin Neurophysiol* **111**: 283–90

Terzano MG, Parrino L, Mennuni GF, eds (1997) *Phasic events and microstructure of sleep*. Consensus Conference, Italian Association of Sleep Medicine (AIMS). Martano Editore, Lecce: 1–161

Terzano MG, Parrino L, Smerieri A, Chervin R, Chokroverty S, Guilleminault C *et al* (2002) Atlas, rules, and recording techniques for the scoring of cyclic alternating pattern (CAP) in human sleep. *Sleep Med* **3**(2): 187–99

Terzano MG, Parrino L, Rosa A, Palomba V, Smerieri A (2002) CAP and arousals in the structural development of sleep: an integrative perspective. *Sleep Med* **3**: 221–9

Terzano MG, Parrino L, Spaggiari MC (1988) The cyclic alternating pattern sequences in the dynamic organization of sleep. *Electroencephalogr Clin Neurophysiol* **69**: 437–47

Thorpy MJ (1992) The clinical use of the Multiple Sleep Latency Test: the Standards of Practice Committee of the American Sleep Disorders Association. *Sleep* **15**: 381

Tyner FS, Knott JR, Mayer WB Jr (1983) *Fundamentals of EEG Technology*. Raven, New York

Walczak T, Chokroverty S (1994) Electroencephalography, electromyography, and electrocardiography: general principles and basic technology. In: Chokroverty S, ed. *Sleep Disorders Medicine: Basic Science, Technical Considerations and Clinical Aspects*. Butterworth-Heinemann, Boston: 97

Weitzman ED, Pollack CP, McGregor P (1980) The polysomnographic evaluation of sleep disorders in man. In: MJ Aminoff, ed. *Electrodiagnosis in Clinical Neurology*. Churchill Livingstone, New York: 496

Wong PKH (1996) *Digital EEG in Clinical Practice*. Lippincott-Raven, Philadelphia

Part II: Clinical aspects of sleep disorders

CHAPTER 5

Snoring and sleep apnea

Huw Davies, Nicholas Antic and Doug McEvoy

Introduction

Snoring and obstructive sleep apnea (OSA) are the most common reasons for referrals to sleep units. Few disorders have passed so rapidly from obscurity to clinical commonplace as OSA. OSA, first described in 1965, was in 1993 described as a leading cause of hypertension, stroke, myocardial infarction, motor vehicle accidents and the stupidity of politicians (Gastaut *et al*, 1966; Phillipson, 1993).

OSA was initially described in morbidly obese subjects with snoring, daytime sleepiness and obstructive apneas during sleep. Similar patients, described in detail in the 1950s, were referred to as suffering from Pickwickian syndrome (Burwell *et al*, 1956) with morbid obesity, hypoventilation during wakefulness and daytime somnolence. However, Gaustaut and colleagues (1966) observed daytime sleepiness in obese patients with normal oxygen and normal CO_2 and hypothesized that it was due to sleep fragmentation caused by recurrent apneas. Subsequent studies confirmed this hypothesis, and the term 'hypersomnia with periodic apneas' (HPA) was used (Lugaresi *et al*, 1980) to refer to what is now established as OSA syndromes.

Definition of terms

The definition of sleep-related disturbed breathing is a controversial subject (American Academy of Sleep Medicine, 1999; Hosselet *et al*, 2001). Most current definitions are intended for epidemiological research and are less useful in clinical practice. From a clinical point of view, it is relevant to distinguish between simple snoring, OSA syndrome and upper airway resistance syndrome (Guillenimault *et al*, 1996).

Snoring is the noise produced by vibration of the soft tissue of the upper airway during sleep. Obstructive sleep apnea is the presence of disturbed breathing during sleep with complete (apnea) or partial (hypopneas) suspension of respiratory flow for at least 10 seconds, usually associated with arousal and/or oxygen desaturation. OSA syndrome is present when OSA is associated with unrefreshed sleep, daytime sleepiness and poor daytime function. These symptoms are reversed by treating the apneas. The term OSA/hypopnea syndrome has been used to highlight the fact that partial obstruction of the airway may lead to sleep fragmentation and unrefreshed sleep .

Episodes of incomplete obstruction of the upper airway occur in obese patients even in the absence of snoring (Gould *et al*, 1988) with intrathoracic negative pressure reaching -50 to -60 cm of water (normal being -10). Patients with this 'incomplete form of sleep apnea' have also been classified as suffering from upper airway resistance syndrome (UARS) (Guilleminault *et al*, 1993). Upper airway resistance syndrome is characterized by snoring, unrefreshed sleep, increased respiratory effort (measured by increased intrathoracic negative pressure) and increased arousals on EEG. It has been argued that UARS is not a separate entity from OSA (Douglas, 2000) and that snoring, UARS and OSA constitute different (increasing) levels of severity of the same process (Lugaresi *et al*, 1983).

The following terminology is often used when dealing with snoring and sleep apnea:

❖ *Pickwickian syndrome:* (Burwell *et al*, 1956) refers to subjects with gross obesity, respiratory failure with CO_2 retention during wakefulness, daytime sleepiness and congestive heart failure. Although the majority of patients with Pickwickian syndrome may have OSA, the term should not be used as a substitute. The majority of patients with OSA do not have respiratory failure and some may not be obese. The use of Pickwickian syndrome is currently being discouraged in favor of sleep hypoventilation syndrome (American Association of Sleep Medicine, 1999).

❖ *Central sleep apnea:* refers to apneas/hypopneas due to a failing of the central respiratory drive. It may resemble Cheyne Stokes respiration (Dowdell *et al*, 1990) or simple periodic breathing. Mixed sleep apnea denotes the presence of a combination of obstructive and central apnea.

❖ *Overlap syndrome:* is sometimes used to refer to the coexistence of moderately severe obstructive airway disease and OSA (Flenely, 1985).

❖ *Ondine's curse:* is seen predominantly in neonates and patients with brainstem pathology (eg. stroke or malignancy). The normal respiratory centre has a dual control, voluntary and automatic drive. In Ondine's curse, the automatic respiratory control malfunctions and subjects stop breathing when they fall asleep (Kuhn *et al*, 1999; Severinghaus *et al*, 1985).

Epidemiology of snoring and obstructive sleep apnea (OSA)

Epidemiological data about a disease provides a measure of prevalence by which to estimate the burden of disease caused in the population and the scale of treatment task the disease represents. It also gives an estimate of the role of risk factors for the disease in the population and which, if any, are modifiable and therefore potential treatment targets (eg. smoking or body weight, as against age and sex). Finally, it estimates the role of the disease in causing death or disability. Existing epidemiological studies of sleep apnea provide some valid and generalizable information on prevalence and outcomes, but their main value is the information about risk factors.

Prevalence of obstructive sleep apnea

There have been several population-based studies of the prevalence of OSA. Most have been relatively small because of the cost of performing sleep studies. All have studied samples potentially affected by volunteer bias — a random sample of the population is approached, but people are more likely to agree to participate if they have symptoms of, or suspect they have, sleep apnea. This means that the observed prevalence is likely to be higher than the true prevalence.

Most studies are compromised by the use of instruments with specificity for the diagnosis of sleep apnea less than 100% (specificity is the proportion of normal or healthy subjects who have a normal test. If a test has a specificity of 90%, it would incorrectly classify 10% as having the disease — false positives). This is important. If a population is studied with an instrument with a disease specificity of 90%, the prevalence estimate will be 10% whether any of the subjects has the disease or not. In most reported epidemiological studies, the specificity of the instruments used is either uncertain or known only in clinic patients. Laboratory polysomnography is the current gold standard for diagnosis of sleep apnea and, therefore, provides a gold standard estimate of prevalence. Studies which have used polysomnography as their diagnostic method are exempt from these comments. However, the comments made elsewhere about the limitations of polysomnography as a gold standard should be kept in mind.

A significant problem with epidemiological studies of sleep apnea is the definition of what is 'normal' and what is 'disease'. The definition of 'disease' is based on the frequency of apneas per hour of sleep; however, the normal value for this frequency is not clearly defined. This is particularly important because epidemiological studies make clear that some apnea during sleep is normal. *Figure 5.1* shows the distribution of apnea/hypopnea frequencies in the Wisconsin Sleep Cohort Study. There is no clear division between normal and abnormal. The prevalence estimate is determined by the selected cut-off and the validity of the prevalence estimate depends entirely on the validity of that cut-off.

The choice of a cut-off for sleep apnea has many parallels with the cut-off used for blood pressure. Normal can be defined in one of the following ways:

1. 95% confidence limits.
2. Evidence of disease.
3. Evidence of the efficacy of treatment.

Using the latter definition, a result on a test can be taken to define disease if: (1) there is good evidence that treatment of patients who have that result is beneficial, or, (2) there

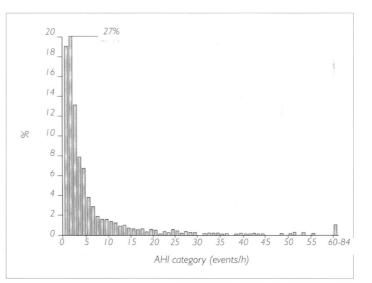

Figure 5.1: Distribution of the apnea/hypopnea index (AHI) in a general adult population sample from the Wisconsin Sleep Cohort Study (N=1299). Reprinted from 'Breathing Disorders in Sleep', McNicholas WT and Phillipson EA. © (2002) Elsevier Ltd.

is good evidence that without treatment the patients' outcomes will be bad. Estimates of the prevalence of mild or threshold sleep-disordered breathing (five to fifteen events per hour) do not define a diseased population in this sense.

OSA, defined as some frequency of apneas and hypopneas, is not really a disease. Among clinic patients, some with only mild sleep apnea and daytime sleepiness appear to improve quite markedly with treatment and it seems likely that mild sleep apnea can be symptomatic. There is a difference of opinion, however, as to whether trials show any consistent benefit in the treatment of mild sleep apnea. Nevertheless, in epidemiological studies, daytime sleepiness is often added to mild sleep-disordered breathing to create an OSA syndrome (OSAS). There is no evidence that, in non-clinic samples, this sleepiness is consistently attributable to sleep apnea or that there is a 'syndrome' at all.

Table 5.1 shows prevalence estimates from a number of studies, in different communities and using different methodologies. The cut-off of thirty apnea/hypopnea per hour was chosen because there is randomized controlled trial evidence that symptomatic clinic patients with this severity of sleep-disordered breathing benefit from treatment. The cut-off of five events per hour, in contrast, is based on selected but widely used data (Young *et al*, 1993; Young and Peppard, 2002).

Table 5.1: Estimated prevalence of sleep apnea in different communities and using different methodologies

Reference	Population	n	Method of monitoring	AHI >5 %	AHI >5 + daytime sleepiness %	AHI >30 %
Lavie (1995)	Israel (men)	78	PSG	5.3	0.9	≈0
Gislason (1988)	Sweden (men)	61	PSG	NR	1.4	≈0
Marin (1997)	Spain (men)	597	Oximetry	15	2.2	<1
Marin (1997)	Spain (women)	625	Oximetry	6	0.8	≈0
Stradling (1991)	England (men)	1001	Oximetry	5.1	1.3	<1
Bearpark (1995)	Australia (men)	311	Respiratory motor	26	3	<1
Young *et al* (1993)	USA (men)	352	PSG	24	4	<1
Young *et al* (1993)	USA (women)	250	PSG	9	2	≈0
Olson (1995)	Australia (men)	247	Respiratory monitor	78.1	NR	12.6*
Olson (1995)	Australia (women)	194	Respiratory monitor	56.7	NR	3.6*

*AHI ≥25

AHI = apnea/hypopnea index; PSG = polysomnography

(modified from Young and Peppard, 2002)

By epidemiological standards, the studies presented in *Table 5.1* are quite small. For this reason, the precision of the prevalence estimates is low and the potential impact of volunteer bias is increased. The small size of the studies is especially important in relation to the higher and better justified cut-off of thirty events per hour because the prevalence of this result is quite low. A guess of 1% for the prevalence of sleep apnea for which randomized controlled trial evidence supports treatment is probably reasonable, but the precision of this estimate is low. This lower estimate still makes sleep apnea a common illness from a clinical point of view, but it would need to have very high impact to be a major problem from a public health point of view.

Another feature of the data is the large variation among studies. Whether this represents real variation among populations, varying degrees of recruitment bias, or the effect of different measuring instruments is unclear. The third key point is the strikingly small proportion of symptomatic subjects among those with low levels of sleep-disordered breathing. It is here that the near-universal instrumental bias of these studies affects the results most significantly. This approach, privileging the instrumentally defined component over the symptomatic component, meant that subjects who were sleepy, but had no sleep-disordered breathing, were simply left out of the table. There are a lot of these subjects and if the question is put the other way around (what is the prevalence of daytime sleepiness and what proportion of subjects with daytime sleepiness have sleep apnea?) the difference is striking. The data shown in *Table 5.2* and *Table 5.3* are from Olson *et al* (1995) of a community study in Newcastle, Australia.

Table 5.2: Proportion of subjects reporting daytime sleepiness

	% answering yes to 'Is daytime sleepiness a problem for you?'	Excluding shift workers
Sleep apnea n = 79	41	32
Snoring n = 289	37	32
No snoring n = 73	37	30

Table 5.3: Proportion of subjects with different severity of daytime sleepiness

	Severe sleepiness n=16	Moderate sleepiness n=70	Mild sleepiness n=151	No sleepiness n=204
AHI 15	4 (25%)	14 (20%)	29 (19%)	32 (16%)
Snoring	9 (56%)	49 (70%)	98 (65%)	133 (65%)
No snoring	3 (19%)	7 (10%)	24 (16%)	39 (19%)
Male	11 (68%)	46 (66%)	86 (57%)	104 (51%)
Sedative use	1 (6%)	2 (3%)	11 (7%)	20 (10%)
Restless legs	0	12 (17%)	26 (17%)	38 (19%)

In this study, sleepiness was situational, defined by asking subjects for the circumstances under which they fell asleep. Severe sleepiness was defined as 'difficulty working or driving because of sleepiness', moderate sleepiness as, 'difficulty staying awake in public', and mild sleepiness as 'difficulty staying awake when comfortable or relaxed'. Similar data were obtained by Young *et al* (1993). Troublesome daytime sleepiness was common in these studies but did not occur more often in people who had sleep apnea and, therefore, only a small minority of sleepy individuals in these studies had sleep apnea. Volunteer bias may be relevant since sleepiness is a symptom likely to lead potential subjects to suspect that they might have sleep apnea and therefore to volunteer.

The paucity of randomized controlled trials of treatment in mild sleep apnea makes it difficult to set a meaningful cut-off for 'abnormal' sleep-disordered breathing. At present, no cut-off lower than thirty events per hour has any firm basis. The frequently quoted estimates of OSAS from the studies of Young *et al* (1993) in *Table 5.1* (4% for males and 2% for females) are really estimates of the prevalence of test results of uncertain significance. On this basis, the prevalence of instrumentally defined sleep apnea (more than fifteen events per hour) may be about 2% of adult men and 1% of adult women. Around half of these individuals will have some degree of daytime sleepiness and they will account for about 20% of the individuals in the community who have daytime sleepiness. Although half of the individuals with sleep apnea will have symptoms, perhaps half again (25% overall) will have sufficiently troublesome symptoms to find long-term treatment with nasal continuous positive airway pressure (CPAP) worthwhile. This makes sleep apnea a common disorder which causes a substantial degree of treatable ill health. The scale of the problem and the gains to be had from large-scale treatment are, however, smaller than has sometimes been suggested.

Risk factors for obstructive sleep apnea

A risk factor is something measured in a study that is statistically associated with the outcome — for the purposes of this discussion, having sleep apnea (Dealberto *et al*, 1994. The point that 'what is not measured cannot be defined as a risk factor' is often neglected. For sleep apnea there are plentiful risk factor data for areas that are easy to measure, such as age and body weight, but much less for those that are harder to assess, but just as likely to be important. This makes it hard to rule out the possibility that the risk factors identified so far are markers for other factors. The most obvious of these is upper airway size and shape. The common view that 'abnormalities' of craniofacial morphology account for only a small proportion of cases of sleep apnea may be a result of epidemiological methods.

The term risk factor implies not merely statistical association but also causation. There should be a plausible mechanism linking the risk factor and the disease, and the temporal relationship between the cause and the outcome must fit this mechanism. Many of the statistical 'risk factors' for sleep apnea discussed below are, on clinical grounds, likely candidates as causal risk factors as well. However, for most there is no mechanism proposed by which they might cause sleep apnea and since most epidemiological studies of sleep apnea are cross-sectional, they do not provide evidence of an appropriate temporal relationship. In most cases, the risk factors discussed below should be thought of as statistical risk factors but not established causal risk factors.

Evidence that something is a risk factor for a disease does not necessarily mean that changing it will treat or prevent the disease. This may be because the identified factor is not part of the causal chain, but merely a marker for something else that is. It may be because the identified risk factors are genuine but minor factors, so that changing them is ineffectual. It may also be because the process leading to disease is, sooner or later, irreversible (stopping smoking does not cure lung cancer).

Obesity is the only risk factor identified so far for sleep apnea that is both important and modifiable. It does not make a great deal of difference, statistically, whether obesity is measured as body mass index, waist circumference or waist/hip ratio, or as neck circumference, although the assumption is that the fat around the upper airway is relevant. The mechanism by which obesity causes sleep apnea is not precisely defined and both local effects, such as interference by upper airway fat on pharyngeal mechanics, and systemic effects, such as hypoxemia caused by obesity, have been implicated. There is little evidence that weight gain precedes the development of clinically significant sleep apnea. In the Wisconsin Sleep Cohort, large weight gains were associated with small increases in apnea/hypopnea frequency, but the vast majority of the observations were at low and clinically insignificant levels of sleep-disordered breathing. In clinic samples, there is no clear relationship between weight gain and severity of sleep apnea. It is common to see patients whose histories suggest strongly that rapid weight gain has caused progression of sleep apnea, but it is important to remember that this has not often been objectively confirmed.

Weight loss is frequently recommended as part of the treatment of sleep apnea. When weight loss is achieved, there is an overall reduction in apnea severity but individual variation is marked: some patients lose their sleep apnea completely with only modest weight loss and others show no change despite large reductions of weight.

Age, *male sex* and a *family history* of sleep apnea are also strongly associated with sleep apnea. These factors are not modifiable so the association is clinically interesting but not useful. One important result of the epidemiological studies is that sleep apnea is more common in women than clinic-based studies have suggested. The male to female ratio is about 4:1 for clinically significant sleep apnea. The discrepancy between community-based and clinic-based studies is due to a different pattern of symptoms in women, leading to their under-diagnosis.

Familial clustering of sleep apnea is also present: a patient with one brother or a parent with sleep apnea will have nearly twice the chance of having sleep apnea. This is not due to obesity alone, but the mechanism is otherwise unknown. It is worthwhile encouraging patients with sleep apnea to tell their families and encourage them to have sleep studies.

By common observation, *alcohol* causes snoring and apnea but daily alcohol consumption is not a risk factor for sleep apnea. It appears there is no hangover effect of alcohol on the upper airway — only alcohol in the blood at bedtime causes snoring and apnea. *Smoking* has been associated with sleep apnea in some studies but not in others. Even in the positive studies the effect is not large and the mechanisms by which it is suggested that smoking might cause sleep apnea are speculative. Benefits to sleep apnea are not a plausible additional argument to offer smokers to encourage them to stop. The most important thing about smoking and sleep apnea is that concern about weight gain should not be an argument against smoking cessation in smokers with established sleep apnea.

History-taking and examination

The following symptoms and signs are common in OSA and have predictive value (Olson *et al*, 1995):

- snoring that disturbs the sleep of another person
- report of apnea by the bed partner
- report of gasping or choking during sleep
- finding the bed clothes in disarray in the morning.

Choking episodes are common, but are not limited to obstructive sleep apnea. Once acute pathology, such as angioedema/anaphylaxis, is excluded, the differential diagnosis of recurrent choking episodes includes obstructive sleep apnea, esophageal reflux with micro-aspiration, panic attacks, and upper airway dysfunction. In OSA, the feeling of not being able to breathe is of short duration (few seconds), and usually not associated with anxiety. In esophageal reflux with aspiration, the episodes are long (>30 seconds a minute) and often associated with coughing. In panic attacks and upper airway dysfunction, the patient reports being unable to breathe *in*, contrary to the difficulty of breathing *out* that is typical of asthma. The episodes are prolonged (minutes) with feelings of impending doom, and adrenergic activation (palpitation, pallor). The terms sleep-related laryngospasm and sleep choking syndrome are used to describe these episodes in the international classification of sleep disorders (American Sleep Disorders Association, 1997).

Other symptoms and observations are common in OSA but are less predictive. For example:

- *Unrefreshing sleep:* Waking up feeling unrefreshed in the morning is common to many sleep disorders and other conditions (eg. depression). It should be noted that some patients with severe sleep apnea, by polysomnography criteria, report feeling refreshed in the morning.

- *Excessive daytime sleepiness:* Daytime sleepiness is part of the definition of OSA syndrome but it is less useful as a predictor because sleepiness is common, being reported by 30–50% of the community (Strohl and Redline, 1996). It should be noted that the word 'tiredness' is often used by patients with OSA to mean a combination of increased sleepiness tendency and lack of energy. Women, particularly, are more likely to report morning tiredness rather than sleepiness (Ambrogetti *et al*, 1991).

- *Obesity:* Among 3664 patients investigated for OSA between 1995 and 2000 in the Newcastle (AUS) sleep unit, 70% with an apnea/hypopnea above fifteen events per hour had a body mass index greater than 30kg/m^2. This is in keeping with observations in other units (Bearpark *et al*, 1995; Braver *et al*, 1995; Browman *et al*, 1984; Rajala *et al*, 1991; Richman *et al*, 1994). It should be noted that obese patients may complain of excessive daytime sleepiness in the absence of disturbed breathing during sleep (Vgontzas *et al*, 1998).

- *Hypertension:* An association between snoring, OSA and hypertension is recognized but the issue is controversial (Samet *et al*, 2000). Recent studies seem to confirm that OSA is a risk factor for hypertension after adjusting for other confounding variables (Lavie *et al*, 2000; Peppard *et al*, 2000; Worsnop, 1998). The association seems to be higher in subjects under fifty years of age (Strohl and Redline, 1996).

❖ **Headache:** Although a dull headache may be reported in the morning by patients with severe sleep apnea with hypoventilation and CO_2 retention, headache is not a common finding in OSA. In fact, in a population study, headache was more common in patients without sleep-disordered breathing than in patients with sleep apnea (Olson *et al*, 1995). However, an association has been reported between cluster headache and disturbed breathing during sleep (Chervin *et al*, 2000).

❖ **Smoking:** Current smokers appear to have an increased risk of snoring and disturbed breathing during sleep (*Figure 5.2*), presumably related to chronic inflammatory changes in the upper airway (Bloom *et al*, 1988; Franklin *et al*, 2004; Wetter *et al*, 1994).

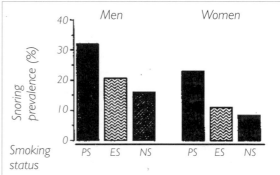

❖ **Cognitive and personality changes:** Increasing irritability, depression or anxiety, memory and concentration deficit and personality changes are often present in OSA and usually improve following treatment (Chugh *et al*, 1996; Engleman and Joffe, 1999; Strohl and Redline, 1996).

Figure 5.2: The effect of cigarette smoking on snoring prevalence. PS = present smokers; ES = ex-smokers; NS = never smokers. Snoring prevalence was significantly different in smoking groups for both men and women (p<.001), except that ex-smokers were not significantly different from never-smokers (Wetter et al, 1994).

❖ **Family history:** Familial clustering of snoring and apnea/hypopnea is documented both in family and twin studies (Jennum *et al*, 1995a; Redline and Tishler, 2000). Familial occurrence of disturbed breathing during sleep may underlie a genetic predisposition even when other inheritable predisposing factors, such as obesity and cranio-facial abnormalities, are taken into consideration.

❖ **Response to napping:** Patients with sleep apnea tend to take planned or unplanned naps through the day because of increased sleepiness. In patients with sleep apnea, napping is usually not refreshing, in contrast to subjects with other causes of daytime sleepiness, such as chronic sleep deprivation and narcoleptic syndrome, who feel refreshed after 15–20-minute naps.

❖ **Decreased libido and impotence:** An association between OSA and decreased libido and impotence is reported even though this type of complaint is not commonly volunteered by the patient (Hirshkowitz *et al*, 1989). In some patients, treatment with nasal CPAP seems to be associated with improvement of the erectile dysfunction. A reduction of androgen levels in sleep apnea is documented and may account for impotence and reduction of libido (Grunstein, 1996).

* ***Alcohol:*** Alcohol consumption is associated with increased snoring and occurrence of apnea even though epidemiological studies have yielded conflicting results (Issa and Sullivan, 1982; Lindberg and Gislason, 2000). Alcohol may increase the probability of snoring and apnea by decreasing the activity of pharyngeal dilator muscles (Krol *et al*, 1984).

* ***Co-existing medical conditions:*** The coexistence of certain medical conditions and physical features can be indicative of OSA (*Table 5.4*).

Table 5.4: Medical conditions that can be indicative of sleep apnoea
⌘ Hypothyroidism
⌘ Acromegaly
⌘ Diabetes
⌘ Renal failure
⌘ Down syndrome
⌘ Marfan syndrome
⌘ Neuromuscular disorders
⌘ Cleft palate
⌘ Left ventricular failure

Hypothyroidism is important to consider as sleepiness can be directly related to thyroid dysfunction and because snoring and OSA seems to be made worse by the lack of thyroid hormone. Although the association between hypothyroidism and OSA is subject to debate (Grunstein and Sullivan, 1988), thyroid stimulating hormone (TSH) should be checked at least once in patients with daytime sleepiness and suspected sleep apnea.

Central sleep apnea is also reported in patients with hypothyroidism (Millman *et al*, 1983). OSA and central sleep apnea are also common in acromegaly and if there is a clinical suspicion, somatomedin C (IGF-1) and growth hormone (GH) levels should be checked. However, routine measurement of these hormones is not indicated.

Patients with mature onset diabetes have an increased risk of OSA, probably through the association with central obesity (Strohl, 1996). Disturbed sleep is also common among patients with end-stage renal failure (*Chapter 8*). Sleep apnea is more prevalent and may contribute to increased cardiovascular morbidity in this group of patients (Kimmel *et al*, 1989; Kraus and Hamburger, 1997). Correction of the metabolic abnormality by haemodialysis has yielded conflicting results (Fein *et al*, 1987; Mendelson *et al*, 1990).

Patients with Down's syndrome appear to have fragmented sleep with high prevalence of sleep apnea (Levanon *et al*, 1999). A combination of central and OSA is documented in these patients (Ferri *et al*, 1997; Marcus *et al*, 1991). A smaller upper airway associated with a large tongue may be a predisposing factor for obstructive episodes in this group of patients (Uong *et al*, 2001).

Other genetic conditions associated with craniofacial abnormalities (Pierre Robin syndrome, Treacher Collins syndrome, Laron syndrome) and floppiness of the airway (Marfan syndrome), should raise suspicion of possible sleep apnea in the appropriate clinical context (unrefreshing sleep and daytime sleepiness) (Cistulli and Sullivan, 1993; Dagan *et al*, 2001). Patients with cleft palate who have undergone corrective surgery (pharyngeal flap) are at increased risk of upper airway obstruction (Orr *et al*, 1987). Left ventricular dysfunction may lead to disturbed breathing during sleep; often central sleep apnea or mixed sleep apnea. Severe OSA however, can aggravate left ventricular failure (Naughton and Bradley, 1998).

Physical examination

Observation during the interview can provide useful information:

- short thick neck: If the neck measurement is made at the level of the cricoid, values greater than 42 cm appear to increase the probability of OSA (Davies and Stradling, 1990; Ferguson *et al*, 1995)
- obesity can be quantified by body mass index. Values above 30 are often present in OSA
- nasal speech (hyponasality) and an adenoidal face suggest nasal obstruction and are often associated with high arched palate
- a small/receding chin: micrognathia and/or retrognathia are predisposing factors for snoring and sleep apnea (*Figure 5.3*).

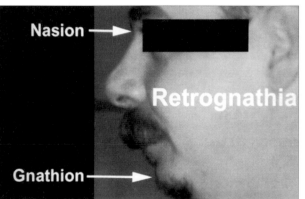

Figure 5.3: From Schellenberg et al, 2000.

Inspection of the nasal passages

Assess nasal patency while asking the patient to breathe through each nostril separately. Inspect the anterior nose for signs of inflammation or a deviated septum. If there is evidence of nasal obstruction, a full examination with a flexible nasendoscopy is useful in assessing the presence of nasal polyps or other nasopharyngeal pathology. The presence of hypertrophied adenoids in adults is relevant and can be indicative of possible human immunodeficiency virus (HIV) infection. The presence of an omega-shaped epiglottis (a sign of laryngeal-malacia), edema and inflammation of the soft tissue is often seen in OSA (*Figure 5.4*).

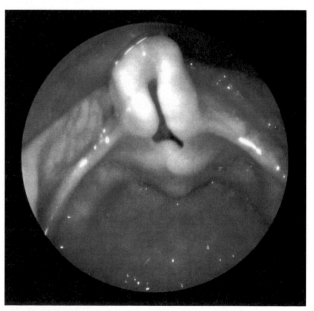

Figure 5.4: An omega-shaped epiglottis is a risk factor for sleep apnea (particularly in children) (courtesy of Professor Paul Walker).

Oral examination

An overall evaluation of the oropharyngeal soft tissue can be obtained using a modified Mallampati score (*Figure 5.5*). The Mallampati score, initially devised for assessing the degree of difficulty of endotracheal intubation, is also correlated with the degree of respiratory disturbance during sleep (Friedman *et al*, 1999).

❖ **Macroglossia:** Macroglossia and hypertrophied tonsils should be noted as surgical correction may be part of the treatment (*Figures 5.6* and *5.7*). A tongue which extends laterally to the dental occlusal plane and tonsils that occupy more than 50% of the posterior pharyngeal space increases the likelihood of OSA (Schellenberg *et al*, 2000).

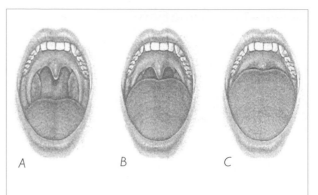

Figure 5.5: Mallampati score correlates with degree of respiratory disturbance during sleep. Reprinted from Friedman M, et al (1999) Clinical predictors of obstructive sleep apnea. Laryngoscope **109**(12): *1901–7.*

❖ **Lateral peritonsillar tissue:** (*Figure 5.8*) tends to narrow the pharyngeal space and is independently associated with apnea and hypopnea (Schellenberg *et al*, 2000).

❖ **An elongated, oedematous soft palate and uvula:** these are often seen in severe snoring and severe sleep apnea.

❖ **Dental bite:** a high, arched palate and an inverted bite are associated with narrow oro-pharynx and increase the likelihood of snoring and OSA.

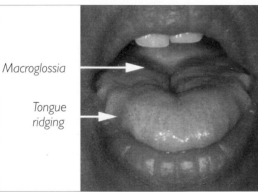

Macroglossia

Tongue ridging

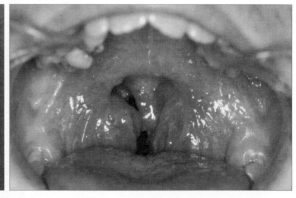

Figure 5.6: Surgical correction of macroglossia may be part of treatment for OSA (from Schellenberg et al, 2000).

Figure 5.7: Tonsillar hypertrophy may be surgically corrected as part of treatment for OSA (courtesy of Professor Paul Walker).

❖ **Dental and periodontal tissue:** this should be examined as poor dentition and dental hygiene preclude the application of dental devices for snoring and mild OSA.

Maneuvers aimed at reproducing snoring while awake are of limited predicted value and not particularly useful. Similarly, cephalometric assessment may have application in research or if mandibular surgery is considered, but it is not part of routine assessment.

Neurological examination

A full neurological examination should be undertaken given the right clinical context. Because respiratory drive is physiologically reduced in sleep and hypotonia is marked during REM sleep, respiratory disturbances and

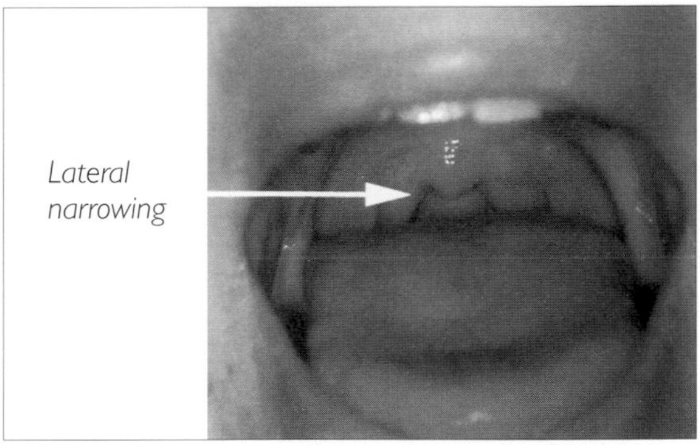

Figure 5.8: Lateral peritonsillar tissue associated with apnea and hypopnea (from Schellenberg et al, 2000).

unrefreshed sleep may be present for weeks or months before a neurological disorder declares itself with full clinical symptoms (eg. motor neuron disease, muscular dystrophy, and myasthenia). A recent onset of symptoms or a pre-existing neurological conditions (stroke, post-polio syndrome) requires full neurological assessment and high index of concern where there is disturbed breathing during sleep (Dean *et al*, 1998).

Clinical presentation and management

Severe obstructive sleep apnea

Case study 1

Mr Frank Tuyau is a 38-year-old taxi driver with a BMI of 38. He is brought reluctantly by his wife for consultation because of loud disruptive snoring and her concern that he stops breathing during sleep. Mr Tuyau says he has sometimes fallen asleep in stationary traffic. He is found to have severe OSA with a respiratory disturbance index (RDI) of 60 per hour and a low nocturnal oxygen saturation with a nadir of 66%. His Epworth sleepiness score (ESS) is 14 (normal < 10).

Mr Tuyau fails to benefit from a 2-month trial of CPAP but has a friend who says surgery cured his snoring. He is keen for a surgical solution.

The polysomnogram (PSG) was discussed with the patient and his wife and the pathophysiology of obstructive sleep apnea was explained in detail with emphasis on clearly evident abnormalities such as oxygen desaturation and sleep fragmentation. A copy of the PSG was then made for the patient to review at home. It is valuable to ensure that the patient and family clearly understands the importance of the therapy to aid compliance.

It is also important to emphasize the consequences of untreated OSA. Differentiating between the concept of 'simple' snoring and OSA needs to be made clear, as do the health consequences of OSA, including: daytime sleepiness and fatigue, hypertension, impaired neurocognitive function, cardiac arrhythmia, and ischemic heart disease and stroke, although the last two are less clearly defined (Davies and Stradling, 1996; Hamilton *et al*, 2004; Marin *et al*, 2005; Parra *et al*, 2004; Roebuck *et al*, 2004; Young *et al*, 2002). Of most significance is the increased risk of motor vehicle accident (MVA), which is two to seven times greater than that of the general population (George, 2001; Horstmann, 2000). However, this risk is normalized with effective CPAP therapy.

Obstructive sleep apnea and driving

There is currently no single test that predicts the risk of MVA in patients with OSA. Tests such as the multiple sleep latency test (MSLT) and maintenance of wakefulness test (MWT) have been used; however, neither of these has been shown to predict the risk of MVA in untreated OSA. The presence of subjective increased daytime sleepiness can be measured by the ESS. The ESS is also an important predictor of the response to specific treatment with CPAP which does not appear to be effective in patients with an ESS of less than 10 (Barbe, 2001).

The document, *Medical Examinations of Commercial Vehicle Drivers* (Austroed, 2003) states that people with established sleep apnea should not drive until treatment is found to be effective. Drivers are legally obliged to notify the driving licensing authority of their condition. The practitioner may need to notify the authority in the situation where patients are known to be non-compliant and continue to drive while sleepy.

These obligations should be explained to the patient. The patient in *Case study 1* is at high risk because he has fallen asleep in stationary traffic. He would be advised not to drive and to notify his condition to the Department of Motor Vehicles. The patient should be reassured that OSA is a treatable condition and that the risk associated with driving returns to normal after effective CPAP therapy. At least 6 weeks of therapy is needed for maximal improvement (Lamphere *et al*, 1996) and patients should not drive during that time. A compliance meter should be added to the patient's CPAP machine and regular review is needed to ensure effective ongoing therapy. After this, a conditional licence may be recommended by a sleep specialist, pending annual review.

Continuous positive airway pressure compliance

There are specific problems that may contribute to poor compliance with CPAP. Common side-effects include nasal congestion, rhinorrhea, dry mouth and difficulty exhaling against the pressure (*Table 5.5*). Nasal congestion and rhinorrhea may be aided by topical nasal corticosteroids. Failing this, humidification may help. Nasal ipratropium bromide may relieve rhinorrhea. Persistent nasal symptoms may require ENT surgical review to address structural abnormalities, such as nasal polyps.

Interface difficulties may lead to mask leaks and flow-on effects such as inadequate pressure, sleep fragmentation or dry mouth. There are many different nasal and oral masks available and a review of the mask fit and exploration of different options may be worthwhile.

Difficulty tolerating the pressure can be a problem although many patients say they acclimatize to this sensation over time. There are 'ramp' devices that increase the pressure gradually over a set time that may help. Bi-level ventilation is another option. These devices provide separate inspiratory and expiratory positive airway pressures, which are lower during expiration. The lowering of mean airway pressure and less resistance to expiration helps overcome what is a commonly reported difficulty in tolerating CPAP. There is no evidence that these devices aid compliance but they may help in individual cases.

A review of the CPAP titration data to check the appropriateness of the pressure prescribed may help. Equally, in those 'failing' CPAP, a review of the baseline PSG may be beneficial to ensure there are no complicating issues, such as the presence of central rather than obstructive sleep apnea, or periodic limb movements that may require different therapy. In some patients there is a strong positional component to OSA, with the disease much worse in the supine position. Jokic *et al* (1999) compared CPAP therapy and avoidance of the supine sleep position (by using a backpack containing a soft ball sewn into the patient's pyjamas) and noted that both therapies were equally effective in reducing ESS and MWT. They also noted a reduction in respiratory disturbance index (RDI) with both therapies, but the fall was greater with CPAP (Jokic *et al*, 1999). It is worthwhile considering if position is a strong contributor of disease severity.

All these issues should be discussed with the patient to minimize potential problems with compliance. A dedicated group of CPAP sleep technicians to aid with these issues is vitally important and is associated with increased compliance (Sin *et al*, 2002). At times, inpatient acclimatization to identify and address these issues is beneficial. It is also useful to note that patients over-report their daily usage of CPAP by approximately one hour (Kribbs *et al*, 1993; Rauscher *et al*, 1993).

The cost of equipment can be prohibitive. In Australia, some patients are eligible for government funded programmes, such as pensioners and healthcare cardholders. For others, the cost of equipment may exceed $1000. Rental machines, rent-to-buy programmes, second-hand machines or social assistance packages may help. These issues must be explored, especially in situations such as in *Case study 1*, where the patient's livelihood is at stake.

Table 5.5: Potential side-effects from nasal CPAP treatment

- ⌘ Mask discomfort
- ⌘ Nasal dryness, congestion or rhinorrhoea
- ⌘ Mouth leaks, open mouth and mouth dryness
- ⌘ Epistaxis
- ⌘ Noise disturbing patient or partner
- ⌘ Early wakening
- ⌘ Eye irritation
- ⌘ Inability to sleep
- ⌘ Claustrophobia
- ⌘ Difficulty exhaling against mask pressure

Effective continous positive airway pressure

The amount of time CPAP needs to be used to achieve a treatment benefit has not been well described. Improvements in daytime sleepiness and neurocognitive function can be seen from as little as 4 hours use per night (Engelman *et al*, 1994). Patients with more severe disease, greater BMI and more subjective daytime sleepiness are more likely to be compliant (Engelman *et al*, 1994; McArdle *et al*, 1999). This is thought to be because these patients are more likely to be symptomatic and, therefore, receive an immediate treatment benefit from CPAP. The average nightly use of CPAP over the first 3 months is also a strong predictor of long-term usage (McArdle *et al*, 1999).

Alternatives to continous positive airway pressure

Mandibular advancement splint (MAS)

If long-term use of CPAP is not possible, alternative therapies are needed. One option is a mandibular advancement splint (MAS). These devices need to be accurately made, and work by fitting over the upper and lower teeth, positioning the mandible more anteriorly by gradual adjustment. It is believed that by moving the mandible forward the tongue and pharyngeal muscles are also moved forward to increase the posterior airspace and reduce sleep-disordered breathing. These devices are able to reduce the RDI by on average 50% (American Sleep Disorders Association, 1995). They have a therapeutic role in mild and moderate OSA and are successful at eliminating snoring. However, CPAP is more effective at normalizing the RDI and reducing daytime sleepiness (American Sleep Disorders Association, 1995; Engelman *et al*, 2002).

The MAS is generally well tolerated with only minor side-effects, including jaw discomfort, excessive salivation or bruxism. The patient needs careful review prior to making the device which may not be suitable if they have upper and lower dentures, or a history of significant temporomandibular pain (*Table 5.6*). It is, however, a lesser therapy in severe OSA. If it is to be used in severe OSA, a repeat PSG would need to be scheduled within 3 months to document the effect of the MAS in the reduction of sleep-disordered breathing. Combining the MAS with loss of weight is more likely to be successful than using the MAS as a stand-alone therapy.

Table 5.6: Contraindications to MAS
⌘ Dentures or insufficient teeth to provide support
⌘ Active periodontal problems
⌘ Active temporomandibular joint disorder
⌘ Limited maximal protrusive distance (<6 mm)

Weight loss

Weight loss should always be discussed in the management of the overweight patient with OSA. A variety of approaches are worth considering, including dietary, exercise, pharmacological agents and gastric banding and other surgical procedures. An adjustable gastric banding procedure has been associated with significant, sustained weight loss for up to 6 years, with highly significant improvements in snoring, daytime sleepiness, sleep quality and observed apneas up to twenty-8 months (Dixon *et al*, 2001; Guardiano *et al*, 2003). However, surgical options are limited and all have poor long-term success rates. Weight loss should be encouraged using the first two measures initially. The long-term goal is to lose enough weight, to repeat the PSG and possibly change the need for therapy for OSA. This should be pursued with the patient but is rarely possible.

Surgical options

It is likely that the friend referred to in *Case study 1* had an uvulopalatopharyngoplasty (UPPP) to treat his snoring. This procedure involves enlarging the upper airway by removing distal palatal tissue. It can be effective at controlling snoring, at least in the short term, and success rates are quoted at around 75% although there is a paucity of long-term data (Ryan, 1997). There is evidence that patients show short-term significant subjective improvement in the perception of snoring and quality of sleep and improvements are noted by both the patient and bed partner. However, there is no significant improvement in PSG data postoperatively (Miljeteig *et al*, 1994).

This operation has limited application in treating OSA. In many patients with sleep apnea there is more than one site of upper airway obstruction and UPPP only treats obstruction at one site. Up to 60% of patients continue to have significant OSA after the procedure (Sher *et al*, 1996). Clinical experience suggests that the more severe the sleep apnea, the higher the risk of treatment failure or recurrence of the disturbed breathing. This is an operation with some role in simple snoring but it is not an effective therapy for OSA.

Other surgical procedures (Sher *et al*, 1996) aimed at enlarging the retropharyngeal space, are listed in *Table 5.7*. From a functional point of view, the site(s) of pharyngeal obstruction is/are identified as retropalatal (type 1), retrolingual (type 3) and more diffuse, both retropalatal and retrolingual (type 2). When the site(s) of obstruction can be identified and other treatments (nasal CPAP, weight reduction, mandibular advancing devices) are unsuccessful or not accepted, more intrusive surgical interventions can be considered. One major practical problem is the lack of accuracy of current diagnostic tests in identifying the site of pharyngeal narrowing. Another is the absence of evidence of the effectiveness of surgery, especially surgery beyond UPPP.

The Stanford University Group uses a two-phase approach to surgery for OSA. They advocate a physical examination, lateral cephalometric measurement and fibreoptic nasopharyngoscopy prior to surgery (Riley *et al*, 2000). These measurements may identify a single site of upper airway obstruction that can be surgically corrected.

Phase 1 operations include nasal reconstruction, UPPP and limited mandibular osteotomy with genioglossus advancement (*Figure 5.9*). The phase 2 operation involves advancement of the maxilla and mandible (*Figure 5.10*). The latter operation can be particularly successful in people with significant craniofacial disorders (maxillomandibular deficiency). This should be considered both on clinical examination and with lateral cephalometric radiology, particularly in the non-obese patient with significant or disproportionate OSA. A surgical approach is usually the last resort for those intolerant of CPAP and in whom other therapies are not suitable.

It should be noted that the role of surgical procedures in the management of OSA is based on case series' and uncontrolled observations (Bridgman *et al*, 1997).

Table 5.7: Upper airway surgical treatments for OSA

Nasal surgery (eg. septoplasty, turbinectomy, polypectomy)	Aimed at improving nasal patency and breathing, it is of limited value on its own
Uvulopalatopharyngoplasty (UPPP)	There are a variety of techniques aimed at increasing the retropalatal space. Overall, success is ~40% when defined as reduction in apnea to 50% or less of base line. Slightly better outcome when the site of obstruction can be identified at the retropalatal level (type 1). The rate of failure increases with time after surgery, particularly if the patient puts on weight
Uvulopalatopharyngoplasty with glossoplasty (UPPPGP)	Similar to UUUP with resection of part of the posterior and lateral portion of the base of the tongue
Laser midline glossectomy (LMG) and lingual plasty	Techniques aimed at reducing the size of the tongue by removing 2.5 cm x 5 cm of tissue from the base of the tongue in the midline (LMG) as well as the lateral part (lingualplasty), when the narrowing is thought to be localised to the retrolingual space
Inferior sagittal mandibular osteotomy (ISO) and genioglossal advancement with hyoid myotomy (GAHM)	Considered usually after other surgery (UPPP) has failed, and when retrolingual space narrowing is considered important. Success rate in reducing apneas and hypopneas to <50%, in small case series is reported up to 79%
Maxillomandibular osteotomy and advancement	Aimed at providing maximal enlargement of the retropharyngeal space by advancing both mandible and maxilla (and the tongue)
Tracheotomy	The procedure of choice in severe sleep apnea patients with respiratory and heart failure, before the advent of nasal CPAP. Not used as a routine procedure

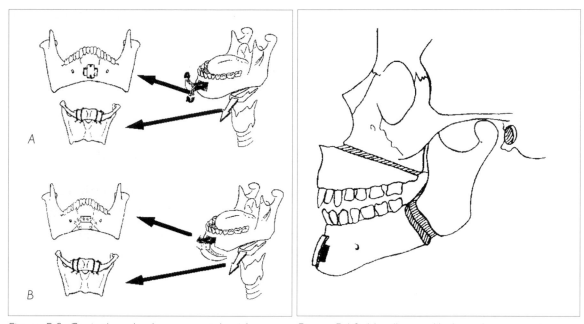

Figure 5.9: Genioglossal advancement, hyoid myotomy, and hypothyroidopexy (GAHT). (A) The genioglossus advancement is usually performed using an inferior rectangular sagittal osteotomy. (B) The osteotomy can also begin at the inferior border of the mandible and is then followed under visual control by trapezoidal osteotomy for advancement of the genioglossus muscle. The late modifications involve stabilization of the hyoid bone inferiorly by attachment to the superior border of the thyroid cartilage (A and B). Reprinted from Bettega et al 2000, 'Obstructive sleep apnea syndrome. Fifty-one consecutive patients treated by maxillofacial surgery'. American Journal of Respiratory Critical Care Medicine 162: 641–9. Official journal of the American Thoracic Society. © American Thoracic Society.

Figure 5.10: Maxillomandibular advancement osteotomy (MMO). Bilateral sagittal split osteotomy and maxillary advancement by Le Fort I osteotomy. Reprinted from Bettega et al 2000, 'Obstructive sleep apnea syndrome. Fifty-one consecutive patients treated by maxillofacial surgery'. American Journal of Respiratory Critical Care Medicine 162: 641–9. Official journal of the American Thoracic Society. © American Thoracic Society.

Simple snoring

Case study 2

Mr Jeff Bowan is a 38-year-old steelworker who attends clinic with his wife because of heavy snoring that is interfering with the sleep of other members of the family, in particular his wife's. Their two children, however, have told their father that they can hear his snoring from the other end of the house. Jeff smokes fifteen cigarettes a day and admits an alcohol intake of ten standard drinks a week, mostly on Friday and Saturday evenings. He has frequent heart burn and mild asthma for which he uses bronchodilators intermittently. He is obese with a body mass index of 32. He has a patent nose, his oropharynx is of normal size with slightly elongated uvula, and he has a full dentitian with mild periodontal disease. His BP is slightly elevated at 140/90.

Jeff's bedtime is around 11.00PM and he falls asleep within 10 minutes. He wakes up once or twice a night briefly but doesn't experience choking sensations. He gets up at 6.00AM on working days and 7.00AM on weekend days. On awakening he feels refreshed. He does not take naps through the day or fall asleep in unusual circumstances. His wife says Jeff snores loudly in any body position and if he falls asleep first, she cannot get to sleep because of the noise and often has to sleep in another room due to the noise. His snoring has worsened over the last 10 years during which time he has put on about 11kg in weight. His snoring is worse on evenings when he drinks.

The overnight polysomnography confirmed loud snoring through the night. Apnea/hypopnea index was less than one per hour with eight arousals per hour.

Snoring is commonly perceived to be a major social problem in the absence of symptoms on the part of the snorer. This patient would not have sought a consultation if it were not for the insistence of his spouse. In some instances the pressure from the spouse to obtain help with snoring goes beyond 'insistence'. Simple snoring (snoring without disturbed breathing) should be seen as a social problem for the couple and the discussion should involve both the snorer and partner.

The following points were discussed with this patient:

❖ Risks associated with snoring: There is no firm evidence that simple snoring, by itself, is a risk factor for cardiovascular diseases (hypertension, stroke, coronary artery disease). This is a controversial issue (Hoffstein, 1996). Since the early 1980s, epidemiological studies have reported an association between snoring and cardiovascular morbidity. However, many studies were based on self-reported snoring without objective measurement of sleep and some did not adjust for important confounding factors such as weight, age, alcohol intake and gender. Because many studies assess snoring without objective measurement (such as overnight polysomnography and measurement of snoring), it is likely that some of the association with cardiovascular risk was related to snoring in the presence of OSA.

❖ Some snorers can have disturbed sleep in the absence of measurable apneas or hypopneas, and upper airway resistance syndrome (UARS) (Guilleminault *et al*, 1993). It should be noted that the measurement of snoring is not standardized. Self-reporting is not reliable as the patient is often unaware of it (Stradling, 1990). Snoring and its loudness are not strong predictors of the presence of apnea/hypopnea severity (Crocker *et al*, 1990). This is due to the prevalence of snoring in people without sleep apnea.

❖ There is no evidence that patients with pure snoring are likely to develop sleep apnea later on in life. However, it should be emphasized that increased weight is an important risk factor for a snorer to develop sleep apnea (*Figure 5.11*).

Treatment of snoring

Conservative measures should be encouraged as the first step in a long-term strategy. Couples are often aware of the connection between increases in weight and alcohol intake and worsening of snoring. Avoiding alcohol in the evening should be recommended. The suggestion of weight reduction is often received with scepticism as often past multiple attempts have been unsuccessful. However, it should be emphasized that any weight reduction will be of some benefit.

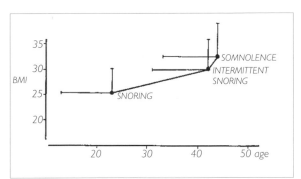

Figure 5.11: Intermittent snoring refers to snoring interrupted by apneas. Lugaresi E et al (1988) 'Snoring: Pathophysiology and clinical consequences'. Seminars Respiratory Medicine 9(6): 577–583. Reprinted by permission.

❖ ***Improvement of nasal patency:*** This can be achieved in the appropriate patient by inhaled steroids in case of allergic rhinitis. The use of mechanical nasal dilators has been tried with variable success. Mechanical nasal dilators include devices which are applied inside the nasal valve (Nozovent™) or external nasal strips (Breathe Right™). Although individual patients report beneficial effects, objective measures have not shown any change in the loudness of snoring (Hoffstein *et al*, 1993; Liistro *et al*, 1998).

❖ ***Mandibular advancing splint (MAS):*** MAS mouthguards have been shown to be effective at reducing snoring in approximately 80% of patients, by the spouse's report as well as by objective measurement. MASs are useful devices for an immediate reduction in snoring. However, they are somewhat uncomfortable, can cause extra salivation and if the bite is not properly accounted for, the MAS can lead to temporal mandibular discomfort. Fitting of a MAS also requires good dentition and dental hygiene. The presence of a dental prosthesis is usually a contraindication to MAS. There is also some evidence suggesting that long-term use of MAS may lead to changes in the dental bite (Pantin *et al*, 1999).

❖ **Palatal surgery:** Surgical intervention involving soft tissue of the pharyngeal area was initially considered an attractive operation for both snoring and sleep apnea (Fairbanks *et al*, 1987; Saunders *et al*, 1989). The initial procedure involved downsizing of the uvula and soft palate as well as lateral pharyngeal structure (*Figure 5.12*). A variety of techniques as well as different degrees of reshaping have been proposed over the years (Saunders *et al*, 1989).

One major problem with surgical intervention is assessing precisely the site of vibration and collapse at pharyngeal level. Uvulopalatopharyngoplasty (UPPP) (Saunders *et al*, 1989) has been shown to be effective in patients in whom vibration occurs predominantly at the uvulopalatal level. A variation to the surgical procedure is laser-assisted uvulopalatopharyngoplasty, whereby a minor downsizing of the uvula and soft palate is performed by laser treatment. This results in stiffening of the soft tissue with reduction in vibration level. A more recent variant is the use of microwave photocoagulation of the soft palate, and sometimes of the base of the tongue (Somnoplasty™) (Fischer *et al*, 2000; Nelson, 2000). All these procedures have the potential to reduce the loudness of snoring but do carry substantial risks of which the patient should be aware (Boudewyns *et al*, 2000; Cartwright *et al*, 2000) (*Table 5.8*). Surgery for snoring should be considered a cosmetic intervention given that there is no evidence that snoring alone is harmful to the patient's health.

Surgical intervention to the pharyngeal structures is not a permanent cure for snoring. The patient should be made aware that there is at least a 50% chance of recurrence at 3–5 years and this is probably a conservative estimate. As noted in *Table 5.8*, important side-effects of pharyngeal surgery include perioperative bleeding and pharyngeal insufficiency with difficulty swallowing. Change in vocal pitch is an issue that may be relevant to people who use their voices for professional reasons.

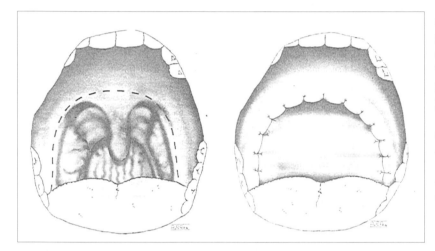

Figure 5.12: Uvulopalato-pharyngoplasty (UPPP). A variety of technical variations have been proposed through the years. Saunders NA et al. 'Uvulopalatopharyngoplasty as a treatment for snoring'. MJA 1989 150: 177–82. © 1989. The Medical Journal of Australia — reproduced with permission.

Mild obstructive sleep apnea

Case study 3

Mrs Anjuli Singh is a 45-year-old clerical assistant with a past history of depression, treated hypertension and seasonal rhinitis. She presents with a history of several years of snoring, witnessed apneic episodes, difficulty initiating sleep and, more recently, excessive daytime tiredness, problems concentrating at work and unrefreshing sleep. She feels that her condition has become worse in the past 2 years since gaining weight. She is a non-smoker and consumes 'social' quantities of alcohol. Her only current medication is atenolol 50mg once daily. Upon examination, Mrs Singh is overweight with a BMI of 33. Her blood pressure is 135/85. She has a minor degree of dental malocclusion and a slightly undershot jaw. Her ESS is 16/24 (normal <10).

A diagnostic polysomnogram shows an RDI of 14 episodes per hour (normal <5 per hour), an arousal index (AI) of 20 per hour (normal for this age <12/hour), and minor oxygen desaturation to a nadir of 88% in REM sleep. These findings are consistent with a diagnosis of mild OSA.

There are a number of important therapeutic issues that should be discussed with the patient before treatment decisions are made. It is likely that Mrs Singh will show some improvement in her daytime sleepiness following effective treatment if OSA is the cause of her symptoms. Mrs Singh should be offered therapy for her OSA as she meets the current Australian criteria of symptomatic OSA with an AHI ≥ 10. In the absence of other pathologies, it is probable that Mrs Singh would notice an improvement in her quality of life and ability to function at work, following successful treatment of her OSA. As Mrs Singh has objectively mild OSA, the disproportionately high ESS suggests that there may be additional causes for her daytime sleepiness beyond OSA. Alternative diagnoses include periodic leg movement disorder (PLMD), other undiagnosed sleep disorders, chronic sleep restriction, depression, etc. If Mrs Singh fails to show an adequate response to effective nasal CPAP therapy, a search for these alternative causes may be necessary.

Table 5.8: Potential side-effects of UPPP
⌘ Perioperative obstruction (due to oedema)
⌘ Perioperative bleed
⌘ Velopalatal insufficiency (manifesting with difficulty, swallowing and nasal regurgitation of fluid)
⌘ Throat dryness
⌘ Change in the voice quality
⌘ Operative death

(Sher *et al*, 1998)

Mrs Singh would be advised to lose weight in an attempt to normalise her BMI. She should also avoid excessive alcohol consumption and attempt to avoid the supine position for sleep. Treatment of her seasonal rhinitis with intranasal corticosteroids may also be of some benefit.

Mrs Singh may benefit from CPAP therapy, despite her relatively mild OSA. However, side-effects are frequent and these, and any potential remedies, need to be discussed with her prior to commencing CPAP therapy. The issue of compliance should also be raised. These options should be discussed with Mrs Singh, as should the potential benefit from either a MAS or surgery. The presence of dental malocclusion and an undershot jaw suggest that there may be surgically correctable anatomical abnormalities present. Both options should be regarded as second- or third-line therapy for use in patients unable or unwilling to use nasal CPAP.

After a thorough discussion of the issues described, consideration would be given to initial management by conservative measures (weight loss, treatment of rhinitis) alone. However, in view of the degree of daytime symptoms as evidenced by the high ESS, nasal CPAP is probably the initial treatment of choice.

Assessment of mild OSA

Objective assessment of severity is based upon the results of polysomnography (PSG) with consideration of the number of arousals per hour (the arousal index, AI), the number of respiratory events per hour (respiratory disturbance index, RDI; or apnea/hypopnea index, AHI) and oxygen desaturation. The PSG results are considered in conjunction with clinical assessment and subjective estimates of sleepiness (eg. the ESS) (Johns, 1991) to determine the severity of OSA. An RDI of 5 to 15 per hour is considered to be mild, 16 to 30 per hour is moderate and >30 per hour is severe. The prevalence of each of these levels of objective severity is not known (National Health and Medical Research Council, 2000).

Morbidity and mortality

OSA is widely considered to be a risk factor for the development of hypertension (Hoffstein *et al*, 1991; Peppard *et al*, 2000; Young *et al*, 2002) and there may an association between myocardial infarction and snoring or OSA (Jennum *et al*, 1995b; Newman *et al*, 2001; Young *et al*, 2002). There is some evidence suggesting a greater risk of early mortality for patients with untreated OSA, apneas greater than twenty events per hour (He *et al*, 1988), but data is lacking for patients with mild to moderate disease (Young *et al*, 2002). It is not yet known whether long-term CPAP therapy can reduce hypertension or other cardiovascular risk factors (National Health and Medical Research Council, 2000; Young *et al*, 2002).

Sleepiness

Excessive daytime sleepiness (EDS) is one of the cardinal features of OSA. However, sleepiness is, at least in part, a subjective state and many individuals with an AHI of ≥ 5 per hour do not report EDS (Kapur *et al*, 2005; Young *et al*, 1993). Conversely, many individuals without OSA also report EDS. Excessive sleepiness in OSA is believed to be due to fragmentation of the normal sleep by repeated arousals due to respiratory events. The factors responsible for the variation in susceptibility to daytime sleepiness remain uncertain, but severe snoring, high sleep efficiency, and increased arousals in the overnight polysomnography, seem to predict EDS (Seneviratne and Puvanendran, 2004). Undiagnosed sleep-disordered breathing has been associated with daytime hypersomnolence (Young *et al*, 1993) but the relationship between daytime sleepiness and objective severity is complicated and incompletely understood (Davies *et al*, 1996; Hack *et al*, 2000).

Cognitive function

There is some evidence of impaired cognitive function and daytime function in patients with OSA (Adams *et al*, 2001; Cheshire *et al*, 1992). It appears to be associated with diminished psychomotor efficiency, a finding not explained by daytime sleepiness (Kim *et al*, 1997; Young *et al*, 1993). This may occur with even mild OSA (Stoohs and Dement, 1993). There may also be some effect on memory (Adams *et al*, 2001) although this is uncertain (Kim *et al*, 1997).

Undiagnosed OSA appears to have a deleterious effect on quality of life (Baldwin *et al*, 2001; Finn *et al*, 1998; Young *et al*, 2002). Mild to moderate OSA appears to be associated with reduced vitality, and subjective symptoms are strongly associated with poorer quality of life (Baldwin *et al*, 2001). It is not clear whether these functional changes are due to hypoxemia, sleep fragmentation or increased effort of breathing (Baldwin *et al*, 2001).

Treating mild OSA

The current Australian consensus regarding mild OSA is that treatment should be considered in patients with an AHI of 10–20 and other significant pathological factors such as EDS (National Health and Medical Research Council, 2000). It is unclear whether there is any benefit to be gained from the treatment of asymptomatic mild OSA, although attention to weight and other factors may prevent progression to more severe or symptomatic disease (Peppard *et al*, 2000).

A number of controlled trials have demonstrated reduced daytime sleepiness after successful treatment of OSA, generally with nasal CPAP therapy (Kiely *et al*, 1999; Montserrat *et al*, 2001). There is conflicting evidence on whether treatment is as effective in mild OSA as it appears to be in moderate to severe OSA (National Health and Medical Research Council, 2000; Wright *et al*, 2002).

Milder forms of symptomatic OSA may show less subjective responses to CPAP, despite normalization of the RDI and correction of hypoxaemia. This may be due to the presence of other factors and causes of excessive daytime sleepiness. These alternative causes need to be considered in assessing failure to respond to treatment of OSA (*Table 5.9*) (Billiard and Dauvilliers, 2001).

Table 5.9: Causes for persistent symptoms in OSA despite CPAP therapy

Chronic sleep restriction/insufficient sleep syndrome

Non-effective CPAP
Non-compliance with therapy
Inadequately adjusted/fitted mask
Inadequate CPAP pressure

Poor sleep quality
Pain and other syndromes responsible for fragmented sleep
Undiagnosed periodic limb movement disorder (PLMD)

Daytime problems
Depression
Chronic fatigue syndrome

Delayed sleep phase syndrome

Long sleepers — 'healthy hypersomniacs'

Hypersomnia:
~ Primary hypersomnias: narcolepsy, Kleine–Levin syndrome, menstrual-associated hypersomnia, idiopathic hypersomnia
~ Secondary hypersomnias: post-traumatic, post-viral

(modified from Billiard and Dauvilliers, 2001)

Treatment should be aimed primarily at managing the complications of the disease (Davies and Stradling, 1996). The main indication for treatment is EDS and related symptoms. There is no good evidence that simple non-invasive lifestyle changes improve OSA, but there is some suggestion that lifestyle modification may be of benefit in treating mild OSA (Shneerson and Wright, 2002). It is estimated that there is a 3% change in AHI for each 1% change in weight (Peppard *et al*, 2000).

Smoking cessation, reduction of alcohol intake and improving nasal patency may be beneficial, as discussed earlier in this chapter.

Body positioning during sleep and, particularly, the supine position is known to have a major effect upon the frequency and severity of breathing disturbance during sleep in OSA patients (Oksenberg *et al*, 1997). Head extension, or cervical positioning using custom-fitted cervical pillows in mild to moderate OSA has been reported to produce some improvement in RDI and reduction in arousals, with a non-significant improvement in sleep efficiency and subjective depth of sleep (Ballester *et al*, 1999; Kushida *et al*, 2001). Other devices have also been suggested (such as the Jokic 'backpack'; Jokic *et al*, 1999).

Nasal CPAP therapy

Nasal CPAP appears to be of benefit even in mild cases of symptomatic OSA and its effect appears to be long-lasting (Engleman *et al*, 1997; Engleman *et al*, 1999; Monasterio *et al*, 2001; Redline *et al*, 1998). It is reversible as therapy can be stopped without adverse consequences (except reversion to the patient's baseline state). Nasal CPAP therapy is superior to placebo in improving quality of life and measures of depression, but the evidence is not convincing on the beneficial effect on blood pressure control and quality of sleep (Ballester *et al*, 1999; Barnes *et al*, 2002; Engleman *et al*, 1997; Engleman *et al*, 1998; Engleman *et al*, 1999; Hack *et al*, 2000; Jenkinson *et al*, 1999; Kiely *et al*, 1999; Monasterio *et al*, 2001; Montserrat *et al*, 2001; NHMR Council, 2000; Redline *et al*, 1998; Sanner *et al*, 2000; Scharf *et al*, 1999; Wright *et al*, 2002) (*Table 5.10*).

Table 5.10: Recent trials of CPAP in OSA	
Intervention	**Outcome**
CPAP and conservative therapy *vs* conservative therapy alone[a]	Favored CPAP (OR 6.53, 95% CI 2.51–17.6)
CPAP *vs* oral placebo[b]	Favored CPAP for objective and subjective sleepiness
Therapeutic *vs* subtherapeutic CPAP[c]	Favored therapeutic CPAP
CPAP *vs* conservative therapy[d]	Favored CPAP in mild OSA

[a]Ballester *et al*, 1999
[b]Kiely *et al*, 1999; Engelman *et al*, 1997, 1998, 1999; Scharf *et al*, 1999; Monasterio *et al*, 2001
[c]Jenkinson *et al*, 1999; Hack *et al*, 2000; Montserrat *et al*, 2001; Barnes *et al*, 2002
[d]Redline *et al*, 1998
CI - confidence interval; OR = odds ratio

However, CPAP can be uncomfortable, side-effects are frequent and a considerable proportion of patients are unable to tolerate nasal CPAP. A number of patients will continue to have residual daytime sleepiness despite apparent compliance with therapeutic CPAP (Kingshott *et al,* 2001). The etiology is unknown, but probably multifactorial. The significance of persisting sleepiness despite adequate CPAP therapy is uncertain. Modafinil has been suggested as a possible therapy for this condition (Black and Hirshkowitz, 2005; Kingshott *et al,* 2001). Other causes of excessive sleepiness will require exclusion in these cases (*Table 5.9*).

In patients without daytime sleepiness the effect of CPAP is uncertain (Barbe *et al,* 2001; Engleman, 2002; Loube *et al,* 1999; Sanner *et al,* 2000).

Not all patients can tolerate CPAP therapy. The commonest reasons for non-compliance are related to nasal or pharyngeal side-effects or a lack of subjective benefit (Janson *et al,* 2000). Patients with less severe OSA appear to be more likely to stop CPAP (Janson *et al,* 2000; McArdle *et al,* 1999; Popescu *et al,* 2001). The side-effects of CPAP are frequent (*Table 5.5*) but, despite this, a high rate of compliance has been reported in some studies (Kalan *et al,* 1999). Partners of patients report poor sleep quality and self-reported health status prior to CPAP and an improvement in subjective sleep quality and sleep disturbance with therapy (Doherty *et al,* 2003; McArdle *et al,* 2001). CPAP generally appears to be well tolerated by the patients' partners.

Compliance may be an issue. Early compliance with treatment is predictive of long-term compliance (McArdle *et al,* 1999; Popescu *et al,* 2001). Poor compliance may be a major cause of treatment failure (McArdle *et al,* 1999; Popescu *et al,* 2001; Kalan *et al,* 1999) and failure to comply may be as high as 25–50%, typically within 2–4 weeks of commencing therapy (Zozula and Rosen, 2001). If patients are able tolerate CPAP for the first month or so, they are generally able to continue long-term therapy.

Dental appliances

There are a number of dental devices aimed at advancing the mandible (American Sleep Disorders Association Report, 1995) that appear to be well accepted by patients, mostly those with mild to moderate OSA (Gotsopoulos *et al,* 2002; Lindman and Bondemark, 2001; Lyons *et al,* 2001; Mehta *et al,* 2001; Tegelberg *et al,* 1999; Wilhelmsson *et al,* 1999). The devices promote significant improvement in RDI and adverse effects are relatively rare. Although CPAP appears to be more effective in improving RDI, both methods improve ESS equally (Flemons, 2002; Wright *et al,* 2002). While many patients prefer the oral devices, the choice is up to the individual, with a recent study showing patients with mild OSA preferring CPAP over use of a MAS (Engleman *et al,* 2002). Contraindications with MASs are frequent (up to 50%) and may preclude their use (*Table 5.6*) (Petit *et al* 2002).

Drug therapy

To date, there is no convincing case for the routine use of any pharmacologic agent in the management of OSA. The drug modafinil appears to improve the MWT but has no effect on sleepiness, MSLT, cognitive function or quality of life (Black and Hirshkowitz, 2005; Kingshott *et al*, 2001). Modafinil can be given once or twice daily (morning and midday), at doses between 100 mg and 400 mg.

Surgery

As discussed elsewhere in this chapter (*Surgical options, p.139*), some forms of surgery may be of benefit in the management of OSA, particularly in those with normal BMI and evidence of anatomical abnormality (maxillomandibular deficiency). Many patients only consider surgery as a last resort, but a few will express a preference for surgery as their treatment of choice for OSA. However, surgery should generally be regarded as a therapy of last resort (Bridgman *et al*, 1997).

Monitoring treatment

CPAP is the longest established and best documented of the therapeutic options and is known to provide long-lasting benefits to patients. CPAP therapy should commence with a formal therapeutic overnight CPAP titration with the intent of establishing the appropriate pressure setting. Once this is established, a domiciliary trial of 6 weeks (or longer) should be instituted following a period of patient education, with subsequent ongoing clinical review. An occasional patient may require inpatient admission for initiation of CPAP therapy. Side-effects should be dealt with as and when they occur. Follow-up and monitoring of clinical response may involve repeated ESS or other formal instruments, and reviewing the patient's self-reported symptoms. If the patient continues to experience excessive daytime sleepiness, consideration should be given to non-compliance, mask leaks or other technical problems, or the existence of another cause for daytime sleepiness.

Additional investigations may be necessary if there are problems with the clinical response to CPAP. If there is concern about compliance, a compliance meter can be fitted to the CPAP unit to check on pump usage.

Gender differences

There may be some gender-based differences in symptoms (*Chapter 3, Figure 3.1*), and women appear to be more likely to report difficulties in initiating sleep (Ambrogetti *et al*, 1991; Jordon and McEvoy, 2003; Shepertycky *et al*, 2005; Stoohs and Dement, 1993), morning headaches and fatigue at similar levels to OSA but hypertension may be less common (Ambrogetti *et al*, 1991). Women seem less likely to use CPAP therapy (McArdle *et al*, 1999) and more likely to discontinue CPAP after one year (McArdle *et al*, 1999; Popescu *et al*, 2001). The menopause may be of some importance in OSA. Several studies have suggested that menopause is independently related to OSA and that hormone replacement therapy (HRT) may be protective (Bixler *et al*, 2001; Edwards *et al*, 1998; Young *et al*, 1993).

Residual sleepiness

Case study 4

Mr Nick Cicolini is a 42-year-old engineer. He was initially assessed for daytime sleepiness and found to have severe sleep apnea (apnea/hypopnea index of 42 per hour), with marked oxygen desaturation during REM sleep and twenty-eight arousals per hour. His body mass index was 37 at the time of the initial assessment. Nasal CPAP successfully corrected the disturbed breathing, oxygen saturation was normalized, arousals reduced and there was improvement in his daytime symptoms. As part of his job, Mr Cicolini has to drive to different locations within a 50 km radius of his office, four to five days a week. During these trips of 30–60 minutes' duration, he still feels drowsy while driving despite nasal CPAP treatment.

Mr Cicolini has a repeated polysomnography assessment on nasal CPAP and MSLT, 2 weeks after wearing an actigraphy. When reviewed, his CPAP machine is checked to assess compliance with treatment and usage time. On average he uses the machine 6 hours per night. Polysomnography reveals improved sleep structure, control of disturbed breathing and seven arousals per hour (improved from the diagnostic study of twenty-eight arousals per hour). The actigraph (see *Chapter 3*) shows a regular rest and activity pattern, with a resting period beginning around 10.30PM until about 6.00AM, with a slight delay on weekends (resting time beginning between 11.30PM and midnight, waking up between 6.30AM and 7.00AM). The MSLT shows a mean sleep latency of 6.5 minutes with no REM abnormalities.

Further review of his history reveals no REM-related symptoms to suggest classical narcolepsy, eg. hypnogogic hallucinations, sleep paralysis, cataplexy or automatic behavior. The onset of sleepiness has been slow, over a period of a few years, but was not present as a teenager. The patient is concerned about his job security but does not display symptoms suggestive of depression.

After discussion with Mr Cicolini, and given the above findings, he is started on methylphenidate 10 mg twice daily, to be taken predominantly when he has to drive. He also agrees to undertake a weight reduction programme. It is arranged that reassessment should occur within the following 12 months.

Persistence of drowsiness and lethargy in patients with OSA is not uncommon and it is a difficult clinical situation, where the use of stimulant medications have a selected role (Guillenimault *et al*, 1996). Non-amphetamine stimulant medication (modafinil) and methylphenidate, like in the above case, can be used (Schwartz *et al*, 2003). There are a few possibilities for this patient's residual daytime sleepiness, despite what appears to be optimal treatment with the nasal CPAP (*Table 5.9*). The clinician needs to re-evaluate the patient's condition over time, maintaining a high index of suspicion for secondary causes of sleepiness and, in particular, poor compliance with OSA treatment and chronic sleep deprivation. It is essential to document that treatment and compliance are adequate.

Snoring and apnea in the elderly

Case study 5

Mr Jim MacDonald is a 76-year-old retired teacher referred for investigation of snoring and apnea reported by his wife. He is an ex-smoker with coexisting hypertension which he has had for 15 years and is well controlled on beta-blockers and diuretics. He is otherwise a healthy, active man.

Mr MacDonald goes to bed around 10.30PM–11.00PM, falling asleep within 30 minutes. He wakes once per night to urinate. He is awake by 5.30AM when he takes his dog for a walk. He feels refreshed and well most of the time and rests for 30–60 minutes after lunch, but not every day. His wife says Mr MacDonald falls asleep while in the lounge room watching television in the evening. She is concerned that he stops breathing at night and she has counted up to 16 seconds before he starts again. She has heard that sleep apnea can be harmful and asked her husband to be investigated.

On examination, Mr MacDonald has a body mass index of $27kg/m^2$, his nose is patent, pharynx is of normal size with mild erythema, and he has an upper dental prosthesis.

A sleep study shows a sleep efficiency of 75% with a reduction in slow-wave sleep (12%), (normal ~ 20%) and REM sleep (10%), (normal ~ 20%). There were thirteen apneas/hypopneas per hour with minimal oxygen desaturation of 88% and 1% of the time recorded below 90%.

The following points were discussed with the patient and his spouse.

It was explained that the finding of thirteen apneas/hypopneas per hour, in a person who sleeps well and has no daytime symptoms (daytime sleepiness, cognitive disturbances) and normal oxygen, does not require treatment. More specifically, there is no evidence that this finding increases the risk of cardiovascular accident (eg. stroke). Importantly, there is no evidence to date that treatment of minor disturbances in breathing, as in this man, is effective in preventing stroke (*Chapter 8*).

General advice about attention to weight and alcohol was given, emphasizing that if weight increase occurs he should be reassessed. In particular, the occurrence of unrefreshed sleep or daytime lethargy would warrant a full reassessment.

Information about OSA is widely available through newspapers, television and the internet. The reports, however, are often incomplete and not critical. The potential for cardiovascular risk of OSA is often emphasized without any reference to severity of OSA and, in particular, to the degree of oxygen desaturation. The initial criteria for OSA (five or more apneas per hour) were based on a population below the age of 60. The significance of mild sleep apnea, as in this man, is not clear. When healthy, asymptomatic elderly people are studied with overnight polysomnography, disturbed breathing (at least fifteen events per hour) can be found, with significant night to night variability (Lord *et al*, 1991; Mant *et al*, 1995) (*Figure 5.13*). These findings do not appear to be associated with increased morbidity or mortality over time (Phillips *et al*, 1996). It is possible that an increase in disturbed breathing is a biomarker of aging rather than a distinct pathological process

(Bliwise, 1996). This, of course, does not contradict the fact that clinically symptomatic severe OSA can be present at any age.

Central sleep apnea

Case study 6

Mr Paul Andrews is a 52-year-old train driver, presently on a disability pension, who is awaiting cardiac transplantation. He has a severe ischemic cardiomyopathy with a left ventricular ejection fraction of 21%. He is severely restricted in his activities (Class III NYHC). He is on maximal medical therapy, including carvedilol 25 mg twice daily, frusemide 250 mg daily, digoxin 250 μg daily, atorvastatin 40 mg daily. Mr Andrews has type II diabetes, well controlled with diet and metformin. His body mass index is 29.3 kg/m².

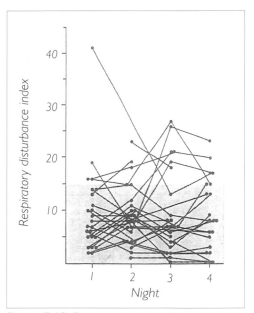

Figure 5.13: Respiratory disturbance index (events/hour sleep) on each of the nights studied. Note that some subjects do not have data for all nights. The shaded area indicates RDI ≤ 15.

Mr Andrews tells his cardiologist he is having a lot of difficulty sleeping and is chronically tired during the day. On specific questioning he says that within a minute or two of falling asleep he suddenly wakes with an intense sense of breathlessness and anxiety. The sensation of breathlessness dissipates within half a minute. He is now very anxious about going to sleep because of this and believes that the anxiety is leading to further difficulty with getting off to sleep. His wife reports that prior to his second operation for coronary artery revasularization 5 years ago he snored, but this has decreased markedly in the last year or two. Mrs Andrews describes a waxing and waning pattern of her husband's breathing when he is asleep, and even sometimes when he is sitting quietly watching television.

Mr Andrews' cardiologist organizes a polysomnography which shows a pattern of cyclical breathing (apnea/hypopnea index 56 per hour) and very disturbed sleep architecture. The breathing pattern is one of slowly waxing and waning efforts with central sleep apneas interspersed with periods of hyperventilation (*Figure 5.14*). Oxygen desaturations are relatively modest with SaO$_2$ fluctuating between approximately 95% and 90%.

Mr Andrews is anxious to know what is causing this breathing disturbance at night and if it is likely to cause his heart function to deteriorate. He asks whether anything can be done to improve his sleep.

It is apparent that Mr Andrews has developed considerable anxiety regarding his experiences of sudden gasping arousals at sleep onset. This may have led to a degree of secondary insomnia which could limit the effectiveness of any treatment. Mr Andrews is offered a trial of CPAP. If this is poorly tolerated and does not resolve his symptoms, one of the newer approaches described below would be used and the therapeutic effectiveness measured by sleep study.

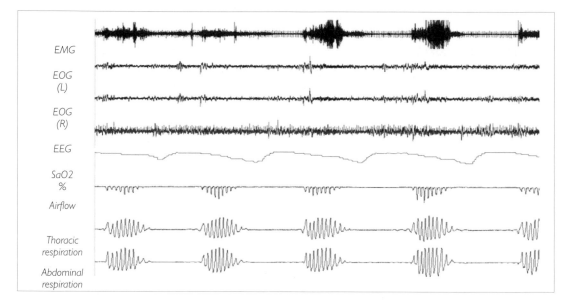

Figure 5.14: Cheyne–Stokes respiration.

Cheyne–Stokes respiration (CSR)

The gradually waxing and waning pattern of breathing is classical of Cheyne–Stokes respiration (CSR). What initiates and perpetuates this form of sleep-disordered breathing has been the subject of much speculation and considerable recent investigation. The central apneas occur in patients who have a high level of resting ventilation (Naughton *et al*, 1993). The cause for increased ventilation is probably a combination of stimulation of juxtacapillary or C-afferent nerve endings in the lung by pulmonary venous congestion and interstitial edema plus an increased chemosensitivity to $PaCO_2$ (Javaheri, 1999).

CSR has been found to be far more common among congestive heart failure (CHF) patients with high pulmonary wedge pressures compared with those with normal pulmonary wedge pressures (Solin *et al*, 1999). Increased resting ventilation causes arterial $PaCO_2$ to be low both awake and during sleep (Naughton *et al*, 1993). In non-REM sleep, if $PaCO_2$ falls below a critical level, ventilation suddenly ceases. This level of $PaCO_2$ is referred to as its apneic threshold (Bradley, 2002). Normally this will be 5–7 mmHg below resting $PaCO_2$ value and require a large preceding increase in ventilation to induce apnea. But, with patients in heart failure and high resting ventilation, the apneic threshold may be only 2–4 mmHg below the resting level. A sigh or two to three slightly larger breaths following say a brief 3–10-second arousal from sleep may be sufficient to trigger a central apnea.

During apnea arterial PO_2 falls, $PaCO_2$ rises and pH decreases. These changes in arterial blood chemistry during apnea might be expected subsequently to stimulate peripheral and central chemoreceptors and cause a gradual resumption of normal breathing patterns (*Figure 5.15*). However, in about 40–50% of patients with CHF (Javaheri *et al*, 1998), a waxing and waning pattern of breathing persists, sometimes for most of the night. This suggests increased 'loop gain' in some patients with CHF.

In control systems that are regulated by feedback loops, theory predicts that when a perturbation in ventilation (eg. central apnea) induces a response (eg. hyperpnea) that is greater than the original perturbation, loop gain will exceed 1 and respiratory control will become unstable. Loop gain of the respiratory control system could be increased in patients with CHF for a number of reasons. For example, increased sensitivity of chemoreceptors, decreased lung volume and therefore lung oxygen stores, prolonged circulation time and delay in feedback to chemoreceptors, and heightened arousal or alerting responses might exaggerate hyperpnea episodes. Patients with CHF and CSR have a higher central chemoreceptor responsiveness to arterial $PaCO_2$ than CHF patients without CSR (Javaheri *et al*, 1999).

CSR is associated with high peripheral and central chemoreceptor sensitivity or high respiratory loop gain (Solin *et al*, 2000). It was long thought that prolonged circulation time might cause CRS in heart failure patients, but recent evidence has thrown doubt on this possibility (Hanly *et al*, 1996: Sin *et al*, 1999). The apneic threshold is higher in men than women (Zhou *et al*, 2000) — that is, men require a smaller fall in $PaCO_2$ to induce apnea and it appears that men also have a larger ventilatory response to brief arousals from sleep than women (Jordan *et al*, 2003). These observations may help explain why CSR is far more common among men than women with heart failure (Hanly *et al*, 1996; Sin *et al*, 1999).

Sleep arousal in CSR occurs at the time of maximal respiratory effort during the hyperpnea phase (Trinder *et al*, 2000). Patients may wake with a start and a sensation of 'air hunger' at this time. Full awakenings are most likely to occur in the transition from wakefulness to sleep. More commonly, arousals are not appreciated by the patient but may cause feelings of tiredness or fatigue on waking. CSR (and arousals) are common in lighter stages of non-REM sleep but rarely occur in REM sleep or 'deep' (stages 3/4) non-REM sleep. However, sleep disruption is

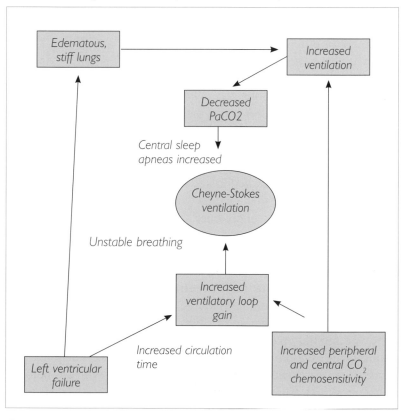

Figure 5.15: Loop gain of the respiratory control (see text).

often so severe that patients do not progress to deeper stages of sleep.

There is evidence of increased sympathetic activity during sleep among patients who have CSR that decreases with CPAP treatment (Naughton *et al*, 1995b). The heightened activity appears to result from an increased frequency of sleep arousals (Naughton *et al*, 1995b). Increased sympathetic activity in chronic heart failure carries with it a poor prognosis (Hanly *et al*, 1996; Lanfranchi *et al*, 1999; Sin *et al*, 1999). Complex arrythmias are more prevalent among patients with CSR and are one potential cause for early death. There is evidence that a reduction of CSR with CPAP, which reduces markers of sympathetic hyperactivity (Naughton *et al*, 1995b), increases left ventricular function (Naughton *et al*, 1995a) and reduces breathlessness and peripheral chemosensitivity. It is not certain whether these improvements with CPAP are attributable to the reduction in sleep-disordered breathing, that is usually incomplete (Naughton *et al*, 1994), or to prolonged mechanical unloading of the left ventricle (reduced LV afterload) during sleep (Naughton *et al*, 1995a) in CSR patients, who usually have worse LV function than those without CSR (Sin *et al*, 2000). A trial of CPAP treatment in patients with CHF and CSR is currently underway to determine whether mortality is reduced by this treatment (Bradley *et al*, 2001). At this time it is not possible to say with certainty whether CSR is an independent risk factor for deterioration in cardiac function or early death in CHF.

Treatments of Cheyne–Stokes respiration

A number of different treatments have been tried to reduce CSR and, therefore, sleep disruption. If better control of heart failure can be achieved by optimizing drug treatment this should be tried first. Reducing pulmonary capillary wedge pressure by more aggressive heart failure treatment has been shown to reduce CSR (Solin *et al*, 1999). Also, the clinical impression from those systematically testing patients with CHF for CSR is that the prevalence of CSR has decreased significantly from the usually quoted figure of 45–50%, since the introduction of the powerful anti-failure drug carvedilol.

Patients should be carefully examined for signs of pulmonary venous congestion or peripheral edema and, if present, consideration given to increasing diuretic dose, then adding spironolactone or further increasing carvedilol. If there is no room to maneuver by adjusting anti-failure drug therapy, the options that can be considered to control CSR include overnight supplemental oxygen, CPAP or bi-level pressure support ventilation.

Supplemental oxygen is easy to administer and is relatively well tolerated by patients. However, it may be difficult to increase the inspired oxygen concentration sufficiently via nasal prongs to eliminate SaO_2 swings. Studies suggest that supplemental oxygen ameliorates, but by no means eliminates, the CSR pattern (Javaheri *et al*, 1999).

Nasal CPAP has been used by the authors to treat CSR in CHF and there is evidence of benefit in terms of left ventricular function, breathlessness and markers of sympathetic hyperactivity, however, but only partial benefit in terms of the CSR pattern and the associated sleep disruption. Compliance is a problem and while some patients will tolerate CPAP for a time, many do not perceive an immediate symptomatic benefit and will not persevere. The application of a nasal CPAP mask to a patient who continues to have central apneas and respiratory-related arousals can lead to further deterioration in sleep architecture.

Other treatments, such as theophylline, a weak respiratory stimulant, and the addition of

CO_2 to the inspirate have been tried, but these approaches appear to be, at best, only partially successful in altering CSR. Two new approaches appear to have considerable promise. First, is a non-invasive servoventilator that detects breath-by-breath effort/flow, and increases the pressure assist via a face or nose mask during periods of apnea or low respiratory effort, while backing off the assist when the patient makes large respiratory efforts. This has been shown to smooth out the breathing patterns of patients with CSR and improve sleep and sleep oxygenation (Teschler *et al*, 2001). Second, is the application of instrumental dead space during sleep to increase $PaCO_2$ and thereby prevent central apneas (Xie *et al*, 1997), which might be highly effective treatment for CSR associated with CHF. The attraction of this method is that, while it will require the patient to wear a mask during sleep, positive pressure does not need to be applied to the airway. Cost of treatment would therefore be minimal. Perhaps, more importantly, if it did eliminate CSR, it would allow studies to be conducted to determine whether CSR is a negative prognostic factor in CHF. Other treatments (eg. positive airway pressure, theophylline) for CSR cannot convincingly demonstrate this since they can have effects on cardiac function independent of changes in CSR. Non-invasive servoventilation seems to be highly effective in eliminating CSR. It may therefore prove to be better tolerated by patients than CPAP, and could be highly effective because of the additional benefits of cardiac afterload and preload reduction.

References

Adams N, Strauss M, Schluchter M, Redline S (2001) Relation of measures of sleep-disordered breathing to neuropsychological functioning. *Am J Respir Crit Care Med* **163**: 1626–31

Ambrogetti A, Olson LG, Saunders NA (1991) Differences in the symptoms of men and women with OSA. *Aust NZ J Med* **21**: 863–6

American Academy of Sleep Medicine Task Force (1999) Sleep-related breathing disorders in adults: Recommendations for syndrome definition and measurement techniques in clinical research. *Sleep* **22**(5): 667–89

American Sleep Disorders Association (1997) *International Classification of Sleep Disorders, Revised: Diagnostic and Coding Manual.* Rochester, Minnesota

American Sleep Disorders Association Report (1995) Practice parameters for the treatment of snoring and OSA with oral appliances. *Sleep* **18**: 511–13

Ancoli-Israel S, Kripke DF, Klauber MR, Fell R, Stepnowsky C, Estline E *et al* (1996) Morbidity, mortality and sleep-disordered breathing in community-dwelling elderly. *Sleep* **19**(4): 277–82

Austroad (2003) *Assessing Fitness to Drive.* Austroad Inc, Sydney

Baldwin CM, Griffith KA, Nieto FJ *et al* (2001) The association of sleep-disordered breathing and sleep symptoms with quality of life in the Sleep Heart Health Study. *Sleep* **24**: 96–105

Ballester E, Badia JR, Hernandez L *et al* (1999) Evidence of the effectiveness of continuous positive airway pressure in the treatment of sleep apnea/hypopnea syndrome. *Am J Respir Crit Care Med* **159**: 495–501

Barbe F, Mayoralas LR, Duran J *et al* (2001) Treatment with continuous positive airway pressure is not effective in patients with sleep apnea but no daytime sleepiness: a randomised, controlled trial. *Ann Intern Med* **134**: 1015–23

Barnes M, Houston D, Worsnop CJ *et al* (2002) A randomised controlled trial of continuous positive airway pressure in mild obstructive sleep apnea. *Am J Respir Crit Care Med* **165**: 773–80

Bearpark H, Elliott L, Grunstein R, Cullen S, Althons W, Sullivan C (1995) Snoring and sleep apnea: a population study in Australian men. *J Res Crit Care Med* **151**: 1459–65

Benumof JL (2002) Obstructive sleep apnea in the adult obese patient: implications for airway management. *Anesthesiology Clin N Am* **20**: 789–811

Bettega G, Pépin J-L, Veale D, Deschaux C, Raphaël B, Lévy L (2000) Obstructive sleep apnea syndrome. Fifty-one consecutive patients treated by maxillofacial surgery. *Am J Respir Crit Care Med* **162**: 641–9

Billiard M, Dauvilliers Y (2001) Idiopathic hypersomnia. *Sleep Med Rev* **5**: 351–60

Bixler EO, Vgontzas AN, Lin HM *et al* (2001) Prevalence of sleep-disordered breathing in women. *Am J Respir Crit Care Med* **163**: 608–13

Black JE, Hirshkowitz M (2005) Modafinil for treatment of residual excessive sleepiness in nasal continuous positive airway pressure-treated obstructive apnea/hypopnea syndrome. *Sleep* **28**(4): 464–71

Bliwise DL (1996) Chronologic age, physiologic age and mortality in sleep apnea. *Sleep* **19**(4): 275–6

Bliwise DL, Nekich JC, Dement WC (1991) Relative validity of self-reported snoring as symptom of sleep apnea in a sleep clinic population. *Chest* **99**: 600–8

Bloom JW, Kaltenborn WT, Quen SF (1988) Risk factors in a general population for snoring. Importance of cigarette smoking and obesity. *Chest* **93**: 678–83

Boudewyns A, Van de Heyning P (2000) Temperature-controlled radiofrequency tissue volume reduction of the soft palate (somnoplasty) in the treatment of habitual snoring: results of a European multicenter trial. *Acta Oto-Laryngol* **120**(8): 981–5

Bradley TD (2002) Crossing the threshold: implications for central sleep apnea. *Am J Res Crit Care Me*d **165**(9): 1203–4

Bradley TD, Logan AG. Floras JS (2001) The CANPAP investigators. Rationale and design of the Canadian Continuous Positive Airway Pressure Trial for congestive heart failure patients with central sleep apnea. *Can J Cardiol* **17**(6): 677–84

Braver HM, Block AJ, Perri MG (1995) Treatment of snoring. Combined weight loss, sleeping on side, and nasal spray. *Chest* **107**(5): 1283–8

Bridgman SA, Dunn KM, Ducharme F (1997) *Surgery for OSA* (updated 12/11/97). The Cochrane Database of Systematic reviews: Cochrane Collaboration, Update Software, Oxford

Browman CP, Sampson MG, Yolles FS, Gujavarty SK, Weiler SJ, Walsleben JA *et al* (1984) Obstructive sleep apnea and body weight. *Chest* **85**: 435–6

Burwell C, Robin E, Whaley RB, Kelman A (1956) Extreme obesity associated with alveolar hypoventilation: A Pickwickian syndrome. *Am J Med* **21**: 811–18

Cartwright R, Venkatesan TK, Caldarelli D, Diaz F (2000) Treatments of snoring: a comparison of somnoplasty and an oral appliance. *Laryngoscope* **110**(10 pt 1): 1680–3

Chervin Rd, Zallek SN, Lin X, Hall JM, Sharma N, Hedger KM (2000) Sleep disordered breathing in patients with cluster headache. *Neurology* **54**: 2302–6

Cheshire K, Engleman H, Deary I *et al* (1992) Factors impairing daytime performance in patients with sleep apnea/hypopnea syndrome. *Arch Intern Med* **152**: 538–41

Chugh DK, Weaver TE, Dinges DF (1996) Neurobehavioural consequences of arousals. *Sleep* **19**(10): S198–S201

Cistulli PA, Sullivan CE (1993) Sleep disordered breathing in Marfan's syndrome. *Am Rev Respir Crit Care Med* **147**: 645–8

Crocker BD, Olson GL, Saunders NA, Hensley MJ, McKeon JS, Murree-Allen K *et al* (1990) Estimation of the probability of disturbed breathing during sleep before a sleep study. *Am Rev Respir Dis* **142**: 14–18

Dagan Y, Abadi J, Lifschitz A, Laron Z (2001) Severe obstructive sleep apnea in an adult patient with Laron syndrome. *Growth Horm IgF Res* **11**(4): 247–9

Davies RJO, Stradling JR (1990) The relationship between neck circumference, radiographic pharyngeal anatomy, and the OSA syndrome. *Eur Respir J* **3**: 509–14

Davies RJO, Stradling JR (1996) The epidemiology of sleep apnea. *Thorax* **51**(suppl 2): S65–S70

Dealberto M-J, Ferber C, Garma L, Lemoine P, Alperovitch A (1994) Factors related to sleep apnea syndrome in sleep clinic patients. *Chest* **105**: 1753–8

Dean AC, Graham BA, Dalakas M, Sato S (1998) Sleep apnea in patients with postpolio syndrome. *Ann Neurol* **43**: 661–4

Dixon JB, Schacter LM, O'Brien PE (2001) Sleep disturbance and obesity. Changes following surgically induced weight loss. *Arch Intern Med* **161**(1): 102–6

Doherty LS, Kiely JL, Lawless G, McNicholas WT (2003) Impact of nasal continuous positive airway pressure therapy on the quality of life of bed partners of patients with obstructive sleep apnea syndrome. *Chest* **124**(6): 2209–14

Douglas N (2000) Upper airway resistance syndrome is not a distinct syndrome. *Am J Respir Crit Care Med* **161**: 1413–16

Dowdell WT, Javaheri S, McGinnis W (1990) Cheyne–Stokes respiration presenting as sleep apnea syndrome. *Am Rev Respir Dis* **141**: 871–9

Edwards N, Wilcox I, Sullivan CE (1998) Sleep apnea in women. *Thorax* **53**(suppl 3): S12–S15

Engleman HM (2002) When does 'mild' obstructive sleep apnea/hypopnea syndrome merit continuous positive airway pressure treatment? *Am J Respir Crit Care Med* **165**: 743–5

Engleman HM, Joffe D (1999) Neuropsychological function in OSA. *Sleep Med Rev* **3**: 59–78

Engleman HM, Kingshott RN, Wraith PK *et al* (1999) Randomized placebo-controlled crossover trial of continuous positive airway pressure for mild sleep apnea/hypopnea syndrome. *Am J Respir Crit Care Med* **159**: 461–67

Engleman HM, Martin SE, Dreary IJ, Douglas NJ (1997) Effect of CPAP therapy on daytime function in patients with mild sleep apnea/hypopnoea syndrome. *Thorax* **52**: 114–9

Engleman HM, Martin SE, Deary IJ *et al* (1994) Effect of CPAP treatment on daytime function in sleep apnea/hypopnoea syndrome. *Lancet* **343**: 572–5

Engleman HM, Martin SE, Kingshott RN *et al* (1998) Randomised placebo controlled trial of daytime function after continuous positive airway pressure (CPAP) therapy for the sleep apnea/hypopnoea syndrome. *Thorax* **53**: 341–5

Engleman HM, McDonald JP, Graham D *et al* (2002) Randomized crossover trial of two treatments for sleep apnea/hypopnea syndrome. *Am J Respir Crit Care Med* **166**: 855–9

Fairbanks NF, Fujita S, Ikematsu T, Simmons FB (1987) *Snoring and OSA*. Raven Press, New York

Fein AM, Niederman MS, Imbriano L, Rosen H (1987) Reversal of sleep apnea in uremia by dialysis. *Arch Intern Med* **147**: 1355–6

Ferguson KA, Lowe AA, Ryan F, Fleetham JA (1995) The relationship between obesity and craniofacial structure in obstructive sleep apnea. *Chest* **108**: 375–81

Ferri R, Curzi-Dascalova L, Del Gracco S, Elia M, Musumeci SA, Stefanini MC (1997) Respiratory patterns during sleep in Down's syndrome: the importance of central apneas. *J Sleep Res* **6**(2): 134–41

Finn L, Young T, Palta M, Fryback DG (1998) Sleep-disordered breathing and self-reported general health status in the Wisconsin Sleep Cohort Study. *Sleep* **21**: 701–6

Fischer Y, Hafner B, Mann WJ (2000) Radiofrequency ablation of the soft palate (somnoplasty). A new method in the treatment of habitual and obstructive snoring. *HNO* **48**(1): 33–40

Flemons WW (2002) Obstructive sleep apnea. *N Engl J Med* **347**: 498–504

Flenely DC (1985) Sleep in chronic obstructive lung disease. *Clin Chest Med* **6**: 651–61

Franklin KA, Gíslason T, Omenaas E, Jõgi R, Jensen EJ, Lindberg E *et al* (2004) The Influence of Active and Passive Smoking on Habitual Snoring. *Am J Resp Crit Care Med* **170**: 799–803

Friedman M, Tanyeri H, La Rosa M, Landsberg R, Vaidyanathan K, Pieri S, Caldarelli D (1999) Clinical predictors of obstructive sleep apnea. *Laryngoscope* **109**(12): 1901–7

Gaustaut H, Tassinari CA, Duron B (1966) Polygraphic study of the episodic diurnal and nocturnal (Hypnic and respiratory) manifestations of the Pickwick syndrome. *Brain Res* **2**: 167–86

George CFP (2001) Reduction in motor vehicle collisions following treatment of sleep apnea with nasal CPAP. *Thorax* **56**: 508–12

Gislason T, Almqvist M *et al* (1988) Prevalence of sleep apnea syndrome among Swedish men — an epidemiological study. *J Clin Epidemiol* **41**(6): 571–6

Gotsopoulos H, Chen C, Qian J, Cistulli PA (2002) Oral appliance therapy improves symptoms in obstructive sleep apnea. *Am J Respir Crit Care Med* **166**: 743–8

Gould GA, Whyte KF, Rhind GB, Airlie MAA, Cotterall JR, Shepiro CM, Douglas NJ (1988) The sleep hypopnoea syndrome. *Am Rev Respir Dis* **137**: 885–98

Grunstein R (1996) Metabolic aspects of sleep apnea. *Sleep* **19**(10): S218–S220

Grunstein R (2002) Hormonal and metabolic disturbances in sleep apnea in breathing disorders. In: McNicholas WT, Philipson EA, eds. *Sleep*. Saunders, London

Grunstein R, Sullivan CE (1988) Sleep apnea and hypothyroidism: mechanisms and management. *Am J Med* **85**: 775–9

Guardiano SA, Scott JA, Ware JC, Schechner SA (2003) The long-term results of gastric bypass on indexes of sleep apnea. *Chest* **124**(4):1615–9

Guillenimault C, Chowdhuri S (2000) Upper airway resistance syndrome is a distinct syndrome. *Am J Respir Crit Care Med* **161**: 1412–6

Guillenimault C, Philip P (1996) Tiredness and somnolence despite initial treatment of obstructive sleep apnea syndrome (what to do when an OSAS patient stays hypersomnolent despite treatment). *Sleep* **19**(9): S117–S122

Guillenimault C, Stoohs P, Clerk A, Cetel M, Maistres P (1993) A cause of excessive daytime sleepiness: the upper airway resistance syndrome. *Chest* **104**: 781–7

Hack M, Davies RJO, Mullins R *et al* (2000) Randomised prospective parallel trial of therapeutic versus subtherapeutic nasal continuous positive airway pressure on simulated steering performance in patients with OSA. *Thorax* **55**: 224–31

Hamilton GS, Solin P, Naughton MT (2004) Obstructive sleep apnoea and cardiovascular disease. *Internal Med J* **34**: 420–6

Hanly PJ, Zuberi-Khokhar NS (1996) Increased mortality associated with Cheyne–Stokes respiration in patients with congestive heart failure. *Am J Respir Crit Care Med* **153**: 272–6

He J, Kryger MH, Zorick FJ *et al* (1988) Mortality and apnea index in obstructive sleep apnea: experience in 385 male patients. *Chest* **94**: 9–14

Hiremath AS, Hillman DR, James AL, Noffsinger WJ, Platt RP, Singer SL (1998) Relationship between difficult tracheal intubation and obstructive sleep apnea. *Br J Anaesth* **80**: 606–11

Hirshkowitz M, Karakan I, Gurakar A, Williams RL (1989) Hypertension, erectile dysfunction and occult sleep apnea. *Sleep* **12**(3): 223–32

Hoffstein V (1996) Snoring. *Chest* **109**: 201–22

Hoffstein V, Chan CK, Slutsky AS (1991) Sleep apnea and systemic hypertension: A causal association review. *Am J Med* **91**(2): 190–6

Hoffstein V, Mateika S, Metes A (1993) Effect of nasal dilation on snoring and apneas during different stages of sleep. *Sleep* **16**(4): 360–5

Horstmann S, Hess CW, Bassetti C, Gugger M, Mathis J (2000) Sleepiness-related accidents in sleep apnea patients. *Sleep* **23**(3): 383–9

Hosselet JJ, Ayppa I, Normal RG, Krieger AC, Rapoport DM (2001) Classification of sleep-disordered breathing. *Am J Respir Crit Care Med* **163**: 398–405

Hu FB, Willett WC, Colditz GA *et al* (1999) Prospective study of snoring and risk of hypertension in women. *Am J Epidemiol* **150**: 806–16

Issa FG, Sullivan CE (1982) Alcohol, snoring and sleep apnea. *J Neurol Neurosurg Psychiatry* **45**: 353–9

Janson C, Noges E, Svedberg-Randt S, Lindberg E (2000) What characterises patients who are unable to tolerate continuous positive pressure (CPAP) treatment? *Respir Med* **94**:145–9

Javaheri S (1999) A mechanism of central sleep apnea in patients with heart failure. *N Engl J Med* **341**(13): 949–54

Javaheri S, Ahmed M, Parker TJ, Brown CR (1999) Effects of nasal O_2 on sleep-related disordered breathing in ambulatory patients with stable heart failure. *Sleep* **22**(8): 1101–6

Javaheri S, Parker TJ, Liming JD *et al* (1998) Sleep apnea in 81 ambulatory male patients with stable heart failure. Types and their prevalences, consequences, and presentations. *Circulation* **97**: 2154–9

Jenkinson C, Davies RJ, Mullins R, Stradling JR (1999) Comparison of therapeutic and subtherapeutic nasal continuous positive airway pressure for OSA: a randomised prospective parallel trial. *Lancet* **353**: 2100–05

Jennum P, Hein HO, Suadicani P, Gyntelberg F (1995b) Risk of ischemic heart disease in self-reported snorers. *Chest* **108**: 138–42

Jennum P, Hein HO, Suadicani P, Sorenson H, Gyntelberg F (1995a) Snoring, family history and genetic markers in men. The Copenhagen Male Study. *Chest* **107**: 1289–93

Johns MW (1991) A new method for measuring daytime sleepiness. *Sleep* **14**: 540–5

Jokic R, Klimaszewski A, Crossley M, Sridhar G, Fitzpatrick MF (1999) Positional treatment vs CPAP in patients with positional OSA. *Chest* **115**: 771–81

Jordan AS, Eckert DJ, Catcheside PG, McEvoy RD (2003) Ventilatory response to brief arousal from non-rapid eye movement sleep is greater in men than in women. *Am J Respir Crit Care Med* **168**: 1512–9

Kalan A, Kenyon GS, Seemungal TA, Wedzicha JA (1999) Adverse effects of nasal continuous positive airway pressure therapy in sleep apnea. *J Laryngol Otol* **113**: 888–92

Kapur VK, Baldwin CM, Resnick HE, Gottlieb DJ, Nieto FJ (2005). Sleepiness in patients with moderate to severe sleep-disordered breathing. *Sleep* **28**(4): 472–7

Kiely JL, Murphy M, McNicholas WT (1999) Subjective efficacy of nasal CPAP therapy in OSA syndrome: a prospective controlled study. *Eur Respir J* **13**: 1086–90

Kim HC, Young T, Matthews CG *et al* (1997) Sleep-disordered breathing and neuropsychological deficits. *Am J Respir Crit Care Med* **156**: 1813–9

Kimmel PL, Miller G, Mendelson WB (1989) Sleep apnea syndrome in chronic renal disease. *Am J Med* **86**: 308–14

Kingshott RN, Venelle M, Coleman EL *et al* (2001) Randomized, double-blind, placebo-controlled crossover trial of modafinil in the treatment of residual excessive daytime sleepiness in the sleep apnea/hypopnea syndrome. *Am J Respir Crit Care Med* **163**: 918–23

Kleitman N (1963) *Sleep and Wakefulness*. The University of Chicago Press, Chicago: 48–50

Koskenvuo M, Kaprio J, Telakivi T *et al* (1987) Snoring as a risk factor for ischaemic heart disease and stroke in men. *Br Med J* **294**: 16–19

Koskenvuo M, Partinen M, Kaprio J (1985) Snoring and disease. *Ann Clin Res* **17**: 247–51

Kraus MA, Hamburger RJ (1997) Sleep apnea and renal failure. *Adv Peritoneal Dialysis* **13**: 88–92

Kribbs NB, Pack AI, Kline LR *et al* (1993) Objective measurement of patterns of nasal CPAP use by patients with OSA. *Am Rev Respir Dis* **147**: 887–95

Krol, RC, Huuth SC, Bartlett D (1984) Selective reduction of genioglossal muscle activity by alcohol in normal human subjects. *Am Rev Respir Dis* **129**: 242–50

Kuhn M, Lutolf M *et al* (1999) The eye catcher. Ondine's curse. *Respiration* **66(3)**: 265

Kushida CA, Rao S, Guilleminault C *et al* (1999) Cervical positional effects on snoring and apneas. *Sleep Res Online* **2**: 7–10

Kushida CA, Sherill CM, Hong SC *et al* (2001) Cervical positioning for reduction of sleep-disordered breathing in mild-to-moderate OSAS. *Sleep Breath* **5**: 71–8

Lanfranchi PA, Braghiroli A, Bosimini E, Mazzuero G, Colombo R, Donner CF, Giannuzzi P (1999) Prognostic value of nocturnal Cheyne–Stokes respiration in chronic heart failure. *Circulation* **99**(11): 1435–40

Lamphere J, Roehrs T, Wittig R *et al* (1996) Recovery of alertness after nasal CPAP in apnea. *Chest* **96**(6): 1364–7

Lavie P (1993) Incidence of sleep apnoea in a presumably healthy working population. *Sleep* **6**: 312–8

Lavie P, Herer P, Hoffstein V (2000) OSA syndrome as a risk factor for hypertension: population study. *Br Med J* **320**: 479–82

Lavie P, Herer P, Peled R, Berger J, Yoffe N, Zomer J, Rubin AE (1995) Mortality in sleep apnea patients: a multivariate analysis of risk factors. *Sleep* **18**(3): 147–57

Lehmukhl P, Prarss D, Pilchmayr I (1987) General anaesthesia and postnarcotic sleep disorders. *Neuropsychobiology* **18**(1): 37–42

Levanon A, Tarasuk A, Tal A (1999) Sleep characteristics in children with Down's syndrome. *J Paediatr* **134**(6): 755–60

Lindberg E, Gislason T (2000) Epidemiology of sleep-related obstructive breathing. *Sleep Med Rev* **4**: 411–33

Lindman R, Bondemark L (2001) A review of dental devices in the treatment of habitual snoring and OSA. *Swed Dental J* **25**: 39–51

Liistro G, Rombaux P, Dury M, Pieters T, Aubert G, Rodenstein DO (1998) Effects of Breathe Right™ on snoring: a polysomnographic study. *Respiratory Med* **92**(8): 1076–8

Loadsman JA, Hillman DR (2001) and sleep. *Br J Anaesthesia* **86**(2): 254–66

Lord S, Sawyer B, O'Connell D, King M, Pond D, Eyland A *et al* (1991) Night-to-night variability of disturbed breathing during sleep in an elderly community sample. *Sleep* **14**(3): 252–8

Loube, DI, Gay PC, Strohl KP *et al* (1999) Indications for positive airway pressure treatment of adult obstructive sleep apnea patients: a consensus statement. *Chest* **115**: 863–5

Lugaresi E, Cirignotta F, Coccagna G *et al* (1980) Some epidemiological data on snoring and cardiocirculatory disturbances. *Sleep* **3**: 221–4

Lugaresi E, Cirignotta F, Montagna P, Zucconi M (1988) Snoring: Pathophysiology and clinical consequences. *Semin Respiratory Med* **9**(6): 577–85

Lugaresi E, Mondini S, Zuicconi M. Montegna P, Cirignotta F (1983) Staging of heavy snorers' disease. A proposal. *Bull Europ Physiopath Resp* **19**: 590–4

Lyons MF, Cameron DA, Banham SW (2001) Snoring, sleep apnea and the role of dental appliances. *Dental Update* 28: 254–6

Mant A, King M, Saunders NA, Pond CD, Goode E, Hewitt H (1995) Four-year follow-up of mortality and sleep-related respiratory disturbance in non-demented seniors. *Sleep* **18**(6): 433–8

Marcus CL, Keens TG, Bautistad B, Von Pechman WS, Ward SL (1991) OSA in children with Down's syndrome. *Paediatrics* **88**(1): 132–9

Marin J, Gascon J, Gispert J (1997) The prevalence of sleep apnoea syndrome in the Spanish adult population. *Int J Epidemiol* **26**: 381–6

Marin JM, Carrizo SJ, Vicente E, Agusti AG (2005) Long-term cardiovascular outcomes in men with obstructive sleep apnoea-hypopnoea with or without treatment with continuous positive airway pressure: an observational study. *Lancet* **365**: 1046–53

McArdle N, Devereux G, Heidarnejad *et al* (1999) Long-term use of CPAP therapy for sleep apnea/hypopnea syndrome. *Am J Respir Crit Care Med* **159**: 1108–14

McArdle N, Kingshott R, Engleman HM *et al* (2001) Partners of patients with sleep apnea/ hypopnoea syndrome: effect of CPAP treatment on sleep quality and quality of life. *Thorax* **56**: 513–18

Mehta A, Qian J Petocz M *et al* (2001) A randomized, controlled study of a mandibular advancement splint for obstructive sleep apnea. *Am J Respir Crit Care Med* **163**: 1457–61

Mendelson WB, Wadhawa NK, Greenberg HE, Gujavarty K, Bergofsky E (1990) Effects of haemodialysis on sleep apnea syndrome in end stage renal disease. *Clin Nephrol* **33**(5): 247–51

Miljeteig H, Hateika S, Haight JS *et al* (1994) Subjective and objective assessment of uvulopalatoplasty for treatment of snoring and OSA. *Am J Respir Crit Care Med* **150**: 1286–90

Millman RP, Bevilacqua J, Peterson DD, Park AI (1983) Central sleep apnea in hypothyroidism. *Am Review Resp Dis* **127**: 504–7

Monasterio C, Vidal S, Duran J *et al* (2001) Effectiveness of continuous positive airway pressure in mild sleep apnea-hypopnea syndrome. *Am J Respir Crit Care Med* **164**: 939–43

Montserrat JM, Ferrer M, Hernandez L *et al* (2001) Effectiveness of CPAP treatment in daytime function in sleep apnea syndrome: a randomised controlled study with an optimised placebo. *Am J Respir Crit Care Med* **164**: 608–13

National Health and Medical Research Council (2000) *Effectiveness of nasal continuous positive airway pressure (nCPAP) in OSA in adults*. National Health and Medical Research Council, Canberra, Australia

Naughton MT, Benard DC, Liu PP, Rutherford R, Rankin F, Bradley TD (1995a) Effects of nasal CPAP on sympathetic activity in patients with heart failure and central sleep apnea. *Am J Respir Crit Care Med* **152**(2): 473–9

Naughton MT, Benard DC, Rutherford R, Bradley TD (1994) Effect of continuous positive airway pressure on central sleep apnea and nocturnal PCO_2 in heart failure. *Am J Respir Crit Care Med* **150**(6 Pt 1): 1598–604

Naughton MT, Bernard D, Tam A, Rutherford R, Bradley TD (1993) Role of hyperventilation in the pathogenesis of central sleep apneas in patients with congestive heart failure. *Am Rev Respir Dis* **148**(2): 330–8

Naughton MT, Bradley TD (1998) Sleep apnea in congestive heart failure. *Clin Chest Med* **19**: 99–114

Naughton MT, Liu PP, Bernard DC, Goldstein RS, Bradley TD (1995b) Treatment of congestive heart failure and Cheyne-Stokes respiration during sleep by continuous positive airway pressure. *Am J Respir Crit Care Med* **151**(1): 92–7

Nelson LM (2000) Radiofrequency treatment for obstructive tonsillar hypertrophy. *Arch Otolaryngol Head Neck Surg* **126**(6): 739–40

Newman AB, Nieto FJ, Guidry U *et al* (2001) Relation of sleep-disordered breathing to cardiovascular disease risk factors — the Sleep Heart Health Study. *Am J Epidemiol* **154**: 50–9

Oksenberg A, Silverberg DS, Arons E, Radwan H (1997) Positional vs nonpositional obstructive sleep apnea patients. *Chest* **112**: 629–39

Olson LG, King MT, Hensley MJ, Saunders NA (1995) A community study of snoring and sleep-disordered breathing. *Symptoms Am J Respir Crit Care Med* **152**: 207–10

Orr WC, Levine NS, Buchanan RT (1987) The effect of cleft palate repair and pharyngeal flap surgery on upper airway obstruction during surgery. *J Plastic Reconstruction Surg* **80**(20): 226–32

Ostermeier AM, Roizen MF, Hautkappe M, Klock PA, Klafta JM (1997) Three sudden postoperative respiratory arrests associated with epidural opioids in patients with sleep apnea. *Anesth Analg* **85**: 542–60

Pantin CC, Hillman DR, Tennant M (1999) Dental side-effects of an oral device to treat snoring and obstructive sleep apnea. *Sleep* **22**(2): 237–40

Parra O, Arboix A, Montserrat JM, Quintó L, Bechich S, Garcia-Eroles L (2004) Sleep-related breathing disorders: impact on mortality of cerebrovascular disease. *Eur Respir J* **24**: 267–72

Peppard PE, Young T, Palta M, Sketrud J (2000) Prospective study of the association between sleep-disordered breathing and hypertension. *N Engl J Med* **342**: 1378–84

Peppard PE, Young T, Palta M *et al* (2000) Longitudinal study of moderate weight change and sleep-disordered breathing. *JAMA* **284**: 3025–21

Pepin JL, Veale D, Mayer P, Bettega G, Wuyam B, Levy P (1996) Critical analysis of the results of surgery in the treatment of snoring, upper airway resistance syndrome (UARS), and obstructive sleep apnea (OSA). *Sleep* **19**(9): S90–S100

Petit F-X, Pepin J-L, Bettega G *et al* (2002) Mandibular advancement devices; Rate of contraindications in 100 consecutive sleep apnea patients. *Am J Respir Crit Care Med* **166**: 274–8

Phillips BA, Berry DTR, Lipke-Molby TC (1996) Sleep-disordered breathing in healthy, aged persons. Fifth and final year follow-up. *Chest* **110**: 654–8

Phillipson EA (1993) Sleep apnea — a major public health problem. *N Engl J Med* **328**(17): 1230–5

Popescu G, Latham M, Allgar V, Elliott MW (2001) Continuous positive airway pressure for sleep apnea/hypopnoea syndrome: usefulness of a 2-week trial to identify factors associated with long term use. *Thorax* **56**: 727–33

Rajala R, Partinen M, Sane T, Pelkonen R, Huikuri K, Seppalainen AM (1991) Obstructive sleep apnoea syndrome in morbidly obese patients. *J Internal Med* **230**(2): 125–9

Rauscher H, Formanek D, Popp W *et al* (1993) Self-reported vs measured compliance with nasal CPAP for OSA. *Thorax* **48**: 529–33

Redline S, Adams N, Strauss ME *et al* (1998) Improvement of mild sleep-disordered breathing with CPAP compared with conservative therapy. *Am J Respir Crit Care Med* **157**: 858–65

Redline S, Tishler PV (2000) The genetics of sleep apnea. *Sleep Med Rev* **4**(6): 583–602

Richman RM, Elliott LM, Burns CM, Bearpark HM, Steinbeck KS, Caterson ID (1994) The prevalence of obstructive sleep apnoea in an obese female population *Int J Obesity Related Metabolic Disorders; J Int Assoc Study of Obesity* **18**(3): 173–7

Riley RW, Powell NB, Li KK, Guilleminault C (2000) Surgical therapy for OSA-hypopnea syndrome. In: Kryger MH, Roth T, Dement WC, eds. *Principles and Practice of Sleep Medicine*. Saunders, Philadelphia

Roebuck T, Solin P, Kaye DM, Bergin P, Baily M, Naughton MT (2004) Increased long-term mortality in heart failure due to sleep apnoea is not yet proven. *Eur Respir J* **23**: 735–40

Ryan CF (1997) Laser assisted uvulopalatoplasty in sleep-disordered breathing. *Thorax* **52**: 5–8

Samet JM, Nieta FJ, Pungabi NM (2000) Sleep-disordered breathing and hypertension. *AJRCCM* **161**: 1409–11

Sanner BM, Klewer J, Trumm A *et al* (2000) Long-term treatment with continuous positive airway pressure improves quality of life in OSA syndrome. *Eur Respir J* **16**: 118–22

Saunders NA, Vandeleur T, Deves J, Salmon A, Gyulay S, Crocker B, Hensley M (1989) Uvulo palatopharyngoplasty as a treatment for snoring. *Med J Australia* **150**: 177–82

Scharf MB, Stover R, McDannold MD *et al* (1999) Outcome evaluation of long-term continuous positive airway pressure therapy in obstructive sleep apnea. *Am J Therapeut* **6**: 293–7

Schellenberg JB, Maislin G, Schwab RJ (2000) Physical findings and risk for obstructive sleep apnea. The importance of oropharyngeal structures. *Am J Respir Crit Care Med* **162**(2 Pt 1): 740–8

Schwartz JR, Hirshkowitz M, Erman MK, Schmidt-Nowara W (2003) Modafinil as adjunct therapy for daytime sleepiness in obstructive sleep apnea: a 12-week open-label study. *Chest* **124**(6): 2192–9

Seneviratne U, Puvanendran K (2004) Excessive daytime sleepiness in obstructive sleep apnea: prevalence, severity and predictors. *Sleep Med* **5**: 339–43

Severinghaus JW, Mitchell R (1985) Ondine's curse. Failure of respiratory center automaticity while awake. *Clin Res* **10**: 122

Shahar E, Whitney CW, Redline S *et al* (2001) Sleep-disordered breathing and cardiovascular disease. *Am J Respir Crit Care Med* **163**: 19–25

Shepertycky MR, Banno K, Kryger M (2005) Differences between men and women in the clinical presentation of patients diagnosed with obstructive sleep apnea syndrome. *Sleep* **28**(3): 309–14

Sher AE, Schectman KB, Piccirillo JF (1996) The efficacy of surgical modifications of the upper airway in adults with OSA syndrome. *Sleep* **19**: 156–77

Shneerson J, Wright J (2002) *Lifestyle modification for OSA* (updated 30/05/01). The Cochrane Database of Systematic Reviews: Cochrane Collaboration, Oxford. Update Software, Issue 2

Sin DD, Fitzgerald F, Parker JD, Newton G, Floras JS, Bradley TD (1999) Risk factors for central and obstructive sleep apnea in 450 men and women with congestive heart failure. [See comments]. *Am J Respir Crit Care Med* **160**(4):1101–6

Sin DD, Logan AG, Fitzgerald FS, Liu PP, Bradley TD (2000) Effects of continuous positive airway pressure on cardiovascular outcomes in heart failure patients with and without Cheyne-Stokes respiration. *Circulation* **102**(1): 61–6

Sin DD, Mayers I, Man GC, Ghahary A, Pawluk L (2002) Can continuous positive airway pressure therapy improve the general health status of patients with obstructive sleep apnea?: a clinical effectiveness study. *Chest* **122**(5): 1679–85

Solin P, Bergin P, Richardson M, Kaye DM, Walters EH, Naughton MT (1999) Influence of pulmonary capillary wedge pressure on central apnea in heart failure. *Circulation* **99**: 1574–9

Solin P, Roebuck T, Johns DP, Walters EH, Naughton MT (2000) Peripheral and central ventilatory responses in central sleep apnea with and without congestive heart failure. *Am J Respir Crit Care Med* 162: 2194–200

Stoohs RA, Dement WC (1993) Snoring and sleep-related breathing abnormality during partial sleep deprivation. *N Engl J Med* **328**: 1279

Stradling JR (1990) Clinical presentation of sleep apnoea. *Eur Respiratory J* **11**: 548s–549s

Stradling JR, Crosby JH (1991) Predictors and prevalence of obstructive sleep apnoea and snoring in 1001 middle-aged men. *Thorax* **46**: 85–90

Strohl KP (1996) Diabetes and sleep apnea. *Sleep* **19**(10): S225–S228

Strohl KP, Redline S (1996) Recognition of obstructive sleep apnea. *Am J Respir Crit Care Med* **154**: 279–89

Tegelberg A, Wilhelmsson B, Walker-Engstrom ML (1999) Effects and adverse events of a dental appliance for treatment of OSA. *Swed Dental J* **23**: 117–26

Teschler H, Dohring J, Wang YM, Berthon-Jones M (2001) Adaptive pressure support servo-ventilation: a novel treatment for Cheyne–Stokes respiration in heart failure. *Am J Respir Crit Care Med* **164**(4): 614–9

Trinder J, Merson R, Rosenberg JI, Fitzgerald F, Kleiman J, Bradley TD (2000) Pathophysiological interactions of ventilation, arousals, and blood pressure oscillations during Cheyne-Stokes respiration in patients with heart failure. *Am J Respir Crit Care Med* **162**(3 Pt 1): 808–13

Uong EC, McDonough JM, Tayag-Kier CE, Zhao H, Hazelgrove J, Mahboubi S *et al* (2001) Magnetic resonance imaging of the upper airway in children with Down's syndrome. *Am J Resp Crit Care Med* **163**(3C PTI): 731–6

Vgontzas AN, Bixler EO, Tan T-L, Kantner D, Martin F, Kales A (1998) Obesity without sleep apnea is associated with daytime sleepiness. *Arch Intern Med* **158**: 1333–37

Wetter DW, Young TB, Bidwell TR, Badr MS, Palta M (1994) Smoking as a risk factor for sleep disorders breathing. *Arch Intern Med* **154**: 2219–24

Wilhelmsson B, Tegelberg A, Walker-Engstrom ML *et al* (1999) A prospective randomised study of a dental appliance compared with uvulopalatoplasty in the treatment of OSA. *Acta Oto-Laryngol* **119**: 503–9

Worsnop CJ, Naughton MT, Barter ED, Morgan TO, Anderson IA, Pierce RJ (1998) The prevalence of OSA in hypertension. *Am J Resp Crit Care Med* **157**: 111–15

Wright J, White J, Ducharme F (2002) *Continuous positive airways pressure for OSA* (updated 01/03/98). The Cochrane Database of Systematic Reviews: Cochrane Collaboration, Oxford. Update Software, Issue 2

Xie A, Rankin F, Rutherford R, Bradley TD (1997) Effects of inhaled CO_2 and added dead space on idiopathic central sleep apnea. *J Appl Physiol* **82**(3): 918–26

Young T, Palta M, Dempsey J *et al* (1993) The occurrence of sleep-disordered breathing among middle-aged adults. *N Engl J Med* **328**: 1230–5

Young T, Finn L, Kim H (1997) Nasal obstruction as a risk factor for sleep-disordered breathing. The University of Wisconsin Sleep and Respiratory Research Group. *J Allergy Clin Immunol* **99**(2): S757–62

Young T, Palta M, Dempsey J, Skatrud J, Weber S, Badr S (1993) The occurrence of sleep-disordered breathing among middle-aged adults. *N Engl J Med* **328**(17): 1230–5

Young T, Peppard PE (2002) Epidemiology of obstructive sleep apnea. In: McNicholas WT, Phillipson EA, eds. *Breathing Disorders During Sleep*. WB Saunders, London

Young T, Peppard PE, Gottlieb DJ (2002) Epidemiology of OSA: A population health perspective. *Am J Respir Crit Care Med* 165: 1217–39

Zhou XS, Shahbuddin S, Zahn BR, Babcock MA, Badr MS (2000) Effect of gender on the development of hypocapnic apnea/hypopnea during NREM sleep. *J Appl Physiol* **89**: 192–9

Zozula R, Rosen R (2001) Compliance with continuous positive airway pressure therapy: assessing and improving treatment outcomes. *Curr Opin Pulm Med* **7**: 391–8

Appendix: Obstructive sleep apnea and anesthesia

Patients are increasingly being referred for assessment of sleep apnea prior to surgical procedures because of the increased risk of perioperative complications (Benumof, 2002).

Patients with difficult perioperative airway management, intubation at induction of general anesthesia and at extubation time, show anatomical features which are present in patients with obstructive sleep apnea (short neck, small receding chin, large tongue, edema of the pharyngeal soft tissue) (Hiremath *et al*, 1998).

The use of anesthetic drugs, neuromuscular blocking agents, benzodiazepines, barbiturates, propofol and analgesic opioids can directly increase airway collapsibility, decrease hypoxic and hypercapnic responses, as well as increased severity of postoperative hypoxemia by reducing central respiratory drive (Benumof, 2002; Hiremath *et al*, 1998; Loadsman and Hillman, 2001).

The risk may apply to the use of peridural opioids as well (Ostermeier, 1997).

Intubation may be difficult because patients with sleep apnea are frequently obese with a thick neck and edema of the epiglottis. Failed intubation can be as high as 5% (Benumof, 2002). At extubation time prolonged apnea, respiratory arrest and negative pressure pulmonary edema are potential complications. Given the prevalence of obstructive sleep apnea inquiry about snoring and disturbed breathing during sleep should be part of the routine preoperative assessment. The presence of obesity (body mass index, BMI, > 30) and male gender should increase the index of suspicion and an overnight oximeter is a practical and valuable screening test. When indicated an overnight polysomnography may have to be performed.

In the presence of severe sleep apnea (apnea/hypopnea index > 30 with marked oxygen desaturation) treatment with nasal CPAP may need to be instituted before surgery.

At intubation time provision should be made as for any 'difficult to intubate patient', including the option of minimizing preoperative sedation and intubation under local anesthesia with the patient awake (Benumof, 2002).

At extubation time anesthetic agents need to be completely reversed and the patient extubated when awake. Careful monitoring with oximeter and staff supervision should be continued in the recovery room. Nasal CPAP should be resumed on the same postoperative night. A postoperative analgesic protocol, other than opioids needs to be considered (Lehmkuhl *et al*, 1987).

It should be noted that in the first few days after surgery sleep structure is grossly disturbed with a rebound increase in rapid eye movement sleep which increases the risk of obstructive sleep apnea.

CHAPTER 6

Abnormal movements during sleep

Antonio Ambrogetti and Michael Hensley

Introduction

Motor activity during sleep is normal with a change of position occurring every 10–15 minutes. Before EEG technology, body movements were extensively observed as part of sleep research. Greater motility was noted in the second half of the night. There was large variability in motor activity between individuals or the same subject on different nights, in part explained by alcohol and caffeine intake. Observational studies concluded that virtually nobody has motionless sleep (Kleitman, 1963).

Abnormal movements during sleep, or parasomnias, are defined as clinical disorders that are not abnormalities of the processes responsible for sleep and awake states per se, but rather undesirable physical phenomena that occur predominantly during sleep (American Academy of Sleep Medicine, 2005). Referral for evaluation of abnormal movements and abnormal behavior during sleep which disturbs the patient or, more commonly, the bed partner, constitutes only 5% of the referrals to sleep units. Some movements are associated with EEG evidence of arousals, but the person is rarely awakened or is aware of them.

It is clinically useful to consider two groups of abnormal movement conditions; simple movements and complex behavior (*Table 6.1*).

Presenting symptoms

Patients present for evaluation with one of the following problems:

1. The patient has injured himself or caused harm to a bed partner.
2. The family has witnessed abnormal behavior or movement and is concerned even though the person is unaware of it.
3. The person presents complaining of unrefreshed sleep and daytime tiredness without any witnessed history of abnormal behavior.

Table 6.1: Disorders of movement and behavior during sleep

Simple movements:

- Restless leg syndrome and periodic limb movement disorder

- Propiospinal myoclonus

- Excessive hypnic jerks (sleep starts)

- Partial sleep myoclonus

- Sleep bruxism (tooth grinding)

- Nocturnal leg cramps

Complex behaviors:

- REM behavior disorders

- Disorders of arousal: sleep-walking, sleep-talking, sleep terrors, confusional arousal

- Nightmares

- Head banging, body rocking

- Nocturnal epilepsy: generalized tonic-clonic seisure, partical complex seizure

- Psychiatric syndromes: dissociative disorders, panic attacks

History and investigations

Apart from a general enquiry regarding sleep and wake patterns (*Chapter 3*), there are aspects of the history which need specific attention. An interview with a family member or friend who has witnessed the abnormal behavior is also essential.

- *Time of sleep when abnormal behavior occurs:* Sleep-walking or -talking commonly occur in the first part of sleep when stages 3 and 4 predominate. Partial complex seizures, which could be mistaken for other parasomnias, may occur through the night without specific predilection. Grand mal seizures (tonic clonic seizures) also occur predominantly during slow-wave sleep (stages 3 and 4), but are not likely to be mistaken for parasomnia. A form of epilepsy that is common in young adults, juvenile myoclonic epilepsy, usually tends to occur in the morning on awakening (*Chapter 10*).
- *Associated events:* Associated events such as tongue biting, incontinence or cyanosis are more in keeping with seizure activity.
- *Family history of abnormal behavior:* Sleep-walking, sleep epilepsy, restless leg syndrome and periodic limb movement disorder do sometimes have a family clustering, and asking about similar abnormal behavior in other family members can be of help.
- *Repetitive nature of the abnormal behavior:* This is an important feature that suggests

partial complex seizure as a possible etiology (see *Case study 7, p 190*). The family will report that the patient's behavior is similar each night (eg. sitting up, rubbing his nose, vocalizing and then lying quietly again).

❖ *Medications:* The use of tricyclic antidepressants and selective serotonin reuptake inhibitors (SSRIs) can be associated with a worsening of periodic limb movement disorder. SSRIs are associated with bruxism; betablockers and ACE inhibitors can cause nightmares.

Investigations are not always needed, but overnight polysomnography with videotaping is often useful in clarifying the diagnosis between primary parasomnias and other forms of complex behavior (sleep epilepsy, dissociative disorders, malingering). More than one night is often required. Modified EEG montage is needed for epilepsy. Another investigation is sometimes requested for metabolic screening (iron, thyroid study).

Simple movements during sleep

Restless leg syndrome (RLS) and periodic limb movement disorder (PLMD)

Restless leg syndrome (RLS) and periodic limb movement disorder (PLMD) are often associated as the majority of patients with restless leg also show periodic limb movement, and approximately a third of patients with periodic limb movement disorder also have restless leg (American Academy of Sleep Medicine, 2005; Stiasny *et al*, 2000). However, it should be pointed out that RLS is essentially a clinical diagnosis, while PLMD is a polysomnographic diagnosis as the patient is often unaware of lower or upper limb movement.

Case study 1

Mrs Reba Martin is a 66-year-old woman with a long-standing history suggestive of RLS and PLMD. She is fairly healthy with no significant background history. She does not smoke and only drinks occasionally. She has suffered a period of depressive illness following a death in the family for which she has been on sertraline (Zoloft™) once daily intermittently.

Mrs Martin normally goes to bed around 10.30PM to 11.00PM but she is unable to fall asleep for two to three hours, mostly due to unpleasant sensations in both calves which require her to move her legs around. She usually has to get out of bed and walk around the house although, sometimes, the discomfort is relieved simply by removing the bed covers.

Mrs Martin's symptoms started during her second pregnancy, 35 years ago. The complaint has been intermittent for many years but constant and occurring most days over the last 2–3 years. She was treated with the L-dopa preparation (Madopar™) which was initially successful. However, despite changes in dosage and formulation, the L-dopa has failed to relieve her discomfort over the last 6 months. She does not feel that the use of sertraline has worsened her symptoms.

Mrs Martin is a widow and her history of sleep-related limb movement is uncertain due to lack of witness. There is no family history of RLS. Prior investigation revealed no evidence of metabolic abnormality, specifically no evidence of iron deficiency, thyroid problem or vitamin B_{12} deficiency.

Mrs Martin has a sleep study while off medications which shows delayed sleep onset with a sleep latency of 75 minutes. Through the night there are 47 leg movements/hour of which 7 are associated with arousals.

Given that the L-dopa was not useful, the patient was started on 5 mg of slow-release morphine (MS-Contin™) increased to 10 mg after a few days with good symptomatic results. She was advised to continue the MS-Contin™ for approximately 4 weeks and then try to use it every second night and eventually to stop. However, following withdrawal of the medication, her symptoms reappeared so she remained on 10 mg of morphine daily.

Case study 2

Mr Jeff Lara is a 42-year-old man referred because of daytime sleepiness and episodes of having 'blacked out' while driving. He has a history of Q fever and transverse myelitis at age 13 which required prolonged hospitalization. He made a slow recovery and was left with lower limb weakness and bladder disturbance. Some sensory deficits were also present below T4. Jeff works in a local abattoir which was the likely source of his previous Q fever infection. He does not take any regular medication.

Jeff goes to bed between 10.00PM and 11.00PM with a sleep latency of between ten to fifteen minutes. He wakes up occasionally through the night but does not snore. He is a restless sleeper and rises at 5.30AM on working days feeling unrefreshed. He does not take naps on purpose but falls asleep if not busy. He says he gets drowsy when driving and visiting people. His bed partner gives a history consistent with periodic limb movement disorder, but nothing suggestive of restless leg syndrome.

Formal neurological examination reveals some degree of leg muscle weakness with no evidence of hyperreflexia, minimally increased tone and down-going toes. Given his background, Jeff's history is consistent with PLMD secondary to previous spinal injury (Yokota et al, 1991). The daytime sleepiness, however, could also be explained by post-infectious hypersomnolence following Q fever (Ayres et al, 1996).

Jeff has an overnight sleep study which shows a reduction in sleep efficiency to 71% (normal value >85%) and reduction in REM sleep (6.3%, normal value 20–24%). There is no significant disturbance in breathing. There are 210 leg movements per hour of which seventeen are associated with arousals. A multiple sleep latency test reveals no evidence of daytime sleepiness with no sleep during any of the four naps.

The possible therapeutic options were discussed with the patient and he was eventually started on temazepam 10 mg, 30 minutes before bedtime. This was increased to 20 mg after one week. At follow-up 2 months later, there was improvement in his daytime sleepiness, as well as reduction in the overall number of leg movements on repeated polysomnography with sixty leg movements per hour, two of which were associated with arousals.

Restless leg syndrome

Restless leg syndrome, also known as Ekbom syndrome (Ekbom, 1945) is a common condition occurring in 5–15% of the population with increased incidence among older people (*Figure 6.1*). Although the cause of RLS is not known, there are a few well-established associations which include iron deficiency, pregnancy, end-stage renal failure, rheumatoid arthritis, spinal injury and extrapyramidal syndromes such as Parkinson's disease (American Academy of Sleep Medicine, 2005, Lee *et al*, 1996; Matthews, 1976; O'Keefe *et al*, 1994; Stiasny *et al*, 2002; Wetter *et al*, 2000; Yokota *et al*, 1991).

Diagnosis

A family history of RLS and PLMD should be asked about as familial aggregation is reported in some series in up to 63% of cases, with a suggested autosomal dominant transmission (Montplaisir *et al*, 2000; Montplaisir *et al*, 1985; Winkelmann, 2000).

The diagnosis of RLS is not difficult, given a typical description from the patient. Symptoms are usually bilateral, but can be more severe on one side. It usually affects the legs, although the arms can be involved. The patient usually describes discomfort in terms of crawling, pins and needles, cramping or toothache. The sensations are unpleasant but not painful. There is an intense urge to move the limbs. The lack of pain is important in the differential diagnosis (see below). Moving the legs, walking around the room or cooling the limbs usually relieves the symptoms of RLS.

The diagnostic effort should aim at establishing if RLS and PLMD are primary or secondary to an associated condition (*Table 6.2*), some of which are reversible, such as iron deficiency and certain medications. The link between iron deficiency and RLS may be related to the role of iron within the central nervous system (Krieger and Schroeder,

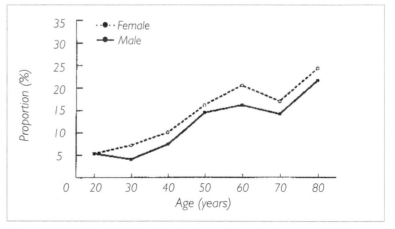

Figure 6.1: Unpleasant leg muscle sensation during sleep (RLS) (Lavigne and Montplaisir, 1991).

2001). Iron seems to be a modulator of dopaminergic (D_2) receptors and a cofactor of tyrosine hydroxylase, a rate-limiting enzyme in the synthesis of dopamine.

Restless leg syndrome can be severe enough to interfere with sleep onset and it is often a cause of difficulty in initiating and maintaining sleep (insomnia). Overnight polysomnography is not necessary for the diagnosis of RLS, which is based on clinical criteria (*Tables 6.3* and *6.4*). An overnight sleep study should be considered when daytime sleepiness is prominent and if other sleep disorders, which often coexist with PLMD and RLS, are suspected, such as obstructive sleep apnea or narcolepsy. When sleep studies are performed, patients with RLS often have associated PLMD (*Figure 6.2*).

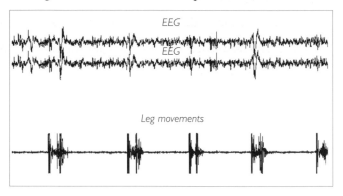

Figure 6.2: Two minutes recording showing brief contractions of the tibialis anterioris muscle.

Table 6.2: Restless leg syndrome and periodic limb movement disorder secondary to:
• Iron deficiency
• Pregnancy and estrogen
• Rheumatological disorders (rheumatoid arthritis, fibromyalgia)
• Extrapyramidal syndrome (Parkinson's disease, and its variants)
• Spinal cord injury
• Peripheral neuropathy (diabetic, uremic neuropathy)
• Levodopa
• Tryciclic antidepressants
• Serotonin reuptake inhibitors
• Olanzapine
• Lithium
• Withdrawal from benzodiazepines or alcohol

The differential diagnosis of RLS includes peripheral neuropathy, which can be characterized by painful sensation. It should be suspected in the appropriate setting (eg. diabetes, nutritional deficiency, uremia, alcohol abuse).

Table 6.3: Diagnostic criteria for RLS

Minimal criteria

1   Desire to move the legs usually associated with paresthesia/dysesthesias

2   Motor restlessness as characterized by foot pacing, leg rubbing, stretching and flexing

3   Worse or exclusively at rest, with relief by activity

4   Worse in the evening/night

Additional criteria

5   Sleep disturbances. Difficulty in sleep onset and maintaining sleep, daytime fatigue and somnolence

6   Involuntary movements
     a) Periodic limb or leg movements in sleep
     b) Periodic or aperiodic limb movements while awake

7   Neurological examination. Normal in idiopathic RLS

8   Clinical course. May begin at any age but most severely affected patients are middle to older age

9   Family history. Autosomal dominant family history present in a third of the cases

(Walters, 1995; Stiasny *et al*, 2002)

Akathisia

Akathisia (Lugaresi *et al*, 1986; Walters *et al* 1991) can be present in extrapyramidal syndromes and in psychiatric patients on chronic treatment with phenothiazine, and is characterized by a compulsion to move which is relieved by rest and relaxation, contrary to RLS which is made worse by inactivity. Also in akathisia the entire body is involved, not just the limbs.

Nocturnal leg cramps

Nocturnal leg muscle cramps are characterized by painful contraction of the calf and the sole of the foot muscles waking the person through the night. They are easily differentiated from RLS: a condition of relaxed wakefulness that is not painful. Nocturnal cramps are described in all ages including children (American Academy of Sleep Medicine, 2005; Montplaisir *et al*, 2000; Weiner and Weiner, 1980) but are common in the elderly and during pregnancy. Although they are often idiopathic, they can be associated with electrolytes and fluid imbalance, dialysis, diuretic therapy, steroid use and oral contraceptive. Familial cases of nocturnal cramping are also described (Jacobsen *et al,* 1986).

Table 6.4: Severity scale for RLS

I   Overall, how would you rate the RLS discomfort in your legs or arms?
      4 = very severe, 3 = severe, 2 = moderate, 1 = mild, 0 = none

II   Overall, how would you rate the need to move around because of your RLS symptoms?
      4 = very severe, 3 = severe, 2 = moderate, 1 = mild, 0 = none

III   Overall, how much relief of your RLS arm or leg discomfort do you get from moving around?
      4 = no relief, 3 = slight relief, 2 = moderate relief, 1 = either complete or almost complete relief, 0 = no RLS symptoms to be relieved

IV   Overall how severe is your sleep disturbance from your RLS symptoms?
      4 = very severe, 3 = severe, 2 = moderate, 1 = mild, 0 = none

V   How severe is your tiredness or sleepiness from your RLS symptoms?
      4 = very severe, 3 = severe, 2 = moderate, 1 = mild, 0 = none

VI   Overall, how severe is your RLS as a whole?
      4 = very severe, 3 = severe, 2 = moderate, 1 = mild, 0 = none

VII   How often do you get RLS symptoms?
      4 = very severe, (this means 6 to 7 days a week), 3 = severe (this means 4 to 5 days a week), 2 = moderate (this means 2 to 3 days a week), 1 = mild (this means 1 day a week or less), 0 = none

VIII   When you have RLS symptoms how severe are they on an average day?
      4 = very severe (this means 8 h per 24-h day or more), 3 = severe (this means 3–8-h per 24-h day), 2 = moderate (this means 1–3-hours per 24-hour day), 1 = mild (this means less than 1 hour per 24-hour day), 0 = none

IX   Overall, how severe is the impact of your RLS symptoms on your ability to carry out your daily affairs, for example carrying out a satisfactory, family, home, social, school or work life?
      4 = very severe, 3 = severe, 2 = moderate, 1 = mild, 0 = none

X   How severe is your mood disturbance from your RLS symptoms – for example angry, depressed, sad, anxious or irritable?
      4 = very severe, 3 = severe, 2 = moderate, 1 = mild, 0 = none

Mild	Moderate	Severe	Very severe
1—10	11–20	21–30	31–40

(Stiasny *et al*, 2002; Hening *et al*, 2001)

Cramps seem to be brought on by the tendency to keep the feet in a relaxed plantar flexion (*Figure 6.3*) which keeps the calf muscles in a passively shortened state. The contraction of the muscle from an already shortened position is thought to be responsible for the painful sensation that can last from a few seconds to a few minutes. Based on this hypothesis, it is recommended that the feet are kept in a more neutral position by the use of a pillow to keep the feet dorsiflexed, and also by stretching the calf muscles before bedtime (Weiner and Weiner, 1980).

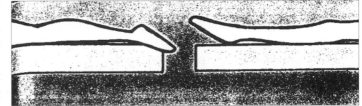

Figure 6.3: The relaxed dorsi-flexion of the feet maintains the calf muscles in a passive shortened position. Active contraction of this state can lead to painful cramps which wake the person through sleep (Weiner and Weiner, 1980).

The medication with best evidence for efficacy is quinine bisulphate 300 mg, one or two tablets at bed time (Man-Son-Sing and Wells, 1995). Quinine may have to be considered when symptoms are frequent and should be administered before bedtime as a preventative therapy. Given the potential serious side-effects of quinine (blood dyscrasia, hypersensitivity reactions) and numerous interactions with other drugs, close monitoring is required.

A more specific form of leg and foot cramp occur in patients with Parkinson's disease toward the end of the night, probably related to a wearing off effect of anti-Parkinson medication. In this setting, the use of controlled-release L-dopa may be useful.

Periodic limb movement disorder

Periodic limb movement disorder was also named nocturnal myoclonus by Sir Charles Symonds who initially thought it was a form of epilepsy (Symonds, 1953). However, PLMD is not epileptic in nature, nor is it myoclonic since the movements last from 0.5–5 seconds compared to a few milliseconds in true myoclonus (*Figure 6.2*). The periodic nature of the movement is codified by the scoring criteria of the International Classification of Sleep Disorders (American Academy of Sleep Medicine, 2005), which requires a minimum of four movements over a period of 5–90 seconds. More than 5 limb movements per hour in children and more than 15 in adults are considered normal.

The presence of PLMD is usually reported by the bed partner, who is aware of the motor activity which predominantly involves the legs but occasionally also the upper limbs. The movement is often stereotyped with extension of the big toes and dorsiflexion of the ankle and sometimes the knee and hip. It is predominantly a polysomnographic finding, but there are three main types of complaints caused by periodic limb movement disorder:

1. Insomnia with difficulty initiating sleep.
2. Excessive daytime somnolence when the leg movements are associated with arousals.
3. Disruption of the bed partner's sleep (Rosenthal *et al*, 1984; Saskin *et al*, 1985).

PMLD may not cause any symptoms and may be an accidental finding associated with other primary sleep disorders, such as obstructive sleep apnea and narcolepsy (Coleman *et al* 1980).

Periodic limb movement during sleep increases with age, with a prevalence of up to 34% in people over the age of 60 years (American Academy of Sleep Medicine, 2005). On overnight polysomnography there is evidence of repetitive contractions lasting between 0.5–5 seconds usually recorded from the leg muscles (tibialis anterioris). The leg jerks usually recur every 20–40 seconds. A complicating factor in the evaluation of these patients is the night-to-night variability in the frequency of limb movements (Edinger *et al*, 1992; Bliwise *et al*, 1988).

Leg movements recorded on polysomnography are usually reported as total number per hour as well as total number per hour associated with arousals (periodic limb movement-arousal index). The fact that the leg movement is or is not associated with arousals is relevant to the interpretation of the findings. For example, the patient in *Case study 1* had forty-seven leg movements per hour, but only seven were associated with arousals. The arousal associated with the movement may be a more meaningful parameter to consider in the evaluation of the patient's symptoms of unrefreshed sleep and daytime tiredness, since the fragmentation of sleep associated with the limb movements may be the cause of the insomnia and daytime tiredness/sleepiness.

The differential diagnosis of PLMD includes limb movement associated with arousals due to other sleep disorders including obstructive sleep apnea.

Similar conditions

❖ Hypnic jerks (see below) only occur during the transition between wakefulness and falling asleep, they are not present through sleep.

❖ Levodopa-induced myoclonus (Klawans *et al*, 1975) can occur during drowsiness and during sleep; it can involve limb and axial body muscle. It is associated with an increased dose of levodopa and tends to improve if the levodopa can be reduced.

❖ Painful legs and moving toes (Spillane *et al*, 1971) is an unusual syndrome characterized by aching in the legs with involuntary movement of the toes. The condition is predominantly present during the day and the discomfort is actually described as a severe pain rather than aching. In this syndrome, the movements are involuntary and increase the intensity of the pain. Patients with this condition usually have a history of back injury, sometimes with previous leg pain and lumbar spine operation (Klawans, 2000).

❖ Another condition that could be confused with PLMD is propriospinal myoclonus (see below), which is associated with limb and body restlessness occurring during periods of relaxation. However, the propriospinal myoclonus tends to disappear during sleep unlike PLMD.

Pathophysiology

The pathophysiology of PLMD is mostly unknown, although there is some evidence of possible peripheral axonal neuropathy (Iannaccone *et al*, 1995) as well as possible striatal dopamine receptors defects (Staedt *et al*, 1995). However, certain associations are well established, such as renal failure, iron deficiency, use of tricyclic antidepressants, selective serotonin reuptake inhibitors, withdrawal from benzodiazepines and spinal cord pathology.

Treatment of restless leg syndrome and periodic limb movement disorder

Treatment of RLS and PLMD is symptomatic as there is no cure (Hening *et al*, 1999). Iron deficiency should be evaluated and corrected if present, and a trial of iron should be considered even in subjects with low to normal levels (Davis *et al*, 2000; Krieger and Schroeder, 2001). The use of medication depends on local availability, expertise, severity of the complaint and costs.

Benzodiazepines

A benzodiazepine or a dopamine agonist is usually the first line of treatment. Among the benzodiazepines, clonazepam (0.5–1 mg) has been often used. However, clonazepam has a long half-life and is likely to accumulate over time causing daytime drowsiness. The use of a short-acting benzodiazepine, such as temazepam, is usually as effective with a dose of up to 10–30 mg about 30 minutes before bedtime (Mitler *et al*, 1986). It should be noted that benzodiazepine medication tends to prevent the arousal associated with PLMD rather than reducing the leg movements.

Dopamine agonists — levodopa

The most commonly used dopamine agonist, levodopa (a precursor of dopamine) has been shown to be effective in improving RLS and PLMD (Brodeur *et al*, 1988). However, because of the short half-life, there is the risk of rebound of symptoms 2–6 hours after the dose requiring a further dose through the night, an increase in dose or the concomitant use of a slow-release formulation (Collado-Siedel *et al*, 1999). Another common complication with prolonged use and increase in dose of levodopa is the worsening and spreading of restless leg syndrome during the day — the *augmentation effect*. This refers to the occurrence of symptoms of restless leg progressively earlier in the evening, and it is associated with increasing doses of levodopa in 59% of cases (Allen and Earley, 1996). It resolves upon cessation of the medication and is minimized by keeping the dose low.

Patients should be warned that L-dopa can cause mild nausea and hypotension, which is particularly relevant in elderly subjects and if other antihypertensive agents are used.

Levodopa with carbidopa (Sinemet 100/25™) or levodopa with benserizide (Madopar 100/25™) can be started as one tablet 30 minutes before bedtime and increased to two tablets a few days later. Side-effects associated with levodopa can limit its use, in particular postural hypotension, nausea and vomiting. Dyskinesia, a problem in the treatment of Parkinson's disease, is not seen with prolonged use of levodopa for RLS and PLMD. Levodopa with benserazide is also shown to effective and safe in uremic patients (Trenkwalder *et al*, 1995).

Synthetic dopamine agonists

Synthetic dopamine agonists (pergolide, pramipexole, ropinirole) are also effective in controlling restless leg (Comella, 2002). One problem with these agents is that they are often not available for the treatment of restless leg so the patient has to bear the full cost of treatment. Augmentation can occur with these agents, but not as commonly as with levodopa.

Pergolide (Permax ™) is a D_1 and D_2 dopamine receptor agonist shown to be effective in RLS and PLMD (Earley *et al*, 1998; Staedt *et al*, 1997; Wetter *et al*, 1999). Predominantly excreted by the kidney, it is administered at bedtime starting with a low dose, 0.05 mg, and increased every two to three days up to 0.5–0.75 mg. Common side-effects include hypotension, insomnia, daytime fatigue and particularly nausea and vomiting, which may require the use of domperidone (Motilium™). Domperidone is a dopamine antagonist with predominantly peripheral action, a reduced ability to pass the blood-brain barrier compared with metoclopramide (Maxolon™) and is not likely to reduce the agonist effect of pergolide. Hallucinations, a common side-effect when these medications are used in patients with Parkinson's disease, are not a problem in this setting.

Pramipexole, a D_2 and D_3 non-ergot dopamine agonist has also been shown to be effective in the treatment of RLS. It is predominantly excreted through the kidneys with a half-life of 8–12 hours, and peak absorption at 2 hours. It is administered about two hours prior to intended bed time starting at the dose of 0.125 mg and titrated upward up to 0.5 mg (Siong-Chi *et al*, 1998). Augmentation is said to be less than with pergolide (Comella, 2002). Ropinirole has been shown to be effective in the management of RLS and PLMD (Bliwise *et al*, 2005; Ondo, 1999; Trenkwalder *et al*, 2004).

Opioids

Opioids in the form of slow-release formulation morphine, or controlled-release of oxycodone, are also very effective treatments (see *Case study 1*) (Hening *et al*, 1986; Montplaisir *et al*, 2000). Codeine is not a recommended agent because of its short half-life, which often results in rebound and worsening of symptoms in the second part of the night. Opioids are usually associated with constipation and concern on the part of the patient about the possibility of addiction and dependency. However, in practice, the use of opioids is very effective, particularly if other agents have failed to control the symptoms and addiction and tolerance are not significant problems. Augmentation is not seen with opioids.

Other medications

Other medications used in the treatment of RLS and PLMD include cabergoline, carbamazepine, bromocriptine, baclofen, clonidine and gabapentin with variable responses (Guilleminault and Flagg, 1984; Handwerker and Palmer, 1985; Hening *et al*, 1999; Mellick and Mellick, 1996; Stiasny *et al*, 2000; Telstad *et al*, 1984).

Treatment during pregnancy

Management of RLS in pregnancy is difficult as the safety of current medications is not established. Restless leg is reported by 19% of pregnant women, particularly in the second and third trimester, with severe symptoms in 7%. However, symptoms abate in 96% of cases, four weeks after delivery. Management includes correction of iron deficiency and anaemia, and folate supplementation (Hening *et al*, 1999). Of the medications shown to be effective, opioids and benzodiazepines can cause neonatal withdrawal syndrome and sedation in breast-fed infants. Dopaminergic medication reduces lactation by inhibiting prolactin.

Abnormal movements at the beginning of sleep

Propriospinal myoclonus

Case study 3

Mr Samuel Seivers is a 30-year-old man presenting with a history of difficulty initiating sleep due to jerking movements involving the legs, arms and head in different combinations. He is a university student who does not take any medications and does not smoke or drink alcohol on a regular basis.

He describes jerking movements involving the lower limbs on both sides and upper limbs, sometimes also involving his head and shoulders. Movements can occur during the day but they are particularly troublesome at bedtime when he is in a resting and relaxed state. They have been present since age 12 but have become a significant problem over the last few years. It was his perception that these abnormal movements are responsible for the failure of relationships.

He goes to bed between 10.00PM and midnight and has difficult falling asleep for up to 2 hours because of the abnormal movements. However, he is able to stop the movements at will, so an epileptic myoclonus is unlikely. He does not snore and gets up between 7.30AM and 9.30AM, depending on the day of the week, feeling mostly unrefreshed. He does not take naps through the day.

Neurological examination reveals no focal abnormalities. An overnight sleep study shows a reduced sleep efficiency of 66% (normal value >85%), with prolonged sleep latency of 80 minutes and jerking movements of his arms and legs during wakefulness. There was no recurrence of abnormal movement through the night and no disturbed breathing.

The diagnosis in this case is suggestive of propriospinal myoclonus. The differential diagnosis would include 'excessive sleep starts'. However, the repetitive nature of the jerks and the pattern of multisegmental involvement is more in keeping with the initial diagnosis.

The site of origin of myoclonic movements can be anywhere in the central nervous system. At the level of the spinal cord, two types of myoclonus are recognized: segmental myoclonus and propriospinal myoclonus (Brown *et al*, 1994; Chokroverty *et al*, 1992; Montagna *et al*, 1997).

In segmental myoclonus, the movement involves the muscle innervated by the same spinal segment. In contrast, in propriospinal myoclonus, the myoclonic activity spreads either upwards or downwards involving multiple segments. Propriospinal myoclonic movements can be monolateral or bilateral and can be idiopathic or symptomatic of spinal cord pathology, including multiple sclerosis, trauma, herpes zoster or spinal compression from any cause. Propriospinal myoclonus typically abates during sleep, including light sleep, differentiating it from periodic limb movement disorder ('nocturnal myoclonus'). It can also be suppressed by any mental activity, such as mental arithmetic, noise or speaking (Montagna *et al*, 1997).

Hypnic jerks (sleep starts) could be responsible for a similar presentation. However, sleep starts occur during light sleep rather than wakefulness (see below).

Treatment can be undertaken with the use of benzodiazepines, such as temazepam 10–20 mg an hour before intended bedtime or clonazepam 0.5–1 mg. Opioids are also effective.

Excessive hypnic jerks (sleep starts)

Hypnic jerks are sudden movements occurring at sleep onset particularly in a drowsy state. They are a common occurrence reported at some stage by 60–70% of the population (American Academy of Sleep Medicine, 2005; Broughton *et al*, 1985). They are sometimes associated with feelings of falling, imbalance or a floating feeling. These sensations need to be distinguished from hypnagogic (at the beginning of sleep) hallucinations, which are vivid and well formed dream-like experiences, more commonly reported in narcolepsy. Hypnic jerks need to be differentiated from startled arousals, which can occur soon after sleep onset in cases of sleep apnea and PLMD. Hypnic jerks are increased in intensity by physical tiredness, emotional stress and caffeinated beverages. On monitoring, there is no evidence of EEG, electrocardiographic or respiratory abnormalities.

Hypnic jerks need to be differentiated from PLMD, which normally occurs during sleep rather than at the beginning of it. PLMD is also characterized by more intense muscle movement with periodicity. As mentioned above, propriospinal myoclonus occurs during relaxed wakefulness with multiple jerks which are repetitive, contrary to hypnic jerks.

Partial-sleep myoclonus

Another uncommon condition is partial-sleep myoclonus (fragmentary myoclonus) where there are short contractions of part of the muscle, resembling fasciculation, in the limbs and the face at sleep onset (Montagna *et al*, 1988; Montagna, 2000). Partial myoclonus, if persistent, could be a cause of daytime tiredness. However, this is rarely encountered in clinical practice (American Academy of Sleep Medicine, 2005).

Treatment

Except for sleep hygiene advice, treatment for abnormal movements at the beginning of sleep is usually not necessary. However, when the motor activity is frequent and intense it can induce increased bedtime anxiety and cause difficulty initiating sleep. In this case, a brief course of a short-acting benzodiazepine, such as temazepam 10–20 mg, about an hour before intended bedtime can be useful. The medication should be discontinued after a few days. Education of the benign nature of these conditions is also useful in reassuring the patient, together with general sleep hygiene measures.

Sleep bruxism (tooth grinding)

The paroxysmal clenching of the jaws associated with a grinding noise is referred to as sleep bruxism. Because similar behavior can occur during wakefulness, referring to sleep (rather than nocturnal) bruxism seems a better choice. The diagnosis of tooth grinding is usually not difficult, however its etiological role when associated with poor sleep quality, headache or myalgia is more difficult to establish.

Orofacial muscle activity is common in asymptomatic people with a frequency of 1.6 episodes per hour, compared to 5.4 per hour in bruxism (Bader and Lavigne, 2000; Lavigne and Montplaisir, 1994). Although bruxism is an occasional experience in most people, approximately 5% of the population between the ages of 33 and 60 report tooth grinding often, and 17%, sometimes (Hublin *et al*, 1998). Bruxism is often present in childhood and continues in adulthood, suggesting a persistent trait related to a genetic influence (Hublin *et al*, 1998) even though its prevalence seems to decrease linearly with age (Lavigne and Montplaisir, 1994) (*Figure 6.4*). Gender differences present with slightly more prevalence in females (American Sleep Disorders Association, 1997: Hublin *et al*, 1998).

Although tooth grinding is commonly reported during sleep interviews, it is not usually a primary reason for referral to a sleep unit. Bruxism can be associated with palpitations, sweating and morning headache, features suggestive of anxiety and muscle tension (Bader *et al*, 1997). The reason for evaluation and treatment is often related to the following:

1. Grinding that disturbs the bed partner.
2. Significant dental damage noticed by the dentist or temporal mandibular pain.
3. Unrefreshed sleep associated with other symptoms.

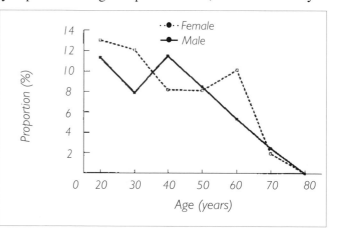

Figure 6.4: The prevalence of bruxism decreases with age (Lavigne and Montplaisir, 1994).

While the etiology is unknown, the following associations are described apart from the genetic predisposition mentioned above (Bader and Lavigne, 2000; Ellison and Stanziani, 1993; Por *et al*, 1996: Yustin *et al*, 1993):

- dental malocclusion
- anxious personality and somatization
- ongoing stress
- selective serotonin reuptake inhibitors (SSRIs).

Bruxism is also often associated with other sleep disorders, such as PLMD and RLS, obstructive sleep apnea, increased body movements and myofacial pain (fibromyalgia).

Diagnosis

Diagnosis does not require overnight polysomnography unless other sleep abnormalities are suspected, which should be the case if the patient's main complaint is daytime sleepiness or unrefreshing sleep. When overnight polysomnography is performed, modified sleep recording montage is needed with extra electromyogram (EMG) leads over the masseters (jaw muscles). In this situation, sleep studies show increased motor activity of the jaw muscle predominantly in stage 1 and 2 (light sleep) associated with a grinding noise. Other non-specific findings are brief bursts of alpha rhythm (8–13 Hz), an alpha-delta pattern (a combination of slow-wave sleep, 0.75–4 Hz, and alpha rhythm) and associated with bruxism, K complexes all characteristic of light sleep.

Treatment

Treatment is symptomatic and only partially successful. Orthodontic management should be considered if dental malocclusion is present. In this situation, treatment may vary in complexity from modification of the person's bite, usually lengthy and expensive, to an occlusal plate (mouthguard). However, follow-up of occlusal plate treatment seems to suggest the compliance over time is less than 20% (Bader and Lavigne, 2000).

General rules of sleep hygiene, such as avoidance of stimulant caffeinated beverages, regular sleep and wake time, and relaxation techniques are useful. Psychotherapy should be considered when bruxism coexists with other symptoms of anxiety disorders or ongoing stressful situations.

Pharmacological interventions have an appropriate role for short periods and in conjunction with the above measures. Short-acting benzodiazepines (temazepam, tricyclic antidepressants) and centrally acting beta-blockers, such as propranolol, have been reported to be useful. It should, however, be noted that propranolol is associated with nightmares and that SSRIs can actually worsen bruxism, as mentioned earlier.

Complex abnormal behavior during sleep

Patients are sometimes referred for evaluation of complex motor activity during sleep. Often the patient is unaware of the motor activity and the referral occurs either because of family or bed partner's concern, injury to the patient or members of the family, or as an investigation of disturbed sleep. Four main groups of conditions should be considered (*Figure 6.5*), but there is often considerable clinical overlap.

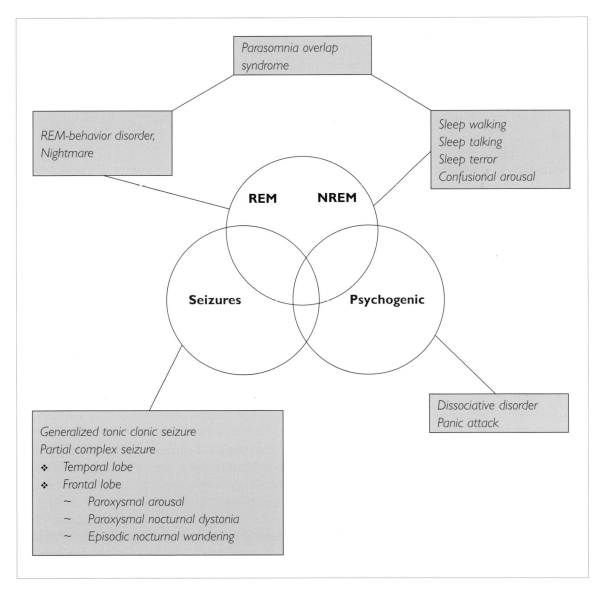

Figure 6.5: Complex abnormal behavior during sleep (modified from Mahowald and Schenck, 2000).

REM-behavior disorder

Case study 4

Mr Conrad Portius is a 76-year-old man referred for evaluation of violent behavior during sleep. He had a history of hypertension which is well controlled on medication and a 12-year history of intermittent depressive illness for which he takes sertraline (Aropax™).

He goes to bed between 10.30PM and 11.30PM with a sleep latency of about 30 minutes. He wakes up once a night to go to the toilet. He snores but not every night. Apneas are not reported by the family. He is a restless sleeper and demonstrates intermittent violent activity, involving thrashing arms and throwing fists which has resulted in self-bruising. On 3 occasions he has grabbed his wife for a prolonged period of time until he woke up. After waking he said he had dreamt of being chased by someone. He is also a regular sleep-talker and will talk for up to 30 minutes at a time.

Neurological examination shows no evidence of abnormalities. There is no cognitive impairment and he is otherwise a well-functioning man. An overnight oximeter reveals no evidence of oxygen desaturation. A formal overnight polysomnography was not performed as the history was strongly suggestive of REM-behavior disorder.

The patient was managed with a short-acting benzodiazepine (temazepam 10 mg at bedtime). The medication was continued for about 10 weeks and then slowly withdrawn with the plan of restarting the medication if the abnormal behavior recurred. It was also requested that the diagnosis of depression should be reviewed in view of considering withdrawing sertraline, a medication which is known to increase the likelihood of REM-behavior disorder (see below).

It should be noted that the coexistence of REM-behavior disorder and other parasomnia, in this case sleep-talking, is a frequent finding referred to as *overlap parasomnia syndrome* (Schenck *et al*, 1997).

Nocturnal epilepsy

Case study 5

Mrs Claudia D'arcy is a 45-year-old woman who presents with a history of daytime tiredness over the past 3 years and abnormal behavior during sleep. She has had a history of idiopathic epilepsy since the age of 11, which is well controlled on carbamazepine (Tegretol™). She is a non-smoker, non-drinker and on no other medications. She is not a shift worker.

Mrs D'arcy goes to bed between 8.30PM and 9.00PM with a sleep latency of about 5 minutes. She does snore but not every night. There are no other features of disturbed breathing. She is a restless sleeper and sleep-talker. She has abnormal behavior perhaps once or twice a fortnight where she sits up in bed making grunting noises with stiffening of her left arm which lasts 10–20 seconds and then she goes to sleep again. On occasions, she has violent clonic jerks.

An overnight polysomnography shows a normal sleep structure both in terms of length and stage distribution. The EEG shows recurrent episodes of 3–4 seconds of spiking wave discharge, but no abnormal behavior was recorded on the night of the study. A previous daytime EEG was reported as normal.

In this case, the diagnosis offered no major difficulties given her pre-existent known grand mal epilepsy from a young age. The behavior at night was suggestive of partial-complex seizure despite treatment. Following neurological review, clonazepam (Rivotril™) was added to her carbamazepine. However, this brought about an increase in her daytime sleepiness. She was slowly withdrawn from the clonazepam and the carbamazepine, and lamotrigine was slowly built up, which resulted in better control of the nocturnal seizure activity (in this particular patient).

Sleep-walking and night terrors

Case study 6

Ms Violet Davies is a 21-year-old woman referred for assessment of episodes of sleep-walking and night terrors, which is causing social problems even though the condition appears to have minimal impact on the patient's function.

Violet goes to bed between 9.30PM and 10.00PM with a short sleep latency. She does not wake through the night. Her boyfriend describes two to three episodes each month where she wakes up with loud vocalization and her eyes wide open with a very anxious appearance. She is difficult to arouse but settles down after a few minutes. She is also a regular sleep-talker. She has walked in her sleep since childhood and this has persisted in adulthood. She often finds herself in the kitchen or bathroom without full awareness of what has happened. However, she has never injured herself or others.

There is no history of head trauma or meningitis and no history of epilepsy in the family.

The importance of the regularity of sleep and wake and avoidance of sleep deprivation was emphasized to the patient. Given the intermittent nature of the problem, no pharmacological intervention was suggested. However, it was agreed that if the sleep-walking was frequent, pharmacological intervention with a short-acting benzodiazepine would be appropriate, particularly if there was any risk of injury.

Dissociative disorder

Case study 7

Ms Ruth Barrett is a 19-year-old woman referred for assessment of increasingly frequent episodes of abnormal behavior during drowsy and sleep states. She has a background of history of mild asthma, glandular fever and a diagnosis of attention deficit disorder going back to the age of 12 when she was started on methylphenidate (Ritalin™). However, as this caused aggressive behavior, the methylphenidate was stopped and she was started on moclobemide (Aurorix™). At age 14, she was also started on sodium valproate (Epilim™) for what was felt to be a mood disorder. She remained on both medications until the age of 18 when both medications were gradually withdrawn at the patient's request.

Ruth was enrolled in year 12 but she did not finish the higher school certificate. At the time of assessment she has been attending a religious education college away from home. The Dean at the college has become increasingly concerned about her health since she arrived on the premises.

The patient reports vivid nightmares concerning death, injury and suicide. At times she vocalizes incomprehensible words. On a few occasions she has injured herself walking into doors and walls. Sometimes she falls asleep on the lounge in the evening but is still able to continue talking or even knitting while her eyes are closed with fluttering eyelids. She is able to be helped to bed and sometimes has restless behavior with vocalization, fist clenching or speaking with a strange voice. This somewhat bizarre behavior has no repetitive feature; apart from the fist clenching, there is no episode of tonic or clonic movements. College staff have been unable to rouse her from this state which could continue for up to 2 hours.

Ruth's bedtime is usually between 8.00PM and 9.00PM and she does not wake up through the night. She has no history suggestive of REM-related symptoms, hypnagogic hallucinations, sleep paralysis or cataplexy. At the time of assessment she is on no medications. There is a significant psychiatric family history with schizophrenia in one uncle and depressive illness with suicide in one grandfather.

Previous investigations including standard and sleep-deprived EEG were reported as normal, including a normal CT of the head.

The diagnosis in this case would include the following:

- nightmares
- sleep-walking and sleep-talking
- probable dissociative disorder
- possible complex partial seizure
- depressive illness.

Overnight polysomnography with videotaping showed abnormal behavior at the beginning of sleep recording with the patient sitting up in bed, rocking back and forwards with incomprehensible vocalization. The technician supervising her sleep recording was unable to interact meaningfully with the patient. During this period, the polysomnography was in keeping with an awake state both in terms of EEG and EMG. After sleep onset, sleep was undisturbed until the morning.

The findings were strongly in keeping with dissociative disorder, as well as body rocking, sleep walking, and nightmares. The patient was further investigated with a 24-hour EEG monitoring in a specialized epilepsy unit and no evidence of epileptic activity was documented.

A formal psychiatric review revealed a complex family dynamic and a difficult upbringing, even though specific details were not available to us. Her diagnosis of dissociative disorder was confirmed and the patient was started on psychotherapy.

The fact that the complex behavior occurred predominantly during a drowsy state and at the beginning of sleep episode with no recurrence through the night was against a diagnosis of complex partial seizure (frontal lobe epilepsy or temporal lobe epilepsy). The highly variable nature of her abnormal behavior was also against an epileptic nature.

Diagnosis of complex abnormal behavior during sleep

A detailed description of the patient's motor activity from a family member or bed partner is essential for diagnosis of complex behavior and motor activity during sleep. The onset of the abnormal behavior and the way it terminates, its duration and recurrence through the same night are important elements to the diagnosis. The frequency over time and the impact on the patient's function and bed partner's sleep are relevant when treatment needs to be discussed.

The term parasomnia refers to the occurrence of unusual events or undesirable behavior while a person is asleep, or at the transition of wakefulness and sleep. The clinical presentation, particularly in cases of complex behavior, often has overlapping features among the different entities and a firm diagnosis is sometimes not possible, or more than one diagnosis needs to be considered.

REM-behavior disorder (RBD)

REM-behavior disorder results from dysregulation of muscle atonia, which is physiologically maximal during REM. The persistence of muscle tone in REM-behavior disorder is likely to be related to alteration in the peri-locus caeruleus area in the brainstem (*Chapter 1*), which allows the person effectively to 'act out' his dream (Olson *et al*, 2000; Schenck *et al*, 1986; 1992).

The referral for investigation is usually triggered by injury suffered by the patient or the bed partner (*Case study 4*). It is more common in the second part of the night when REM episodes are more prolonged and consolidated. The treatment of REM-behavior disorder is symptomatic (see below) and the clinician's effort is directed to ascertain if REM-behavior disorder is idiopathic, part of a neurodegenerative process or an acute, isolated episode (*Table 6.5*). RBD can precede the onset of a neurodegenerative syndromes (eg. Parkinson's disease) by months or years and only follow-up over time can clarify this issue.

RBD predominantly occurs in males over the age of 55, even though it is seen sporadically in younger populations and even reported in children (*Chapter 10*).

The history is usually sufficient to make the diagnosis. However, if there is uncertainty, overnight polysomnography with videotaping is useful in differentiating RBD from other complex behavior. RBD arises during REM sleep without atonia, while seizures usually have no specific stage preferences even though they are more common in stages 1 and 2 (*Table 6.6*).

Table 6.5: REM-behavior disorder

Chronic	Acute transient
Symptomatic of:	Toxic-metabolic
• Parkinson's disease	Tricyclic antidepressants
• Alzheimer's disease	Serotonin re-uptake inhibitors
• Lewy body dementia	Withdrawal from ethanol or sedative
• Encephalitis	Withdrawal from amphetamine or cocaine
• Other neurodegenerative conditions	
• Multiple sclerosis	
• Cerebrovascular disease (brainstem)	
• Subarachnoid hemorrhage	
• Cerebral trauma	

Table 6.6: Distinguishing features of nocturnal events

	NREM parasomnia	REM behavior disorder	Nocturnal seizures	Psychogenic events
Time of occurrence	First third of night	During REM	Any time	Any time
Memory of event	Usually none	Dream recall	Usually none	None
Stereotypical movements	No	No	Yes	No
Polysomnography findings	Arousals from delta sleep	Excessive EMG tone during REM	Potentially epileptiform activity	Occur in awake state

(Vaughn, 2002)

Disorders of arousal (wakefulness, slow-wave sleep overlap)

It is useful to consider sleep-walking, sleep terrors and confusional arousals as motor and autonomic manifestations of 'state boundary' dysregulation (Mahowald and Schenck, 1992) (*Figure 6.5*). Wakefulness, slow-wave sleep and REM sleep have EEG, physiologically and behaviorally distinct characteristics, which by convention help identify them as specific states. In practice, the boundaries between wakefulness, slow-wave sleep and REM are not always distinct, and some degree of overlap occurs. This can lead to substantial motor and behavioral dysregulation, which results in abnormal behavior.

Confusional arousals, sleep-walking and night terrors (*Pavor nocturnus*) are common in children and are discussed in more detail in *Chapter 10*. They can persist or occur *de novo* in adulthood. Cases of sleep terrors can be difficult to differentiate from epilepsy (Lombroso, 2000). The motor activity can be complex and in some instances lead to injury. More than one parasomnia can be present in the same patient, such as in *Case study 6*, where sleep-walking and night terrors coexisted. Parasomnias often start during arousals, the period of transition from slow-wave sleep (stages 3 and 4) and wakefulness, either spontaneously or triggered by some other events, and therefore more common in the first half of the night. External stimuli such as noise, or internal ones, such as esophageal reflux, apneas, and limb movements can facilitate the onset of parasomnias. Spontaneous oscillation during slow-wave sleep, the cyclic alternating pattern (CAP), could also facilitate their onset in predisposed subjects (Terzano and Parrino, 2000) (see *Chapter 4* for CAP).

Any condition that increases fragmentation of sleep such as stress, over-tiredness, caffeinated beverages or fever is also likely to increase the likelihood of parasomnia. There is often a positive family history, which suggests a genetic predisposition.

Disturbance of arousals share a set of characteristics; being more common in the first part of the night, lack of recollection of the events and inability to communicate meaningfully between the observer and patient. The behavior can have different degrees of purposefulness, such as in complex sleep-walking and confusional arousals, or be predominantly characterized by intense autonomic discharge such as in sleep terrors, with loud vocalization, tachycardia, palpitations and violent motor activity (*Chapter 10*).

Parasomnias are more common in patients with narcolepsy, idiopathic hypersomnolence where arousals are often partial and prolonged, and also in sleep apnea syndrome (Pressman *et al*, 1995). These parasomnias need to be differentiated from sleep associated epilepsy, nightmares, panic attacks and dissociative disorders (*Table 6.7*).

The impression that sleep walking and night terrors starting in adulthood are more common among the psychiatric population is a subject of controversy (Gau and Soong, 1999; Maholwald and Schenck, 2000).

Treatment

Treatment of sleep-walking, sleep-talking, sleep terror and confusional arousal is conservative, with reassurance, stress reduction, and encouragement of good sleep practices. Prevention of possible injury can be achieved by simple modifications such as locking the door, securing the windows and removing dangerous objects from the bedroom. When pharmacological treatment is necessary, a short-acting benzodiazepine such as temazepam (10–20 mg), or a low dose tricyclic antidepressant (imipramine, clomipramine 10–25 mg) can be used for short periods intermittently.

Nightmares

Patients experiencing a nightmare often wake up or are easily woken up and able to recall a frightening dream in contrast to sleep terrors where attempts to wake the patient are usually unsuccessful and can worsen the behavior. In sleep terrors, the patient does not report any dream content. Nightmares arise in REM sleep and are more common in the psychiatric population (eg. in post-traumatic stress disorder; *Chapter 9*). Certain medication may be associated with increased reports of nightmares (*Table 6.8*).

Management of nightmares is required when they are persistent and the focus of the patient's concern. Avoidance of medication associated with nightmares can be a first step. However, anxiety dreams are often a part of an underlying psychiatric disturbance that requires in depth analysis of the emotional factors involved (eg. post-traumatic stress disorder) and psychotherapy. Pharmacological intervention is only partially successful and relies on medications that suppress REM, such as tricyclic antidepressants and monoamine oxidase inhibitors (MAOIs).

Panic attacks

Panic attacks can occur exclusively during sleep (American Academy of Sleep Medicine, 2005). Patients may wake with a feeling of impending doom with a choking sensation (prolonged, sometimes minutes in length), autonomic activation, looking pale, and perspiring with tachycardia. They are usually aware of these feelings. After a few minutes the condition settles down, even though they may have difficulty resuming sleep because of hyperarousal. Comorbidity with anxiety and depression is often found. The diagnosis poses no difficulty in typical cases. However, choking arousal can also occur with obstructive sleep apnea (brief, ie. seconds) and in esophageal reflux with aspiration (prolonged with coughing).

Treatment should address the underlying anxiety problem, with reassurance of the benign nature of the episode of choking sensation. Instead of trying to breathe 'harder' patients should be instructed to hold their breath and breathe out very slowly.

Benzodiazepines can be used for brief periods (a week or two) for fast symptomatic control. The choice of benzodiazepine depends on the patient's background. If the panic attack occurs as part of an underlying generalized anxiety disorder, a long-acting benzodiazepine like diazepam is a better choice, as its long action will continue during the day. A short-acting benzodiazepine like temazepam is otherwise sufficient.

Table 6.7: Differential diagnosis of common parasomnias and nocturnal complex partial seizures

Clinical data	Confusional arousals	Nightmares	Sleep terrors	Complex partial seizures
Typical age	Toddler/pre-school	Pre-school	3–10 years, but may occur in teens	All ages
Time of night	First third	Last third	First third	Around sleep onset or arousal
Usual sleep stage	Slow wave	REM sleep	Slow-wave	Stage 1 or 2
Character of movements	Not distinctive	Rarely includes walking or talking	Increased muscle tone	Stereotypic, may involve elaborate automatisms
Character of behavior	Confused/inappropriate	Rare vocalizations	Severe panic and confusion	Altered consciousness
Autonomic activation	Mild/moderate	Mild/moderate	Severe	Variable
Response to stimulation	Variable	Often awakens	Poor	Poor
Duration	Minutes, rarely hours	Variable, usually minutes	Minutes	Seconds to minutes
Recall of event	Poor	Excellent	Poor	Poor
State on awakening	Confused	Usually alert	Confused	Confused
Family history	May be strong	Not strong	May be strong	Variable
EEG	Normal	Normal	Normal	Often abnormal
Neuroimaging	Normal	Normal	Normal	Variable

(Wise, 2002)

Sleep-related seizures

Approximately 5–25% of epilepsy attacks occur exclusively during sleep (American Academy of Sleep Medicine, 2005; Gibberd and Bateson, 1974). The majority are cryptogenic in origin and EEG is often normal, even following hyperventilation and sleep deprivation (Janz, 1962). Within the sleep cycle inter-ictal epileptogenic activity is more likely to be recorded during non-REM sleep, particularly stages 1 and 2, and they are rare or abate during REM (Meierkord, 1994; Sammaritano and Therrien, 2002).

Generalized tonic clonic seizures

Generalized tonic clonic seizures do not usually present any difficulty for diagnosis if the event is witnessed or video-recorded during polysomnography. Some forms appear to be more common during periods of relaxation or on awakening (Juvenile myoclonic seizure of Janz, *Chapter 10*) (Malow, 1996).

Epileptiform discharges can also be recurrent through the sleep episode without seizure activity but be responsible for arousal/awakening (paroxysmal awakening) leading to fragmentation of sleep which can result in daytime tiredness and sleepiness (Malow, 1996; Peled and Lavie, 1986).

Table 6.8: Drugs associated with nightmares
• Sertraline
• Paroxetine
• Propranolol
• Metoprolol
• Atenolol
• Pindolol
• Nicotine patches
• Nitrazepam
• Simvastatin
• Methyldopa
• Captopril
• Prazosin
• Topical beta-blockers (eye drops)

(ADRAC, 2000; Nagi *et al*, 2000; Thompson and Pierce, 1999)

Partial complex seizures

This group of epilepsy is particularly challenging to the sleep physician for two reasons:

1. The clinical manifestation can be difficult to differentiate from other parasomnias.
2. The surface EEG is often normal during the ictal episodes.

Both frontal and temporal lobe epilepsy may occur, at least initially, only during sleep. Nocturnal frontal-lobe epilepsy (NFLE), in particular, occurs predominantly during sleep and is often associated with lack of post-ictal confusion and sometimes with preservation of awareness. The clinical presentation is variable both in terms of complexity of motor activity and duration.

Within the frontal lobe, the supplementary sensory–motor area (SSMA) and the fronto-orbital areas appear to be the site of origin of complex presentation (Dinner, 2002; Malow, 1996). The SSMA is an area in the medial aspect of frontal lobe (*Figure 6.6*) which contains both motor and sensory body representation. Seizures from these areas often occur during sleep and are brief in duration with bilateral tonic isometric posturing of theupper and lower limbs ('fencing posture') sometimes associated with vocalization. Sensory symptoms may also be associated with, or precede, the motor activity in the form of tingling, pulling or heaviness of the limbs.

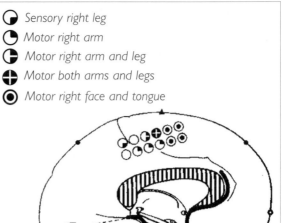

Figure 6.6: Supplementary sensory–motor area which is a source of complex partial seizures (Dinner, 2002).

The behavior and manifestation of frontal lobe epilepsy ranges from brief paroxysmal arousals (PA), to more prolonged episodes (paroxysmal nocturnal dystonia, PND) and agitated sleep walking episodes (episodic nocturnal wandering, ENW), (Lugaresi and Cirignotta, 1981; Montagna, 1992; Montagna *et al*, 1990; Pedley and Guilleminault, 1977; Provini *et al*, 1999, 2000). These entities have been described over the last 25 years and their epileptic nature has only been confirmed and accepted recently, hence their name which is only descriptive. Epileptic nocturnal wandering of temporal lobe origin is also described (Nobili *et al*, 2002).

The difference between these entities, PA, PND and ENW is predominantly related to the complexity and length of the behavior:

❖ Paroxysmal arousals (*Figure 6.7*) are usually brief, lasting 2–20 seconds, with brief dystonic posture and stiffening of upper and lower limbs. Sometimes the movement can be minimal such as scratching of the nose or face or chewing movements. They are probably underdiagnosed. PA can be associated with awakenings and paroxysmal awakenings (Peled and Lavie, 1986).

❖ In paroxysmal nocturnal dystonia, the episodes tend to be longer, up to 1–2 minutes. The patient can be aware of the movements (*Figure 6.8*).

❖ In episodic nocturnal wandering (*Figure 6.9*) the motor activity is more complex, similar to agitated sleep walking, sometimes with violent behavior and vocalization and can last up to 3 minutes. During ENW, retrograde amnesia is present and the patient has no knowledge of the happenings (Kushida *et al*, 1995).

Frontal lobe epilepsy tends to recur through the night, the motor pattern tends to be repetitive in the same subject and two-thirds of cases arise in stage 1 and 2. These clinical features, together with a preferential response to antiepileptic medications, help differentiate these entities from primary parasomnia, as well as dissociative state (*Table 6.9*)

Confirming the diagnosis can be difficult, although special montage for epilepsy as well as specific derivations may be useful (surface and intracranial recordings). However, even then, EEG interpretation can be made difficult by the limitation of scalp derivations and frequent motor artefacts (Malow and Varma, 1995).

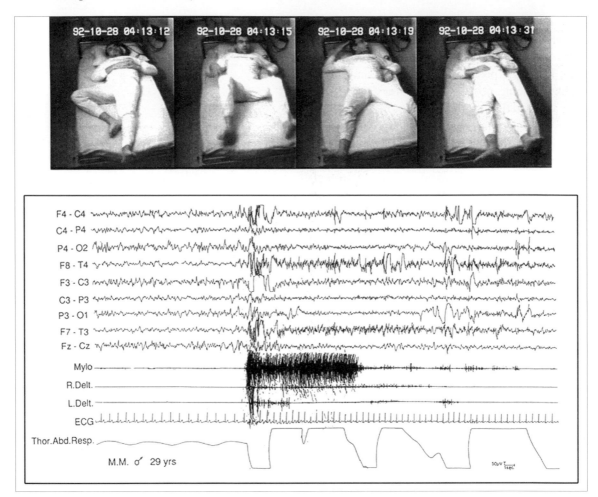

Figure 6.7: Paroxysmal arousal. The episode is brief, lasting only a few seconds (Provini et al, 1999).

Treatment

Treatment of frontal lobe epilepsy and complex partial seizure is based on antiepileptic medications. Carbamazepine has been widely used with doses of 200–1000 mg as a single dose. Phenytoin, sodium valproate, lamotrigine and clonazepam have also been used, as monotherapy or a combination therapy. The treatment can completely abolish seizures (in 20%) or only partially control them (Provini *et al*, 1999).

When focal abnormalities are found on neuroimaging, surgery for epilepsy can be considered an alternative option.

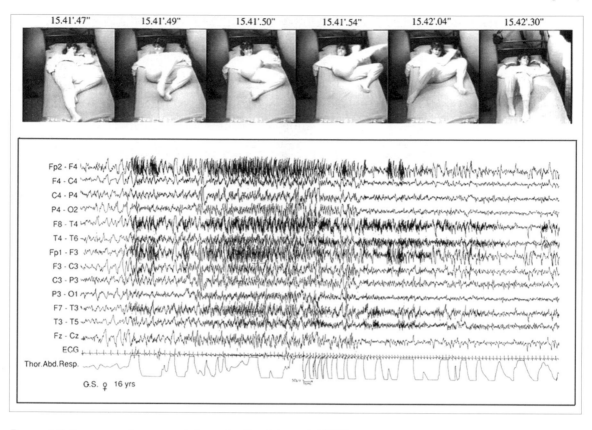

Figure 6.8: Paroxysmal nocturnal dystonia (Provini et al, 1999).

Psychogenic abnormal behavior during sleep

Some psychiatric illnesses are associated with complex motor behavior during sleep, which can make the differential diagnosis difficult with primary sleep parasomnias and sleep epilepsy. Panic attacks can present only during sleep even though the clinical features (see above) usually do not pose diagnostic difficulties.

In post-traumatic stress disorder, night time is grossly disturbed (*Chapter 9*) with anxiety dreams which may arise both from REM and sometimes from slow-wave sleep. There is restless sleep and repetitive body movements sometimes with violent jerks possibly due to coexistent REM-behavior disorders.

Case study 7 (p. 190) shows that it can be very difficult to differentiate clinically dissociative disorders from complex seizures (Fleming, 1987). Dissociative disorders are defined by the diagnostic and statistical manual of mental disorders (DSM IV, 1995) as a consequence of disruption in the integrated functions of consciousness, memory, identity and perception of the environment. Dissociative disorders can present at night-time and in a dramatic form, as in the case described. They seem to be more predominant in women and there is frequently a history of physical or sexual abuse during childhood.

The diagnosis is greatly helped by being able to have a polygraphic recording during one of the episodes. When this is available it shows onset of abnormal behavior during wakefulness and no evidence of epileptic activity.

Another important distinguishing feature is the length of the behavior, which can last hours rather than minutes, as in complex partial seizure and primary sleep parasomnia. Antiepileptic medications are not effective. Psychogenic epileptic seizures are rare between midnight and 6.00AM and do not arise during sleep (Roberts, 1998).

Table 6.9: Comparative features of parasomnias versus nocturnal frontal-lobe epilepsy

	Parasomnias (sleep-walking/ sleep terrors)	Nocturnal frontal-lobe epilepsy
Age at onset (mean ± standard deviation)	Usually <10 years	14 ± 10
Family history positive for parasomnias	62–96%	39%
Episode frequency/month (mean ± standard deviation)	From <1 to 4	20 ± 10
Episode frequency/night (mean ± standard deviation)	1	3 ± 10
Clinical course through the years	Tend to disappear	Increased frequency
Disease duration	7 years	20 ± 12 years
Episode duration	From 15s to 30 min	From 2s to 3 min
Movement semiology	Complex, non-stereotypic	Violent, stereotypic
Triggering factors	Sleep deprivation, febrile illness, stress, alcohol consumption	None in 78%
Ictal EEG	High amplitude slow waves	Normal in 44%: epileptic activity in 8%
Autonomic activation	Present	Present
Episode onset after sleep onset	First third of the night	Any time
Sleep stages during which episodes appear	3–4 REM	2 REM in 60%

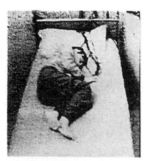
3 09'08"

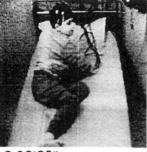
3 09'26"

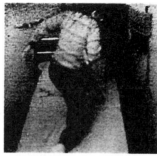
3 09'29"

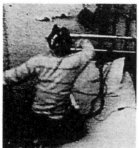
3 09'41"

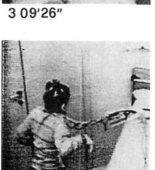
3 09'42"

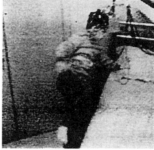
3 09'51"

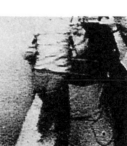
3 10'29"

3 10'35'

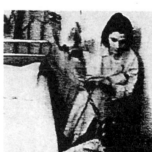
3 10'38"

3 10'42"

3 10'53"

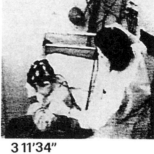
3 11'34"

Figure 6.9: Episodic nocturnal wandering (Plazzi et al, 1995)

(Provini *et al*, 1999)

Yawning

It is uncommon for a patient to be assessed because of yawning, but the question of 'excessive' yawning is often raised. Yawning is a semi-voluntary act which occurs before or after sleep, but not during sleep itself, as well as in other settings (Daquin *et al*, 2001). Yawning is the result of a coordinated action involving the brainstem, respiratory centres and respiratory muscle and cranial nerves. It is characterized by a prolonged inspiratory phase of 4–6 seconds, a brief inspiratory suspension of breathing at maximal inspiration, sometimes associated with lacrimation and eye closure and the rapid expiratory phase.

Yawning behavior is observed in many animals and, in humans, it is documented also in the fetus. The significance is uncertain, but it is hypothesized that yawning may have an alerting action in passive situations and a communicative aim in group setting (non-verbal communication of boredom or lack of interest).

Animal studies suggest that dopamine (D_2 post-synaptic receptors) and cholinergic (muscarinic 1 receptor) pathways are associated with yawning, together with other neuropeptides.

Yawning is clinically relevant to the clinician because apart from being a physiological response to drowsiness and boredom, it is sometimes associated with migraine, neurodegenerative disease, focal brain lesions, renal and hepatic insufficiency, hypoglycaemia, thyroid and hypothyroidism together with other medication conditions (*Table 6.10*). Sopite syndrome (Lawson and Mead, 1998) refers to the combination of yawning, lethargy, apathy, mood changes and sleep disturbances in the context of motion sickness. Sopite is derived from the Latin 'sopire' which means 'to promote sleep'.

Table 6.10: Yawning can be associated with other conditions and medications

- **Physiological**
  Drowsiness, boredom
  Imitation, thinking about
  Hunger

- **Pathological**

- **Neurological**
  Dopaminergic dysfunction: Parkinson's disease (unfrequent yawns), Huntington's disease, supranuclear palsy, migraine (frequent yawns)
  Focal lesions of the frontal lobe, mesodiencephalic or bulbar lesion
  Tumor
  Multiple sclerosis
  Stroke
  Intracranial hypertension
  Myasthenia
  Narcolepsy
  Epilepsy

Table 6.10 continued: Yawning can be associated with other conditions and medications

- **Psychiatric**
  Hysteria
  Schizophrenia
  Depression
- **Iatrogenic**
  Opiate withdrawal
  Antidepressants (clomipramine, imipramine)
  Sodium valproate
  Estrogens
- **Infectious**
  Fever by itself
  Trypanosomiasis, typhoid fever
  Various encephalitic drowsiness: herpes virus encephalitis, measles encephalitis, etc
  Meningitis: listeria, tuberculosis
- **Metabolic disorder**
  Acidocetosis
  Renal insufficiency
  Severe hepatic failure
  Thyroid insufficiency
  Hypoglycemia
- **Sopite syndrome**
- **Gastrointestinal disease**
  Gastroduodenal ulcer
  Gastroesophageal reflux
  Acute pharyngeal obstruction

(Daquin *et al*, 2001)

References

Adverse Drug Reactions Advisory Committee (ADRAC) (2000) Drug-induced nightmares. *Austral Adverse Drug React Bull* **19**(1): 2

Allen RP, Earley CJ (1996) Augmentation of the restless legs syndrome with carbidopa/levodopa. *Sleep* **19**: 205–13

American Academy of Sleep Medicine (2005) *The International Classification of Sleep Disorders. Diagnostic & Coding Manual.* 2nd edn. American Academy of Sleep Medicine, Westchester, IL

American Psychiatric Association (1995) *DSM-IV. Diagnostic and Statistical Manual of Mental Disorders*, 8th edn. American Psychiatric Association, Washington DC

American Sleep Disorders Association (1997) *International Classification of Sleep Disorders revisited: Diagnostic and Coding manual.*ASDA, Rochester, Minnesota

Ayres JG, Smith EG, Flint N (1996) Protracted fatigue and debility after acute Q fever. *Lancet* **347**: 978–9

Bader G, Kampe T, Tagdae T, Karlsson S, Blomqvist M (1997) Descriptive physiological data on a sleep bruxism population. *Sleep* **20**(11): 982–90

Bader G, Lavigne G (2000) Sleep bruxism; an overview of an oromandibular sleep movement disorder. *Sleep Med Rev* **4**(1): 27–43

Bliwise DL, Carskadon MA, Dement WC (1988) Nightly variation of periodic leg movements in sleep in middle-aged and elderly individuals. *Arch Gerontol Geriatr* **7**(4): 273–9

Bliwise DL, Freeman A, Ingram CD, Rye DB, Chakravorty S, Watt RL (2005) Randomized, double blind, placebo-controlled, short term trial of ropinirole in restless leg syndrome. *Sleep Med* **6**(2): 141–7

Brodeur C, Montplaisir J, Godbout R, Marinier R (1988) Treatment of restless leg syndrome with periodic movements during sleep with L-dopa: A double-blind, controlled study. *Neurol* **38**: 1845–8

Broughton R, Tolentino MA, Krelina M (1985) Excessive fragmentary myoclonus in NREM sleep: a report of 38 cases. *Electroenceph Clin Neurophysiol* **61**: 123–33

Brown P, Rothwell JC, Thompson PD, Marsden CD (1994) Propriospinal myoclonus: evidence for spinal 'pattern' generators in humans. *Movements Disorders* **9**(5): 571–6

Chokroverty S, Walters A, Zimmerman T, Picone M (1992) Propriospinal myoclonus: A neurophysiologic analysis. *Neurology* **42**: 1591–5

Coleman RM, Pollak CP, Weitzman ED (1980) Periodic movement in sleep (nocturnal myoclonus): relation to sleep disorders. *Ann Neurol* **8**: 416–21

Collado-Seidel V, Kazenwadel J, Wetter TC, Kohnen R, Winkelmann J, Selzer R *et al* (1999) A controlled study of additional sr-L-dopa in L-dopa-responsive restless legs syndrome with late-night symptoms. *Neurology* **52**(2): 285–90

Comella C (2002) Restless legs syndrome. Treatment with dopaminergic agents. *Neurol* **58** (suppl 1): S87–S92

Daquin G, Micallef J, Blin O (2001) Yawning. *Sleep Med Rev* **5**(4): 299–312

Davis BJ, Rajput A, Rajput ML, Aul EA, Eichhorn GR (2000) A randomized, double-blind placebo-controlled trial of iron in restless legs syndrome. *Eurn Neurol* **43**(2): 70–5

Dinner DS (2002) Supplementary sensorimotor area epilepsy. In: Bazil CW, Malow BA, Sammaritano MR, eds. *Sleep and Epilepsy: the Clinical Spectrum.* Elsevier, New York

Earley CJ, Yaffee JB, Allen RP (1998) Randomized, double-blind, placebo-controlled trial of pergolide in restless legs syndrome. *Neurology* **51**(6): 1599–602

Edinger JD, McCall WV, Marsh GR, Radtke RA, Erwin CW, Lininger A (1992) Periodic limb movement variability in older DSM patients across consecutive nights of home monitoring. *Sleep* **15**(2): 156–61

Ekbom K (1945) Ekbom Syndrome (PLMD). *Acta Medica Scand* (supp 158)

Ellison JA, Stanziani P (1993) SSRI-associated nocturnal bruxism in four patients. *J Clin Psychiatry* **54**: 432–4

Fleming J (1987) Dissociative episodes presenting as somnambulism: a case report. *Sleep Res* **16**: 263

Gau SF, Soong WT (1999) Psychiatric comorbidity of adolescents with sleep terrors or sleepwalking, a case-control study. *Aust NZ J Psychiatry* **33**(5): 734–9

Gibberd FB, Bateson M (1974) Sleep epilepsy: its pattern and prognosis. *Br Med J* **2**: 403–5

Guilleminault C, Flagg W (1984) Effect of baclofen on sleep-related periodic leg movements. *Ann Neurol* **15**(3): 234–9

Hening WA, Walters A, LeBroca C *et al* (2001) The International RSL Study Group Rating Scale: a reliable instrument for assessing severity of the restless leg syndrome. *Neurology* **56** (suppl 3): A4

Hening W, Allen R, Earley C, Kushida C, Picchietti D, Silber M (1999) The treatment of restless legs syndrome and periodic limb movement disorder. *Sleep* **22**(7): 970

Hening WA, Walters A, Kavey N, Gidro-Frank, Cote L, Fahn S (1986) Dyskinesias while awake and periodic movements in sleep in restless legs syndrome: Treatment with opioids. *Neurology* **36**: 1363–6

Hublin C, K aprio J, Partinen M, Koskenvuo M(1998) Sleep bruxism based on self-report in a nationwide twin cohort. *J Sleep Res* **7**: 61–7

Iannaccone S, Zucconi M, Marchettini P, Ferini-Strambi L, Menmi R, Quattrini A *et al* (1995) Evidence of peripheral axonal neuropathy in primary restless legs syndrome. *Movement Disorders* **10**(1): 2–9

Jacobsen JH, Rosemberg RS, Huttenlocher PR, Spire J-P (1986) Familial nocturnal cramping. *Sleep* **9**(1): 54–60

Janz D (1962) The grand mal epilepsies and the sleeping–waking cycle. *Epilepsia* **3**: 69–109

Klawans HL (2000) *Defending the Cave Woman*. WW Norton and Company, New York

Klawans HL, Goetz C, Bergen D (1975) Levodopa-induced myoclonus. *Arch Neurol* **32**: 331–4

Kleitman N (1963) *Sleep and Wakefulness*. The University of Chicago Press, Chicago

Krieger J, Schroeder C (2001) Iron, brain and restless legs syndrome. *Sleep Med Rev* **5**(4): 227–86

Kushida CA, Clerk AA, Kirsch CM, Hotson JR, Guilleminault C (1995) Prolonged confusion with nocturnal wandering arising from NREM and REM sleep: a case report. *Sleep* **18**(9): 757–64

Lavigne GJ, Montplaisir JY (1994) Restless legs syndrome and sleep bruxism: prevalence and association among Canadians. *Sleep* **17**(8): 739–43

Lawson BD, Mead AM (1998) The Sopite syndrome revisited: drowsiness and mood changes during real or apparent motion. *Acta Austronautica* **43**(3–6): 181–92

Lee MS, Choi YC, Lee SH, Lee SB (1996) Sleep-related periodic leg movements associated with spinal cord lesions. *Movement Disorders* **11**(6): 719–22

Lombroso CT (2000) Pavor nocturnus of proven epileptic origin. *Epilepsia* **41**(9): 1221–6

Lugaresi E, Cirignotta F (1981) Hypnogenic paroxysmal dystonia: epileptic seizure or a new syndrome? *Sleep* **4**(2): 129–38

Lugaresi E, Cirignotta F, Coccagna G, Montagna P (1986) Nocturnal myoclonus and restless legs syndrome. *Adv Neurol* **43**: 295–307

Mahowald MW, Schenck CH (1992) Dissociated states of wakefulness and sleep. *Neurology* **42**(suppl 6): 44–52

Mahowald MW, Schenck CH (2000) *Parasomnia Purgatory: Epileptic/Non-Epileptic Parasomnia Interface. Non-Epileptic Seizures*. 2nd edn. In: Gates JR, Rowan AJ, eds. Butterworth Heinemann, Boston

Matthews WB (1976) Letter: iron deficiency and restless legs. *Br Med J* **1**(6014): 898

Malow BA (1996) Sleep and epilepsy. Sleep disorders II. *Neurol Clin* **14**(4): 765–89

Malow BA, Varma NK (1995) Seizures and arousals from sleep — which comes first? *Sleep* **18**(9): 783–6

Man-Son-Sing M, Wells G (1995) Meta-analysis of efficacy of quinine for treatment of nocturnal leg cramps in elderly people. *Br Med J* **310**: 13–17

Meierkord H (1994) Epilepsy and sleep. *Curr Opinion Neurol* **7**: 107–12

Mellick GA, Mellick LB (1996) Management of restless legs syndrome with gabapentin (Neurontin). *Sleep* **19**(3): 224–6

Mitler MM, Browman CP, Menn SJ, Gujavarty K, Timms RM (1986) Nocturnal myoclonus: treatment efficacy of clonazepam and temazepam. *Sleep* **9**(3): 385–92

Montagna P (1992) Nocturnal paroxysmal dystonia and nocturnal wandering. *Neurol* **42** (suppl 6): 61–7

Montagna P (2000) Motor disorders of sleep. In: Culebras A, ed. *Sleep Disorders and Neurological Disease*. Marcel Dekker, New York

Montagna P, Liguori R, Zucconi M, Sforza E, Lugaresi A, Cirignotta F, Lugaresi E

(1988) Physiological hypnic myoclonus. *Electroenceph Clin Neurophysiol* **70**: 172–6

Montagna P, Provini F, Plazzi G, Liguori R, Lugaresi E (1997) Propriospinal myoclonus upon relaxation and drowsiness: a cause of severe insomnia. *Movement Disorders* **12**(1): 66–72

Montagna P, Sforza E, Tinuper P, Cirignotta F, Lugaresi E (1990) Paroxysmal arousals during sleep. *Neurol* **40**: 1063–6

Montplaisir J, Godbout R, Boghen D, DeChamplain J, Young SN, Lapierre G, Ing M (1985) Familial restless legs with periodic movements in sleep: Electrophysiologic, biochemical, and pharmacologic study. *Neurology* **35**: 130–4

Montplaisir J, Nicolas A, Godbout R, Walters A (2000) *Restless legs syndrome and periodic limb movement disorder. In: Principles and Practice of Sleep Medicine*. 3rd edn. WB Saunders Company, London

Negi A, Thoung D, Dabbous F (2000) Nightmares with topical beta-blocker. *Eye* **14**(5): 813–4

Nobili L, Francione S, Cardinale F, Lo Russo G (2002) Epileptic nocturnal wanderings with a temporal lobe origin: a stereo-electroencephalographic study. *Sleep* **25**(15): 669–71

O'Keefe ST, Gavin K, Lava JN (1994) Iron status and restless legs syndrome in the elderly. *Age Aging* **23**: 200–3

Olson EJ, Boeve BF, Silber MH (2000) Rapid eye movement sleep behavior disorder: demographic, clinical and laboratory findings in 93 cases. *Brain* **123**: 331–9

Ondo W (1999) Ropinirole for restless legs syndrome. *Movement Disorders* **14**(1):138–40

Pedley TA, Guilleminault C (1977) Episodic nocturnal wanderings responsive to anticonvulsant drug therapy. *Ann Neurol* **2**: 30–5

Peled R, Lavie P (1986) Paroxysmal awakenings from sleep associated with excessive daytime somnolence: A form of nocturnal epilepsy. *Neurol* **36**: 95–8

Plazzi G, Tinuper P, Montagna P, Provini F, Lugaresi E (1995) Epileptic nocturnal wanderings. *Sleep* **18**(9): 749–56

Por CH, Watson L, Doucette D, Dolovich l (1996) Sertraline — associated bruxism. *Can J Clin Pharmacol* **3**: 123–5

Pressman MR, Meyer TJ, Kendrick-Mohamed J, Figueroa WG, Greenspon LW, Peterson DD (1995) Night terrors in an adult precipitated by sleep apnea. *Sleep* **18**(9): 773–5

Provini F, Plazzi G, Montagna P, Lugaresi E (2000) The wide clinical spectrum of nocturnal frontal lobe epilepsy. *Sleep Med Rev* **4**(4): 375–86

Provini F, Plazzi G, Tinuper P, Vandi S, Lugaresi E, Montagna P (1999) Nocturnal frontal lobe epilepsy. A clinical and polygraphic overview of 100 consecutive cases. *Brain* **122**: 1017–31

Roberts R (1998) Differential diagnosis of sleep disorders, non-epileptic attacks and epileptic seizures. *Curr Opin Neurol* **11**: 135–9

Rosenthal L, Roehrs T, Sicklesteel J, Zorick F, Wittig R, Roth T (1984) Periodic movements during sleep, sleep fragmentation and sleep–wake complaints. *Sleep* **7**(4): 326–30

Sammaritano MR, Therrien M (2002) Epilepsy and the 'sleep–wake cycle'. In: Bazil CW, Malow BA, Sammaritano MR, eds. *Sleep and Epilepsy: The Clinical Spectrum*. Elsevier, Amsterdam

Saskin P, Moldofsky H, Lue FA (1985) Periodic movements in sleep and sleep–wake complaint. *Sleep* **8**(4): 319–24

Schenck CG, Boyd JL, Mahowald MW (1997) A parasomnia overlap disorder involving sleepwalking, sleep terrors, and REM sleep behavior disorder in 33 polysomnographically confirmed cases. *Sleep* **20**(11): 972–81

Schenck CH, Bundlie SR, Ettinger MG, Mahowald MW (1986) Chronic behavioral disorders of human REM sleep: a new category of parasomnia. *Sleep* **9**(2): 293–308

Schenck CH, Mahowald MW (2000) On the reported association of psychopathology with sleep terror in adults. *Sleep* **23**(4): 448–9

Schenck CH, Mahowald MW, Suck Won Kim, O'Connor KA, Hurwitz TD (1992) Prominent eye movements during NREM sleep and REM sleep behavior disorder associated with fluoxetine treatment of depression and obsessive-compulsive disorder. *Sleep* **15**(3): 226–35

Siong-Chi Lin, Kaplan J, Burger CD, Fredrickson PA (1998) Effect of pramipexole in treatment of resistant restless legs syndrome. *Mayo Clin Proc* **73**: 497–500

Spillane JD, Nathan PW, Kelly RE, Marsden CD (1971) Painful legs and moving toes. *Brain* **94**: 541–56

Staedt J, Stoppe G, Kogler A, Riemann H, Hajak G, Munz DL *et al* (1995) Single photon emission tomography (SPET) imaging of dopamine D2 receptors in the course of dopamine replacement therapy in patients with nocturnal myoclonus syndrome (NMS). *J Neural Transm* **99**(1–3): 18–93

Staedt J, Wassmuth F, Ziemann U, Hajak G, Ruther E, Stoppe G (1997) Pergolide: treatment of choice in restless legs syndrome (RLS) and nocturnal myoclonus syndrome (NMS). A double blind randomised crossover trial of pergolide versus L-dopa. *J Neural Transm* **104**: 461–8

Stelstad W, Sorensen O, Larsen S, Lillevold P, Stensrud P, Nyberg-Hansen R (1984) Treatment of the restless legs syndrome with carbamazepine: a double blind study. *Br Med J* **288**: 444–6

Stiasny K, Robbecke J, Schuler P, Wolfgang H (2000) Treatment of idiopathic restless legs syndrome (RLS) with the D2-agonist cabergoline — an open clinical trial. *Sleep* **23**(3): 349–54

Symonds CP (1953) Nocturnal myoclonus. *J Neurol Neurosurg Psychiat* **16**: 166–71

Telstad W, Sørensen Ø, Larsen S, Lillevold PE, Stensrud P, Nyberg-Hansen R (1984). Treatment of the restless legs syndrome with carbamazepine: a double blind study. *Br Med J* **288**: 444–6

Thompson DF, Pierce DR (1999) Drug-induced nightmares. *Ann Pharmacother* **33**: 93–8

Terzano MR, Parrino L (2000) Origin and significance of the cyclic alternating pattern (CAP). *Sleep Med Rev* **4**(1): 101–23

Trenkwalder C, Garcia-Borreguero D. Montagna P, Lainey E. de Weerd AW, Tidswell P *et al* (2004) Ropinirole in the treatment of restless legs syndrome: results from the TREAT RLS 1 study, a 12 week, randomised, placebo controlled study in 10 European countries. *J Neurol Neurosurg Psychiatry* **75**(1): 92–7

Trenkwalder C, Stiasny K, Pollmacher TH, Wetter TH, Schwarz J, Kohnen R *et al* (1995) L-dopa therapy of uremic and idiopathic restless legs syndrome: a double-blind, crossover trial. *Sleep* **18**(8): 681–8

Vaughn BV (2002) Differential diagnosis of paroxysmal nocturnal events. In: Bazil CW, Malow BA, Sammaritano MR, eds. *Sleep and Epilepsy: The Clinical Spectrum*. Elsevier, New York

Walters AS (1995) Toward a better definition of the restless legs syndrome. The International Restless Legs Syndrome Study Group. *Movement Disorders* **10**(5): 634–42

Walters AS, Hening W, Rubinstein M, Chokroverty S (1991) A clinical and polysomnographic comparison of neuroleptic-induced akathisia and the idiopathic restless legs syndrome. *Sleep* **14**(4): 339–45

Weiner IH, Weiner HL (1980) Nocturnal leg muscle cramps. *JAMA* **244**(20): 2332–3

Wetter TC, Collado-Seidel V, Pollmacher T, Yassouridis A, Trenkwalder C (2000) Sleep and periodic leg movement patterns in drug-free patients with Parkinson's disease and multiple system atrophy. *Sleep* **23**(3): 361–7

Wetter TC, Stiasny K, Winkelmann J, Buhlinger A, Brandenburg U, Penzel T *et al* (1999) A randomized controlled study of pergolide in patients with restless legs syndrome. *Neurol* **52**: 944–50

Winkelmann J, Wetter TC, Collado-Seidel V, Gasser T, Dichgans M, Yassouridis A, Trenkwalder C (2000) Clinial characteristics and frequency of the hereditary restless legs syndrome in a population of 300 patients. *Sleep* **23**(5): 597–602

Wise MS (2002) Differential diagnosis of paroxysmal nocturnal events in infants and children. In: Bazil CW, Malow BA, Sammaritano MR, eds. *Sleep and Epilepsy: The Clinical Spectrum*. Elsevier, New York

Yokota T, Kirose K, Tanabe H, Tsukagoshi H (1991) Sleep-related periodic leg movements (nocturnal myoclonus) due to spinal cord lesion. *J Neurolog Sci* **104**: 13–18

Yustin D, Neff P, Rieger MR, Hurst I (1993) Characterization of 86 bruxing patients and long term study of their management with occlusal devices and other forms of therapy. *J Orofacial Pain* **7**: 54–60

CHAPTER 7

Insomnia

Delwyn Bartlett and Antonio Ambrogetti

Introduction

Insomnia is a symptom of sleep disorder experienced by virtually everybody at some stage in life. Surveys conducted in different countries suggest that, with a few exceptions, the prevalence of insomnia is 25–35% of the total population, with 9–13% reporting severe insomnia which occurs at least three times per week and affects daytime function (Ancoli-Israel *et al*, 1999; Angst *et al*, 1989; Bixler *et al*, 1979; Brebbins *et al*, 1993; Lack *et al*, 1988; Leger *et al*, 2000; Mellinger *et al*, 1985; Ohayon, 1996; Olson, 1996; Quera Salva *et al*, 1991; Simon and Vonkorff, 1997; Weyerer and Dilling, 1991).

Complaints of insomnia increase with age and are more frequent in women (*Figure 7.1*). Insomnia appears to be more common in married people, divorcees and city dwellers. The effect of social demographic status and white- versus blue-collar employment is uncertain.

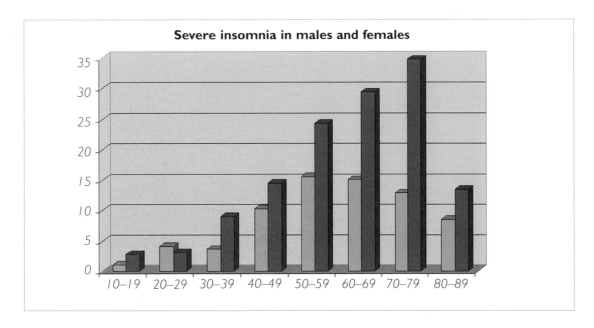

Figure 7.1: Prevalence of insomnia by age group (years) and gender (Weyerer and Dilling, 1991). Males dark gray; females, light gray.

Insomnia is especially prevalent in patients with physical and psychiatric disorders (*Figure 7.2*). Patients with chronic insomnia and no pre-existing psychiatric disorder are at increased risk of developing symptoms of major depression and anxiety in the following 12 months (Bixler *et al*, 1979; Weissman *et al*, 1997).

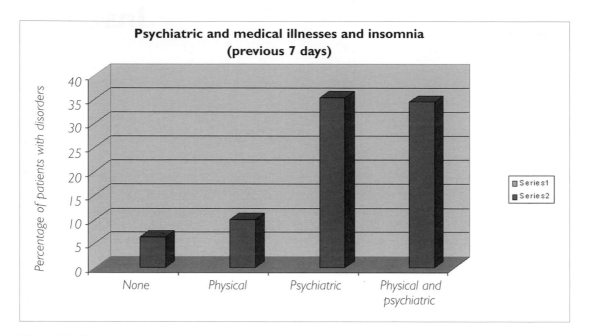

Figure 7.2: Chronic insomnia is more common in patients with medical and psychiatric conditions.

Insomnia can have a significant negative impact on the sufferer's quality of life. Patients with insomnia report memory and concentration problems as well as interpersonal and job-related difficulties. They are 2.5 times more likely to be involved in vehicle accidents than people without, or with only occasional, insomnia (Roth and Ancoli-Israel, 1999).

Despite insomnia being the most commonly reported symptom of sleep disturbance, only one in four patients discusses the problem with their medical practitioner, and only one in twenty consults a doctor specifically about insomnia (Ancoli-Israel and Roth, 1999; Leger *et al*, 2000). Insomnia has a significant impact on both a personal and societal level, however assessment and management of insomnia is poorly understood and rarely taught in medical school.

Part of the problem stems from the incorrect labeling of insomnia as a 'purely psychological' problem. Patients may be unwilling to discuss their insomnia with a practitioner for fear that they will be told the problem is 'all in your mind' and, as such, not worthy of the gravity afforded other common syndromes such as chest pain, wheezing or shortness of breath (Pressman, 1991). This attitude, however, is entirely unjustified given the prevalence of insomnia and the personal and social impact on the sufferers (*Table 7.1*) (Kales *et al*, 1984). Chronic insomnia can persist for a long time, usually years. This time-span may be related to the nature of the complaint but poor management may also be a significant factor.

Factor[2]	Insomnia patients		Control subjects	
	N	**%**	**N**	**%**
Mental health				
More nervous than others	107	50	11	12
Ready to go to pieces	109	51	11	12
Feel life is a strain	99	46	7	7
Less happy than others	111	52	19	20
Lack self-confidence	94	44	19	20
Lonely much of the time	92	43	7	7
Brood a great deal	88	41	8	8
Feel blue	75	35	2	2
Feel future is hopeless	36	17	0	
Physical health				
Poor in childhood	19	19	11	11
Poor currently	43	43	3	3
Under a doctor's care	55	55	11	11
Psychosomatic illnesses	126	59	29	31
Work limited by illness	49	49	17	17

Table 7.1: Health factors reported by insomniac patients and control subjects[1]

[1] Percents for all mental health factors and 'psychosomatic' illnesses are based on the responses of 214 insomniac patients and their 94 control subjects; the remaining physical health factors are based on 100 insomniac patients and their 100 control subjects.

[2] Significantly more of the insomnia patients reported all of the factors, except poor physical health, during childhood.

(Kales *et al*, 1984)

Fundamental concepts

Important points that the practitioner should consider and explain to the patient should include the following:

❖ Insomnia can be defined as the subjective perception of non-restorative sleep and the subsequent poor daytime functioning. The subjective nature of the problem needs to be emphasized as many people who show a pattern of sleep, by history and polysomnography, similar to subjects with insomnia, have no sleep complaints and function well during the day.

❖ Insomnia is a symptom not a disease, except on very rare occasions. Therefore, although it is appropriate to provide symptomatic relief (eg. with medications) the underlying causes of the symptom need to be clarified and addressed.

⌘ Insomnia is a symptom of night-time and daytime malfunction. This statement is important for two practical reasons:

1. The practitioner needs to pay particular attention to, and take a detailed history of, the patient's daytime function, and not just focus on night-time behavior.
2. Patients need to shift their attention away from bedtime and take a critical look at their daytime activity.

It is important that early in the consultation you introduce this concept: 'while it is true that a good night's sleep will make you feel well during the day, it is equally true that by functioning well during the day, you will sleep well at night'. Behavioral interventions need to address bedtime as well as daytime activity. It is likely that the psychological and physiological disturbances associated with insomnia are directly responsible for the poor sense of well being during the day, rather than being the exclusive result of the reduction in the quantity and quality of sleep.

❖ Insomnia (particularly chronic insomnia) is symptomatic of a problem with more than one function. It is always a combination of genetic, physical, emotional and often primary sleep disorders, such as sleep apnea, restless legs or poor sleep habits, which contribute to the clinical presentation of insomnia. It is necessary to identify and treat each factor involved to achieve successful management of insomnia. For example, a patient who presents with poor sleep habits with irregular sleep patterns, depression, heavy smoking and alcohol intake, needs to be told how each of these contribute to the difficulty of initiating and maintaining sleep. Trying to ameliorate sleep hygiene by recommending reduction of smoking and alcohol, but without addressing the depressive illness, will prove ineffective. By the same token, treating the depression without addressing the need for regular sleep habits and without removing the false idea that alcohol helps sleep, is also likely to fail.

❖ The multifactorial nature of chronic insomnia should be explained to patients so they can change their understanding of insomnia and develop realistic expectations of the work needed to improve their well being.

❖ Assessment and management of chronic insomnia requires that an adequate consultation time is allocated for each patient. The current situation in general practice, with 15–20 minutes being allotted for normal consultations, does not provide adequate time to deal with insomnia. Also, as multiple sessions are needed, it is important that the same practitioner sees the patient each time.

❖ Assessment of a person presenting with insomnia follows the general rules applied to other medical problems, but the use of a structured interview can be helpful. An example of a clinically useful interview is located at the end of this chapter.

History-taking

History-taking follows the same general line applied to any other medical condition with questions aimed to clarify three main areas.

❖ **The patient's background:** identify any predisposing factors: genetic, premorbid emotional or interpersonal, which may make the person more susceptible to developing persistent sleep problems.

❖ **Trigger events:** these are events which have precipitated the onset of insomnia. This can be a difficult part of the history as often the patient has forgotten, or actively repressed, certain trigger events and specific questioning is needed.

❖ **Perpetuating factors:** these are behaviors, situations or preconceived ideas about sleep that perpetuate insomnia. These are also difficult to assess because the multiple factors interact with each other and can be difficult for the individual to isolate.

The interview

Start the assessment with open questions, allowing the patient to explain their view of the problem with minimal interaction from you the practitioner: 'Tell me the problem as you see it' or 'Tell me what concerns you regarding your sleep'. However, it is useful to establish early on whether the insomnia is associated with daytime sleepiness.

> *Patients with insomnia who fall asleep during the day*
> *versus*
> *Patients with insomnia who cannot sleep during the day*

This is a clinically important distinction and it points to which conditions are more likely to be behind the sleep problem, narrows down the diagnostic possibilities and allows you to investigate certain parts of the history more closely (*Table 7.2*).

Table 7.2: Insomnia and daytime sleepiness	
Insomnia with daytime sleepiness	**Insomnia without daytime sleepiness**
• Restless leg syndrome and periodic limb movement disorder (PLMD) • Sleep apnea • Circadian sleep disorder (eg. delayed sleep phase syndrome) • Narcolepsy • Depression (uncommon) • Alcohol/drug abuse	• Sleep misperception • Anxiety disorder • Depression • Psychophysiological insomnia • Short sleeper • Idiopathic insomnia (childhood onset insomnia)

Leave personal inquiries, such as early childhood experiences, personality type and previous episodes of anxiety and depression, until towards the end of the interview. If these questions are introduced too early during the first clinical encounter, it can cause the patient to become defensive, which may hinder honest discussion on the origin of the symptoms. Once patients have told you about their problems, you need to systematically cover the points outlined in *Table 7.3*, either directly or with the use of a structured form (*Appendix A, Chapter 3*).

Table 7.3: Important questions in history-taking in insomnia	
Topic to be inquired about	**Comments**
Allow the person to describe his problem	Use open questions: 'Tell me what the problem is as you see it'. This gives an insight into the patient's ideas and expectations regarding sleep and how realistic, or otherwise, they are
How the problem is affecting the patient during the day	This gives a measure of severity of the insomnia problem. It may reveal that the patient is functioning well, but is worried and overly concerned about the effect that lack of sleep may eventually have on his health
How the patient's family and friends perceive the patient's problem	This is useful to give an idea of how insomnia is affecting the people close to the patient. It also gives insight as to what level of support the person may receive from their family or friends. Perhaps the family is, indeed, part of the patient's problem (relationship problems)
Detail history of the insomnia	When did it start? Any triggers? Any stressors? Was the insomnia continuous or intermittent? What treatment has the patient received (medication, counselling)? What was the result of those treatments? This may allow you to judge adequacy of (or lack of) previous intervention which may not be tried again
Current sleep habit: ~ Are bedtime and wake-up time regular during the week and on weekends?	Sleeping in on weekends may suggest insufficient sleep due to poor sleep habit which needs correction
~ How does the patient decide that he is ready to go to sleep? ~ What kind of pre-sleep activities is he engaged in (reading, watching television, relaxation)? ~ Does the patient feel tense or worried when he is going to bed?	This gives the opportunity to educate the patient towards sleep-promoting attitudes and behavior
Current medical problems	Particular notice should be taken of chronic painful conditions, chronic respiratory, cardiovascular or rheumatological diseases, which may interfere with continuity of sleep

Table 7.3 continued: Important questions in history-taking in insomnia	
Medications, including sleep medications used in the past	Specific questions about alcohol, caffeine, smoking, recreational drugs should be elicited in all patients. The use of previous sleeping tablets or current sleeping tablets is relevant as it may indicate hypnotic-dependent sleep disorder and possible problems due to withdrawal
Primary sleep disorders	Specific questioning should be undertaken to elicit a history of obstructive sleep apnea, restless legs and periodic limb movement disorder, abnormal behavior during sleep as well as circadian sleep disorders
What the patient thinks is the cause of the insomnia	This will give an idea of the likely attitude of the patient towards a more physiological or more psychological explanation for his problem, which may suggest an initial management strategy. A patient with a firm view of a physiological ('biochemical') view of the cause of the insomnia is not likely to accept, at least at the beginning, a behavioral and psycho-dynamic treatment.
Form a view of the patient's personality and possible psychiatric comorbidity	Is the patient a chronic worrier, over-concerned with lack of sleep? Is he a perfectionist with rigid and firm views of how much sleep a person should have? The use of a screening questionnaire can be helpful in ascertaining possible psychiatric comorbidity
Form a view about whether the patient has any secondary gain from insomnia	Secondary gain at personal or job level may cause resistance to treatment unless dealt with and clarified
Form a view of the level of education as well as how motivated the patient is	Certain forms of treatment particularly (eg. psychotherapy) require a degree of education and psychological sophistication to be understood fully and undertaken by the patient

Description of the complaint

It is important to clarify what the patient means by insomnia. Is it difficulty initiating sleep, staying asleep, and waking up too early in the morning, or a combination of these? Sometimes the patient simply states that 'I do not get enough sleep' or 'I haven't woken up refreshed for as long as I can remember'.

Other important aspects

These include how insomnia interferes with the patient's daytime function. Does it interfere with work, family, mood, concentration or memory? Is the patient likely to sleep during the day? Are the symptoms continuous or intermittent? Does poor sleep quality occur every night or only once a week? Answers to these question help establish how severe the problem is, although a sleep diary and/or an actigraphy recording may give a more reliable record as patients tend to exaggerate the worst case scenario. If the insomnia is intermittent, are there any particular triggers or associations, such as seasonal variation work or school factors, or does it occur during perimenstrual periods?

Onset of insomnia

Did it have an acute onset or was the onset of insomnia gradual? Can the patient recall a specific time when the symptoms began? Was there a specific trigger: a death in the family, a problem or change at work, a health problem or the introduction of a new medication?

Past treatments

If this is the first time the patient has sought help for the problem, what has changed to cause this contact? If the patient had previous interventions, was it medication or non-pharmacological treatment or a combination of both? Has the patient used 'alternative substances'? During this part of the interview, the patient's perceptions and beliefs about the condition may become apparent. For example, patients may use homeopathic treatments or minerals supplements, because they are convinced that the insomnia is 'caused by chemical imbalances in the brain' or they wish to strengthen 'an immune system weakened by the lack of sleep'. If patients have seen a psychiatrist or psychologist, this is a good time to ask whether anxiety or depression have ever been diagnosed. Ask if the patient thinks that emotional problems may be contributing to the insomnia.

Sleep and wake routine

This is part of the usual sleep history-taking (*Chapter 3*). Bedtime routine should be clarified: do patients read or watch television in bed, do they keep the light on, how long does it take them to fall asleep, how many times do they wake during the night, and for how long do they stay awake? If a person wakes during the night and stays awake for a long time, they may be suffering from anxiety, depression or a general state of hyperarousal; while subjects who wake many times for brief periods are more likely to have an intrinsic sleep disorder, such as periodic limb movement disorder (PLMD) sleep apnea or are affected by environmental factors (eg. noise).

Wake-up time on workdays as well as weekend days should be clarified. A difference between weekdays and weekend daysis an important clue. If the person wakes at 5.30AM on weekdays, and 8.00AM at the weekends, it may suggest a state of chronic sleep deprivation which can explain the tiredness (which is due to lack of sleep).

Sleep quality

The way patients feel when they wake in the morning should also be noted. Feeling consistently unrefreshed and groggy may suggest an intrinsic sleep disorder, such as obstructive sleep apnea or PLMD. Do they nap through the day? Specific inquiries should be made about planned naps as well as involuntary napping. This is relevant as dozing off even for brief periods in the evening, for example, while sitting in the lounge watching television or reading, may be sufficient to disturb sleep onset later in the evening.

Work and exercise

Do patients take work home and continue working in the evening until retiring to bed or do they allow for a cooling down period? Do patients stay in front of the computer until late in the evening? There is some evidence that even a small amount of light, in predisposed individuals, may lead to delayed sleep onset, which presents with difficulty initiating sleep.

Details of times of the day when recreational and physical exercise are undertaken should also be sought. Intense physical activity in the 2–3 hours before intended bedtime is not advisable if the patient has difficulty falling asleep, as the rise in body temperature from an increased metabolic rate may interfere with sleep onset.

Recreational substances

Take a detailed history of the amount of alcohol, coffee, marijuana or any other recreational drugs that the patient uses as these can be responsible for insomnia. In certain predisposed individuals there is evidence that coffee may disturb sleep even when taken in the morning (Landolt *et al*, 1995). The combination of alcohol and caffeine can be particularly disruptive in the second part of the night (*Figure 7.3*). Ask about the use of any recreational drugs in the past, as well as at the time of the consultation, as sleep disturbances may persist for months after abstinence from alcohol abuse.

Medical conditions and medications

A review of co-existing medical illnesses may reveal contributing factors to fragmentation of sleep. Poorly controlled asthma, gastroesophageal reflux, heart failure, chronic painful conditions, degenerative neuro-logical problems, such as Parkinson's disease, Alzheimer's disease and prostatism can all contribute to the fragmentation of sleep and complaints of insomnia.

Medications like cortisone, theophylline, selective serotonin reuptake inhibitors (SSRIs), lipophilic beta-blockers (eg. propranolol), diuretics, some new anti-epileptic agents, such as lamotrigine and felbamate (Leppik, 1995; Sadler, 1999) can all cause disruption of sleep. Medications can affect sleep differently during periods of acute ingestion, chronic use and withdrawal phase, so enquiries should include current and recent prescriptions.

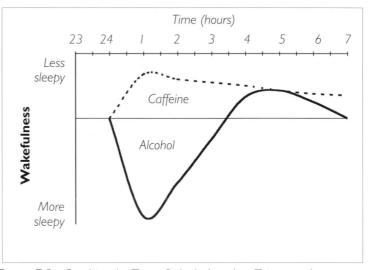

Figure 7.3: Combined effect of alcohol and caffeine on sleep onset and sleep maintenance.

Psychological and psychiatric assessment

Given the fact that psychiatric conditions are the most common cause of chronic insomnia, psychological and psychiatric assessment should be an integral part of insomnia evaluation (Kales *et al*, 1976; Tan *et al*, 1984). Insomnia is a diagnostic criterion for many psychiatric disorders as defined by DSM-IV, in particular depression and dysthymic disorders, generalized anxiety, post-traumatic stress disorder (PTSD), and substance abuse sleep disorders. However, it is advisable to leave psychiatric assessment to the second part of the interview to allow time to develop an initial doctor-patient relationship which is fostered by an attitude of empathy and openness on the part of the physician. This will encourage the patient to express feelings and emotions which might otherwise remained internalized.

Assessment of personality characteristics, beliefs and attitudes regarding sleep occurs throughout the clinical interview. An appraisal of early childhood development, family circumstances, early adulthood, personal and job-related issues and stresses should be undertaken. Family disruption and difficulty during childhood may have resulted in a reduced ability to manage stressful situations later in life, or a diminished ability to cope with events such as separation, death or professional setbacks. As mentioned above, probing the emotional aspect of the patient requires substantial tact, even though occasionally it is made easier if a patient suggests that anxiety or depression may be an important contributor.

A practical approach to this part of the examination is to use a questionnaire which is filled out by the patient, such as the Depression Anxiety Stress Scale (DASS; Lovibond and Lovibond, 1995) or Brief Patient Health Questionnaire (PRIME-MD; Spitzer *et al*, 1999). You can then discuss the findings and, if appropriate, arrange for formal psychiatric and psychological assessment and counselling (see *Appendices E* and *F* in *Chapter 3* for details of the questionnaires).

Patients who are more likely to worry excessively ('worriers'), in particular regarding the negative consequences of bad sleep, to internalize problems and ruminate more commonly complain of insomnia (Tan *et al*, 1984). These people say they cannot 'switch off' or 'stop thinking'. This feeling of lack of control negatively conditions sleep by increasing anxiety. This is typical of psychophysiological insomnia, which is characterized by a state of hyperarousal and of negative associations with bedtime. Physical expression of hyperarousal often translates into increased pulse rate, hyperventilation and elevated core body temperature.

Input from the family or bed partner, if available, should be sought to clarify symptoms and signs suggestive of a primary sleep disorder, such as obstructive sleep apnea, periodic limb movement disorder or REM-behavior disorder, of which the person may not be aware.

Physical examination

Physical assessment will involve a general examination focusing on the upper airway (for possible features of sleep apnea), cardiovascular, neurological and endocrine assessments, to exclude common conditions which may be contributing to sleep disturbance, such as hyperthyroidism, diabetes, peripheral neuropathy, asthma, and left ventricular failure.

Objective assessment of insomnia

Ask patients to keep a sleep diary, or log, for 1–2 weeks before their first or follow-up interview. A sleep diary allows a more precise assessment of the sleep and wake pattern over an extended period of time and, also, directly involves patients in their own management, giving them a better insight into the problem. The sleep diary is also a useful tool for planning management, in particular restricting time in bed, and for providing assessment of improvement over time. Occasionally, a sleep diary may not be advisable. For patients with hypochondriac and obsessive–compulsive traits, the sleep diary may actually increase their anxiety and preoccupation with sleep.

Whereas a sleep diary may be subject to some degree of bias recall, actigraphy is a useful way to assess objectively sleep and wake patterns (Sadeh *et al*, 1995). Both the sleep diary and actigraphy results can be easily understood by the patient, and they are often the first therapeutic intervention for insomnia, particularly in cases of sleep misperception and difficulty initiating sleep, in cases of delayed sleep phase syndrome (see 'Clinical cases' below and *Chapter 3*).

A more controversial issue is the use of overnight polysomnography in the assessment of insomnia. In a primary care setting, the routine use of polysomnography in the evaluation of insomnia is not supported. However, polysomnography should be considered when there is suspicion of a primary sleep disorder (eg. OSA, PLMD) in cases of sleep misperception or when patients do not respond to initial behavioral and pharmacological interventions. Recent recommendations for the use of polysomnography in the evaluation of insomnia (*Table 7.4*) seems to reflect current clinical practice (Standards of Practice Committee of the American Sleep Disorders Association, 1995).

Table 7.4: Indications for polysomnography in the evaluation of insomnia
• When other primary sleep disorders are considered in the differential diagnosis, eg. obstructive sleep apnea, periodic limb movement disorder, other abnormal behavior during sleep
• When the diagnosis is unclear and the patient has failed to respond to initial management
• To help clarify certain conditions, such as sleep misperception and circadian rhythm sleep disorders

Overnight polysomnography is useful for confirming other primary sleep disorders, such as obstructive sleep apnea and periodic limb movement disorder, particularly in older patients where these conditions are more prevalent and in the case of sleep misperception. It is also valuable in situations where the diagnosis is uncertain, or following an unsuccessful trial of treatment based on clinical diagnosis, as it may uncover the primary sleep disorder (Edinger *et al*, 1989; Jacobs *et al*, 1988; Reite *et al*, 1995).

Polysomnography, however, is not useful in differentiating different types of insomnia. For example, in circadian rhythm sleep disorders, actigraphy is a much more informative procedure. Overnight polysomnography also suffers from technical limitation mostly related to the current methodology of scoring sleep stages based on 20–30-second sleep epochs, in particular when the diagnostic issue is one of insomnia. Other techniques of continuous analyses of EEG, based on mathematical modeling, still lack standardization and are not as yet as clinically useful.

Clinical cases

It should be noted that each of the following cases has more than one diagnosis and the heading is only indicative of the major contributing factor.

Case study 1: Psychophysiological insomnia

Abigail Green is a 39-year-old woman who works as a part-time lecturer in a tertiary institution. She is currently taking two temazepam 10mg (Normison™) tablets to initiate sleep, in conjunction with Prothiaden® 25mg tabs. She is in a stable, married relationship and has two children aged 2 and 5 years.

There are no significant factors from her childhood or teenage years that may have precipitated sleep difficulties. Her current sleep and wake pattern evolved over a number of months. In the last month of her second pregnancy she experienced extreme physical discomfort and was aware of not being able to 'switch off' her brain. She was prescribed temazepam 10 mg by her GP to 'break' the pattern. Abigail had normal delivery of a full-term baby girl but continued with her hypnotic medication. The baby was sleeping through the night by 3 months but Abigail's sleep pattern had deteriorated. She was diagnosed with postnatal depression and prescribed prothiaden 150 mg (75 mg twice daily) and her sleep difficulties abated after a few weeks.

Abigail's ideas about her sleep relate to her belief that she is unable to initiate sleep without hypnotic medication. She also feels that she needs at least 7 hours sleep per night in order to function well the next day. If she is unable to achieve this amount of sleep she says she is more irritable with her children and finds it difficult to get out of bed in the morning. She does not, however, describe herself as an insomniac.

Abigail's sleep and wake pattern consists of an evening meal around 7.00PM. She does not drink alcohol due to the antidepressant medication. She watches television to relax at night when the children are in bed. Her bedtime is 10.00PM and she takes both the temazepam (20 mg) and the prothiaden (25 mgs) at this time. Initiation generally occurs within 30 minutes. She usually sleeps for 3.5–4 hours before waking, but is only aware of this one wake period. If she is unable to return to sleep after 30–40 minutes she takes another temazepam (10 mg). Her morning waking time is 5.00AM to 6.30AM and she lies quietly until rising at between 7.00AM and 7.30AM. She does not nap and there is little difference in her sleep patterns between weekdays and the weekend, except that she finds it easier to return to sleep on Friday and Saturday nights when she wakes. Although she sleeps better when on holidays, she is aware that she still needs to manage her small children and their needs. There were no 'other sleep disorder' symptoms. There was no significant medical or surgical history.

Abigail has a moderate to high intake of caffeine, consuming three strong cups of percolated coffee per day and diet coke 3–4 times per week. She has never smoked. Although she enjoys her work she often feels quite overwhelmed by it when she does not sleep well. She is not in any regular exercise program as there is little time for 'just her' between looking after two small children and working part-time. She lives in a quiet street in a free-standing house and has a comfortable bed with a relatively new mattress. She is asked to keep a diary and to complete some baseline questionnaires relating to mood (Depression Anxiety Stress Scale; DASS,;*Chapter 3*), to daytime sleepiness (Epworth Sleepiness Scale; ESS), fatigue (Fatigue Severity Scale; FSS; *Appendix B*), and to sleep quality (Pittsburgh Sleep Quality Index; PSQI; *Appendix C*) and to return in 2 weeks for review.

It appears that Abigail has a longstanding psychophysiological insomnia (>2 years) which is likely to have been triggered by the physical discomforts of late pregnancy and further exacerbated by the onset of postnatal depression. Loss of confidence in her ability to initiate and maintain sleep appears to be associated with her continued use of hypnotic medication.

At the first follow-up consultation, Abigail's diary showed that she was spending 8 hours in bed and averaging 5–6 hours of sleep, showing an average sleep efficiency of 70–75%. (Sleep efficiency consists of hours of sleep divided by time in bed and multiplied by 100. Good sleep efficiency is thought to be greater than 85%.) It is suggested that she slowly reduces the number of hours spent in bed, thereby increasing her sleep debt, which is similar to a partial sleep deprivation regimen. She decides that she would rather go to bed later and only get out of bed a little earlier to instigate the sleep restriction or bedtime restriction programme (Bootzin and Nicassio, 1978). It is important for individuals to choose which end of sleep they would like to curtail first. Some individuals are more morning-orientated (larks), while other individuals are evening-orientated (owls). The need for a constant waking time should also be considered within this framework.

The rationale for sleep hygiene measures is discussed in detail with Abigail. Special emphasis is placed on the importance of her taking control of her sleep. Implementing a constant getting up time, in conjunction with exposure to early morning light, is necessary to 'reset' the body clock in relation to both the environment and the time of year. Light exposure requires the individual to be outside for at least 30–40 minutes without wearing either sunglasses or a hat. Walking in the morning potentially has a number of benefits, including light exposure, time for exercise and also 'time out' for Abigail. These issues are discussed in detail.

Other important behavioral changes relate to removing the frustration and anxiety associated with being unable to sleep away from the bedroom and bed. This programme, called stimulus control therapy, is one of the most effective means of changing sleep behavior and improving sleep confidence (Edinger *et al*, 2001; Morin *et al*, 1994; 1999). Stimulus control therapy is also one of the most difficult behavioral measures to implement, as individuals find it hard to get out of bed when all they want to do is stay in bed and go to sleep. The actual parameters for both sleep restriction and stimulus control therapy are set out later in this chapter (*p. 244–245*).

The baseline questionnaires show that Abigail has considerable sleep disturbance with a PSQI score of 14 (>5 shows sleep disturbance); an ESS of 3, suggest no daytime sleepiness (>10 shows excessive sleepiness); an FSS of 45 (>36 shows excessive daytime fatigue); and the scores on the DASS showing mild depression (>9), moderate anxiety (>9), and no significant stress (<13).

Abigail has three more consultations over a 3-month time frame. At the second follow-up visit she has stopped taking the temazepam when she wakes in the middle of the night and is generally able to return to sleep. At the third follow-up she is taking temazepam (10 mg ie. one tablet) to initiate sleep and is achieving a relatively consolidated sleep of 6–7 hours. At this visit it is suggested that she further reduce her hypnotic medication to half a tablet and have one 'no temazepam' night per week of her choosing. At the fourth visit she is not taking hypnotic medication on a regular basis. She finds it too tedious to break the tablets in half and says she would rather manage by herself. Generally, she is feeling more confident about her ability to sleep but she will take the odd sleeping tablet if she needs to. The follow-up questionnaires show some reduction in her overall sleep disturbance with a PSQI global score of 9 (>5 shows sleep disturbance). Her ESS is still three indicating no significant daytime sleepiness, her FSS is also reduced at 26 (>36 shows excessive daytime fatigue), and her scores on the DASS show mild depression (>9), mild anxiety (>9), and no significant stress (<13). Although these mood scores continue to show some significant disturbance there was an overall general improvement.

Comments

Gaining confidence about one's ability to gain and maintain control over sleep is an important component of insomnia treatment. When hypnotic medication is being used on a regular basis, the individual tends to believe that it is the medication which is making the improvement and not the combination of the behavioral and pharmacological treatment (Morin *et al*, 1999).

Case study 2: Insomnia in major depression/anxiety

Sari Ross is a 41-year-old woman referred because she has had chronic difficulty initiating and maintaining sleep for many years. Separated from her husband, she lives by herself. She has a background history of Cushing's syndrome, requiring an adrenalectomy, and is on cortisone replacement. She has been treated for depression and is currently on paroxetine. She describes her childhood in unfavorable terms, reporting sexual interference at the age of 12.

Her sleep difficulty started 15 years prior to the consultation. At that time she had a rather acrimonious separation from her husband. She continued her home business until 1987 when, at the time of the economic recession, the business folded and she lost all her assets including her family home. At that time she attempted suicide and she received intermittent psychiatric counselling and different antidepressants, including sertraline, fluoxetine and moclobemide. She smokes thirty cigarettes and drinks two cups of coffee per day.

Her bedtime varies from 10.00PM to midnight, with a sleep latency of up to 1 hour. She has used a short-acting benzodiazepine (temazepam) at least 4 times per week, initially 10 mg with variable success, but more recently she has increased this to 20 mg because there is no effect with the smaller dose.

After falling asleep she says she wakes every hour to an hour and a half and is awake between thirty minutes and 1 hour. She smokes a few cigarettes, watches television and then tries to sleep again. At about 4.00AM–5.00AM she is unable to go back to sleep. During the day she does not fall asleep, even though she feels profoundly tired with poor concentration and has difficulty holding a job, even part-time, adding to her financial problems.

During the interview she shows a range of emotions in keeping with her poor sense of well being. Although she asked her local medical officer to refer her for the consultation, she has a negative attitude about the possible outcome of her sleep problem given the previous unsuccessful attempts. The sleeping tablets have been only variably successful and she has had to increase her medication to 20 mg of temazepam. When she tries to stop the medication her sleep deteriorates. There are no features suggestive of obstructive sleep apnea or periodic limb movement disorder.

An overnight polysomnography confirms reduced sleep efficiency (66%; normal value >85%), recurrent prolonged arousals after sleep onset (120 minutes), and reduction in slow-wave sleep (9%; normal value 20–24%).

The diagnosis includes:
- major depression
- inadequate sleep hygiene
- hypnotic-dependent sleep disorder.

Treatment involves explaining how all the above elements are contributing to her poor sense of well being and how intervention is needed, both for her sleep habits and her depression. An important point in the management of cases like this is to take the person's attention away (at least in part) from bedtime and night-time, and refocus on daytime function as a determinant of sleep quality.

The paramount importance of a regular bedtime and wake-up time is explained, together with rules of sleep hygiene (see later in this chapter). The effect of nicotine as a stimulant and its contribution to sleep fragmentation is also discussed.

Restriction of time in bed was instituted (see later in the chapter). Sari's sleep diary is kept for 2 weeks and suggests that she is having 4 hours of sleep on average, and the polysomnography shows just below five hours of total sleep time. She agrees to a bedtime of midnight, rising not later than 6.00AM by the clock. No naps are allowed during the day. The importance of not sleeping in the morning is explained, as this will defeat the purpose of restricting time in bed. Sari is told that her daytime tiredness will increase initially. Temazepam is continued every night at midnight for the first week, every second night for the second week, and is subsequently stopped. It is not advisable to stop the benzodiazepine while implementing restriction of time in bed as the patient may not be able to cope and is likely to abandon the programme. The rationale of withdrawing benzodiazepines and their potential role in perpetuating insomnia should be explained in detail (see later in this chapter).

The fact that Sari's depression is affecting her sleep quality is emphasized and she is urged to continue counselling and her antidepression medication. However, she is instructed to take the paroxetine in the morning, rather than at night, as the mild stimulatory activity of the SSRI may add to sleep fragmentation. Sari is asked to keep in touch by telephone twice per week to discuss any problems. The availability of the clinician is an essential part of the treatment.

Two months after the initial consultation, Sari's overall function has improved. She is sleeping from 11.00PM to 6.00AM with only one to two brief awakenings through the night. However, she remains tired through the day. She has discontinued the benzodiazepine. Her perception of her sleep problem has improved and she is continuing her psychiatric counselling and treatment.

Comments

This case exemplifies the multifactorial nature of chronic insomnia, even when a leading diagnosis can be identified (in this case, depressive illness). Insomnia associated with psychiatric illnesses (Barkovec, 1982; Ford and Kamerov, 1989; Ohayon, 1997; Vollrath *et al*, 1989) is common with high prevalence in both patients attending sleep disorders centres (35%) and those in the general population (40%).

Affective disorders may range from major depression to patients with depressed moods, who are often affected by somatized anxiety about the effect of lack of sleep. More challenging are cases of atypical depression, where the patient may deny being depressed. Maladaptive sleep behavior, sleep perceptions and chronic abuse of hypnotics are common complicating factors requiring attention in the management of these patients. Patients with insomnia associated with depression often report a pattern of recurrent arousals and early morning awakening.

Polysomnographic changes commonly associated with affective disorders, such as early onset of REM (<50 minutes), are often not recorded as patients are usually taking antidepressants or benzodiazepines or both, which are strong REM suppressants. Poor sleep efficiency, reduction in slow-wave sleep (SWS), and increase in stages 1 and 2 are often present.

It should be noted that the relationship between depression and insomnia is complex and the two conditions may be interdependent (*Figure 7.4*), requiring management of both depression and insomnia at the same time (Jindal and Thase, 2004), even when depression is the primary diagnosis, as in *Case study 2*.

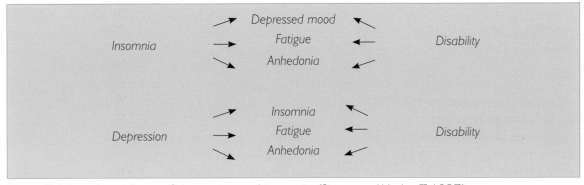

Figure 7.4: Interdependency of depression and insomnia (Simon and Vonkorff, 1997).

Treatment of underlying depression constitutes the mainstay of management using both medications and psychodynamic intervention. Tricyclic antidepressants have been used extensively in the past to exploit both the antidepressant activity and hypnotic action. Given the anticholinergic side-effects of tricyclics, selective serotonin reuptake inhibitors (SSRIs) are more commonly used. However, these antidepressants have an arousing effect which may exacerbate insomnia. These undesirable side-effects can be managed with short-term (2–3 weeks) and intermittent use of non-benzodiazepine hypnotics, such as zolpidem 10 mg, zopiclone 7.5 mg, or zaleplon 10 mg at bedtime. Atypical antidepressants, such as nefazodone and mirtazapine, may have less impact on sleep structure in some patients.

Antidepressant treatment needs to be combined with interventions aimed specifically at improving sleep hygiene, promoting a more regular sleep routine, and reducing ruminative thoughts and negative feelings at bedtime (*Table 7.5*). Long-term follow-up is needed because of the likely recurrence of insomnia with future episodes of depression.

Table 7.5: Feelings, thoughts and activities before going to sleep reported by 100 insomnia patients and 100 control subjects

	Insomnia patients (%)	Control subjects (%)
Feelings		
'Mind racing'[a]	48	15
Tense/anxious	44	2
Worried	35	6
Depressed[a]	24	2
Desperate[a]	10	0
Mentally tired[a]	56	39
Sleepy[b]	31	71
Thoughts		
About getting enough sleep[a]	77	12
About personal problems[c]	49	30
About work[c]	47	29
About health[a]	36	16
About death[c]	14	3
Activities		
Reading[c]	53	37
Eating[a]	31	7
Drinking water, milk, etc[a]	31	13
Drinking alcoholic beverages[c]	15	3
Taking sleep medication[a]	52	0
Trying hard to sleep[a]	48	17
Turning on light[a]	21	5
Getting out of bed[a]	43	21
Going to bathroom[a]	61	28

[a] Significantly more of the insomnia patients reported this item ($p<.01$)
[b] Significantly more of the control patients reported this item ($p<.01$)
[c] Significantly more of the insomnia patients reported this item ($p<.05$)

(Kales *et al*, 1984)

Case study 3: Sleep misperception

Maxine Cooper is a 36-year old woman who has had difficulty maintaining sleep for the past 11 years. She has two children, aged 11 and 5 and works in the family business. A non-smoker with occasional alcohol intake, she drinks 5–6 cups of coffee per day, the last one at dinner time. She takes no medication except for the contraceptive pill.

Maxine goes to bed between 9.00PM and 10.00PM and falls asleep in 5–10 minutes. She wakes at 1.00AM or 2.00AM and cannot go back to sleep and remains in bed unable to sleep until around 6.30AM–7.00AM when she gets up for the day. She says she is not overly sleepy and does not take naps through the day. Her work is not affected.

The problem started 11 years ago after the birth of her first child when she had to breast feed through the night and continued during his toddler years as he was a difficult sleeper. Prior to his birth, Maxine's sleep was undisturbed from 10.00PM until about 7.00AM. The disrupted sleep pattern was reinforced with the birth of the second child 5 years ago. However, for the past 2 years, both children have slept through the night but her pattern of sleep has persisted. While she feels tired during the day, she is most concerned that her lack of sleep may affect her immune system. She has used herbal remedies including kava kava and valerian with only minimal success.

She is a thin lady with micrognathia but no history of snoring or restless legs. Her thyroid function is normal. She is concerned about lack of sleep but has no symptoms suggestive of anxiety or depression. She says that there are no current or recent stresses in the personal, family or business areas of her life.

The possible diagnosis includes:
- sleep misperception
- effect of excessive caffeine
- malingering.

The clinical presentation is strongly suggestive of sleep misperception, compounded by an excessive use of caffeine. An actigraph was recorded for 1 week (*Figure 7.5*) and shows a regular resting period of 8 hours between 11.00PM and 7.00AM, in keeping with the suggested diagnosis of sleep misperception.

In discussing the actigraphy with Maxine, she says that she is resting in bed at night but is not asleep. Indeed, the actigraphy is a measure of resting activity which is then extrapolated as wakefulness and sleep (*Chapter 3*). The prediction of sleep period by the actigraphy is fairly accurate in 'normal sleepers', but not well correlated in patients complaining of insomnia.

Maxine has an overnight polysomnography which shows bedtime at 10.30PM with a sleep latency of 18 minutes and a total sleep time of just below 6 hours. When questioned the morning after, Maxine says that she hardly slept at all. When the sleep study was discussed she remains reluctant to accept the finding of 6 hours total sleep time. She is assured that sleep misperception is a 'real' and not an 'imagined' sleep disorder, even though it is poorly understood. There was nothing in the history or the finding suggesting malingering and no obvious secondary gain.

Maxine is reassured that she is getting a sufficient amount of sleep. She is encouraged to reduce her coffee intake to two cups per day and avoid any caffeine in the afternoon to minimize sleep fragmentation. She is told to go to bed later, around 11.00PM–11.30PM but to keep the same rising time of 6.30AM–7.00AM. As in *Case study 2*, some degree of sleep restriction is helpful in consolidating sleep. A melatonin 3 mg capsule at 9.00PM is used empirically for 4 weeks. Maxine is also educated about sleeping tablets and the benzodiazepine, particularly, which is contraindicated and may actually lead to drug dependence (American Sleep Disorders Association, 1997).

At follow-up 6 weeks later, Maxine says that she feels better about her sleep. However, she feels that after since stopping melatonin, after the initial 4 weeks, her sleep has somewhat deteriorated. She remains off melatonin at further follow-up.

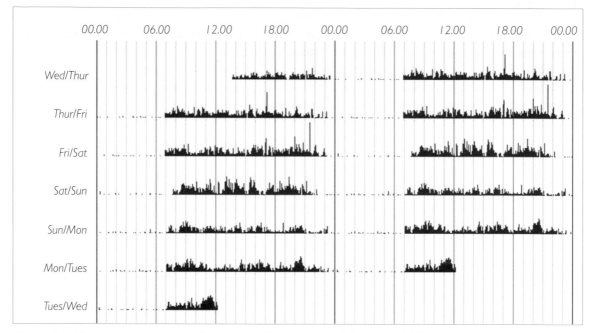

Figure 7.5: Note a regular onset of rest period between 11.00PM and 11.30PM, and get-up time around 7.00AM.

Comments

Sleep misperception (or pseudo-insomnia) is a subjective complaint of difficulty falling and staying asleep in the absence of objective evidence of disturbed sleep (American Academy of Sleep Medicine, 2005). Sleep misperception, in terms of underestimation of sleep latency and sleep length, is common in all patients with insomnia, but a primary diagnosis is rare (two per 1000 patients in our unit). Even after an overnight polysomnography, which shows evidence of normal or near-normal sleep, patients with sleep misperception often maintain that they have not slept at all. In this patient, actigraphy did not show increased motor activity during the resting period as has been reported in some cases (Hauri and Wisbey, 1992).

The reason for the discrepancy between objective and subjective findings is unclear. It is accepted that patients with sleep misperception have a genuine problem, but one which current investigation techniques are unable to clarify. Recent studies suggest that patients with primary insomnia have an increased amount of high frequency EEG activity in the beta (14–35 Hz) and gamma (35–45 Hz) range compared to normal controls and patients with insomnia secondary to mood disorder. The increase in high frequency activity was positively correlated with sleep misperception in term of total sleep time (TST), and to a lesser degree with sleep onset latency (Perlis *et al*, 2001). In this case, the use of a stimulant (caffeine) was a contributing factor to her problem, although not the primary cause.

Case study 4: Idiopathic insomnia (childhood onset insomnia)

Stacey Finch is a 42-year-old woman with a lifelong history of difficulty falling asleep and early morning arousal. A non-smoker with occasional alcohol intake, she was diagnosed with fibromyalgia and chronic fatigue a few years earlier and uses amitriptyline 25 mg at night to help the fibromyalgia and her sleep pattern, but with minimal success.

She says she cannot remember ever having a satisfactory sleep. She had disrupted sleep as a teenager but cannot remember anything from her earlier years except that her mother said she was a poor sleeper as a child. Her relationship with her father was distant but she had a good relationship with her mother although they were never very close (apart from a period 10 years ago when her mother was dying of pancreatic cancer).

Stacey has been happily married since she was 23 and has one child aged 12. Stacey's sleep disturbances deteriorated after the birth of her child who suffered from severe esophageal reflux until the age of 2. Her bedtime is any time between 10.30PM–12.30AM, with a sleep latency of between 45 minutes and 2 hours. She wakes up any time between 3.00AM and 5.00AM and cannot fall asleep again. She says she doesn't take naps through the day but that she is profoundly tired and has difficulty concentrating. She has tried conventional and alternative treatments, all of which were unsuccessful. She is currently consulting a biochemist who has prescribed a bowel detoxification programme. Because of her tiredness, poor daytime functioning and the failure of different treatments, Stacey is anxious and disheartened but has no symptoms of depression.

An overnight sleep study (*Figure 7.6*) confirms prolonged sleep latency to persistent sleep, a sleep efficiency of 56% with 4 hours of total sleep time, significant sleep fragmentation with poor sleep structure while off any medication including herbal substances. There is no recorded periodic limb movement and no alpha intrusion on the EEG, a finding sometimes associated with fibromyalgia.

The diagnoses to be considered are:
- primary insomnia (childhood-onset insomnia)
- poor sleep hygiene
- psychophysiological insomnia
- sleep disturbance associated with fibromyalgia.

The nature of the above problems and how they are contributing to Stacey's poor sleep quality is explained to her in detail. Although psychophysiological insomnia is the result of her long-standing sleep problem, rather than its cause, it is contributing to increased anxiety and concern over her inability to fall asleep, and this is compounding the problem.

She is advised to establish a regular bed- and wake-up routine and to avoid any naps through the day. She is told to maintain a bedtime between 11.30PM and midnight and is prescribed a melatonin 3 mg capsule at 10.00PM for 4 weeks. With this strategy her sleep onset improves, usually within 15 minutes, but she still complains of fragmented sleep and early arousal.

Zolpidem 5 mg (half a tablet) is added at bedtime with a subjective report of good quality sleep up until 6.00AM. An attempt to stop the zolpidem is followed by a recurrence of sleep fragmentation. The medication is re-introduced. A sleep study performed 3 weeks later, while on treatment (*Figure 7.7*), shows a sleep onset latency of 29 minutes, total sleep time 6 hours with an efficiency of 84% and a normal sleep structure.

Although it is generally recommended that hypnotic medications are not taken for longer than 4 weeks, Stacey elects to continue zolpidem daily, together with regular bed and wake-up times. The documented benefit is still present 12 months after treatment was started.

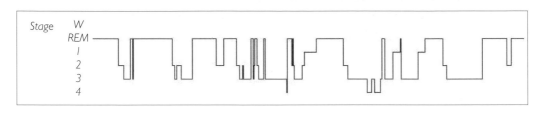

Figure 7.6: Initial overnight polysomnography without any medication — note recurrent periods of wakefulness and fragmentation of sleep. W = wake; REM = rapid eye movement sleep; S1 = Stage 1 sleep; S2 = stage 2 sleep; S3 = stage 3 sleep; S4 = stage 4 sleep.

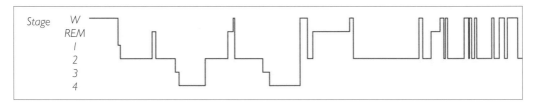

Figure 7.7: Overnight polysomnography on zolpidem 5 mg. W = wake; REM = rapid eye movement sleep; S1 = stage 1 sleep; S2 = stage 2 sleep; S3 = stage 3 sleep; S4 = stage 4 sleep.

Comments

Idiopathic insomnia (childhood-onset insomnia) is a rare condition said to have a possible familial association and an association with difficult birth and prematurity (American Academy of Sleep Medicine, 2005). The diagnosis requires a longstanding history of insomnia in the absence of psychopathology, even though, depending on the impact on daily function, the patients may show a depressed mood and, as in this case, a component of psychophysiological insomnia. Because of the longstanding nature of idiopathic insomnia, patients have often tried a multitude of treatments from antidepressants to relaxation techniques. Management requires individual consideration of not only the principal disorder (idiopathic insomnia), but also learned maladaptive sleep habits including the use of stimulant substances used to improve daytime performance. This patient responded well to the use of a non-benzodiazepine hypnotic (zolpidem). Other case reports support the use of opioids and/or benzodiazepines (Regenstein, 1987; Regenstein and Reich, 1983).

This case study raises the issue of sleep disturbances associated with fibromyalgia. Fibromyalgia is a rheumatic disorder characterized by chronic tiredness, diffuse aches and pains with specifically recognized painful soft tissue points. It is more commonly diagnosed in women. Only recently, fibromyalgia has been recognised as a 'real' clinical entity by the medical community (Csillag, 1992; Woolfe *et al*, 1990), but not without controversy (Cohen and Quintner, 1998).

Fibromyalgia and depression share many aspects, such as chronic fatigue, sleep disturbances and cognitive dysfunction. Patients with fibromyalgia complain of chronic, unrefreshing sleep with increased sleep fragmentation and difficulty initiating and maintaining sleep (Jennum *et al*, 1993; Moldofsky, 1995). It remains unclear as to whether the sleep disturbances are due to the chronic diffuse aches and pains, or, if the fragmentation of sleep is the primary disturbance responsible for the daytime symptoms. Studies seem to support both possibilities (Smith and Haythornwaite, 2004), but none of the pathophysiological theories put forward has resulted, so far, in better or more successful treatments.

Objective measures of sleep confirm, to a variable degree, subjective reports of sleep fragmentation (Branco *et al*, 1994) and the frequent occurrence of alpha intrusion during non-REM sleep EEG. Alpha waves are EEG frequencies of 7.5–11 Hz seen in 'normal' people who are awake with their eyes closed and in a relaxed state. The description of delta-alpha rhythm as an alpha rhythm overriding slow-wave sleep EEG (1.5–4 Hz) has been described in psychiatric patients, other rheumatological conditions and also in normal subjects. There is no strong evidence that alpha intrusion has an aetiological role in fibromyalgia, in general, nor in the associated sleep disturbances. In the patients with fibromyalgia who respond positively to small doses of amitriptyline (the minority), the response is not correlated with changes in alpha intrusion (Carette *et al*, 1995).

The role of overnight polysomnography in the investigation of fibromyalgia is limited and the indications are the same as for any other sleep disorder. Specifically, polysomnography is indicated if there is a suspicion of sleep fragmentation from other primary sleep disorders, such as periodic limb movement disorder or sleep apnea, which may be contributing to the fibromyalgia symptoms. The recognition of alpha intrusion is of value as a research tool, and does not have clinical value for the diagnosis.

Management of sleep disturbances in fibromyalgia requires a multimodal approach: a combination of physical therapy and medication to control the pain and adoption of regular sleep routine. It is important, however, to avoid prolonged time in bed, which is counterproductive to sleep quality.

There is a need to define the nature of the chronic fatigue state which is universally present in fibromyalgia and overlaps with chronic fatigue syndrome. When there is evidence of increased daytime sleepiness as an underlying mechanism of the chronic fatigue (eg. by multiple sleep latency test), a small dose of stimulant medication may be indicated (dexamphetamine, methylphenidate, modafinil).

Significant sleep deprivation should be ascertained by history and a sleep diary, as insufficient sleep is a frequent cause of symptoms similar to fibromyalgia. When the proper sleep routine is implemented, the use of medication may be considered on an individual basis. Amitriptyline (10–25 mg) at bedtime, a short-acting hypnotic (temazepam 10 mg, zoplicone 7.5 mg) can be useful. Because of the often coexistent depressed moods, the new group of antidepressants (fluoxetine, venlafaxine and nefazodone) have been used with some beneficial effects (O'Malley *et al*, 2000; Slawson and Meurer, 2001).

Case study 5: Chronic painful conditions and insomnia

Davina Goodchild is a 69-year-old woman with a 3-year history of difficulty in falling asleep, awakening through the night and daytime tiredness. She has Wenkenbach's heartblock, hyperparathyroidism requiring parathyroidectomy, severe osteoarthritis and osteoporosis with left total knee replacement, total right shoulder replacement and stable ischemic heart disease.

Her bedtime is irregular, usually between 10.00PM and midnight, but at least twice a week she stays up, sometimes until after 1.00AM. Sleep onset is up to 1½ hours after bedtime. She wakes two to three times a night with shoulder and lower back pain. Her final wake-up time is about 6.00AM. She dozes on and off until 7.30AM when she gets up feeling tired. She has no history of snoring or choking arousals. She has mild episodes of restless legs at least two to three nights a week. She complains of tiredness during the day but she doesn't fall asleep in unusual circumstances.

She has used temazepam and zolpidem with limited success. Davina has tried various non-steroidal anti-inflammatory medications and now takes celecoxib (Celebrex™) 200mg twice a day but with only partial pain relief.

Actigraphy (*Figure 7.8*) reveals a pattern suggestive of delayed sleep onset with fragmentation of the resting period, presumably related to musculoskeletal pain.

The diagnosis includes:
- delayed sleep onset
- fragmentation of sleep secondary to chronic pain due to osteoporosis and osteoarthritis
- restless leg syndrome.

Davina is asked to maintain a regular bedtime around 11.30PM and wake-up time of 6.30AM–7.00AM irrespective of how much sleep she has had and to avoid naps through the day. She is given melatonin 3mg to take between 9.00PM and 10.00PM, and 5mg of slow-release morphine to take at about 10.00PM. At follow-up a week later, she says that her sleep quality has improved.

Melatonin is continued for 4 weeks and when Davina is reviewed at 6 weeks she says that her sleep quality has improved greatly and that she falls asleep easily by 11.30PM, only wakes occasionally through the night, and sleeps soundly until 7.00AM. Her restless legs are well controlled. Davina remains off melatonin and manages her chronic pain with panadeine before bedtime and morphine 5mg for brief periods when the pain is worse.

Comments

This case highlights the importance of appropriate symptomatic relief in patients with chronic medical conditions, in this case, chronic pain. It is also a good example of the usefulness of morphine both for chronic pain control and management of restless legs (see below). It should be noted that the amount of slow-release morphine, 5 mg, was, although a very small dose, quite effective. The melatonin was useful in the first few weeks to advance sleep onset to earlier hours.

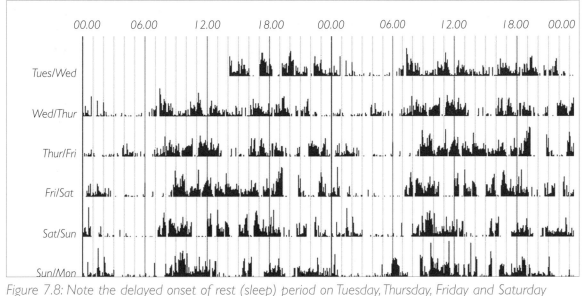

Figure 7.8: Note the delayed onset of rest (sleep) period on Tuesday, Thursday, Friday and Saturday nights. Time scale: 0:00 = midnight.

Case study 6: Insomnia and substance abuse

Serina Enright is an 18-year-old university student referred due to daytime tiredness and an inability to fall asleep and stay asleep. She has a history of tiredness since the age of 13 and her symptoms, consistent with depression and anorexia nervosa, were recognized at the age of 16 when she was treated with antidepressants. She shares a house with her boyfriend and takes cipramil and the contraceptive pill.

Serina goes to bed between midnight and 1.00AM and can take up to 2–3 hours to fall asleep. She wakes once or twice a night briefly and gets up between 8.00AM and midday, depending on commitments. According to her family, Serina has been a 'poor sleeper' since she was a toddler and suffered frequent night terrors.

When Serina is interviewed alone (without her family present) answering direct questions, she admits to smoking marijuana heavily over the last 6 months (four cones a day, usually in the evening). She also drinks about 500 ml of cola drink first thing in the morning and another 3 litres during the day, usually in the afternoon. She feels that she cannot fall asleep at night without marijuana. She says that once every 10 days or so she stays awake in bed all night without being able to fall asleep. She displays no symptoms of depression.

An overnight polysomnography shows evidence of prolonged sleep onset latency (2 hours after bedtime at 11.00PM) but no other abnormalities. No daytime sleepiness is documented on multiple sleep latency testing.

The diagnosis includes the following:
- substance-induced sleep disorder
- delayed sleep phase syndrome
- prior depression and eating disorder.

Management includes explaining in detail how the above diagnoses are interacting to cause her sleep problems. Serina is guided through a gradual withdrawal of caffeine, starting by reducing the night-time amount and also reducing her marijuana use over a period of 6 weeks. The reduction has to be slow to prevent withdrawal symptoms, in particular headache and worsening of sleep patterns.

Serina is requested to maintain a regular bed and wake-up time, of between midnight and 7.00AM, and to avoid napping through the day. Her psychiatrist has told her of the potential risk of the reappearance of depression once she is completely substance free.

At follow-up, Serina has reduced her marijuana intake to six cones over a 4-week period and 1 litre of cola drink at weekends. She does not feel as tired and falls asleep before midnight each night. She is encouraged to stop all caffeine beverages and cannabis. The deleterious effect of caffeine is well known, causing a reduction of sleep time, prolonged sleep onset latency and REM suppression.

Marijuana extracts have variable effects depending on the individual and the social circumstances in which the drug is taken. At high doses it is shown to delay sleep onset, reduce total sleep time and the percentage of REM, and possibly increase stage 4. sleep Upon withdrawal, there is an increase in REM (REM rebound). The effects of marijuana usually last between 2–6 hours (Feinberg et al, 1976).

Comments

This case highlights the importance of taking an accurate history on possible use of substances which interfere with sleep. Inquiring about the intake of coffee, tea, chocolate, caffeinated beverages and recreational drugs should be routine in any sleep history. A similar effect on sleep occurs when other stimulants, such as amphetamines and cocaine, are used.

Case study 7: Difficulty staying asleep and early morning arousals (advanced sleep phase syndrome)

Charles Bowman is a 74-year-old retired mechanic presenting with difficulty staying asleep. He is a non-smoker, non-drinker, with a history of hypertension, coronary artery bypass surgery and a prostate operation 5 years ago. He is overweight and has maturity onset diabetes which is poorly controlled on diet. There were no other abnormalities; his oropharynx is normal.

Charles goes to sleep between 7.00PM and 7.30PM and falls asleep within half an hour of retiring. He wakes around midnight with a dry mouth and drinks apple juice which he keeps at the bedside. He falls asleep again until between 2.00AM and 3.00AM when he wakes and struggles to fall asleep again until 5.00AM when he gets up for the day. He says he doesn't sleep through the day. His wife says he is a noisy breather but she has not noticed apneas. He has taken temazepam (Normison™) intermittently with no significant change in his sleep pattern.

Polysomnography shows reduced sleep efficiency to 70% with a total sleep time of 5 hours and 25 minutes, and a total bedtime of 7 hours 30 minutes between 8.00PM and 4.30AM. He has to get up three times during the night to urinate.

The diagnosis includes the following:
- advanced sleep phase syndrome
- sleep fragmentation due to polyuria secondary to poorly controlled diabetes
- possible prostatism (despite previous prostate surgery).

It is explained to Charles that a total sleep time of 6–6½ hours is normal for someone of his age.

As he is going to bed at 7.00PM–7.30PM he is fulfilling most of his sleep requirements by 3.00AM at the latest. Part of his problem is a timing issue for which sleeping tablets are not helpful. Normison™ is stopped and he is advised to move his bedtime 30 minutes later every 3–4 days, with the aim of going to bed around 10.00PM–11.00PM. He is also advised to keep his living room well lit up until 9.00PM.

Fragmentation of sleep due to polyuria secondary to poorly controlled diabetes is associated with urinary frequency and with dry mouth. Charles is referred back to his family doctor for further management of his diabetes. Prostatism is not felt to be a problem for Charles although it is a frequent problem for sleep fragmentation in this setting.

Comments

The multiple problems in this case are used to highlight a common cause of early morning arousals in elderly people. Although advanced sleep phase syndrome (ASPS) is frequent in institutionalized patients (eg. in nursing homes and hostels) it is also seen in elderly patients living independently, usually due to poor mobility and reduced social contact which exacerbates a phase advance of the endogenous circadian pacemaker seen in this age group (Lack *et al*, 1996).

Difficulty staying asleep through the night, and early morning arousals are often made worse by other aspects of poor sleep hygiene. It is common for patients to go to bed around 8.00PM, wake around 1.00AM, make a cup of tea or coffee and watch television, then try to sleep again, usually dozing lightly until 5.00AM or 6.00AM. For these people the day starts early, at 3.00AM or 4.00AM, and they often feel tired and sleepy during the day.

Using hypnotics in this setting is contraindicated as it adds to the risk of falling when the patient gets out of bed in the middle of the night. Sleeping tablets are uniformly unsuccessful. In particular, using sleeping tablets in the middle of the night, at 2.00AM or 3.00AM, is not advised as it will adversely affect the patient during the day.

Management includes moving bedtime to later in the evening and using bright light in the evenings. Keeping the living area well lit is sufficient for many patients, together with exposure to outdoor light during the 'daylight saving' period of the year. Although there are light-boxes available for this specific purpose, these are expensive and a halogen lamp diverted to the ceiling to avoid eye damage may be sufficient.

Case study 8: Night-time eating or nocturnal-eating syndrome (NES)

Liana Vercoe is a 22-two-year-old nurse, who slept well for most of her life until she started travelling with her boyfriend. While overseas, she would often wake up in the middle of the night feeling hungry and she and her boyfriend would go out to eat. Eating when she woke became a habit which continued even after she returned home. Her weight has subsequently increased by approximately 12 kg. This is distressing for her and she has stopped eating during the daytime in order to lose weight. At night, her boyfriend locks her in the bedroom to stop her eating. However whenever the door is left unlocked (usually two to three times per week) Liana gets up and eats.

Liana's sleep and wake pattern consists of a bedtime between 10.00PM and 11.00PM on weekdays and around midnight at the weekend. Her sleep latency is 10–15 minutes and she sleeps until approximately 2.00AM to 3.00AM when she gets up and goes to the kitchen. She is aware of getting up and being in the kitchen, but is not aware of eating. She estimates that she is up for approximately 20 minutes. She is also aware of being back in bed and that it takes her about 15 minutes to return to sleep. Her final waking time is 6.15AM with an alarm on weekdays and 7.00AM to 8.00AM on weekend days.

There are no significant symptoms of other sleeping disorders, such as obstructive sleep apnea, restless leg syndrome, periodic limb movements, bruxism or narcolepsy. Liana has a low intake of caffeine, does not smoke and rarely drinks alcohol during the working week. However, on weekends she can consume up to eight vodkas at a time. She is on an intense, regular exercise programme, working out at the gym at least 5 days per week from 5.00PM to 7.00PM.

Liana is asked to complete a number of baseline questionnaires and to keep a sleep diary over the following 2 weeks. It is suggested that her boyfriend leaves the door unlocked on at least 2 nights per week but not to tell her which nights. Liana is reassured that although eating in the middle of the night is not common, it is an acknowledged disorder associated with sleep.

Liana returns for review 2 weeks later. Her baseline sleep diary shows that her bedtime continues to be around 10.00PM or 11.00PM weeknights and midnight to 1.00AM on weekends. The first week of the diary shows that she got up and ate 2 out of the 3 nights when the bedroom door was unlocked. In the second week, the door was always left unlocked as Liana's sister was staying with them and sleeping on the sofa. Liana knew that getting up would disturb her sister. Interestingly, during this second week, Liana only got up twice even though the door was unlocked. She was able to return to sleep on the nights that she woke and had a total sleep time of 7–9 hours.

During this consultation the rationale for sleep hygiene measures was explained and Liana is encouraged to adhere to a behavioral regimen where she incorporates both bed restriction and light therapy to reset her circadian rhythm on a daily basis and builds up a sleep debt to decrease her waking at night. She is also encouraged to increase her calories at breakfast time, and on the days that she goes to the gym she is to have afternoon tea, plus a small carbohydrate snack half an hour prior to bedtime. Her baseline questionnaires show some daytime sleepiness with an ESS of 8, but no significant mood changes on the DASS, and a relatively low fatigue score of 18. Her PSQI is almost normal with a global score of 6. She is asked to return for further review in a month and to keep up with the sleep diary.

Liana does not return for review but sends a letter describing her sleep and eating patterns. She no longer wakes in the middle of the night to eat and has a consolidated sleep of 7–9 hours. She is eating a larger breakfast and enjoys the structure of her early morning with light exposure and walking.

Comments

The criteria for night-eating disorders (Allen, 2000) require individuals to have morning anorexia and eat more than 50% of their daily food intake after the evening meal and before the end of the sleep period. There is usually amnesia associated with night eating. Liana was aware of getting up and being back in bed, but not of actually eating. In a research study involving two separate protocols for NES, ten NES patients and ten matched controls (mostly female) were monitored for nocturnal awakenings, mood and calories consumed, while twelve NES subjects and twenty-one controls (all female) were evaluated for neuroendocrine characteristics over 24 hours with 2-hourly blood sampling for glucose, insulin, melatonin, leptin and cortisol. The behavioral assessment of patients with NES suggest that they consume 74% of their calories after dinner and have more awakenings from sleep with depressed mood than the controls. They also have significantly lower melatonin levels and leptin throughout the night (Birketvedt *et al*, 1999). NES patients appear to be experiencing a circadian rhythm disorder more than an arousal disorder. It is also unclear as to whether the neuroendocrine changes occurred as a result of, or were a trigger for, the night-time eating (Allen, 2000). Overall, it appears that night-time eating patterns should be enquired about when treating individuals with sleep maintenance insomnia. Modification of the patient's eating pattern seems an important treatment strategy, because food intake and induction of satiety appear to decrease sleep latency (the patient falls asleep faster), to increase slow-wave sleep and to consolidate sleep (Lauer and Krieg, 2004).

Treatment of insomnia

It cannot be over-emphasized that management of chronic insomnia requires a multimodal strategy, tailored to individual patients. The key words here are 'multimodal' and 'individual'. The management will be somewhat different in each individual with varied emphasis on behavioral/cognitive, pharmacological and psychodynamic intervention.

The aim of treatment should be to provide the patient with a strategy to be used in the future if symptoms recur, which is often the case (Angst *et al*, 1989; Mendelson, 1995). An important management issue relates to retraining and learning control over sleep. The underlying message is that sleep is controllable. People suffering from chronic insomnia often have a sense of hopelessness from repeated treatment failures. The overall management aim is to restore a sense of control and confidence that something can be done, albeit complete remission or improvement. Certain basic instructions are common to any intervention:

- education about sleep and wake function
- regularity of bedtime and wake-up time
- avoiding prolonged time in bed
- creating a positive environment for sleep, including reduction of any stimulant medication.

The decision to employ a particular management strategy should be based on the individual patient, keeping in mind the following:

- level of education and intelligence
- level of psychological sophistication and willingness to participate in their own treatment
- individual preferences.

Cognitive and physiological arousal is present in insomnia, with variable effects on the individual (Gross and Borkovec, 1982; Lushington and Lack, 2002; Morin, 1993). At the end of the initial assessment, the clinician should have an idea of how well the patient will be able to undertake and benefit from cognitive behavioral therapy intervention, to what extent, and to what level of detail. Individual preference should be respected as this is likely to influence the outcome positively (Vincent and Lionberg, 2001).

Patient education

Providing information on sleep is essential for any intervention and forms the basis on which to motivate changes in thinking about sleep and sleep behavior. The degree of detail will vary between patients and whether the information is directed to an individual or a group. The following topics are examples of the education process.

Sleep and sleep stages

For individuals to change their sleep behavior and adopt new strategies, a general understanding of sleep performance and circadian rhythm (cycles that fluctuate on a daily basis) is necessary (*Chapters 1* and *2*).

Background: We spend almost a third of our lives sleeping but find it difficult to determine either the length or the quality of sleep when compared with objective measures.

Measuring sleep: Brain waves can be measured by the use of electroencephalograms (EEG). During sleep, the different stages of sleep (using EEG) can be recorded and this is called polysomnography (PSG). Sleep is an active process made up of non-rapid eye movement (NREM) sleep of which there are four stages, moving from light (stage 1) to deep (stage 4), and rapid eye movement (REM) sleep or dream sleep (*Figure 7.9*).

Our sleep needs: We cycle through the stages of sleep approximately every 90 minutes achieving the most amount of deep sleep (NREM states 3 and 4) in the first 180 minutes of sleep. Deep sleep or slow-wave sleep is when the electrical activity of the brain is slowed down, referred to as the restorative part of sleep, whereas REM is more associated with cognition and memory.

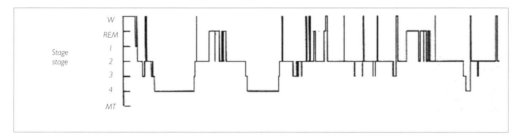

Figure 7.9: Normal hypnogram showing sleep stage distribution. W = wake; REM = rapid eye movement sleep; 1 = stage 1 sleep; 2 = stage 2 sleep; 3 = stage 3 sleep; 4 = stage 4 sleep; MT = movement time.

These facts can be reassuring for individuals with insomnia: knowing that no matter what time the individual goes to sleep, even a few hours will provide enough deep sleep to maintain baseline function the following day. A diagram of overnight sleep (hypnogram) helps patients to visualize the above ideas (*Figure 7.9*). Emphasizing that most deep sleep is achieved in the first 180 minutes of sleep is important (although an oversimplification) and, in conjunction with the information that most REM sleep (dream sleep) occurs towards the morning, helps correct the common misperception that deep sleep occurs just before waking.

It is important to introduce the concept that a shortened sleep time does not always result in poor performance. Poor sleep usually results in a compensatory mechanism where cortisol and adrenocorticotrophin-releasing hormone (ACTH) are increased to allow individuals to function adequately during the daytime (Vgontzas *et al*, 2001). Individuals with long-standing insomnia generally respond and relate well to this information.

Insomnia and hyper-arousal response

It takes little to over-arouse someone physiologically. From an evolutionary point of view, arousal is what permits survival to react to threat. It can take less than a second to become fully alert if a potential danger is perceived to be present (eg. an unusual noise in the house) but a long time to relax after this (Spielman and Glovinsky, 1991). People with insomnia are often excessively aroused (hyper-aroused), and even so-called 'normal sleepers' can be physiologically over-aroused and have the quality of their sleep reduced by consuming increased amounts of caffeine or experiencing a week of induced insomnia (Bonnet and Arand, 1992).

Although physiological arousal is found in many individuals with insomnia (Vgontzas *et al*, 2001) there are many people who have poor sleep (objectively) but do not perceive themselves as having insomnia (Lushington and Lack, 2002). There is also the converse situation of sleep state misperception, where individuals are extremely inaccurate at being able to assess either the quantity or quality of their sleep. They perceive that they have not slept when EEG shows near normal sleep.

The discrepancy between objective assessment and subjective perception of sleep quality may be explained by limitations of current EEG technology. Using more complex EEG assessment (fast Fourier analysis) subtle changes within sleep stages can be identified. This information may, in time, provide an explanation for the sense of not sleeping, and daytime fatigue found in individuals with insomnia (Ferrara *et al*, 2002; Vgontzas *et al*, 2002). At present it is unclear whether physiological hyper-arousal causes insomnia, or vice versa.

Insomnia and performance

Individuals with insomnia perform as well on objective tasks (reaction time tests and executive function tasks) as those who sleep well (Reidel and Lichstein, 2000). However, subjectively, individuals with insomnia generally do not feel that they are able to function adequately the next day.

Falling asleep

Falling asleep is driven primarily by two factors:

- prior wakefulness (sleep debt)
- the time of the day in the 24-hour sleep-wake cycle.

We go to sleep because we have built up a sleep debt and we stay asleep because it is the right time of the day night cycle for us to sleep (Horne, 1988). Environmental conditions also influence our sleep. We live in a 24-hour environment yet the human daily rhythm (circadian rhythm) is a slightly longer period (or sometimes shorter) and, therefore, requires resetting on a daily basis by environmental cues (*Chapter 2*).

The light–dark cycle, the body clock and melatonin

The most powerful environmental cue is the light–dark cycle, which helps synchronize body functions by sending light messages via the retina to the body clock at the base of the brain, the suprachiasmatic nucleus (SCN). The SCN interacts with many other parts of the brain (*Figure 2.5, Chapter 2*), in particular, the pineal gland which produces the hormone melatonin. During the day, bright light helps suppress the production of melatonin and increases the corticotrophic hormones, such as cortisol, which promote wakefulness. At night, melatonin is released in response to darkness and has two functions (Lewy *et al*, 1996):

- a slightly hypnotic action
- causing a fall in the core body temperature.

Sleep onset and the maintenance of sleep are associated with a decrease in core body temperature. Exposure to morning light and a constant waking time, regardless of the quality or length of night-time sleep, are important cues to maintaining a healthy sleep–wake pattern. This relatively simple explanation of sleep forms the rationale for sleep hygiene measures that are described below.

Individually sleep hygiene measures are not particularly successful but, in combination, they are more effective in the long term than pharmacotherapy (Morin *et al*, 1994). Not all sleep hygiene measures need to be explained on the first follow up visit as the patient will already have been given a great deal of information. It is important to have written instructions outlining three or four recommendations tailored to the individual's needs, with explanations as to why these proposals are made. Giving patients a list of general sleep hygiene rules is usually not successful (Hauri, 1991).

Sleep hygiene measures

Sleep hygiene is a term which covers a number of approaches aimed at improving sleep patterns through behavioral changes (Hauri, 1991). The behavioral measures described below are aimed not only at consolidating and improving the quality of sleep, but also at regaining and maintaining control over sleep.

Reduce time in bed

Many people compensate for their poor sleep–wake pattern by spending long periods of time in bed. This generally results in increased sleep anxiety and deterioration in the quality of sleep. The aim of this programme is to curtail time in bed to approximately match sleep time, or have sleep time as 85% of the period spent in bed. Keeping a sleep diary is a useful method of assessing both time in bed and total sleep time. However a sleep diary is counterproductive in patients with compulsive obsessive traits because it tends to increase focus on the sleep problem and consequent anxiety.

Consistent waking time

Getting out of bed at the same time each day is more important than going to bed at the same time at night. Going to bed at the same time each night does not guarantee sleep, as there must be a sleep need for sleep onset to occur. Therefore, any changes to sleep behavior patterns must occur with changes in getting up times. This is not an easy task, especially when many individuals feel that their best sleep occurs in the last sleep cycle. To begin this programme, it is often necessary for individuals to decrease the time spent in bed.

Early morning light exposure

The most powerful cue for resetting the brain sleep clock is light around dawn. This light is not necessarily sunlight. Exposure to bright light in the morning tends to advance the sleep cycle (the person is ready to go to sleep earlier in the evening). This is achieved by resetting melatonin production earlier in the evening. There is also an associated increased release of corticosteroid which allows the individual to function more effectively during the day. The patient is advised to be outside for at least 30 minutes, and not to wear sunglasses, tinted glasses or hats with a brim during the day.

Bed activities and sleep

Bed needs to be a safe and comfortable place for sleeping. Noise from the environment, from television or other sources, such as radio and CDs, disrupts sleep. Music is not static but changes considerably, resulting in constant arousals during sleep.

Clock-watching and sleep

Watching the clock at night tends to increase anxiety about sleep. Good sleepers see 2.00AM on the clock when they wake and think 'Wonderful, four more hours in bed'. Poor sleepers see the same time and think 'Disaster — I am never going to get back to sleep!' Keep the clock in your room but turn it to the wall; put it on the floor or even outside the bedroom door.

Alcohol, coffee and smoking

Alcohol, coffee and smoking should be avoided by people with difficulty initiating and maintaining sleep. Alcohol may help in achieving sleep but it generally causes people to wake in the second half of the night. The last alcoholic drink of the evening should be consumed at least 3 hours prior to bedtime. Caffeine can affect sleep in predisposed individuals, even if it is taken 12 hours prior to bedtime. Nicotine, particularly in high doses, has a stimulant effect and is counterproductive to sleep.

Temperature control and sleep

A falling core body temperature is crucial for the onset and maintenance of sleep. To enhance the onset of sleep, raising the core body temperature some hours prior to sleep onset is a useful trigger and can be achieved by active or passive means, for example:

- *exercise* — it may take up to 5 hours for the body to cool and slow down sufficiently for sleep onset to occur following aerobic exercise. More gentle exercise, such as walking, may only require a cooling down time of one to two hours.
- *baths* — a warm deep bath of at least 20 minutes, 1.5 hours prior to bedtime will raise the core body temperature. It is important to stay out of bed for at least 1 hour after the bath to enhance the fall in core body temperature, which promotes sleep onset.

Diet and sleep

A carbohydrate snack: a malted milk drink, toast, a small portion of rice or pasta 30 minutes prior to bedtime is considered by some to be a useful 'sleep enhancer'. It is not clear why a snack appears to promote sleep in some people and convincing evidence is lacking. However, it is possible that a release of tryptophan, a precursor of melatonin, may be involved. Avoid high-protein foods (with the exception of milk) and large meals a few hours prior to bedtime.

Stimulus control therapy

This programme has two specific aims:

1) To regulate the individual's sleep and wake pattern.
2) To change behavior patterns and thought processes.

The individual learns to re-associate bed with sleep as opposed to the anxiety and frustration experienced through lying awake in bed for long periods of time. The rules of the behavior programme include the following:

- do not go to bed early

- go to bed only when sleepy or relaxed
- get out of bed if unable to initiate sleep within 15–20 minutes
- go into another room
- do some non-stimulating activity such as reading, watching TV, listening to music, or gentle breathing or relaxation exercises
- do not use bright light but learn to feel comforted in the dark
- avoid smoking, coffee or tea.

When the individual feels less tense or a little sleepy they should return to bed and try to sleep again. This pattern of changing sleep and wake behavior generally requires many trials over a number of consecutive nights. These measures need to be reassessed at each session and changes made as necessary, reinforcing success and helping troubleshoot failure. A crucial message to give a patient with insomnia is that many small changes lead to the development of a behavior-strength.

Background

Stimulus control therapy evolved from the premise that insomnia results from the association of being awake in bed at night (the environment), with the time (night), and sleep-incompatible behaviors. By removing the stimuli (bed, bedtime and behavior) the individual can reassociate the bed with regular sleeping (Bootzin *et al*, 1991; Bootzin and Nicassio, 1978). Reducing the time spent awake in bed can be achieved by a combination of behavioral therapies. Stimulus control therapy is the most successful behavioral treatment and is one of the few treatments to show an overall effectiveness (Edinger, 2001; Morin *et al*, 1994). In combination with other treatments, stimulus control therapy strengthens the idea that many small changes are required to regain a good sleeping pattern. Stimulus control therapy is, however, a difficult concept for many people to accept which may require that they address some incorrect beliefs.

This programme to change sleep–wake behavior needs to be repeated generally over a number of consecutive nights to be effective.

Many individuals with insomnia go to bed early or stay in bed for long periods of time, believing that they:

- are at least resting
- can take their time to go to sleep as they feel less pressurized.

The reality, however, is that they tend to use the time to over-arouse themselves cognitively by worrying, planning and having long internal monologues that increase their anxiety and frustration about not being asleep. They may also go to bed because they feel tired but are not actually sleepy. Explaining the difference between being sleepy (the desire to close your eyes and go to sleep), and being physically tired or fatigued (lacking in energy) is a useful step.

Being fatigued is different from being sleepy. People can be tired and fatigued from playing sport but not ready to go to sleep. Being sleepy is when someone finds it very difficult to stay awake; they have an overwhelming need to sleep. Many individuals with chronic insomnia have not experienced feeling sleepy for a long time as the stronger feeling associated with sleep is one of being anxious, over-aroused or 'wired'. Starting a behavior pattern (stimulus control therapy) of getting out of bed when they are unable to sleep is difficult, especially in winter, and requires not only a mindset change but also preparation for the likelihood/possibility of getting up.

The following advice can help the patient implementing stimulus control.

Preparation for stimulus control therapy

Preparation for getting out of bed during the night may include leaving a book in the sitting room or lounge to read, putting a blanket out (not for sleeping) or a heater to keep warm in winter, and organizing a lamp which can be used to read instead of using an overhead light. Making these preparations is part of the commitment to this programme.

No matter how many times people get up during the night; it is of paramount importance that they still get up in the morning at the same time, regardless of the quality or quantity of their sleep. A constant getting-up time and exposure to early morning light is crucial in resetting circadian rhythm on a daily basis. A little change in the getting-up time is acceptable one day in the week but it must be within a 1–2-hour range, or the outcome is similar to the effects of jet lag and all the hard work during the week will be disrupted.

The patient should be made aware that when these measures are implemented, performance during the day may initially deteriorate, because sleep may be quite curtailed. This is a common reason given for failing to persevere with treatment. In these cases, strategic napping during the day may be allowed.

Napping

Napping is a useful method of managing overwhelming daytime sleepiness. Short naps (10–30 minutes) improve performance better than longer naps (Tietzel and Lack, 2002). Napping longer than 35 minutes allows the individual to go into slow-wave sleep or deep sleep, which decreases the amount of sleep debt and may be detrimental to sleep onset in the evening (Webb and Agnew, 1975). All naps must be stopped by 3.00PM, which is again related to building up a sleep debt in order to achieve a consolidated period of slow-wave sleep. Even a brief involuntary nap for a few minutes (watching television after dinner) can interfere with sleep onset later in the evening and should be avoided.

Bed restriction therapy

Restriction of time spent in bed is an effective technique by itself and strengthens the effects of stimulus control therapy (Spielman *et al*, 1987). Bed restriction is based on the premise that an excessive time spent in bed both exacerbates and maintains the symptoms of insomnia.

Individuals inadvertently train themselves to be awake in bed through a combination of either physical arousal, cognitive arousal, or a combination of the two. Estimating sleep efficiency is a good determinant of the degree of bed restriction required to induce mild sleep restriction and, thereby, increase sleep debt and sleepiness. The formula for sleep efficiency is as follows:

$$\text{Sleep efficiency} = \frac{\text{time asleep} \times 100}{\text{time in bed}}$$

$$\text{Example: } \frac{\text{six hours asleep} \times 100}{\text{eight hours in bed}} = 75\%$$

The aim of bed restriction therapy is for a sleep efficiency of more than 85%. This goal is achieved by slowly decreasing the time spent in bed by rising earlier, going to bed later or a combination of the two. It is important for people to select which is the most appropriate for them as this will increase their adherence. This therapy requires a verbal contract between the patient and doctor and, therefore, the sleep routine has to be realistic and fit in with the patient's lifestyle. In the example above, the aim would be to gradually reduce the time in bed to 6 hours only for the number of nights or weeks it takes until the individual is sleeping for that length of time. The time in bed is then gradually increased, but always with the underlying principle that sleep efficiency is being maintained at a level of greater than 85%.

Relaxation strategies

Relaxation strategies are important in reducing hyperarousal (rush of thoughts, worrying) and promoting sleep onset. To learn to relax, patients must first be aware of when they are tense or stressed. Many people feel too pressured by their environment, work, relationships or social factors to take the time to examine the effects of these factors on themselves and their sleep patterns. Stress is the emotional interpretation of an event that results in anxious feelings. The anxiety translates into tension which manifests itself in tightening muscles and becoming physically alert. This response is a protective mechanism against potential danger but when associated with sleep, it leads to further anxiety about not being able to sleep (Lushington and Lack, 2002; Wicklow and Espie, 2000).

The combination of maladaptive sleep habits or poor sleep hygiene and physiological and cognitive-emotional hyper-arousal inevitably leads to a cycle that maintains the insomnia (Morin, 1993). Breaking these factors into workable units or blocks that can be treated individually is a crucial part of retraining patients with insomnia who are emotionally distressed by their poor sleep.

Discuss the factors that favour or hinder relaxation:

* identify events that are usual and safe (known sounds, eg. neighbours coming home)
* recognize anxiety-provoking events, eg. unexpected noises, thinking about 'night-time' and 'not sleeping', and their negative impact on sleep onset
* explain that daytime performance will not be reduced by not sleeping well. Objective daytime performance is not generally compromised even though there may be a subjective interpretation of poor performance and fatigue (Reidel and Lichstein, 2000)

- explain increased muscle tension and thought-processing leads to a physiological arousal response, which is not conducive to sleep.

Eventually, bedtime and the bedroom become associated with arousal and not being able to sleep, an association which persists after the initial stress trigger is no longer present and even forgotten. The individual is left with the hyperarousal response associated with the onset of or difficulty returning to sleep. Thinking about sleep is associated with negative thoughts before even attempting sleep (Van Egeren *et al*, 1983). The cause or the trigger for not sleeping is lost but the belief of an inability to sleep well is maintained.

Relaxation should be practiced during the day when there is less pressure to succeed at a given technique and no pressure to sleep. Relaxation, initially, should be practiced regularly, not only when needed. Many individuals have the mistaken idea that relaxation techniques are for the night only. Emphasize the importance of **not** practising relaxation techniques in bed, as the bed has become a place of not feeling safe or comfortable enough to go to sleep. Many people find that they can learn relaxation techniques lying on the bedroom floor, as it is a 'neutral place' generally not associated with sleep. Practical issues have to be considered and the bedroom may be the only room in the house where the individual with insomnia can find space for themselves.

The goal of sleep relaxation is to create a strong association between the practice of relaxation during the day, and a sense of having 'time out', 'of not thinking' and 'letting go'. Even if these techniques are used for only a few minutes, they are beneficial and can be extended to longer periods and then be used at bedtime.

It is also important to stress that relaxation strategies do not work every time. It is rare for something to have the same effect all the time, yet this mistaken assumption is often made about the ability to relax or go to sleep. The 'no effect' of a given strategy is influenced by the individual's level of arousal and how they feel in terms of mood and other environmental and social factors. Relaxation strategies are generally positively received by patients but used alone do not appear to improve sleep (Harvey *et al*, 2002). Therefore, relaxation techniques need to be used in combination with other strategies such as stimulus control and restriction of time spent in bed.

A good relaxation strategy to start with is diaphragmatic breathing (*Box 7.1*). This involves learning a new way to breathe. By focusing on abdominal movements, intrusive thoughts are shut out, marking the beginning of the relaxation response. Practicing abdominal breathing for 10 minutes at a time is a good starting plan. Another technique for time out is described in *Box 7.2*.

Cognitive restructuring

Many treatment programmes for insomnia promote cognitive behavioral therapy (CBT) when, in reality, the emphasis is only on changing behavior. Cognitive restructuring is sometimes overlooked in insomnia treatment, yet is an integral component of the treatment process (Morin *et al*, 2002). Learning to sleep is a combination of changing inappropriate behavior and misguided or unrealistic thoughts about sleep. What we think affects how we feel and both in turn affect our behavior. People with insomnia have more negative thoughts about sleep than good sleepers do (Van Egeren *et al*, 1983). They worry more about sleep (Watts *et al*, 1994) and believe that they need to sleep for a set number of hours to function well the next day (Morin *et al*, 2002).

Box 7.1: Diaphragmatic breathing

⌘ Make yourself comfortable.

⌘ Take two to three slow, deep breaths.

⌘ Place your hands on the abdominal muscles under your navel.

⌘ As you gently breathe in, push your abdominal muscles out so that they are pressing against your hand.

⌘ Hold that breath and slowly count to three.

⌘ As you let your breath go, pull your abdominal muscles in tightly.

⌘ Count to three and repeat.

Diaphragmatic breathing provides a pleasant way of having time out, which you control.

Box 7.2: Alternative time out technique

⌘ Make yourself comfortable and close your eyes.

⌘ Breathe in and out in a slow, controlled way.

⌘ Imagine a circle or some other shape between your eyes.

⌘ Make that circle change color until you find a color that you like.

⌘ Imagine that you can be drawn into that color.

⌘ Through the color you can 'let go' of where you are — feel a sense of drifting, of feeling deeply relaxed.

Cognitive therapy occurs throughout the entire therapist–patient interaction. Providing information about the nature of sleep, discussing the rationale for stimulus control, sleep hygiene measures, and restriction of time in bed is part of cognitive restructuring. This information provides the foundations of modifying dysfunctional attitudes and beliefs about sleep. However, a more structured cognitive programme, with or without pharmacotherapy, can produce beneficial results in insomnia (Morin *et al*, 2002). Changes in beliefs and attitudes about sleep can be addressed by considering the five areas described in the dysfunctional beliefs and attitudes sleep scale (Morin, 1993; Morin *et al*, 1994; 2002). These relate to:

1. Misconceptions about sleep:
    My pineal gland is not producing enough melatonin and therefore I can't sleep.
2. Diminished perception of control and predictability of sleep:
    One night of poor sleep will be the beginning of weeks of insomnia, like before.
3. Unrealistic sleep expectations:
    I can't do anything properly at work without eight hours of good sleep.
4. Misattribution and amplification of the consequences of insomnia:
    My memory is terrible because I only get a few hours sleep a night.

5. Faulty beliefs about sleep-promoting practices:
    At least going to bed early lets me rest even if I can't sleep.

These are examples of core beliefs, which often have a connotation of helplessness. It is important to realise that individuals with insomnia tend to overgeneralize, be catastrophic, magnify events and feelings, excessively ruminate and suffer from selective recall about their sleep (Morin, 1993). These tendencies of 'all or nothing' are also seen with depression (Yapko, 1998). In insomnia retraining, the goal is to challenge incorrect beliefs and provide a more positive and constructive attitude. An individual should be taught to re-evaluate beliefs such as 'poor sleep affects every aspect of my ability to function effectively during the day' which is negative and helpless. A more positive approach being 'even with poor sleep I can still manage to work quite well although I feel tired'. The long-term goal is for the individual to appreciate that one night of poor sleep is only one night of poor sleep. It is neither fatal nor the beginning of a down-hill spiral of poor sleep, poor performance and worsening mood.

Cognitive behavioral therapy programmes are highly effective on a number of sleep measures. Espie *et al* (2001) found that, on average, at 1-year follow up, night-time sleeplessness was reduced by 1 hour per night, with two thirds of the sample population no longer meeting the criteria for insomnia, and of those previously taking hypnotic medication, 80% had ceased (Espie *et al*, 2001). Morin *et al* (2002) found that improved post-treatment scores (lowered) on the dysfunctional beliefs and attitude sleep scale (DBAS) were significantly correlated with increased sleep efficiency. The immediate effects of CBT intervention are not always apparent but there appear to be long-term positive implications. These treatment methods can be integrated into a group educational programme, which is both cost and time effective, especially in a public health system.

Insomnia education in a group setting

The following insomnia group educational programme is based on the successful work by Professor Colin Espie from Glasgow in Scotland (Espie *et al*, 2001). It has been modified by one of the authors (in conjunction with Adelaide-based clinical psychologist, Annette Brock) for an Australian public hospital setting.

The group programme consists of four, 1.5-hour sessions every fortnight (*Appendix E*). Up to twelve individuals with insomnia are enrolled in the group. Each person is assessed by either a sleep physician or sleep psychologist prior to commencement of the group to exclude the possibility of other sleep disorders or medical or psychiatric conditions which would not benefit from a group education programme. In the initial visit to the hospital sleep clinic, insomnia individuals are shown how to keep a sleep diary and are asked to complete the baseline questionnaires, including the Pittsburg Sleep Quality Index (PSQI), daytime fatigue (FSS), situational sleepiness by Epworth Sleepiness Scale (ESS), and mood using the Depression Anxiety Stress Scale (DASS), in addition to the shortened version of the Belief and Attitudes Sleep Questionnaire (*Appendix D*). If any person forgets to bring their questionnaires to the first group session they are asked to complete these questionnaires at the end of that session. These questionnaires are repeated at the end of the intervention period. Espie (1998) organized educational treatment programmes for insomnia in a community setting run by health visitors (registered nurses with additional university training).

These educational programmes are in six, 1-hour sessions.

The programme outlined in *Appendix E* aims to educate participants about effective treatment regimens. Strategies to counterbalance misattributions about sleep are introduced early in the programme, as the 'fear' associated with not sleeping requires considerable restructuring. A group insomnia educational programme has a number of potential benefits. There is a common goal to overcome sleep difficulties, and the small group makes it easier to assimilate information. The boundaries of the group need to be clearly defined in terms of it being an educational group as opposed to a psychotherapy group session. The expectations and goals of the programme should also be defined early on, stressing the need for an active role to be played by each participant.

Pharmacological treatment

Hypnotic medications

The use of hypnotic medications (mostly benzodiazepines) in patients with chronic insomnia, either continuously or intermittently, is a subject of controversy. However, the use of 'sleep-promoting' medications in transient (reactive) insomnia is an accepted and recommended therapy in the short term (3–4 days) (Consensus Conference, 1984; Roth *et al*, 1995). Prescription medications (benzodiazepines have been the most commonly prescribed hypnotic) are, if anything, under-used. In a recent survey, only 15% of patients with insomnia were using prescription medication (Brust, 1993; The Gallup Organisation, 1995; Walsh and Schweitzer, 1999; Wood *et al*, 1988). Those who did use prescription medications reported beneficial results and they often took less than the prescribed dose.

It is unfortunate that questionable use of scientific reports by policy makers, and confusion over drug dependence, withdrawal and addiction, have led to misconceptions among the general public and medical practitioners regarding the appropriate use of hypnotic medications (Salzman 1999) (see also *Chapter 12*).

While there is a group of researchers who believe that no long-term use of hypnotic medication should be allowed (Holbrook *et al*, 2000; Kripke *et al*, 1979, 1998) many clinicians consider the long-term use of hypnotic medication appropriate in qualified cases (Oswald *et al*, 1982; Regenstein, 1987; Scharf *et al*, 1994) and, in the short term, a useful adjunct to other management strategies in chronic insomnia. There is no evidence that benzodiazepines promote self-administrative behavior except in subjects who use drugs for recreational purposes or who are multiple drug users (Fleischhacker *et al*, 1986). The following medications are in clinical use:

- benzodiazepines
- non-benzodiazepine GABA A receptor agonists
- antidepressants
- melatonin
- opioids.

Indications for use of hypnotics (Roth *et al*, 1982) include :

- transient situational insomnia
- chronic insomnia refractory to other forms of treatment (childhood-onset insomnia, some forms of psychophysiological insomnia)
- chronic insomnia associated with conditions such as restless legs, periodic limb movement disorder or anxiety disorders.

Relative contraindications for hypnotics include:

- patients with a history of recreational drug use, including alcohol abuse
- pregnancy, particularly in the first trimester, or if breast feeding (as benzodiazepines cross the placenta and are excreted in the milk)
- severe obstructive sleep apnea, because of the increased risk of respiratory depression
- patients in high-risk occupations, such as commercial drivers, heavy machinery operators, workers on call who may need to attend their work in the middle of the night
- elderly patients because of the increased risk of toxicity (Roth *et al*, 1982), although the short-acting hypnotics, zaleplon and zolpidem, seem to be safe (Ancoli-Israel *et al*, 2005).

Choice of hypnotic medication

The choice of medication should be based on the clinical situation and the pharmacological properties of the drug.

- ❖ In patients with predominantly sleep onset difficulties, who cannot 'switch off' or have increased anxiety at bedtime, the use of short-acting hypnotics with rapid onset of activity is the recommended choice (triazolam, zolpidem, zopiclone and temazepam).
- ❖ In patients with a tendency to wake up after sleep onset, hypnotics with an intermediate length of action, 6–8, are preferable (oxazepam, lorazepam, temazepam). This group of medications is also useful in people with restless legs and periodic limb movement disorder.
- ❖ In subjects with anxiety disorders, a long-acting benzodiazepine with a rapid onset of action (diazepam, nitrazepam) may be a better choice, as the prolonged action will be useful the day after to control the anxiety symptoms.

The pharmacological characteristics of commonly used hypnotic medications are summarized in *Table 7.6*.

Long-acting hypnotics (half-life >24 hours) are likely to accumulate over time leading to an increased risk of side-effects, in particular, residual daytime sedation. Because of the long half- life, efficacy may be delayed for up to 3 days, therefore, this group of medications is not recommended if treatment is needed for only a few days (such as in transient insomnia). However, the clinical action does not strictly correlate with elimination of half-life. For example, diazepam and flunitrazepam, benzodiazepines with a long half-life of more than 24 hours, have a rapid redistribution into the peripheral muscular and adipose tissues after absorption, leading to a short clinical action when used for one or two nights (Greenblatt, 1991).

Table 7.6: Benzodiazepine and non-benzodiazepine hypnotic medications

Medication	Duration of action	Absorption	Dose	Comments
Temazepam (Normison™, Temaze™)	Intermediate (5–15 hr)	30–60 minutes	10–30 mg	Very safe profile, minimal daytime residual effects. Capsules have faster absorption than tablets
Zaleplon (Sonata™)	Short (1–2 hours)	30–60 minutes	5–10 mg	Use the smaller dose in the elderly. Safe profile, with minimal daytime effects
Zolpidem (Stilnox™)	Short (~2.5 hours)	30–60 minutes	5–10 mg	Use the smaller dose in the elderly. Safe profile, with minimal daytime effects
Zopiclone (Imovane™)	Short (~ 5.2 hours)	60–90 minutes	3.25–7.5 mg	Erythromycin increases the zopiclone concentration, requiring a dose reduction (of zopiclone). Zopiclone also causes a metallic taste.
Triazolam (Halcion™)	Short (1.5–5 hours)	< 30 minutes	0.125–0.25 mg	Fast and short action, can be associated with daytime anxiety, anterograde amnesia, and rebound insomnia (rare)
Oxazepam (Serapax™)	Intermediate (4–15 hours)	60–120 minutes	15–30 mg	The slow absorption makes it unsuitable for sleep onset insomnia
Lorazepam (Ativan™)	Intermediate (12–15 hours)	30–60 minutes	1–4 mgr	More commonly used as anxiolytic rather than hypnotic
Diazepam (Valium™, Ducene™)	Long (20–120 hours)	30–60 minutes	2–10 mg	Not indicated for management of chronic insomnia except within the context of anxiety disorder
Flunitrazepam (Rohypnol™)	Long (20–30 hours)	30–60 minutes	1–2 mg	Active metabolites make its sedative action quite prolonged. Not recommended in the management of chronic insomnia

Note: there is wider inter-subject variability in response to individual hypnotic

The speed of onset of hypnotic activity depends on how rapidly the medication is absorbed. For example, diazepam (Valium™) has a rapid absorption and fast hypnotic action which has made it a popular choice in the past as a hypnotic, despite the fact that its long half-life may cause daytime sedation and impaired daytime function when used chronically. Oxazepam (Serepax™) has a slow absorption rate and is therefore not ideal when sleep onset is the main problem. It is useful for sleep maintenance insomnia often seen in the elderly, because it does not have active metabolites.

Other benzodiazepines with intermediate/short action, such as temazepam, lorazepam and triazolam, which also have no active metabolites and minimal daytime residual effects, have been a popular choice because of their safer profile.

Zolpidem, zopiclone, and zaleplon share with benzodiazepines and barbiturates the same GABA-receptor complex but with selectivity for different parts of the molecule which may explain some of the differences in action (*Chapter 11*). Some features of these compounds have made them common first choices as hypnotics. They have rapid onset of action and short duration, minimizing the potential risk of carry-over effects during the day. At clinical doses (10 mg for zolpidem, 7.5 mg for zopiclone, and 5 mg–10 mg for zaleplon) they appear to have a minimal effect on structure of sleep, in particular on slow-wave sleep (Parrino and Terzano, 1996). The use of zolpidem in patients with chronic obstructive airways disease and mild hypercapnia seems also to be safe (Girault *et al*, 1996).

Zolpidem, zopiclone and zaleplon have no muscle relaxant activity, making them a poor choice, compared to benzodiazepines, in patients with restless legs and periodic limb movement disorder.

These compounds have little rebound effect on discontinuation. Although polysomnographic parameters suggest some effects on withdrawal of the medication, clinical symptoms are not prominent compared to benzodiazepines (Lader, 1998). When tapering and withdrawing from a benzodiazepine, it is possible to switch safely to zolpidem and zoplicone in an effort to minimize withdrawal symptoms. There is some evidence that zaleplon and zolpidem are effective in selected patients above the age of 70, even following prolonged use (6–12 months), with no significant side-effects (Ancoli-Israel *et al*, 2005).

Side-effects and contraindications

As with any other medication, there is wide individual variability in both clinical response and susceptibility to undesirable side-effects. It is safe practice to start with a small dose and, in the elderly, even half a standard dose. Side-effects include the following:

* ❖ **Symptoms:** light-headedness, 'dizziness' and occasionally unsteadiness are reported but they are usually of short duration.

* ❖ **Daytime sedation:** is seen predominantly with long-acting medications and after prolonged use because of their accumulation, but is not a common problem with short-acting or intermediate agents such as triazolam, temazepam, and zolpidem. A distinction needs to be made between the effect in normal volunteers and patients with insomnia. In patients with insomnia, including the elderly, alertness may actually be improved by short-acting hypnotics (eg. zolpidem) (Carskadon *et al*, 1982; Leger *et al*, 1999; Morin *et al*, 1999; Nicholson, 1986; Roehrs *et al*, 1986).

* ❖ **Risk of falls and hip fracture:** wide publicity has been given to the report of increased

falls in the elderly in association with the use of psychotropic drugs and, in particular, benzodiazepines. However, it should be emphasized that the risk is linked with benzodiazepines with a long (>24 hours) half-life. The risk of falls is not increased with short-acting and intermediate compounds (eg. temazepam) (Ray *et al*, 1987; 1988).

❖ *Anterograde amnesia:* all benzodiazepines confer some degree of anterograde amnesia when used intravenously, a feature exploited in anaesthesia and anaesthesia premedications. The amnestic affect depends on plasma concentration and the timing of administration. This is occasionally a clinically significant problem in some elderly patients.

❖ *Rebound insomnia:* refers to prolonged sleep latency and worsening of sleep efficiency for one to two nights following the abrupt discontinuation of benzodiazepine hypnotics. It does not contribute to physical dependence. Rebound insomnia occurs after the use of benzodiazepines, as well as placebo (Roehrs *et al*, 1986). Rebound insomnia appears to be a minimal problem with zolpidem and zoplicone, although minor deterioration does occur on polysomnographic parameters with these compounds.

❖ *Daytime anxiety:* has been reported in some patients using triazolam and consists of increased anxiety the day after taking the medication (Morgan and Oswald, 1982) due to its very short half-life.

❖ *Benzodiazepine withdrawal:* symptoms of autonomic activation with sweating, tachycardia, insomnia, and confusion are seen in patients who have used benzodiazepines at high doses for a prolonged period of time as an anxiolytic. However, it is uncommon in the context of insomnia management. Furthermore, the use of benzodiazepines under medical supervision within a therapeutic context should not be construed as addiction.

❖ *Risk of road traffic crashes:* epidemiological and laboratory studies suggest that the use of psychotropic medications (benzodiazepines and tricyclic antidepressants) is associated with impairment of driving performance (Barbone *et al*, 1998; Hemmelgarn *et al*, 1997; Verster *et al*, 2004). However, the effect of different compounds is variable and depends on the reason for their prescription, with a clearer deleterious effect in cases where use is as an anxiolytic rather than as a hypnotic. There appears to be an increased risk at the beginning of treatment compared with more prolonged use (Verster *et al*, 2004). Hypnotic benzodiazepines with a long half-life (eg. >10 hours) are more likely to have residual effects during the day (*Table 7.6* and *Chapter 12*), with temazepam having the best safety profile. The hypnotic non-benzodiazepines, zaleplon and zolpidem, are not associated with an increased risk of accident and appear to have the safest profile. In prescribing hypnotic medication for insomnia, consideration should be given to comorbidity, age, and other medications (multiple psychotropic drugs increase the risk of motor vehicle accidents).

❖ *Effects on sleep structure:* benzodiazepines tend to increase stage 2 and decrease stages 3, 4 and REM. The effect of zolpidem and zoplicone on sleep structure is less pronounced than that of benzodiazepines and depends on the dose and duration of treatment (Parrino and Terzano, 1996).

Prescribing hypnotic medication

It is useful to be familiar with a small number of hypnotics (perhaps two to three) and use them in the context of insomnia management. The choice of individual drugs depends on availability in specific countries. For example, triazolam (Halcion™) is available in Australia but was withdrawn in other countries, including the United Kingdom in the early 1990s, following reports of rebound insomnia, anterograde amnesia and daytime anxiety. Flunitrazepam (Rohypnol™) is also not available in the United Kingdom.

The following principles of prescribing are guidelines for chronic insomnia, although adjustment may be needed in individual patients and specific circumstances:

- give clear instruction on how to use the medication
- at the start of treatment, the hypnotic should be used every night for at least 2–3 weeks to establish a new sleep and wake routine, while other non-pharmacological interventions have time to make an impact
- the use of a hypnotic on alternate days is not advisable in the majority of cases, as the 'night off' may be troublesome if rebound symptoms are prominent
- after a few weeks, when a new pattern of sleep is established and behavioral sleep modifications are implemented, gradually reduce the medication
- close follow-up is necessary at this time.

Timing of administration

Patients should take the medication 30–60 minutes before bedtime. This has the advantage of achieving an effective blood level and avoids a negative association between going to bed and taking medication, which is particularly detrimental if there is pre-existing bedtime anxiety.

Review frequently and be available for counselling. Frequent review, often over the telephone, is necessary (at least twice a week) until a clear response is achieved so that the dose can be modified or, if necessary, the medication changed.

Antidepressants

Sedative tricyclic antidepressants (TCAs, amitriptyline, doxepin) were the medications of choice prior to the introduction of selected serotonin reuptake inhibitors (SSRI) for patients with insomnia-associated with depression. The anticholinergic side-effects of sedative tricyclic antidepressants (TCAs), ie. dry mouth, tachycardia, urinary retention and diffraction errors causing blurred vision, were limiting factors in many patients, even when the dose was increased slowly.

The SSRIs, including fluoxetine, and serotonin-norepinephrine-reuptake inhibitors (SNRIs), eg. venlafaxine (Efexor™) are often associated with worsening sleep quality with increased arousals, decreased stages 3 and 4 and REM suppression, as measured by polysomnography, even though these effects tend to lessen with chronic use. However, the net subjective results vary between individuals as a result of improvement in depressive illness and the sleep-related side-effects of the medications (Oberndorfers *et al*, 2000). Some of the arousal effects of SSRIs can be overcome by taking the medication in the morning and by adding a small dose of benzodiazepine at night-time. Another important sleep-related side-effect of SSRIs and SNRIs is the increased risk of circadian rhythm sleep disorders (*Chapter 11*).

More recently, the atypical antidepressants nefazodone (Serzone™) and mirtazapine (Avanza™) have been advocated as beneficial in insomnia associated with depression. They have a sedative action due to their antagonistic effect on $5-HT_2$ and $5-HT_{1a}$ receptors (Jindal and Thase, 2004; Rush *et al*, 1998; Thase, 1999; Winokur *et al*, 2000). Preliminary studies suggest that nefazodone and mirtazapine, when given at night-time, increase sleep efficiency and reduce sleep fragmentation with minimal effect on polysomnographic parameters. However, like the SSRIs, the net effect is complex and polysomnographic documentation (overnight sleep study) is often necessary (Oberndorfers *et al*, 2000).

Melatonin

Melatonin (Brzezinski, 1997) is a useful agent in the management of certain conditions that present with insomnia. It is used in two ways:

1. In circadian sleep disorders as a body-rhythm regulator.
2. As a hypnotic.

Melatonin use is limited by a series of problems, which should be made clear to the patient (Arendt, 1996). Melatonin is classified as a naturopathic substance and this results in lack of standardization in the preparations available on the market. The uncertainty applies to the actual amount of melatonin present in the tablets or capsules, as well as the pharmacokinetic characteristics, due to poor formulation and poor quality control. In practice, it is difficult to be sure that what is on the label is what the person actually gets. Other problems include uncertainty as to the optimal therapeutic dose and what the duration of treatment should be. There is also a lack of safety data on long-term use.

Use of melatonin

In sleep medicine melatonin has two main applications:

*   in managing difficulty initiating and maintaining sleep associated with circadian rhythm sleep disorders, in particular delayed sleep phase syndrome (*Chapter 11*) (Dagan *et al*, 1998; Dahlitz *et al*, 1991)
*   as a 'sleeping tablet' (Attenburrow *et al*, 1996; Garfinkel *et al*, 1995;Sack *et al*, 1997; Zdhanova, 2000).

Melatonin reduces latency in sleep onset and waking after sleep onset, both in healthy elderly subjects and patients with insomnia. Sleep stages are minimally affected, with some increase in stage 2 and decrease in stage 4.

Dose of melatonin

A variety of doses have been used in research settings, from milligrams to grams. A dose of 0.3 mg produces a physiological level of melatonin. The usual dose in clinical setting ranges between 0.5–6 mg (pharmacological doses). However, the dose–response curve in terms of sleep-promoting action is rather flat, so the sleep-promoting action of 50 mg is not much greater than 0.5 mg. Case reports also suggest the risk of exacerbation of mood disorder symptoms and potential suppression of endogenous melatonin production with high doses (Carman *et al*, 1976; Leibenluft *et al*, 1997). This is likely to be due to melatonin receptor saturation. There is significant intersubject variability in the level of response to the same amount of melatonin in different age groups and also within the same age group. For management of delayed sleep phase syndrome, higher doses (3–5 mg) are preferable.

Timing of administration

For the purpose of sleep phase advancement (advancing sleep onset) in delayed sleep phase syndrome, melatonin should be given in the early evening between 8.00PM and 9.00PM (Avery *et al*, 1998). As a sleep-promoting agent, melatonin is given about 30–60 minutes before bedtime.

Melatonin is rapidly absorbed after oral administration with a peak plasma level within 20–60 minutes. It is metabolized by the liver with a short half-life of forty to fifty minutes. Because of the rapid metabolism, slow release formulation has been advocated, particularly in the elderly with sleep maintenance insomnia, but the reliability of the available products remains a problem (Garfinkel *et al*, 1995).

Duration of treatment

There is no good evidence as to how long melatonin should be used. Practical experience suggests that it should be used for at least a few weeks (4–8) together with non-pharmacological management.

Relapse

In case of delayed sleep phase syndrome, relapse following the discontinuation of melatonin is reported to be high (84%), but this may depend on the severity of the syndrome. Relapse can be minimized if strict adherence to bedtime and wake-up time is maintained.

Clinical response

It is important to explain to the patient that melatonin is a 'sleep-promoting medication' rather than a sleeping tablet (it helps you fall asleep, rather than puts you to sleep) and that it works in conjunction with the other sleep-promoting behaviors which should always be part of chronic insomnia management. The patient should not expect the immediate effect that may be obtained with other hypnotic agents (eg. triazolam, zolpidem), and full assessment of the benefit should be evaluated over a period of 2–3 weeks.

Side-effects and contraindications

Side-effects due to melatonin are minimal, but fatigue, headache and nausea are sometimes reported but are uncommon in low doses (<3 mg).

Melatonin secretion is linked to reproductive function in different species and may have a regulatory role (suppression) of the pituitary gonadal function in humans prior to puberty. The safety of prolonged use of melatonin in children is not known and it should be used with caution until safety data is available. Similarly, the use in pregnant women should be avoided. Melatonin can be used safely with other hypnotic agents such as temazepam or triazolam (Mendelson, 1997).

Opioids

The usefulness of opioids in the management of chronic insomnia is probably under recognized. The concern with physical dependence and addiction has led to reluctance in prescribing by physicians and poor acceptance from patients even in conditions where opioids are beneficial. The availability of slow-release morphine makes it a useful drug for difficulty in initiating and maintaining sleep in common chronic medical conditions, including:

- chronic pain in patients with rheumatological and orthopedic diseases such as osteoporosis, osteoarthritis, rheumatoid arthritis (*Chapter 9*)
- severe heart failure or refractory angina
- restless leg syndrome. Although most attention in the management of restless legs is given to dopamineagonist agents (eg. levodopa, ropinirole), long-acting opioids are effective and under-utilized.

Slow-release morphine at a dose between 5–30 mg results in significant subjective improvement in the above conditions. Although a nightly dose is necessary, on occasions, patients maintain benefit by taking the medication every second or even third day. Empirical evidence suggests that dose escalation does not occur and addiction is not seen in the right clinical context. Side-effects include sedation, nausea, constipation and pruritus. These can be minimized by starting with a small dose and increasing slowly every few days.

Over-the-counter sleep aids for insomnia

The practice of using 'over-the-counter' preparations for insomnia is felt to be widespread, but difficult to quantify. The type of non-prescription sleep aids used varies depending on cultural and traditional factors and local availability (Gyllenhaal *et al*, 2000; Jindal and Thase, 2004; Meoli *et al* 2005; *Chapter 12*) .

Antihistamine-1-receptor antagonists (eg. diphenhydramine 12.5–50 mg, doxylamine 25 mg) by themselves, or in combination with analgesics, are commonly used and effective. The patients report subjective improvement in sleep latency and duration with less awakening. However antihistamines have significant side-effects with daytime drowsiness and sedation, dry mouth, voiding difficulty, increased intraocular pressure and potential overdose risk.

Many 'natural' products are claimed to be beneficial in helping insomnia (*Table 7.7*). With the exception of valerian which may have some mild beneficial effect (*Chapter 12*), for most of the other substances there is no objective evidence of efficacy. One major problem with 'natural' substances is that their preparation varies from root and bark (as decoction), infusion, alcohol-based (tincture), to capsule and tablet. They often contain multiple constituents and the dosage and bioavailability is uncertain, varying from one product to another. For some of these products there are report of adverse reactions: hepatotoxicity (Jamaican dogwood, kava kava, skullcap), hallucination (wild lettuce), *eosinophilia myalgia* syndrome (a particular formulation of L-tryptophan) and interaction with other prescription medications (eg. St John's wort).

Natural sleep aids:
Valerian
Chamomile
Lemon balm
Hops
Passionflower
Skulllcap
Californinan poppy
Jamaican dogwood
Kava Kava
Lavender
Catnip

References

Allen RP (2000) Behavioral and neuroendocrine characteristics of the night eating disorders. *Sleep Med* **1**(1): 67–8

American Academy of Sleep Medicine (2005) *The International Classification of Sleep Disorders. Diagnostic & Coding Manual.* 2nd edn. American Academy of Sleep Medicine, Westchester, IL

Ancoli-Israel S, Richardson GS, Mangano RM, Jenkins L, Hall P, Jones WS (2005) Long-term use of sedative hypnotics in older patients with insomnia. *Sleep Med* **6**: 107–13

Ancoli-Israel S, Roth T (1999) Characteristics of insomnia and the United States: Results of the 1991 National Sleep Foundation Survey I. *Sleep* **22**: S347–S353

Angst J, Vollrath M, Koch R, Dobler-Mikolo A (1989) The Zurich Study: VII. Insomnia: symptoms, classification and prevalence. *Eur Arch Psychiat Neurol Sci* **238**(5–6): 285–93

Arendt J (1996) Melatonin. Claims made in the popular media are mostly nonsense. *Br Med J* **312**: 1242–3

Attenburrow MEJ, Cowen PJ, Sharpley AL (1996) Low dose melatonin improves sleep in healthy middle-aged subjects. *Psychopharmacology* **126**: 179–81

Avery D, Lenz M, Landis C (1998) Guidelines for prescribing melatonin. *Ann Med* **30**: 122–30

Barbone F, McMahon AD *et al* (1998) Association of road-traffic accidents with benzodiazepine use. *Lancet* **352**: 1331–6

Barkovec TD (1982) Insomnia. *J Consult Clin Psychol* **50**(6): 880–95

Birketvedt GS, Florholmen J, Sundsfjord J *et al* (1999) Behavioral and neuroendocrine characteristics of the night-eating syndrome. *JAMA* **282**(7): 657–63

Bixler EO, Kales A, Soldatos CR, Kales J, Healey S (1979) Prevalence of sleep disorders in the Los Angeles metropolitan area. *Am J Psychiatry* **136**: 1257–62

Bonnet MH, Arand DL (1992) Caffeine use as a model of acute and chronic insomnia. *Sleep* **15**(6): 526–36

Bootzin RR, Epstein D, Wood JM (1991) Stimulus control instrtuctions. In: Peter J, Hauri P, eds. *Case Studies in Insomnia*. Plenum Medical, New York

Bootzin RR, Nicassio P (1978) Behavioral treatment for insomnia. In: Hersen M, Eisler RM, Miller PM, eds. *Progress in Behavior Modification* (Vol 6). Academic Press, New York

Branco J, Atalaia A, Paiva T (1994) Sleep cycles and alpha-delta sleep in fibromyalgia syndrome. *J Rheumatol* **21**: 1113–17

Brebbins CJ, Deway ME, Copeland JRM, Davidson A, McWilliam C, Saunders P *et al* (1993) Insomnia in the elderly: Prevalence, gender differences and relationships with morbidity and mortality. *Int J Geriat Psychiat* **8**: 473–80

Brust JCM (1993) *Neurological Aspects of Substance Abuse*. Butterworth-Heinemann, Boston: 115–30

Brzezinski A (1997) Melatonin in humans. *New Eng J Med* **17**: 186–95

Carette S, Oakson G, Guimont C, Steriade M (1995) Sleep electroencephalography and clinical response to amytriptiline in patients with fibromyalgia. *Arthritis Rheum* **38**(9): 1211–17

Carman JS, Post RM, Buswell R, Goodwin FK (1976) Negative effects of melatonin on depression. *Am J Psychiat* **133**(10): 1181–6

Carskadon MA, Seidel WF, Greenblatt DJ, Dement WC (1982) Daytime carryover of triazolam and flurazepam in elderly insomniacs. *Sleep* **5**(4): 261–371

Cohen ML, Quintner JL (1998) Fibromyalgia syndrome and disability: a failed construct for those in pain. *Med J Austral* **168**: 402–4

Consensus Conference (1984) Drugs and insomnia: the use of medications to promote sleep. *JAMA* **251**: 2410–14

Csillag C (1992) Fibromyalgia: the Copenhagen declaration. *Lancet* **340**: 663–4

DaganY, Yovel I, Hallis D, Eisenstein M, Raichik I (1998) Evaluating the role of melatonin in the long-term treatment of delayed sleep phase syndrome (DSPS). *Chronobiol Int* **15**(2): 181–90

Dahlitz M, Alvarex B, Vigman J, English J, Arendt J, Parkes JD (1991) Delayed sleep phase syndrome response to melatonin. *Lancet* **337**: 1121–4

Edinger JD, Hoelscher TJ, Webb MD, Marsh GR, Radtke RA, Erwin CW (1989) Polysomnographic assessment of DIMS: empirical evaluation of its diagnostic value. *Sleep* **12**(4): 315–22

Edinger JD, Wohlgemuth WK, Radtke RA, Marsh GR, Quillian RE (2001) Cognitive behavioral therapy for treatment of chronic primary insomnia: a randomized controlled trial. *JAMA* **285**(14): 1856–64

Espie CA, Brindle S, Tessier S *et al* (1998) Supervised cognitive-behavior therapy for insomnia in general medical practice — preliminary results from the West of Scotland Program. In: Sanavio E, ed. *Behavior and Cognitive Therapy Today: Essays in Honour of Hans J. Eysenck*. Elsevier, Amsterdam: 67–75)

Espie CA, Inglis SJ, Harvey L, Tessier S (2000) Insomniacs' attributions: psychometric properties of the dysfunctional beliefs and attitudes about sleep scale and the sleep disturbance questionnaire. *J Psychosom Res* **48**: 141–8

Espie CA, Inglis SJ, Tessier S, Harvey L (2001) The clinical effectiveness of cognitive behavior therapy for chronic insomnia: Implementation and evaluation of a sleep clinic in general medical practice. *Behav Res Ther* **39**: 45–60

Feinberg I, Jones R, Walker J, Covness C, Floyd T (1976) Effects of marijuana extract and tetrahydro-cannabinol on electroencephalographic sleep patterns. *Clin Pharmacol Ther* **19**(6): 782–94

Ferrara M, De Gennaro L, Curcio G, Cristiani R, Corvasce C, Bertini M (2002) Regional difference of the human sleep electroencephalogram in response to selective slow-wave sleep deprivation. *Cerbral Cortex* **12**: 737–48

Fleischhacker WW, Barnas C, Hackenberg B (1986) Epidemiology of benzodiazepine dependence. *Acta Psychiatrica Scandinavica* **74**(1): 80–3

Ford DE, Kamerov DB (1989) Epidemiologic study of sleep disturbances and psychiatric disorders: an opportunity for prevention? *JAMA* **262**: 1478–84

Gallup Organization (1995) *Sleep in America*. The Gallup Organization, Princeton, NJ

Garfinkel D, Laudon MN, Zisopel N (1995) Improvement of sleep quality in elderly people by controlled-release melatonin. *Lancet* **346**: 541–4

Girault C, Muir JF, Mihaltan F, Borderies P, De La Gicleis B, Verdure A *et al* (1996) Effects of repeated administration of zolpidem on sleep, diurnal and nocturnal respiratory function, vigilance and physical performance in patients with COPD. *Chest* **110**: 1203–11

Greenblatt DO (1991) Benzodiazepine hypnotics: sorting the pharmacokinetic Facts. *J Clin Psychiatry* **52** (suppl 9): 4–10

Gross RT, Borkovec TD (1982) Effects of a cognitive intrusion manipulation on the sleep onset latency of good sleepers. *Behav Ther* **13**: 117–24

Gyllenhaal C, Merritt SL, Peterson SD, Block KI, Gochenour T (2000) Efficacy and safety of herbal stimulants and sedatives in sleep disorders. *Sleep Med Rev* **4**(3): 229–51

Harvey L, Inglis SJ, Espie CA (2002) Insomniac's reported use of CBT components and relationship to long term clinical outcome. *Behav Res Ther* **40**: 75–83

Hauri P, Wisbey J (1992) Wrist actigraphy in insomnia. *Sleep* **15**: 293–301

Hemmelgarn B, Suissa S, Huang A, Boivin JF, Pinard C (1997) Benzodiazepine use and the risk of motor vehicle crash. *JAMA* **278**: 27–31

Holbrook AM, Crowther R, Lotter A, Cheng C, King D (2000) Meta-analysis of benzodiazepine use in the treatment of insomnia. *CMAJ* **162**(2): 225–33

Horne J (1988) *Why We Sleep: The functions of sleep in humans and other mammals*. Oxford University Press, Oxford

Jacobs EA, Reynolds III CF, Kupfer DJ, Lorin PA, Ehrenpreis AB (1988) The role of polysomnography in the differential diagnosis of chronic insomnia. *Am J Psychiat* **145**: 346–9

Jennum P, Drewes AM, Andreasen A, Nielsen KD (1993) Sleep and other symptoms in primary fibromyalgia and healthy controls. *J Rheumatol* **20**: 1756–9

Kales A, Caldwell AB, Preston TA, Healey S, Kales JD (1976) Personality patterns in insomnia. *Arch Gen Psychiatry* **33**: 1228–34

Kales JD, Kales A, Bixler ED, Soldatos CR, Cadieux RJ, Kashurba GJ, Vela-Bueno A (1984) Biopsychobehavioral correlates of insomnia, v: clinical characteristics and behavioral correlates. *Am J Psychiatry* **141**: 1371–6

Kripke Df, Klauber MR, Wingard DL, Fell RL, Assmus JD, Garfinkel L (1998) Mortality hazards associated with prescription hypnotics. *Biol Psychiatry* **43**(9): 687–93

Kripke DF, Simons RN, Garfinkel L, Hammond EC (1979) Short and long sleep and sleeping pills. Is increased mortality associated? *Arch Gen Psychiat* **36**(1): 103–16

Jindal RD, Thase ME (2004) The treatment of insomnia associated with clinical depression. *Sleep Med Rev* **8**(1): 19–30

Lack LC, Mercer JD, Wright H (1996) Circadian rhythms of early morning awakening insomnias. *J Sleep Res* **5**: 211–19

Lack L, Miller W, Turner D (1988) A survey of sleeping difficulty in an Australian population. *Community Health Study* **12**: 200–7

Lader M (1998) Withdrawal reactions after stopping hypnotics in patients with insomnia. *CNS Drugs* **10**(6): 425–40

Landolt HP, Werth E, Boberly AA, Dijk DJ (1995) Caffeine intake (200mg) in the morning affects human sleep and EEG power spectra at night. *Brain Res* **675**: 67

Lauer CJ, Krieg JC (2004) Sleep in eating disorders. *Sleep Med Rev* **8**(2): 109–18

Leger D, Guillaminault C, Dreyfus JP, Delahaye C, Poillard M (2000) Prevalence of insomnia in a survey of 12778 adults in France. *J Sleep Res* **9**: 35–42

Leger D, Scheuermaier K, Roger M (1999) The relationship between alertness and sleep in a population of 769 elderly insomniacs with and without treatment with zolpidem. *Arch Gerontol Geriatr* **29**: 165–73

Leibenluft E, Feldman-Naim S, Turner EH, Wehr TA, Rosenthal NE (1997) Effects of exogenous melatonin administration and withdrawal in five patients with rapid-cycling bipolar disorder. *J Clin Psychiatry* **58**(9): 383–8

Leppik IE (1995) Felbamate. *Epilepsia* **36**(suppl 2): 566–72

Lewy AJ, Ahmed S, Sack RL (1996) Phase shifting the human circadian clock using melatonin. *Behav Brain Res* **73**(1–2): 131–4

Lovibond SH, Lovibond PF (1995) Manual for the Depression Anxiety Scales. In: *Psychology Foundation Monography, Sydney*. The Psychology Foundation of Australia Inc, University of NSW

Lushington K, Lack L (2002) Non-pharmacological treatments of insomnia. *Israel J Psychiat* **39**(1): 36–49

Mellinger GD, Balter MB, Uhlenhut EH (1985) Insomnia and its treatment, prevalence and correlates. *Arch Gen Psychiat* **42**: 225–32

Mendelson W (1995) Long-term follow-up of chronic insomnia. *Sleep* **18**(8): 698–701

Mendelson WB (1997) A critical evaluation of the hypnotic efficacy of melatonin. *Sleep* **20**(10): 916–9

Meoli AL, Rosen C, Kristo D *et al* (2005) Oral non-prescription treatment for insomnia: an evaluation of products with limited evidence. *J Clin SLeep Med* **1**(2): 173–87

Moldofsky H (1995) Sleep, neuroimmune and neuroendocrine functions in fibromyalgia and chronic fatigue syndrome. *Adv Neuroimmunol* **5**: 39–56

Morgan K, Oswald I (1982) Anxiety caused by a short-life hypnotic. *Br Med J* **284**: 942

Morin C (1993) *Insomnia: Psychological assessment and management.* Guilford Press, New York

Morin CM, Blais F, Savard J (2002) Are changes in beliefs and attitudes about sleep related to sleep improvements in the treatment of insomnia? *Behav Res Ther* **40**: 741–52

Morin CM, Colecchi C, Stone J, Sood R, Brink D (1999) Behavioral and pharmacological therapies for late-life insomnia. A randomised controlled study. *JAMA* **281**: 991–9

Morin CM, Cuthbert J, Schwartz S (1994) Non-pharmacological interventions for insomnia: a meta-analysis of treatment efficacy. *Am J Psychiatry* **151**(8): 1172–80

Nicholson AN (1986) Transient insomnia and rapidly eliminated hypnotics. *Sleep* **9**(2): 317–23

Oberndorfers S, Saletu-Zyhlarz G, Saletu B (2000) Effects of selective serotonin reuptake inhibitors on objective and subjective sleep quality. *Neuropsychobiol* **42**(2): 69–81

Ohayon M (1996) Epidemiological study of insomnia in the general population. *Sleep* **3**: S7–S15

Ohayon MM (1997) Prevalence of DSM-IV diagnostic criteria of insomnia. distinguishing insomnia related to mental disorders from sleep disorders. *J Psychiat Res* **31**(3): 333–46

Olson LG (1996) A community survey of insomnia in Newcastle. *Aust NZ J Publ Hlth* **20**(6): 655–7

O'Malley PG, Balden E, Tomkins G, Santoro J, Kroenke K, Jackson JL (2000) Treatment of fibromyalgia with antidepressants: an analysis. *J Gen Intern Med* **15**(9): 659–66

Oswald I, French C, Adam K, Gilham J (1982) Benzodiazepine hypnotics remain effective for 24 weeks. *Br Med J* **284**: 860–3

Parrino L, Terzano MG (1996) Polysomnographic effects of hypnotic drugs; a review. *Psychopharmacology* **126**: 1–16

Perlis ML, Smith MT, Andrews PJ, Orff H, Giles DE (2001) Beta/gamma EEG activity in patients with primary and secondary insomnia and good sleeper controls. *Sleep* **24**(1): 110–7

Pressman M (1991) Whatever happened to insomnia (and insomnia research)? *Am J Psychiat* **148**: 419–20

Quera-Salva MA, Orluc A, Goldenberg F, Guilleminault C (1991) Insomnia and the use of hypnotics: study of a French population. *Sleep* **14**(5): 386–91

Ray WA, Griffin MR, Downey W (1988) Benzodiazepines of long and short elimination half-life and the risk of hip fracture. *JAMA* **262**: 3303–7

Ray WA, Griffin MR, Schaffner W, Baugh DK, Melton LJ (1987) Psychotropic drug use and the risk of hip fracture. *New Eng J Med* **316**: 363–9

Regenstein PK, Reich P (1983) Incapacitating childhood onset insomnia. *Compt Psychiatry* **24**: 244–8

Regenstein QR (1987) Specific effects of sedative/hypnotics drugs in the treatment of incapacitating chronic insomnia. A*m J Med* **83**: 909–16

Reidel BW, Lichstein KL (2000) Insomnia and daytime functioning. *Sleep Med Rev* **4**(3): 277–98

Reite M, Buysse D, Reynolds C, Mendelson W (1995) The use of polysomnography in the evaluation of insomnia. *Sleep* **18**(1): 58–70

Roehrs T, Kribbs N, Zorick F, Roth T (1986) Hypnotic residual effects of benzodiazepines with repeated administration. *Sleep* **9**(2): 309–16

Roth T, Ancoli-Israel S (1999) Daytime consequences and correlates of insomnia in the United States: Results of the 1991 National Sleep Foundation Survey II. *Sleep* **22**: S354–S358

Roth T, Roehrs T, Vogel G (1995) Zolpidem in the treatment of transient insomnia: double-blind randomised comparison with placebo. *Sleep* **18**(4): 246–51

Roth T, Zorich F, Wiltig R, Roehrs T (1982) Pharmacological and medical considerations in hypnotic use. *Sleep* **5**: S46–S52

Rush AJ, Armitage R, Gillin JC, Yonkers KA, Winokur A, Moldofshky H *et al* (1998) Comparative effects of nefozadone and fluoxetine on sleep in outpatient with major depressive disorder. *Biolog Psychiat* **44**(1): 3–14

Sack RL, Hughes RJ, Edgar DM, Lewy AJ (1997) Sleep-promoting effects of melatonin: at what dose, in whom, under what conditions, and by what mechanism? *Sleep* **20**(10): 908–15

Sadeh A, Hauri P J, Kripke D F, Lavie P (1995) The role of actigraphy in the evaluation of sleep disorders. *Sleep* **18**(4): 288–302

Sadler M (1999) Lamotrigine associated with insomnia. *Epilepsia* **40**(3): 322–5

Salzman C (1999) An 87-year-old woman taking a benzodiazepine. *JAMA* **281**(12): 1121–5

Scharf MB, Roth T, Vogel GW, Walsh JK (1994) A multicenter, placebo-controlled study evaluating zolpidem in the treatment of chronic insomnia. *J Clin Psychiat* **55**: 192–9

Simon GE, Vonkorff M (1997) Prevalence, burden and treatment of insomnia in primary care. *Am J Psychiat* **154**: 1417–23

Slawson JG, Meurer L (2001) Are antidepressants effective in the treatment of fibromyalgia, and is this effect independent of sleepiness? *J Fam Pract* **50**(1): 14

Smith MT, Haythornthwaite JA (2004) How do sleep disturbance and chronic pain inter-relate? Insight from the longitudinal and cognitive-behavioral clinical trials literature. *Sleep Med Rev* **8**(2): 119–32

Spielman AJ, Glovinsky PB (1991) Introduction. In: Hauri PJ, ed. *Case Studies in Insomnia*. Plenum Medical, New York

Spielman AJ, Saskin P, Thorpy MJ (1987) Treatment of chronic insomnia by restriction of time in bed. *Sleep* **10**(1): 45–56

Spitzer RL, Kroenke K, Williams JB (1999) Validation and utility of a self-report version of PRIME-MD: the PHQ primary care study. Primary care evaluation of mental disorders. Patient health questionnaire. *JAMA* **282**(18): 1737–44

Standards of Practice Committee of the American Sleep Disorders Association (1995) Practice parameters for the use of polysomnography in the evaluation of insomnia. *Sleep* **18**(1): 55–7

Tan T-L, Kales JD, Kales A, Soldatos CR, Bixler EO (1984) Biopsychobehavioral correlates of insomnia, IV: Diagnosis based on DSM-III. *Am J Psychiat* **141**: 357–62

Tietzel A, Lack L (2002) The recuperative value of brief and ultra-brief naps on alertness and cognitive performance. *J Sleep Res* **11**(3): 213–18

Thase M (1999) Antidepressant treatment of the depressed patient with insomnia. *J Clin Psychiatry* **60**(suppl 17): 28–31

Van Egeren L, Haynes SN, Franzen M, Hamilton J (1983) Presleep cognitions and attributions in sleep-onset insomnia. *J Behav Med* **6**: 217–32

Verster JC, Veldhuijzen DS, Volkerts ER (2004) Residual effects of sleep medication on driving ability. *Sleep Med Rev* **8**: 309–25

Vincent N, Lionberg C (2001) Treatment preferences and patient satisfaction in chronic insomnia. *Sleep* **24**(4): 411–17

Vgontzas AN, Bixler EO, Lin HM, Prolo P, Mastorakos G, Vela-Bueno A *et al* (2001) Chronic insomnia is associated with nyctohemeral activation of the hypothalmic-pituitary-adrenal axis: clinical implications. *J Clin Endocrinol Metab* **86**(8): 3787–94

Vgontzaz AN, Zoumakis M, Papanicolaou DA, Bixler EO, Prolo P, Lin H-M *et al* (2002) Chronic insomnia is associated with a shift of interleukin-6 and tumor necrosis factor secretion from nighttime to daytime. *Metabolism* **51**(7): 887–92

Vollrath M, Werner W, Angst J (1989) VIII insomnia: association with depression, anxiety, somatic syndromes, and course of insomnia. *Eur Arch Psychiatr Neurol Sci* **239**: 113–24

Walsh JK, Schweitzer PK (1999) Ten-year trend in pharmacological treatment of insomnia. *Sleep* **22**(3): 371–5

Watts FN, Coyle MP, East MP (1994) The contribution of worry to insomnia. *Br J Clin Psychol* **33**: 211–20

Webb WB, Agnew HW (1975) Sleep efficiency for sleep–wake cycles of varied length. *Psychophysiology* **12**: 637–41

Weissman MM, Greenweld MA, Nino-Murcia G, Deumont LWC (1997) The morbidity of insomnia uncomplicated by psychiatric disorders. *Gen Hosp Psychiat* **19**: 2445–50

Weyerer S, Dilling H (1991) Prevalence and treatment of insomnia in the community: Results. *Sleep* **14**(5): 392–8

Wicklow A, Espie CA (2000) Intrusive thoughts and their relationship to actigraphic measurement of sleep: towards a cognitive model of insomnia. *Behav Res Ther* **38**: 679–93

Winokur A, Sateia MJ, Hayes JB, Bayles-Dazet W, MacDonald MM, Gary KA (2000) Acute effects of mirtazepine on sleep continuity and sleep architecture in depressed patients: a pilot study. *Biolog Psychiat* **48**(1): 75–8

Wood JH, Kotz JL, Winger (1988) Use and abuse of benzodiazepines issues relevant to prescribing. *JAMA* **260**(23): 3476–80

Woolfe F, Smythe HA, Yunus M *et al* (1990) The Americal College of Rheumatology 1990 criteria for the classification of fibromyalgia. Report of the multicenter criteria committee. *Arthritis Rheum* **33**: 160–72

Yapko MD (1998) *Breaking the Patterns of Depression*. Main Street Books, Mansfield

Zdhanova IV (2000) The role of melatonin. In: Culebres, ed. *Sleep and Sleep Disorders and Neurological Disease*. Marcel Dekker, New York

Appendix A: Fatal familial insomnia

Fatal familial insomnia (FFI) is an autosomal dominant disease characterized by progressive and untreatable insomnia, associated with disregulation of the autonomic nervous system, with hypertension, increased body temperature and tachycardia (sympathetic hyperactivity) (Lugaresi *et al*, 1986). Circadian rhythmicity is progressively lost in the cardiovascular and hormonal function (Portaluppi **et al**, 1994a; Portaluppi *et al*, 1994b).

Early neurophysiological investigation reveal attention and memory deficit (Gallassi *et al*, 1996). Patients with FFI have progressive reduction in night-time sleep. Eventually, the patient fluctuates between a state of wakefulness and light sleep (stage 1) with intrusion of atypical REM (REM without atonia), during which the patient may have dream-like episodes with motor activity resembling REM behavior disorder. As the condition progresses, dysarthria and myoclonic jerks may also appear (Lugaresi *et al*, 1986) until the patient eventually becomes poorly responsive and comatose. The course of the FFI varies from 7 months to 7 years with heterozygotes having a slower progression (Lugaresi and Provini, 2001).

Polysomnography is characterized by loss of spindle and slow-wave sleep. During advanced phase of the disease, the patient appears to fluctuate in a mixed state of sub-wakefulness and atypical REM (wake-REM state) (Lugaresi and Provini, 2001).

FFI was shown to be due to a point mutation of the prion protein (PrP) gene (McLean *et al*, 1997; Medori *et al*, 1992). Prions (protinaceous infectious particle (on) are normal cellular components that have undergone a conformation change, making them resistant to their usual degradation pathway (protease resistant). FFI has been shown to be a transmittable condition (Tateishi *et al*, 1995) like other prion diseases.

Pathological examination of an FFI patient revealed marked degeneration of the anterior and medial dorsal thalamic nuclei. Variable involvement of other area is also present (Manetto *et al*, 1992). A clinical picture similar to FFI is also being described in Morvan's chorea and delirium tremens (acute alcohol withdrawal in chronic alcohol abusers) (Lugaresi and Provini, 2001).

Morvan's chorea is characterized by severe insomnia with hallucinations, motor agitation and sympathetic overactivity. The majority of patients recover spontaneously. No pathological abnormality is found in post-mortem cases. The fact that plasma exchange seems an effective treatment in some cases has led to the theory that Morvan's chorea may be due to autoimmune limbic encephalopathy.

The term agrypnia excitata has been used (Lugaresi and Provini, 2001; Lugaresi *et al*, 2000) to refer to neurological disorders such as FFI, Morvan's chorea and delirium tremens, and is characterized by insomnia (*agrypnia* = agrein [to hunt] and *hypnos* = sleep) and autonomic and motor activation (*excitata*).

Appendix B: Fatigue severity scale

Instructions: Below are a series of statements regarding your fatigue. By fatigue we mean a sense of tiredness, lack of energy or total body give-out. Please read each statement and choose a number from 1 to 7, where # 1 indicates you completely disagree with the statement and # 7 indicates you completely agree. Please answer these questions as they apply to the past **2 weeks**.

Circle the appropriate number on the answer sheet!

Questions:

		Completely disagree						**Completely agree**
1.	My motivation is lower when I am fatigued	1	2	3	4	5	6	7
2.	Exercise brings on my fatigue	1	2	3	4	5	6	7
3.	I am easily fatigued	1	2	3	4	5	6	7
4.	Fatigue interferes with my physical functioning	1	2	3	4	5	6	7
5.	Fatigue causes frequent problems for me	1	2	3	4	5	6	7
6.	My fatigue prevents sustained physical functioning	1	2	3	4	5	6	7
7.	Fatigue interferes with carrying out certain duties and responsibilities	1	2	3	4	5	6	7
8.	Fatigue is among my three most disabling symptoms	1	2	3	4	5	6	7
9	Fatigue interferes with my work, family or social life	1	2	3	4	5	6	7

Score by adding up the responses and dividing by 9. Useful in individual patients to assess progress over time.

(From Krupp *et al*, 1989)

Appendix C: Pittsburgh Sleep Quality Index (PSQI)

Instructions: The following questions relate to your usual sleep habits during the past month only. Your answers should indicate the most accurate replay for the majority of days and nights in the past month. Please answer all questions.

During the past month:

1. When have you usually gone to bed ?
2. How long (in minutes) has it taken you to fall asleep each night?
3. When have you usually got up in the morning?
4. How many hours of actual sleep did you get that night? (This may be different than the numbers of hours you spent in bed)

5.	During the past month, how often have you had trouble sleeping because you:	Not during the past month (0)	Less than once a week (1)	Once or twice a week (2)	Three or more times a week (3)
a.	Cannot get to sleep within 30 minutes				
b.	Wake up in the middle of the night or early morning				
c.	Have to get up to use the bathroom				
d.	Cannot breathe comfortably				
e.	Cough or snore loudly				
f.	Feel too cold				
g.	Feel too hot				
h.	Have bad dreams				
i.	Have pain				
j.	Other reason(s), please describe, including how often you have had trouble sleeping because of this reason(s)				
6.	During the past month, how often have you taken medicine (prescribed or 'over-the-counter') to help you sleep				
7.	During the past month, how often have you had trouble staying awake while driving, eating meals, or engaging in social activity?				
8.	During the past month, how much of a problem has it been for you to keep up enthusiasm to get things done				
		Very good (0)	Fairly good (1)	Fairly bad (2)	Very bad (3)
9.	During the past month, how would you rate your overall sleep quality ?				

Component 1   #9 score
                     C1_____

Component 2   #2 score (≤15min (0); 16-30 min (1); 31–60 min (2);, >60 min (3)
                     + #5a score (if sum is equal 0=0; 1–2=1; 3–4=2; 5–6=3)
                     C2_____

Component 3   #4 Score (>7(0); 6–7(1); 5–6(2); <5(3))
                     C3_____

Component 4   (total # of hours asleep)/total # of hours in bed) x 100
                     >85% =0; 75–84% =1; 65–74% =2; <65% =3)
                     C4_____

Component 5   #sum of scores 5b to 5j (0=0; 1–9=1; 10–18=2; 19–27=3)
                     C5 _____

Component 6   #6 Score
                     C6_____

Component 7   #7 Score
                     + #8 Score (0=0; 1–2=1; 3–4=2; 5–6=3)
                     C7_____

Add the seven component scores together _____ Global PSQI score _____

The PSQI contains nineteen self-rated questions, which cover seven areas of sleep assessment, over the previous month: Subjective sleep quality (C1), sleep latency (C2), sleep duration (C3), sleep efficiency (C4), sleep disturbances (C5), use of sleeping medications (C6), daytime dysfunction (C7). Each component scores from '0' for no difficulty, to '3' for severe difficulty, for a total score (Global PSQI) from 0 to 21. The PSQI also include five questions (not included in the template above) that can be answered by a bed partner or room mate if available, but they are not part of the PSQI score.

(from Buysse *et al*, 1989)

Appendix D: Beliefs and attitudes questionnaire

Beliefs and attitudes questionnaire

What do you believe about the following statements?

		True	Maybe	False

1. I need eight hours of sleep every night to feel refreshed.

2. When I do not get the amount of sleep I need at night, I have to catch up the next day by napping.

3 I am concerned that if I go for two or three nights without sleep I may have a nervous breakdown.

4. By staying in bed longer, I can usually get more sleep and feel better the next day.

5. When I have trouble sleeping, the best thing is to stay in bed and try harder to sleep.

6. If I don't sleep well at night, I know I cannot possibly function well on the following day.

7. When I feel irritable, depressed, or anxious during the day, I know it is because I slept poorly the night before.

8. There is no way I can manage the negative consequences of disturbed sleep.

9. I get overwhelmed by my thoughts at night, and there is no way to control my racing mind.

10. Unless I can lick insomnia there is no way I can enjoy life and be productive.

As the statements are not true, the patient's answers point to areas that may need to be addressed during treatment.

(from Hauri and Linde, 1996)

Appendix E: Insomnia group educational programme

Session 1: Learning about sleep — what this means for you

1. The need for sleep and its functions
2. How much sleep do we need?
3. No sleep versus reduced sleep
4. What is insomnia?
5. Prevalence of insomnia
6. Daytime function and insomnia — objective performance is not compromised
7. Sleep across the life span
8. Sleep as a process with stages/phases
9. The human biological clock — and environmental factors
10. Other sleep patterns – 'owls and larks'
11. Jet lag — treatment of jet lag
12. Measuring sleep and sleep problems — keeping a sleep diary
13. Relaxation

Session 2: Sleep hygiene — how to improve your sleep

1. Regulating sleep patterns
2. Many small changes make a big difference
3. Sleep hygiene measures — define individual sleep requirements
4. Sleep environment I — what to do before bed
5. Sleep environment II — what not to do in bed
6. Exercise
7. Alcohol
8. Caffeine
9. Nicotine
10. Food
11. Over-the-counter medications for sleep difficulties
12. Prescribed medication for sleep difficulties
13. Management of insomnia — reducing arousal levels
14. The environment — same waking time
15. Early-morning light exposure
16. Relaxation

Sessions 3: Insomnia treatments — how you think about your sleep

1. Making small changes — changes in daily behavior. Establish parameters for bedtime period
2. Differentiate rest from sleep, and fatigue from sleepiness
3. Schedule sleep periods with respect to average sleep at baseline
4. Bed restriction therapy — suggest where necessary
5. Establish seven-day per week compliance

6. Stimulus control therapy — remove incompatible activity from bedroom environment
7. Get out of bed if still wakeful after twenty minutes
8. Avoid sleeping in as 'compensation' for poor quality sleep
9. Establish stability from night to night
10. Adjust the sleep period as sleep efficiency improves
11. The role of daytime napping — the dos and don'ts
12. Beliefs about sleep — challenge negative thoughts
13. Develop strategies to stop thinking about sleep — at night (thought-blocking, imagery, distraction)
14. What works for you
15. Factual statements about sleep
16. Managing negative sleep thoughts during the day
17. The rationale behind relaxation therapy
18. Relaxation time

Sessions 4: Consolidation — pulling it all together

1. Consolidation of the information
2. Many small changes make a BIG difference to behavior patterns and thoughts
3. Checking your sleep — your plan of action
4. Summing up of the course and the present research
5. Discussion of sleep hygiene again
6. Things to remember:
   - sleep changes across the life span
   - don't blame sleep for other things in your life
   - readdress misattributions connecting sleep and waking time
7. Dysfunctional beliefs and attitudes questionnaire
8. Eliminate 'effort' to control sleep but reinforce that sleep is controllable
9. Motivate to maintain behavior and cognitive change
10. Utilize relapse prevention techniques — normal process of relearning
11. 'Don't let the setback set you back'
12. Relaxation time

Always allow time for questions and discussion throughout these sessions and keep them informal.

References for appendices

Buysse DJ, Reynolds CF, Monk TM, Berman SR, Kupfer DJ (1989) The Pittsburgh Sleep Quality Index: A new instrument for psychiatric practice and research. *Psychiat Res* **28**: 193–213

Gallassi R, Morreale A, Montagna P, Cortelli P, Avoni P, Castellani R *et al* (1996) Fatal familial insomnia: behavioral and cognitive features. *Neurology* **46**(4): 935–9

Hauri P, Linde S (1996) *No More Sleepless Nights*. Revised edn. John Wiley & Son, New York

Krupp LB, La Rocca NG, Muir-Nash J, Steinberg AD (1989) The Fatigue Severity Scale. Application to patients with multiple sclerosis and systemic lupus erythematosus. *Arch Neurol* **46**: 1121–3

Lugaresi E, Medori R, Montagna, Baruzzi A, Cortelli P, Lugaresi A *et al* (1986) Fatal familial insomnia and dysautonomia with selective degeneration of thalamic nuclei. *New Engl J Med* **315**(16): 997–1003

Lugaresi E, Provini F, Plazzi G (2000) Insomnia in neurology. In: Culebras A, ed. *Sleep Disorders and Neurological Disease*. Marcel Dekker, New York

Lugaresi E, Provini F (2001) *Agrypnia excitata*: clinical and pathophysiological implications. *Sleep Med Rev* **5**(4): 313–22

Manetto V, Medori R, Cortelli P, Montagna P, Tinuper P, Baruzzi A *et al* (1992) Fatal familial insomnia: clinical and pathologic study of five new cases. *Neurology* **42**(2): 312–9

Medori R, Tritschler HJ, LeBlanc A, Villare F, Manetto V, Chen HY *et al* (1992) Fatal familial insomnia, a prion disease with a mutation at codon 178 of the prion protein gene. *New Engl J Med* **326**(7): 444–9

McLean CA, Storey E, Gardner RJ, Tannenberg AE, Cervenakova L, Brown P (1997) The D178N (cis-129M) 'fatal familial insomnia' mutation associated with diverse clinicopathologic phenotypes in an Australian kindred. *Neurology* **49**(2): 552–8

Portaluppi F, Cortelli P, Avoni P, Vergnani L, Contin M, Maltoni P *et al* (1994a). Diurnal blood pressure variation and hormonal correlates in fatal familial insomnia. *Hypertension* **23**(5): 569–76

Portaluppi F, Cortelli P, Avoni P, Vergnani L, Maltoni P, Pavani A *et al* (1994b) Progressive disruption of the circadian rhythm of melatonin in fatal familial insomnia. *J Clin Endocrinol Metab* **78**(5): 1075–8

Tateishi J, Brown P, Kitamoto T, Hoque ZM, Roos R, Wollman R *et al* (1995) First experimental transmission of fatal familial insomnia. *Nature* **376**(6539): 434–5

CHAPTER 8

Tiredness and sleepiness

Antonio Ambrogetti

Introduction

Excessive daytime sleepiness is a common problem and has multiple causes (Thorpy, 2005). When a patient presents complaining of falling asleep or not being able to stay awake in everyday situations (talking to people or sitting at the table) a diagnostic path is not difficult to plot (*Figure 8.1*).

However, many patients do not complain of sleepiness but rather of the 'consequences' of being sleepy. People often think that the act of falling asleep is a consequence of being tired, eg. 'I sleep because I am always tired'. As a result, patients often regard the complaint as one of tiredness rather than sleepiness.

A patient presenting with a complaint of chronic fatigue or chronic tiredness poses a difficult problem as the diagnostic possibilities are wide and, more importantly, there is often more than one cause for the presenting symptom.

Diagnostic approach

This chapter deals with the diagnosis and treatment of the sleep and wake abnormalities that can lead to a state of chronic sleepiness. *Figure 8.1* summarizes one method for reaching a diagnosis in patients presenting with chronic sleepiness, tiredness or fatigue.

Defining sleepiness, tiredness and fatigue

It is useful to clarify what the patient means by fatigue and tiredness. Tiredness may refer to lack of energy, physical exhaustion, tiring early during prolonged activity, or physical or mental fatigue. Some patients also use the terms fatigue and tiredness to refer to lack of motivation or drive. In contrast, sleepiness refers to a tired state where the person has a desire to lie down and go to sleep. And, of course, people can experience a lack of energy, sleepiness, and a lack of motivation simultaneously.

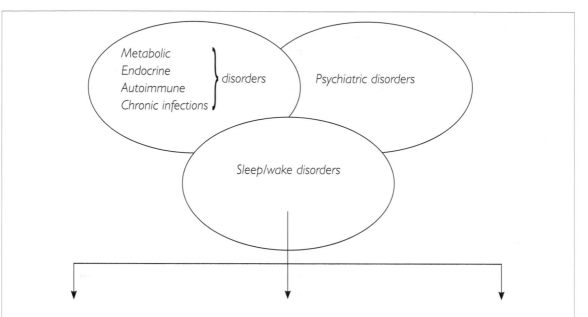

Primary

- Narcolepsy with cataplexy
- Narcolepsy without cataplexy
- Narcoplepsy secondary to medical condition:
  - ~ post-infection
  - ~ post-traumatic
  - ~ brain pathology
  - ~ menstrual-related
  - ~ genetic disorders
- Idiopathic hypersomnia with long sleep time
- Idiopathic hypersomnia without long sleep time
- Hypersomnia due to medical condition:
  - ~ Parkinson's disease
  - ~ post-traumatic
  - ~ hypothyroidism
  - ~ hepatic encephalopathy
  - ~ chronic renal failure
  - ~ adrenal insufficiency
  - ~ industrial toxin (eg. organic solvent)

Secondary

- Obstructive sleep apnea
- Periodic limb movement/ restless leg syndrome
- Shift working
- Delayed sleep phase syndrome
- Insufficient sleep from any cause
  - ~ poor sleep hygiene
  - ~ chronic medical disorders
  - ~ painful conditions, asthma, gastroesophageal reflux, heart failure, severe fractures, brain pathology
  - ~ medications (beta-blockers, sedatives
- Substance abuse including:
  - ~ alcohol
  - ~ caffeine
  - ~ stimulants
- Depression
- Long sleepers

Sub-wakefulness states

- Some chronic fatigue states with subjective sleepiness and cognitive impairment

Figure 8.1: Chronic sleepiness and tiredness

The patient should be encouraged to identify which sensation is the most significant as this distinction is clinically important. A predominant symptom of lack of energy would be suggestive of metabolic, endocrine, autoimmune and chronic inflammatory conditions. A complaint of lack of motivation may indicate a psychiatric component for tiredness (eg. depression). When sleepiness is a prominent symptom, sleep and wake disorders are an important consideration.

Onset of sleepiness/tiredness

Identifying when the onset occurred helps to narrow down diagnostic possibilities. Subacute onset during teenage years or the early forties is common in narcoleptic syndromes; either narcolepsy-cataplexy or idiopathic hypersomnolence. However, insufficient sleep is also a common cause of sleepiness in teenagers. Acute onset following an infective illness or head trauma may suggest a secondary (symptomatic) narcolepsy, post-traumatic or post-infectious hypersomnolence. Onset or exacerbation during pregnancy may suggest narcolepsy, restless leg syndrome, postnatal depression, iron deficiency or thyroid dysfunction.

Time course of sleepiness and fatigue

Is sleepiness/tiredness continuous or intermittent? Intermittent sleepiness/tiredness with symptoms over months or years makes the diagnosis of narcolepsy or idiopathic hypersomnolence less likely, although cases of recurrent hypersomnia have been described. Perimenstrual symptoms are sometimes reported with a remission in between.

Associated symptoms

A history of snoring and apnea, restless legs, shift working or irregular sleep and wake patterns are likely causes or contributors to daytime sleepiness and tiredness. A history (or family history) of hypothyroidism, autoimmune condition (lupus, rheumatoid arthritis, Sjögren's) heart failure, poorly controlled asthma or diabetes, epilepsy, iron or vitamin B_{12} deficiency are all relevant findings. A detailed medication history is also important and should include the use of beta-blockers, anxiolytics/sedatives, antidepressants and recreational drugs.

Objective measurement of sleepiness

Some form of objective measure of sleepiness is useful for both diagnostic purposes and assessing treatment responses. There are a variety of behavioral measures, performance testing (eg. reaction time tests, driving simulator), self-reported questionnaires, and electrophysiological tests, as discussed in *Chapter 3*. Most of these assessments are suited for research or epidemiological studies. In a clinical setting dealing with an individual patient, questionnaires are used as screening tests and to follow up patients over time. Electrophysiological tests are the most reliable and well-validated measures of sleepiness tendency, although they are expensive and time-consuming. The multiple sleep latency test (MSLT) is the standard measure of sleep propensity and the maintenance of wakefulness test (MWT) measures the ability to remain awake. The two tests are not closely correlated as they measure two different functions, sleepiness (with the MSLT) and arousal state (with the MWT) which are closely linked, but distinct processes (Sangal *et al*, 1992).

Genetic testing and hypocretin-1 level

Genetic testing and measurement of hypocretin-1 (orexin A) level in the spinal fluid are research instruments and are not used in the day-to-day differential diagnosis of hypersomnolence syndrome. However, in particular, hypocretin assay may be useful for differentiating narcolepsy–cataplexy from other hypersomnolence conditions, specifically narcolepsy with cataplexy, and narcolepsy due to medical conditions from idiopathic hypersomnolence. Currently the assay requires a lumbar puncture to obtain a spinal fluid sample. In patients with primary narcolepsy-cataplexy with positivity for HLA-DR2, hypocretin-1 is less than 110 pg/ml (or 30% of control value) than in patients with narcolepsy without cataplexy and idiopathic hypersomnolence (Kanbayashi *et al*, 2003). Low level of CSF hypocretin-1 are also found in seriously ill patients with other medical disorders. Although a low hypocretin-1 level is useful in confirming the diagnosis of narcolepsy–cataplexy, a normal level does not exclude the diagnosis, as up to 10% of patients with narcolepsy–cataplexy have normal levels (American Academy of Sleep Medicine, 2005). Until a simpler measurement, perhaps using serum, is available, lumbar puncture in this circumstance is difficult to justify outside a research protocol.

Genetic testing has demonstrated an association between some human leucocytes; antigens (HLA) and narcolepsy–cataplexy (*Table 8.1*). These antigens are found on the surface of lymphocytes B and macrophages and coded by genes in the short arm of chromosome 6. Genes in the DR2, DQB1 (*DRDQ1*0602*) and DQA (*DQA1*0102*) regions are positive in more than 95% of patients with narcolepsy–cataplexy, with minor ethnic variability, compared to 20–30% of positive subjects in the general population (Mignot *et al*, 1998; Overeem *et al*, 2001).

However, there are well-documented cases of narcolepsy–cataplexy with negative genetic findings, so a negative result does not rule out the diagnosis. In practice, genetic tests are not part of the diagnostic investigation of patients with sleepiness outside a research setting,

Laboratory testing

The extent of laboratory investigation is dictated by the clinical findings in the history and examination. Most patients undergo simple laboratory tests, such as full blood count, electrolytes and renal function, thyroid-stimulating hormone (TSH), erythrocyte sedimentation rate (ESR), and perhaps C-reactive protein. Depending on the clinical context, serology for infectious diseases, tests for autoimmune conditions, celiac disease, vitamin B_{12} and folate need to be considered. In the context of headache, or previous head trauma with subacute onset (weeks or months) of hypersomnolence, brain imaging needs to be undertaken.

Table 8.1: HLA allele frequencies in narcoleptic and control subjects		
Human leucocyte antigen (HLA) marker	**Frequency of narcolepsy–cataplexy**	**Controls**
HLA-DR2: Serological typing, the oldest narcolepsy marker		
Caucasians	85–100%	26%
African–Americans	65–75%	31%
Japanese	100%	36%
HLA DR15: DR2 subtype		
Caucasians	85–100%	23%
African–Americans	65–75%	29%
Japanese	100%	35%
HLA-DRB1*1501: DR15 subtype, beta chain		
Caucasians	85–100%	22%
African–Americans	10–20%	7%
Japanese	100%	13%
HLA-DQ1: Serological typing, low specificity		
Caucasians	90–100%	67%
African–Americans	>95%	75%
Japanese	100%	73%
HLA-DQB1*0602: DQ1 subtype, beta chain		
Caucasians	85–100%	22%
African–Americans	90–95%	34%
Japanese	100%	12%
HLA-DQB1*0102: DQ1 subtype, alpha chain		
Caucasians	85–100%	36%
African–Americans	90–95%	48%
Japanese	100%	26%
HLA-DQA1*0102/HLA DQB1*0602: DQ1 subtype		
Caucasians	85–100%	22%
African–Americans	90–95%	33%
Japanese	100%	12%

(from Nishino *et al*, 2000)

Narcoleptic syndromes

The term narcoleptic syndromes encompasses a group of primary hypersomnolence conditions. It refers to hypersomnolence syndromes (eg. narcolepsy, narcolepsy–cataplexy, secondary or symptomatic narcolepsy, and idiopathic hypersomnolence) where sleepiness is the primary problem rather than the consequence or symptom of another disease (eg. obstructive sleep apnea, restless legs, shift work, insufficient resting time, drug use). It is a concept that is clinically useful during the initial evaluation of chronically sleepy/tired patients, when it is difficult to distinguish between the different entities. In cases of monosymptomatic or incomplete narcolepsy (see below) it can take months or years before full diagnostic criteria are met (sometimes they never are). In these situations, which are common in clinical practice, the term narcoleptic syndromes provides a useful working diagnosis and one which can be refined or reviewed as the clinical picture becomes clearer.

Narcolepsy–cataplexy

Case study 1

Jasmine Mohamed is a 17-year-old studying for her higher school certificate examination. She has a history of subacute onset of sleepiness going back to the age of 14 associated with concentration and memory problems. She describes her tiredness as a sleepiness tendency. There is a family history of thyroid problems and some of her relatives are known to be 'sleepy people'. Jasmine does not use medication and has never smoked or used alcohol.

Jasmine goes to bed about 10.00PM with a sleep latency of only a few minutes. She wakes occasionally through the night. She does not snore but is known to talk in her sleep. She gets up between 6.00AM and 8.00AM feeling unrefreshed most of the time. She does not take naps through the day but occasionally falls asleep in the morning as well as the afternoon. If she falls asleep, she sleeps for about 15 minutes and wakes feeling refreshed. She has fallen asleep at school and feels drowsy while driving. She has also fallen asleep at the table and, occasionally, talking to people.

There is a history of visual and auditory hypnagogic (at the beginning of sleep) hallucinations but no sleep paralysis. She describes having a 'jelly-like' feeling go through her body when listening to a joke or if she gets angry. There is no history of automatic behavior.

She is a thin young woman with a normal cardiorespiratory examination. There is no organomegaly. Biochemistry investigations reveal iron deficiency and a normal thyroid function.

A sleep study shows high sleep efficiency (90% — normal value above 85%) with normal sleep structure and sleep stages. There is severe daytime sleepiness, falling asleep with a mean sleep latency of 2.9 minutes and 4 out of 4 early onset stage REM sleep.

Jasmine had a classical presentation of narcolepsy and cataplexy, both in terms of history as well as polysomnography (*Table 8.2*). She was started on dexamphetamine sulfate with good symptomatic response. However, according to Jasmine's family, she became angry and short-tempered. She was changed to methylphenidate, up to six tablets a day. This produced similar effects and she tended not to take her medication. About 3 years after the initial diagnosis, driving the 15-minute trip home from university, Jasmine fell asleep 200 metres away from her house. There were no serious consequences but she has been more compliant with her medication since then. The Road and Traffic Authority requires a 12-month review of her driving licence.

Case study 2

Mrs Elaine Ewing is a 75-year-old woman who presents for assessment of 'collapsing on the ground'. She has a history of hypertension, gastroesophageal reflux and depression. She reports loss of muscle power since the age of 15. She consulted a physician about 30 years ago about the attacks who told her she had cataplexy but did not recommend any treatment.

The attacks involve lower limb weakness and her head slumping forward. Mrs Ewing has fallen off a chair on a number of occasions and feels weak in her legs. The episodes usually last from a few seconds to up to one minute. They occur on a daily basis up to three times a day. They are normally triggered by emotional stimulation; upsets as well as good news, such as the news of the birth of her grandson. She fell to the ground once in a supermarket after meeting a person she had not seen for some time. During this episode, she was fully aware of the surroundings, had no loss of consciousness, but was unable to talk.

She tends to fall asleep during the day at inappropriate times, such as sitting at the table or talking to people, and even with a cup of tea in her hand. There is no history of sleep paralysis or hypnagogic hallucinations. She takes sertraline (Zoloft™) for depression but says this has little impact on her episodes of cataplexy.

A sleep study is performed while on sertraline 50 mg in the morning, as Mrs Ewing feels she cannot stop the antidepressant. Overnight polysomnography shows poor sleep quality with no slow-wave sleep. During the day she has a mean sleep latency of 5.3 minutes and one early onset REM.

Mrs Ewing is started on dexamphetamine sulfate 5 mg three times daily, one at breakfast, one at midday and one at 3.00PM which results in an improvement in her daytime sleepiness. However, the cataplectic attacks continue. Zoloft is withdrawn and she is started on clomipramine (Anafranil™), a tricyclic antidepressant, 25 mg in the morning with marked improvement in the cataplectic attacks.

The two previous case studies are of unequivocal narcolepsy–cataplexy syndrome, a condition with an estimated prevalence of 20–60 cases per 100,000 (Hublin *et al*, 1994; Overeem *et al*, 2001). The diagnosis is straightforward. The first case presented predominantly with profound sleepiness, which was affecting the school performance and daily living of the young patient.

Cataplexy in this patient was an infrequent and less important symptom. In the second patient, cataplexy was a major component of her presentation occurring on average three times a day. It was not controlled by sertraline which, like other selective serotonin re-uptake inhibitors (SSRIs), has a REM suppressant activity and is often used to control cataplexy (see below).

It is important to note that the onset of symptoms in both patients was around the teenage years, however the second patient was not diagnosed with cataplexy until the age of fifty and the diagnosis of narcolepsy/cataplexy was not considered until the age of 75. This is not an uncommon situation as the delay between the onset of symptoms and a final diagnosis of narcolepsy is on average 14–15 years (Ferrans *et al*, 1992). However, cases presenting with pathological sleepiness with or without cataplexy after the age of 40 are recognized in clinical practice (Rye *et al*, 1998).

Case study 3

Ms Cynthia Dimitriou is a 31-year-old mother of two children aged 6 and 2. She presents with a long history of daytime tiredness that she describes as a sleepiness tendency going back to her childhood. She does not smoke or drink and only takes a contraceptive pill. There are no other medical problems. She says she has 'never felt energetic', and would fall asleep coming home from school on the bus as a young teenager. In her work as an accountant, she often takes naps through the day in her office.

After specific questioning, Ms Dimitriou relates a history of visual and auditory hypnagogic hallucinations going back to her childhood when she saw people in her room. At the time, this was dismissed as childhood imagination. She had frightening episodes of sleep paralysis as a young adult, but no symptoms suggestive of cataplexy. She has frequent automatic behavior, particularly while driving.

Soon after her second pregnancy she became particularly tired and she was started on an antidepressant on the assumption that some of her symptoms were related to postnatal depression. The antidepressant was, however, discontinued because it was not beneficial.

Ms Dimitriou has good insight into her condition and has no somatic or psychological evidence of mood and anxiety disorder. She has a sleep study which shows poor sleep efficiency of 60% (normal value more than 85%) but no disturbed breathing. Multiple sleep latency testing shows a mean sleep latency of 16 minutes and no early onset REM. However, she is found to have brief micro-naps all through the daytime napping. The 'microsleeps' being less than 15 seconds did not qualify for the criteria for sleep onset.

This is a more complex case than the previous case studies. The patient had a clear history of daytime sleepiness going back to her teenage years and perhaps even before. She had no metabolic or psychiatric abnormality to explain her symptoms. There was evidence of REM-related symptoms in terms of hypnagogic hallucinations and sleep paralysis with disturbed sleep (often present in patients with narcoleptic syndrome), but no polysomnographic criteria of daytime sleepiness.

The clinical impression was that the patient had a narcoleptic syndrome. Her self-reported degree of sleepiness, as measured by the Epworth sleepiness scale, was 16 out of 24, in keeping with significant severe daytime sleepiness. Her symptoms of sleepiness were affecting her daytime functioning and she could hardly socialize because of constant tiredness. She would not drive more than 10–15 minutes due to a concern of falling asleep.

It was decided that the testing should be repeated and that a trial of stimulant medication was appropriate. The medical and the medicolegal implications of the diagnosis of narcolepsy were explained to her. These include restrictions on driving as well as potential insurance consequences, such as increases in premium.

The diagnosis of narcolepsy

The diagnosis of narcolepsy is based on clinical and polysomnographic criteria (*Table 8.2*). As the initial description of narcolepsy by the French neuropsychiatrist Jean Baptiste E Gélineau included severe sleep attacks and cataplexy triggered by emotions, the first two case studies' clinical criteria are sufficient to establish the diagnosis. It was subsequently recognized that sleep paralysis and hypnagogic hallucinations were common in narcoleptic patients (Daniels, 1934; Yoss and Daley, 1957) and that some polysomnography findings were frequent in narcolepsy.

In the overnight sleep study, latency to sleep onset is typically very short and REM sleep may appear within 30 minutes of sleep onset (normal is between 90 and 120 minutes). Daytime testing by multiple sleep latency test (MSLT) shows increased sleep tendency with mean latency to sleep onset usually, but not always, below 5 minutes and early onset REM in two or more naps (Rechtschaffen *et al*, 1963; Vogel, 1960).

Because some patients may never experience cataplexy, or cataplexy is not recognized (see below), the current classification of sleep disorders includes the diagnosis of narcolepsy without cataplexy (*Table 8.2*) (American Academy of Sleep Medicine, 2005).

Sleepiness

Sleepiness in classic narcolepsy is usually overwhelming and characterized by an irresistible need to fall asleep. A person usually falls asleep for a few minutes and wakes feeling refreshed. Not all cases of narcolepsy are so dramatic. In some people, sleepiness can be resisted most of the time except in boring situations such as lectures, driving on highways or watching television.

Sleepiness also interferes with the person's daytime function. If it occurs during school years it may also interfere with learning. The first case study discussed an average student who had difficulty at school. It is not uncommon for patients with narcolepsy to be labelled 'lazy' or 'unmotivated'. Lack of awareness on the part of the teachers and sometimes the family can lead to serious learning and school difficulties for young people with narcolepsy. The second case study patient was unable to read and write and it is possible that this problem was related to the narcolepsy which started during her teenage years, some 50 years prior to the diagnosis.

Table 8.2: Diagnostic criteria of narcolepsy

1. Excessive daytime sleepiness occurring almost daily for at least 3 months.

2. The hypersomnia is not better explained by other sleep disorders or medical, neurological or psychiatric disorders.

Narcolepsy with cataplexy	Narcolepsy without cataplexy	Narcolepsy due to medical condition
Typical cataplexy	No cataplexy or atypical symptoms	An underlying medical or neurological condition accounts for the sleepiness and one of the following:
MSLT <8min with at least 2 SOREM	MSLT <8 minutes with at least 2 SOREM	Typical cataplexy or MSLT <8 minutes and at least 2 SOREM
or		or
Hypocretin-1 in CSF level <110pg/ml or (30% of normal control value)	Hypocretin-1 in CSF usually normal	Hypocretin-1 in CSF level <110pg/ml or (30% of normal control value)

Cataplexy is defined as sudden and transient episodes of loss of muscle tone triggered by emotions.
MSLT = multiple sleep latency test; SOREM = sleep onset REM; CSF = cerebrospinal fluid.

Cataplexy

The recognition of cataplexy is critical for the diagnosis of narcolepsy. However the identification of cataplexy is difficult. Classic presentation consists of bilateral muscle weakness triggered by emotions. When attacks are frequent, the diagnosis is easier, although direct observation by the physician is rare. However patients with documented cataplexy asked to describe trigger factors and how cataplexy manifests itself, relate a wide range of triggers and clinical presentations (*Tables 8.3* and *8.4*) (Gelb *et al*, 1994) which highlight the difficulty of taking a relevant history.

Sleepiness preceding or following cataplectic attacks does not always occur and is reported by only 48% of patients. Some patients are able to abort an attack using strategies such as talking through it, concentrating on something else or moving vigorously. In some cases, the patients report precataplectic aura in the form of feelings of warmth, nervousness or fear.

The differential diagnosis of cataplexy includes syncope and presyncope, conversion syndrome (hysteria) and hyperekplexia (startle disease). In the case of syncope of any cause there is loss of consciousness which is absent in cataplexy. Even in the most extreme case of cataplectic attack, when the patient collapses, consciousness is maintained. *Gelastic syncope* (*gelos* = mirth, from Greek) is a form of loss of consciousness associated with laughing (Totah and Benbadis, 2002) with pathophysiology similar to cough syncope, whereby an increased intrathoracic pressure due to breath holding leads to low blood pressure, hypoperfusion and syncope. Again, the association with laughing may be misleading, but the loss of consciousness is absent in cataplexy. Some forms of seizure are also associated with laughing (*gelastic seizure*) (Arroyo *et al*, 1993). However, in these cases, usually part of a complex partial epilepsy arising from the cingulate-temporal cortex, laughing is not associated with emotional trigger or content. There are usually focal clonic movements, even though consciousness is maintained.

Cases of *conversion syndrome* (hysteria), where collapsing and unresponsiveness are symptoms of an underlying psychiatric syndrome, need to be considered on the basis of this type of clinical history.

Hyperekplexia can be difficult to differentiate from cataplexy when it is associated with sleepiness/tiredness (Brown *et al*, 1991; Hochman *et al*, 1994). Hyperekplexia is commonly referred to as 'startle disease', which is an exaggerated manifestation of a normal alerting reaction (startle reflex). This consists of increased muscle contraction and tone in response to a sudden unexpected stimulus, visual or auditory. When this response is excessive, patients lose their balance and may fall. The event is similar to a cataplectic attack, except that cataplexy results from loss of muscle tone and hyperekplexia from an exaggerated increase in tone. The distinction is relevant because startle disease is treated with

Table 8.3: Triggers of cataplexy	
• Laughter	65%
• Anger, frustration and annoyance	40%
• Nervousness	19%
• Embarassment	13%
• Sadness	13%
• Fear	6%
Others: being teased, disciplining pets, sexual fantasies, receiving flattery, playing racquetball, hearing religious music	

Table 8.4: Description of cataplexy	
• Collapse	68%
• Twitching, contortion or paralysis of the face	52%
• Head dropping	35%
• Jaw dropping	13%
• Buckling of the knee	32%
• Weakness of the upper body	42%
• Jelly-like feeling (generalized weakness without falling)	35%
Others: wave of dizziness, sudden jolt or interruption of consciousness	

muscle relaxant (clonazepam), while cataplexy requires tricyclic antidepressants or serotonin reuptake inhibitors.

Another rare condition associated with muscle weakness and sleepiness is *hyperkalemic paralysis* (Iranzo and Santamaria, 1999). In this condition, weakness occurs after physical activity with a loss of tendon reflexes and elevation of potassium (>6 mmol/lit). Hyperkalemia can be transient and difficult to document. Emotions do not trigger this condition.

Cataplexy can occur in isolation, without sleepiness or other REM-related symptoms (sleep paralysis and hypnagogic hallucination) (Van Dijk *et al*, 1991). The pathophysiology of cataplexy is thought to be related to a combination of reduced adrenergic drive and cholinergic hypersensitivity involving the cholinergic connection between the limbic system (involved with emotions) and the hypothalamic/brainstem centers (*Chapter 1*).

Hypnagogic and hypnopompic hallucinations

Hypnagogic (at the beginning of sleep) and hypnopompic (at the end of sleep) hallucinations are often present in narcolepsy. They include visual or auditory hallucinations, such as seeing things or hearing noises or voices. Sometimes the patient reports abnormal body positions or even extra-body experiences. These vivid images or sounds occur at the beginning of sleep and when the patient wakes up, usually in the morning, but also in the middle of the night or even during daytime naps. They are related to early intrusion of REM sleep during drowsy state.

It is important to be precise when asking if the hallucinations occur when the patient is sleepy but still awake. It must be stressed that you are referring to the transition from full wakefulness to sleep, when the person is drowsy, rather than asleep and dreaming. Also, the difference between thinking about things while we try to fall asleep (a universal experience) and hallucinations (visual and auditory experiences) should be clarified.

It should be noted that hypnagogic hallucinations may occur in the absence of narcolepsy, particularly in patients who are sleep-deprived by any cause, including people with severe obstructive sleep apnea. It is also reported by 4% of the normal population (American Academy of Sleep Medicine, 2005).

Sleep paralysis

Sleep paralysis refers to a sensation of not being able to move, except for breathing and eye movements, which occurs when the person wakes from sleep or occasionally when falling asleep. Like hallucinations, sleep paralysis is not specific to narcolepsy and can occur in isolation (Buzzi and Cirignotta, 2000; Fukuda *et al*, 1998). However, it is one of the four symptoms often present in narcoleptic syndrome. When asking about sleep paralysis, it is again important to be specific. The sensation is one of being paralysed, rather than not wanting to move.

Sleep paralysis is usually a frightening experience and the patient is normally able to recall the event in detail. The paralysis can last from a few seconds to a minute and resolves spontaneously. However it can be terminated by a person talking to or touching the patient. Sleep paralysis is due to persistence of REM sleep at the time the person is waking up. There is a delay between cortical activation (consciousness) and the resolution of the paralysis, which is a normal occurrence during REM sleep. As a consequence of this dys-synchrony, the person is fully awake but unable to move.

Automatic behavior

Automatic behavior is a common occurrence in everybody at some stage in life. It is an important and frequent, although often underestimated, symptom in narcolepsy. Automatic behavior refers to a situation where the person acts without full awareness of their surroundings. A typical example is drivers who, when they reach their destination, are unaware of what happened during the travel period. Another common situation is where the patient intends to go to the one room but finds themselves in another, unsure as to how or why they got there. Automatic behavior is thought to be related to a microsleep where the person has reduced awareness of their surroundings but remains able to continue their actions.

Daytime sleepiness with or without sleep attacks, hypnagogic and hypnopompic hallucinations, sleep paralysis and cataplexy constitute the tetrad of symptoms typical of narcolepsy. It should be noted that sleepiness and sleep attacks are the fundamental symptoms present in virtually all patients. Cataplexy, when present, is sufficient to make the diagnosis of narcolepsy. However, cataplexy, hallucinations and sleep paralysis may be transient phenomena that occur only once or twice in the lifespan of the patient. It is not uncommon for these REM-related symptoms to present early on in the history of the patient but then resolve spontaneously. However, sleepiness is a persistent symptom. Occasionally, cataplexy may be the presenting symptom and sleepiness develops later on in the patient's life.

Nocturnal sleep in narcolepsy

Nocturnal sleep in narcolepsy patients is often disturbed and it is common for patients to complain of difficulty staying asleep due to sleep fragmentation with recurrent arousal. Insomnia, predominantly difficulty maintaining sleep, is reported in up to 61% of patients (Ferrans *et al*, 1992).

Narcolepsy is better viewed as a disturbance of the sleep and wake distribution over a 24-hour period rather than an increase in the amount of sleep, which is more characteristic of idiopathic hypersomnolence (see below) (Zorick *et al*, 1986). In simple terms, narcoleptic sleep episodes tend to intrude through the day, being responsible for sleep attacks; and wakefulness intrudes through the night, causing recurrent awakening. Increasing the level of alertness during the day using stimulant medication commonly improves sleep quality at night.

Psychosocial consequences of narcoleptic syndromes

Narcolepsy sufferers are often affected by chronic sleepiness and by the fact that diagnosis can be delayed for years. Feelings of depression are reported by up to 51% of patients. These feelings correlate more highly with the negative social impact of narcolepsy than the degree of sleepiness. In children, narcolepsy can affect learning and development with long lasting consequences (*Chapter 10*). In adults, it is associated with personal, interpersonal and family problems (Broughton, 1992). Patients are often unable to hold down a job and have an increased incidence of separation and depressive illness.

Even when the diagnosis is finally made, the people close to the patient often do not understand the associated disability. Social support, or lack of it, is one the most important factors in determining level of function in patients with narcolepsy. Therefore education about narcolepsy should involve both the patient and the immediate family.

Sexual dysfunction

Another problem for men with narcolepsy is sexual dysfunction related to erectile failure, decreased libido due to sleepiness and, occasionally, cataplexy triggered by sexual arousal (Karacan *et al*, 1992). Part of the problem can be related to the medication, as amphetamines, tricyclic antidepressants and serotonin reuptake inhibitors can cause erectile dysfunction. Treatment is therefore difficult, as reduction in sleepiness due to a stimulant may be beneficial in some patients but aggravate the problem in others. Tricyclic antidepressants with less anticholinergic (eg. desipramine) activity may interfere less with erectile function.

Medicolegal implication of narcolepsy

The medicolegal implications of being diagnosed with narcolepsy should always be explained to the patients. In many countries, including Australia, narcoleptic patients have serious restrictions on driving. Often insurance companies require a higher premium for a variety of policies, even though the life expectancy in narcolepsy is no different from the general population. A diagnosis of narcolepsy is an exclusion criterion for certain occupations, such as enrolment in the army, the navy or the airforce.

Polysomnography in narcolepsy

In the overnight polysomnography of narcoleptic patients, the sleep latency is often less than 10 minutes, and it is possible to see early onset of REM within thirty minutes of sleep onset in 25–50% of cases (American Academy of Sleep Medicine, 2005). This is contrary to what normally occurs in adults, whereby the first REM sleep episode occurs between 90 and 120 minutes.

In the multiple sleep latency test (*Chapter 3*), there is evidence of pathological daytime sleepiness (mean sleep latency less than 8 minutes and often less than 5) and the occurrence of REM sleep in two or more naps. Daytime sleepiness on multiple sleep latency test and early onset REM (SOREM) are non-specific of narcolepsy. They can be found in people with severe obstructive sleep apnea, insufficient sleep due to any cause, following withdrawal from a central nervous system sedative, and occasionally in normal subjects with no symptoms (Rosenthal *et al*, 1994). A small proportion of normal sleepers (less than 2%) are also found to have sleep onset REM in the multiple sleep latency test (MSLT) (American Academy of Sleep Medicine, 2005; Bishop *et al*, 1996). Polysomnography is also a useful tool with which to document other sleep disorders, such as obstructive sleep apnea, which appear to be more prevalent in narcolepsy patients (Guilleminault and Dement, 1977) and may aggravate daytime sleepiness. However, this association could be due to ascertainment bias. It should be noted that there is substantial overlap in mean sleep latency in the MSLT between narcoleptic patients (3.1 ± 2.9 min), idiopathic hypersomnia sufferers (6.2 ± 3 min), and healthy controls (10.5 ± 4.6 min) (American Academy of Sleep Medicine, 2005).

Clinical versus research diagnostic criteria for narcolepsy

According to the International Classification of Sleep Disorders (ICSD; American Sleep Disorders Associaton, 1997), the criteria for the diagnosis of narcolepsy, as with all sleep disorders (*Table 8.1*), are intended to be a 'working platform'. They should be seen as an aid to establishing the unequivocal presence of a particular sleep disorder, but there will be situations which do not meet the minimal criteria, when clinical judgment will need to be used (see *Case study 3, p. 284*). This should be kept in mind when assessing individual patients. For example, although pathological sleepiness is defined as a mean sleep latency in the MSLT of <5 minutes, and a requirement in the ICSD criteria for narcolepsy, values of less than 7 or 8 minutes are found in patients who otherwise would meet diagnostic criteria. On occasion, a patient may have subjective sleepiness, cataplexy and mean sleep latency above 10 minutes (normal range) (Gelb *et al*, 1994).

Monosymptomatic narcolepsy and possible/probable narcolepsy

The concept of monosymptomatic narcolepsy is practical because the full picture of narcolepsy–cataplexy is not always present. It is not uncommon for patients to experience sleepiness or sleep attacks without any other REM-related symptoms (hypnagogic hallucinations, sleep paralysis or cataplexy). More rarely the initial presentation is one of isolated hypnagogic hallucination or sleep paralysis or cataplexy, and only later (months or years), a full picture of sleepiness becomes apparent. When hallucinations are the only presenting symptom, the potential of misdiagnosing schizophrenia is a real risk (Douglass *et al*, 1991). In these situations, the possibility of monosymptomatic narcolepsy should be considered, and close follow-up is needed over time. In other circumstances, a firm diagnosis of narcolepsy cannot be made because the full criteria are not met. In these situations it is better to maintain an open diagnosis of possible or probable narcolepsy.

In particular, when sleepiness is the only presenting symptom (often without sleep attacks), a differential diagnosis with idiopathic hypersomnolence can be difficult to make. When sleepiness is the only symptom but there are some polysomnographic features of narcolepsy, such as early onset REM sleep in the overnight sleep study or on the MSLT, the term incomplete narcolepsy has been suggested (Parks *et al, 1998*). The future use of hypocretins as a diagnostic aid should help clarify these issues (*Table 8.2*).

Idiopathic hypersomnolence (non-REM narcolepsy)

Case study 4

Dan Oswald is a 57-year-old man, a self-employed cook with a long history of severe tiredness. He describes his tiredness predominantly as sleepiness tendency and lack of energy. He smokes one to two cigars a week but does not drink alcohol. He remembers feeling sleepy back to his teenage years when he used to fall asleep at school. He finished year ten at school and entered the workforce. At the age of 23 he had a car accident where he hit the back of the car in front of him. He has no recollection of the event and suspects he had fallen asleep. Over the years he has worked for himself as a successful restaurateur and he is known to his family and co-workers by the nickname of 'Nightie', as he falls asleep as soon as he sits down anywhere.

He only ever drives within a 10–15-minute distance of home and his wife drives at all other times. There are no REM-related symptoms and his sleep study shows a sleep efficiency of 90%, with reduction in slow-wave and REM sleep. Multiple sleep latency testing shows a mean sleep latency of 6 minutes (normal > 10 minutes) and no REM sleep in any of the naps.

Dan is started on dexamphetamine sulfate but with only minimal benefit and side-effects consisting specifically of palpitations, sweating and headaches. He is satisfied with the diagnosis which finally explains his state of health (eg. he is not lazy, just sleepy), and decides not to continue treatment given the fact that he has managed reasonably well most of his life and is well adjusted.

The above case is an example of idiopathic hypersomnolence characterized by insidious onset of sleepiness going back to an early age that has continued unabated through the life of the patient. The term non-REM narcolepsy is sometimes used to refer to this syndrome.

The prevalence of idiopathic hypersomnolence is uncertain because of the tendency (Billiard 1996) to lump it under the diagnostic label of hypersomnolent conditions, which did not meet criteria for narcolepsy. It is said that approximately 5–10% of patients being assessed for sleepiness in sleep units may have idiopathic hypersomnolence (American Sleep Disorders Association, 1997). Indirect estimates suggest a prevalence of two to five cases per 100,000 (Bassetti and Aldrich, 1997).

It is possible that cases of monosymptomatic narcolepsy or incomplete narcolepsy are classified as idiopathic hypersomnolence in some series. Some degree of overlap between narcolepsy and idiopathic hypersomnolence is commonly observed clinically and has been referred to as mixed form (Bassetti and Aldrich, 1997). However, there are clinical and laboratory differences which help differentiate narcolepsy from idiopathic hypersomnolence. Recent research on the level of hypocretin-1 may aid in the distinction (*Table 8.5*).

Sleep over a 24-hour period is often increased (< 10 hours) in idiopathic hypersomnolence (idiopathic hypersomnolence with long sleep time), compared to narcolepsy, where the total amount of sleep may be normal but fragmented. In some cases, the total amount of sleep is not increased (idiopathic hypersomnolence without long sleep time) (American Academy of Sleep Medicine, 2005). The nocturnal sleep episode is often reported as deep but unrefreshing. Similarly, daytime naps are longer (one to three hours) than in narcolepsy (minutes), and the person wakes feeling unrefreshed. It should be noted that daytime naps are not always present but microsleep episodes are often documented on continuous EEG recordings.

Sleep drunkenness is a confusional state which occurs during arousal from slow-wave sleep and is said to be common in idiopathic hypersomnolence (Roth, 1980). Symptoms and signs suggestive of autonomic nervous system dysfunction have also been reported, including vascular headaches, labile blood pressure with pre-syncope and cold hands and feet (Guilleminault and Faull, 1982).

Table 8.5: Narcolepsy versus idiopathic hypersomnolence

	Idiopathic hypersomnolence	Narcolepsy
Age of onset	Usually < 30	Usually < 30
Progression over time	Stationary, unremitting	Stationary, unremitting
Daytime naps	Prolonged and unrefreshing	Short and usually refreshing
Irresistible sleep attacks	Rare	Common
REM-related symptoms ~ hypnagogic hallucination ~ sleep paralysis ~ cataplexy	Not present	Present in variable combination
Nocturnal sleep	Prolonged and undisturbed, but unrefreshing	Often fragmented
Sleep drunkenness	Common (50–60%)	Uncommon
Response to stimulant	Variable	Usually good
Hypocretin-1 level in CSF	Normal	Undetectable
MSLT	6.2 (±3) min	3.1±2.9
SOREM	2 or more	Less than 2

CSF = cerebrospinal fluid; MSLT = multiple sleep latency test; SOREM = sleep onset REM.

(modified from Roth, 1980 and American Academy of Sleep Medicine, 2005)

Idiopathic hypersomnolence appears to be a less characterized syndrome than others and particular attention should, therefore, be given to exclude other diagnoses which are secondary causes of hypersomnia (eg. obstructive sleep apnea, periodic limb movement disorder, hypersomnia associated with mood disorders, insufficient sleep, delayed sleep phase syndrome, and post-infection hypersomnia).

The pathophysiology of this condition is not known, even though there is some family clustering which may suggest a genetic predisposition (Billiard, 1996; Poirier *et al*, 1986). Also, although idiopathic hypersomnolence has an insidious onset, at times some triggered events can be identified, such as viral illness or previous minor trauma. The treatment of idiopathic hypersomnolence is with stimulant medication (see below) but responses are not as dramatic as they are in narcolepsy.

Antonio Ambrogetti

Post-infectious hypersomnolence

Case study 5

Bree Larbalestier is a 22-year-old third year medical student who presents with a long-standing complaint of abnormal fatigue. She was well until 5 years ago when she contracted severe glandular fever, confirmed by blood testing. She was incapacitated for 9–10 months and missed almost all of year 10 at school. Her function improved slowly to about 70% of prior to her illness, but was left with profound fatigue and sleepiness. She eventually finished her HSC and was accepted into a medical degree. She has managed to pursue her studies although she has had to give up other activities and pastimes, including cross-country walking, because of her tiredness.

Since the beginning of her symptoms 5 years ago, Bree has experienced episodes of acute exacerbation of fatigue associated with bouts of rhinitis or sinusitis. When questioned directly about the nature of her fatigue she says that sleepiness is a major component of it. She takes two to three naps during the day lasting between 20–30 minutes. She feels sleepy during lectures and does not feel confident driving long distances.

Bree goes to bed around 9.30PM with short sleep latency and she sleeps undisturbed until 7.00AM when she rises feeling unrefreshed. She has had extensive investigations, which show no evidence of metabolic or endocrine abnormalities. She feels depressed at times, but formal psychiatric assessment reveals no clinical depression. On examination, there is nothing relevant except inflamed nasal mucosa.

A sleep study and multiple sleep latency test show 7 hours sleep with short sleep latency of 8 minutes and efficiency of 94%. The sleep structure is normal in terms of stages distribution. Multiple sleep latency testing reveals a mean sleep latency of 5 minutes with no REM abnormalities.

A diagnosis of post-infectious hypersomnia is considered and Bree is started on a small dose of dexamphetamine. However, she experiences palpitations, anxiety and confusion even on a dose of 10 mg twice a day. She is changed to modafinil 200 mg twice a day with an excellent response.

This type of complaint is reasonably common and the salient issue is the identifiable onset of the symptoms of tiredness/sleepiness associated with an infective illness (in this case glandular fever) (Guilleminault and Mondini, 1986). However, similar cases are well documented following a variety of other infective illnesses, including brucellosis, Ross River virus and CMV infection.

Although post-infectious hypersomnolence was the diagnosis considered, the final diagnosis probably needs to remain open. Given the onset of her illness as a teenager, and the occasional report of the onset of narcolepsy or idiopathic hypersomnolence following infective illness, it is possible that her presentation is the first episode of a narcoleptic syndrome rather than post-infectious hypersomnolence. The lack of REM-related symptoms (hypnagogic hallucinations, sleep paralysis, cataplexy) is relevant, but does not exclude narcolepsy as monosymptomatic narcolepsy could present in the same way and only follow-up over time will clarify the diagnosis.

Patients with post-infectious hypersomnolence often have worsening symptoms following episodes of other infection, but tend to improve over time. Conversely, narcolepsy and idiopathic hypersomnolence tend to have a steady, unremitting course through the life of the patient. This was explained to the patient and she was asked to attend a review on a regular basis, every 12–24 months. At each visit she will be taken off the medication and fully reassessed to see if her level of alertness has improved and if the medication can be stopped.

Post-traumatic hypersomnia

Case study 6

Mr George Hubacher is a 37-year-old man referred for assessment of daytime tiredness and cognitive impairment which interferes with his activities as a musician and teacher.

George was involved in a motor vehicle accident a decade ago and experienced anterograde and retrograde amnesia for about 10 days after the accident. He was hospitalized for about 30 days with a slow recovery over a period of 6 months. Initially, he had severe daytime sleepiness, sleeping up to 15 hours a day. After about 6 months, his sleep and wake pattern changed and he had increasing difficulty falling asleep at night and sleepiness during the day.

George says he has daytime fatigue, difficulty concentrating and memory impairment. He has been feeling depressed due to difficulties at work. He does not take any regular medication, apart from short-acting benzodiazepines two to three days a month.

George goes to bed between 10.00PM and 11.00PM and falls asleep within 30 minutes. He wakes briefly once or twice a night. He snores but his wife has not noticed any apnea. George wakes around 8.30AM usually feeling unrefreshed. While he does not nap deliberately through the day, he feels sleepy when he is not busy. There are no focal neurological deficits on examination.

A sleep study shows 6 hours and 30 minutes of sleep with no evidence of apneas. There is reduction in REM sleep to 9% and increase in stage 2. Sleep efficiency is 88%. Multiple sleep latency test reveals a mean sleep latency of 7 minutes and no REM onset episodes. A drug screen at the time of the MSLT is negative.

A diagnosis of post-traumatic hypersomnolence was considered and a trial of a small dose of stimulant was started. However, there was no significant benefit and the medication was discontinued.

In this man, the differential diagnoses, apart from post-traumatic hypersomnolence, would include insufficient sleep syndrome (given his occupation as a musician), hypersomnia secondary to the use of a sedative, as he admitted to the use of benzodiazepines at times to help him sleep, and delayed sleep phase syndrome, sometimes seen after head trauma (Dagan, 2002; Quinto *et al*, 2000).

The patient's history is typical of sleep disturbance following severe head trauma (Guilleminault *et al*, 1983; Lankford *et al*, 1994). This type of patient often goes through a period of severe daytime sleepiness with prolonged sleep episodes of up to 15 hours/day followed sometimes by reversal of the sleep cycle with fragmented sleep at night and daytime naps. In a case like this, where naps do not occur, the underlying mechanism of daytime tiredness/sleepiness can be accounted for by episodes of microsleeps through the day.

Pathologic study to assess the neuroanatomic correlation of sleepiness in these cases are uncommon, even though widespread lesions may be found. Lesions involving the thalamic and hypothalamic area are likely to be associated with these findings (American Sleep Disorders Association, 1997). The response to treatment with stimulant medication is inconsistent.

Recurrent hypersomnia

Kleine–Levin syndrome

Case study 7

Marc Farrah is a 15-year-old boy referred for investigation of episodes of sleepiness lasting from a few days to 2 weeks, and occurring about once or twice every three months. Marc was diagnosed with nephrotic syndrome at age 4 which has been difficult to control and for which he takes prednisone 7.5mg. He does not take any other medication.

Marc describes episodes of acute onset of sleepiness lasting for 2–3 days associated with a craving for food. During these episodes he is able to go to the toilet and also to the pantry and eat whatever is available. After 2–3 days of almost continuous sleeping, he appears to recover for a few days but starts sleeping again. These episodes last for 1–2 weeks at 5–6-week intervals. The last episode occurred three weeks prior to the referral and lasted for 1 week.

During his normal sleep period, Marc goes to bed between 8.00PM and 9.30PM with a sleep latency of about 30 minutes. He wakes occasionally through the night, snores, but not every night, and is a restless sleeper. There is no apnea reported by the family. Marc gets up any time between 6.30AM and midday depending on the day of the week. He naps during the day but not every day. He gets drowsy at school and, at times, while watching television.

On examination, Marc does not appear depressed or anxious and he demonstrates a range of emotion in keeping with the content of the interview. He is quite articulate when describing his symptoms and answering questions. He is overweight for his age and height but has no abnormalities in the oropharyngeal area. There is no evidence of infective illness preceding the onset of this behavior.

The differential diagnosis included:
- Kleine–Levin syndrome (most likely)
- sleep apnea
- inadequate sleep hygiene.

This young patient had put on weight because of the chronic use of steroids. Obstructive sleep apnea or upper airway resistance syndrome needed to be considered as potential contributors to daytime sleepiness. Also, in teenagers, insufficient sleep should always be part of the differential diagnosis.

Overnight polysomnography was conducted while the patient was symptom-free and showed a high sleep efficiency of 89%, a sleep latency of 15 minutes, no respiratory abnormality and no fragmentation of sleep. There was mild daytime sleepiness on multiple sleep latency test with a mean sleep latency of 6.9 minutes and no REM abnormalities.

The nature of the problem, and likely spontaneous resolution of Kleine–Levin syndrome, was explained to the patient, and supportive management only was suggested, as pharmacological intervention with stimulants is usually not successful and does not prevent the attacks of sleepiness.

Kleine–Levin syndrome (KLS) is more common in males with onset usually occurring in adolescence, characterized by recurrent hypersomnia, hyperphagia and spontaneous remission. Occurrence in young women is also recognized (Kesler *et al*, 2000). The epidemiology and pathophysiology of KLS are uncertain. However given the combination of symptoms of sleep attacks, eating disorders and occasional mood changes, hypothalamic dysfunction (Fernandez *et al*, 1990) has been hypothesized.

Occasionally the episodes appear to start after either an infective illness, minor head trauma, physical or emotional stress. The beginning of menstruation has also been put forward as a possible trigger in the few cases occurring in females (Duffy and Davison, 1968), but such cases are better classified under 'menstrual-related sleep disorder'.

The episodes of sleepiness usually have an abrupt onset — within a matter of a few hours — and can last for up to 24 hours or more with the patient only being able to wake partially and eat or void in a semi-awake state. Hyperphagia is one of the features, together with irritability and, on occasion, hypersexuality. Spontaneous resolution is the most common progression in Kleine–Levin syndrome, even though recurrence may occur months or years later.

The differential diagnosis of KLS, although they are rare events, should include less benign intracranial pathology, such as craniopharyngioma, pituitary and hypothalamic tumour and pinealoma.

Periodic hypersomnia (monosymptomatic Kleine–Levin syndrome)

Case study 8

Justine Suitor is a 43-year-old woman who has experienced recurrent episodes of sleepiness occurring about every 4 months and lasting up to 2 days, for the past 7 years. In one of these episodes she says that she felt an urge to sleep on a Saturday morning around lunchtime. She tried to fight the sleepiness but eventually fell asleep between 2.00PM and 3.00PM and slept continuously until 11.00AM Sunday morning. She felt nauseated and depressed for the following few days. Feelings of depression also occurred during previous episodes. There is no relation to her menstrual cycle.

When specific inquiry was made regarding increased sexual desire (a feature often reported in recurrent hypersomnolence of the Kleine–Levin type), Justine recalled her husband saying that they had sexual activity during one of the episodes but she had little memory of this. She has tried amphetamines prior to this presentation with no effect.

There is no history of increased eating during the episodes. On a few occasions Justine says that she has had difficulty falling asleep at night following the episodes of sleepiness. On one occasion she remembers an unusual taste in her mouth for about 30 minutes prior to having an overwhelming need to fall asleep. However there are no other features suggestive of seizure activity and previous EEGs on two occasions have been reported as normal.

An overnight sleep study shows a high sleep efficiency of 88% with no significant disturbed breathing. There is reduction of stage 3 and 4 possibly due to first-night effect and normal REM of 24% (within normal limits). A multiple sleep latency test showed a mean sleep latency of 9.7 minutes and one early onset REM in the first nap.

The differential diagnosis included:
- periodic hypersomnia (monosymptomatic Kleine–Levin syndrome)
- functional hypersomnia (conversion syndrome)
- surreptitious use of sedatives
- epilepsy partialis
- endozepine stupor.

The best chance of narrowing the diagnosis is to examine the patient during one of the episodes of prolonged sleepiness, including an EEG recording. Direct observation would allow the administration of an agent such as flumazenil (a benzodiazepine antagonist), which is effective in waking the person in cases of endozepine stupor or sleepiness due to benzodiazepine intake.

The importance of being seen at the time of the sleep attacks was explained to the patient and she was given an explanatory letter for the local hospital so that we could be contacted in the event of her presenting to casualty. However, this never happened. The sleep episodes became less frequent and she has not returned to follow up.

Atypical forms of Kleine–Levin syndrome are probably more commonly seen as periodic hypersomnia without the other symptoms. Overnight sleep studies usually have no specific features to help the diagnosis. The multiple sleep latency test can be abnormal, as in the case presented, with or without REM abnormalities (Reynolds *et al*, 1980). Treatment is usually supportive only. The use of stimulant medication during prolonged episodes of hypersomnolence is generally not effective.

Endozepine stupor

A differential diagnosis relevant to *Case study 8* is endozepine stupor. This is a recently described condition (Lugaresi *et al*, 1998a) characterized by an increase in endozepine which leads to a prolonged period of sleep episode with confusional arousals. Endozepines are endogenous analogs of benzodiazepine similar to the more widely known endorphins which are the body's equivalent of opioids. Measurement of endozepine-4 is not routinely available. One way to diagnose endozepine stupor is to administer the patient a benzodiazepine antagonist (such as flumazenil) intravenously, which usually results in their prompt awakening even though the effect is of short duration (~90 minutes). The use of flumazenil requires supervision because of the potential risk of triggering an epileptic seizure. An important differential diagnosis is the surreptitious use of benzodiazepines, something which should be excluded by urine testing (Granot *et al*, 2004; Lugaresi *et al*, 1998b).

Insufficient sleep syndrome

Case study 9

Ms Anita Newby is a 30-year-old receptionist referred for investigation of chronic tiredness/sleepiness over the last 10–12 years. She is a single mother of a 10-year-old girl and she is a trained pianist. Piano tutoring does not provide a sufficient income so she also works as a receptionist between 8.00AM and 4.00PM, five days a week. She takes no medication except the contraceptive pill. She does not smoke and has about two to three standard drinks per week.

Anita's tiredness is of subacute onset going back to her teenage years, and is continuous in nature. She describes fatigue both in terms of lack of energy as well as sleepiness and 'fogginess'. Her bedtime is between 11.00PM and midnight, with sleep latency of less than 10 minutes. Overnight sleep is undisturbed but she feels unrefreshed at 7.00AM when she rises. At weekends, she sleeps in until 9.00AM or 10.00AM. On examination, she is an overweight lady with a body mass index of 27, a patent nose and a normal looking pharynx. She snores but does not have choking arousals or apnea. There is no history of REM-related symptoms (hypnagogic hallucinations, sleep paralysis or cataplexy).

An initial diagnosis of possible upper airway resistance syndrome or idiopathic hypersomnolence was considered. A sleep study showed a short sleep latency of less than 5 minutes and normal sleep structure with minimal snoring and no disturbed breathing. A multiple sleep latency test showed pathological daytime sleepiness with a mean sleep latency of 4.6 minutes but no early onset REM naps.

The findings were discussed with the patient. The multiple sleep latency test clearly pointed to severe daytime sleepiness as a major contributor to her tiredness. During the second interview, her day routine was again reviewed. Following prompting it appeared that on occasion she was supplementing her receptionist income as a piano bar musician on weekends. The patient was asked to keep a sleep diary for a week and at the same time wear an actigraphy (*Figure 8.2*). Although in the sleep diary, bedtime seemed to be no later than midnight, the actigraphy showed the patient was active until 1.30AM on Saturday night, Sunday night and Monday night, corresponding to her piano bar activity. On working days she woke up around 7.00AM–7.30AM, and on Saturday morning she would sleep in until midday.

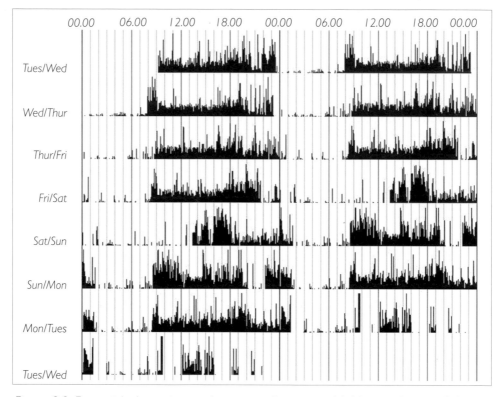

Figure 8.2: Forty-eight-hour time scale at top of actigram. 00:00 = midnight, 12:00 = midday. Note that on Saturday morning the patient got up at 12:30PM, and on Saturday, Sunday and Monday her sleep period did not start until 1:30AM–2:00AM.

It was explained to the patient that the underlying reason for her chronic tiredness and sleepiness was insufficient sleep. This is often the case when restriction in resting time continues for weeks or months. Intervention requires the patient to understand the underlying mechanism and be willing to modify their behavior.

Case study 10

Katie Anthrope is a 16-year-old girl who presents with her mother following a referral for assessment of chronic fatigue. She is in year 10 at school and she describes chronic tiredness and a deterioration in her school performance noticeable over the last 12 months. She is an otherwise healthy teenager who says that she does not smoke or use recreational drugs. She drinks two caffeinated drinks a day. She describes her tiredness predominantly as lack of energy and lack of concentration.

Katie goes to bed between 10.00PM and 11.00PM and falls asleep within half an hour. She sleeps undisturbed until 7.00AM on school day and 8.30AM on weekends. She usually feels tired when she wakes up.

Until prompted by the physician, neither Katie nor her mother mentioned that Katie's sleep and wake pattern on weekends is very different from that during the week. She says she goes out with friends on Friday and Saturday night and does not come home until between 1.00AM and 2.00AM. However, an actigraphy performed for a week (*Figure 8.3*) shows that on Saturday, Katie came home between 3.00AM and 4.30AM and still got up between 6.00AM and 7.00AM.

Katie says she gets into trouble for being a day dreamer at school, not paying attention in lectures, and showing poor enthusiasm for her school work. She does not take naps after school. On examination, she is a thin young lady with no abnormal findings.

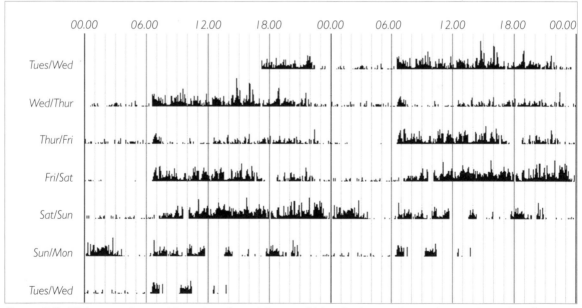

Figure 8.3: 48-hour actigram. Note that for a 16-year-old her bed time during the week is already quite late, between 11.00PM and midnight. However on Saturday, her bedtime was 4.00AM, and she got up at 6:30AM.

The most likely diagnosis here is insufficient sleep due to poor sleep hygiene. Without the precise knowledge of her weekend behavior one might have considered a diagnosis of narcoleptic syndrome.

Case studies 8 and *9* highlight the importance of careful history-taking, which includes not only working days but also weekends. Insufficient sleep from any cause is probably the most common reason for daytime tiredness and sleepiness in our society. Particularly in teenagers and young adults, the possibility of chronic lack of sleep should be pursued meticulously. When possible, objective documentation using instruments such as actigraphy is valuable as even sleep diaries can be subject to bias report or manipulation.

Treatment is difficult unless the patient is willing to cooperate. Teenagers are often brought in for assessment by the family and do not think that they have a problem. Advice that involves modifying their weekend behavior is often ill received by the young patient. It is, therefore, important to provide a full explanation and education, which links the poor sense of well-being and tiredness to the sleep and wake pattern. It should be pointed out that improvement in tiredness and sleepiness will take at least a few weeks, if not a few months, to restore a more regular sleep and wake pattern.

Patients may argue that they have maintained the same behavior for years, but it is only recently that their symptoms of tiredness have emerged. This is not an uncommon situation because young people, in particular, are able to tolerate a degree of sleep deprivation for a long time before symptoms emerge. This usually happens when the person runs out of any physical and mental reserve and this point should be stressed to the patient.

Lack of sleep does not need to be dramatic. It has been shown that even a small reduction in resting time over a prolonged period is sufficient to lead to chronic sleep deprivation. The fact that sleep deprivation accumulates over time has been shown in an experimental protocol (*Figure 8.4*). By the same token, prolongation of resting time, both in terms of increasing amounts of sleep as well as simply resting, is associated with an increase in alertness.

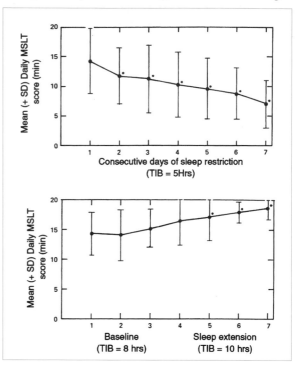

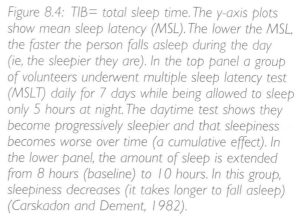

Figure 8.4: TIB= total sleep time. The y-axis plots show mean sleep latency (MSL). The lower the MSL, the faster the person falls asleep during the day (ie, the sleepier they are). In the top panel a group of volunteers underwent multiple sleep latency test (MSLT) daily for 7 days while being allowed to sleep only 5 hours at night. The daytime test shows they become progressively sleepier and that sleepiness becomes worse over time (a cumulative effect). In the lower panel, the amount of sleep is extended from 8 hours (baseline) to 10 hours. In this group, sleepiness decreases (it takes longer to fall asleep) (Carskadon and Dement, 1982).

Hypersomnia associated with mood disorders

The association between mood disorders (depression, bipolar and dysthymic disorders) and insomnia is well known. Less appreciated is the fact that hypersomnia can also be a prominent symptom. Initial studies based on a questionnaire (Detre *et al*, 1972) suggest that sleepiness is a common self-reported complaint in this group of patients. It is difficult to ascertain the effect of medications, weight increase (a common finding) and subjective versus objective documentation of sleep and sleepiness. More specifically, it may be difficult to distinguish between the anergic patient resting in bed for prolonged periods awake (clinophilia) and sleeping (Billiard *et al*, 1994).

However, when polysomnographic recordings are used, the complaint of sleepiness is found to be related to the subjective sensation of lack of interest, decreased energy and psychomotor retardation (Nofzinger *et al*, 1991), as well as objective sleepiness within the moderate to severe range (mean sleep latency < 10 minutes, during the day) in 36% of patients with mood disorder who complained of lethargy (Billiard *et al*, 1994).

Because patients with chronic hypersomnia (narcolepsy, idiopathic hypersomnolence) may have depressed mood as a consequence of sleepiness, it can be difficult to be sure if the depressed mood is the primary or secondary event. Either way, mood disorders should be high on the list of the differential diagnosis in patients with chronic fatigue and sleepiness.

One variant of depressive illness with atypical features, including hypersomnia, is seasonal affective disorder (SAD). This describes recurrent episodes of depression occurring with the beginning of autumn and winter months and remission in summer. The episodes of depression have atypical symptoms; hypersomnia is more prominent than insomnia, and a craving for carbohydrates causing subsequent weight increase.

Case study 11

Mr Joseph Miller is 50-year-old man referred for assessment of episodes of sleepiness lasting 4–6 weeks. He describes a slow onset of depressed mood starting in May (autumn in Australia), and an unwillingness to do anything. He has difficulty with concentration and in making decisions. He depends on his wife and feels unsafe without her around.

He sleeps from 9.00PM until 9.00AM or 12MD if left undisturbed. However, it is difficult for his wife to be sure if he is asleep during this time or just lying motionless but awake. He will not drive for more than 10 minutes because he feels unsafe. At the time of assessment, the end of August, he is feeling better after the local doctor had started him on venlafaxine (Efexor™) 300mg daily. A similar episode had occurred in the previous 2 years and resolved spontaneously a few weeks after moving from New South Wales to Queensland.

The above case is strongly suggestive of SAD. It is more typically described in countries located at high latitude, with onset of symptoms in autumn and winter and remission in spring and summer, but also occurs in more temperate climates (Magnusson and Boivin, 2003; McIntyre *et al*, 1989; Morrissey *et al*, 1996). It is described in children and the elderly, but the peak incidence is in middle age, predominantly among females. SAD is classified as a major depressive episode but the severity is variable and some patients do not meet the full criteria for major depression and are classified as sub-syndromal SAD (s-SAD) (Partonen and Rosenthal, 2001). The combination of SAD and subsyndromal SAD may have an estimated prevalence of 17.2% (male) and 23.9% (female) in the ages of 16–64 years (Eagles, 2001).

Sleepiness, expressed as an increase in total time of sleep in the 24 hours, is reported by 80% of patients with SAD (Shen and Shapiro, 2001). This is confirmed on overnight polysomnography which shows high efficiency with increased total sleep time in winter compared to summer. Multiple sleep latency test, however, does not confirm increased daytime sleepiness. It is felt that SAD may represent a form of circadian rhythm disorder, with features of delayed sleep phase in some predisposed individuals. This would be in keeping with the beneficial effect of light therapy administered in the morning.

Management of SAD includes light therapy and/or pharmacological intervention. Light therapy (Partonen and Rosenthal, 2001) requires an educated, committed patient. About 70% of patients improve after one week of treatment with 2500 lux, 2 hours in the morning between 6.00AM and 10.00AM. Shorter periods of exposure (30 minutes) are effective with higher light intensity (10,000 lux) (see *Table 8.6*).

Light therapy, however, is rather intrusive and cumbersome and pharmacological management seems also to be effective. Antidepressants with noradrenergic mechanism of action, venlafaxine, moclobemide, mirtazapine and reboxetine have been shown to be effective (Kasper *et al*, 2001).

Sub-wakefulness syndromes (hypovigilant state)

There is a group of patients in whom, even after having excluded metabolic, endocrine, autoimmune, psychiatric syndromes, as well as primary and secondary sleep disorders, a complaint of profound tiredness, cognitive impairment and subjective sense of sleepiness remains undiagnosed. Sleep studies and multiple sleep latency testing often do not reveal any objective evidence of daytime sleepiness. However, some of these patients have micro-sleeps, which are brief periods of drowsy states, as documented by continuous EEG over a 24-hour period (American Sleep Disorders Association, 1997). Clinically, they are often labelled chronic fatigue syndrome. Because the patients' state of health is often associated with personal and social disability, mood changes may be present and, not uncommonly, their problem is labelled 'functional'.

Case study 12

Ms Miriam Mitselburg is a 33-year-old woman referred to the sleep unit for assessment to exclude a possible sleep disorder as part of her investigation of chronic fatigue syndrome. She has an 8-year history of a subacute onset of fatigue described both in terms of lack of energy and sleepiness. Although the initial request was for 'exclusion of sleep apnea', the diagnosis could be easily dismissed on clinical grounds given the fact that the patient is slim with no symptoms of sleep apnea and no features suggestive of it on examination. However, the history of chronic fatigue, cognitive impairment, and what she describes as sleepiness, prompted further investigation.

Miriam is a mother of three children, aged 8, 10 and 12 who works part-time in a local gallery. She describes her upbringing in positive terms and she is happily married with no stress at home or work. She is attending university as a part-time student and says she has difficulty maintaining concentration during lectures.

She normally goes to bed around 10.00PM with a sleep latency between 5 and 30 minutes. She wakes up a couple of times during the night but not every night. She is a non-snorer with no history of leg movement. She is not a restless sleeper. She gets up between 7.00AM and 8.00AM depending on the day of the week and feels unrefreshed 50% of the time. She takes a nap in the afternoon if she is not busy.

Miriam considers herself to be unsafe while driving even though she has never fallen asleep at the wheel. She has one sister who was said to have chronic fatigue syndrome.

Over the years she has undergone different treatments for chronic fatigue syndrome, including dietary manipulation with an amine-free and salicylate-free diet, anti-Candida therapy and other, mostly unorthodox treatments offered for chronic fatigue syndrome. She has no REM-related symptoms suggestive of narcolepsy.

A sleep study shows no snoring and no disturbed breathing with six arousals per hour (normal is up to 10). There is normal sleep structure with slightly increased stage 2 and slightly decreased stages 3 and 4 (20% and stage REM 19%). Mean sleep latency on multiple sleep latency test was 14.3 minutes with no REM abnormalities.

Given the fact that she is a mother with three children and working part-time, the possibility of chronic sleep deprivation was considered. However, a sleep diary kept over a period of 3 weeks showed fairly regular sleep and wake periods not suggestive of sleep deprivation. The sleep study is repeated together with a multiple sleep latency test at the end of the 3 weeks of sleep diary. Again sleep efficiency is high (93%), there is still some reduction in stage 3, 4 and REM but no other abnormalities. Mean sleep latency on multiple sleep latency test on the second occasion was 13.6 minutes with no REM abnormalities (comparable to the initial study).

A formal psychiatric interview revealed a well-adjusted woman with no evidence of psychiatric morbidity.

A tentative diagnosis of hypo-vigilant syndrome is considered and, on that basis, a trial of a small dose of stimulant is started. Miriam is eventually stabilized on three tablets of dexamphetamine a day which results in an improvement in her sense of well being, concentration and ability to function during the day. She has remained stable on this treatment for 3 years with no increase in dosage and no side-effects.

Table 8.6: Light therapy

Dose	2500 lux* for 2 hours 10, 000 for 30 minutes	Distance from the light source is critical as the light intensity (light dose) decreases with increasing distance
	Dawn simulator	Dawn simulators are light sources which are activated by a clock so that the bedroom becomes illuminated over a period of thirty minutes in the morning simulating a summer dawn
Time of the day	Morning between 6.00AM and 10.00AM is considered most effective	Other times of the day may be effective
Duration of treatment	2–4 weeks	Treatment need not to be every day. Five out of seven days may be effective. The effect persists for a variable period, with recurrence after a few weeks. However, in some individuals, one treatment period may suppress symptoms for the entire season
Type of light	White light with ultraviolet (UV) radiation filtered (<1%), and reduced blue light (<10%)	Light box is the standard device. UV and blue light are deleterious to the lens and retina
Position of the patient	Facing the light directly through a diffuser	The patient can engage in other activity, such as exercise, provided that the light intensity in the room is appropriate
Safety recommendations	Light box should respect safety standards (low UV and low blue light)	Transparent eye glasses which filter high frequency radiation can be employed if the nature of the light source is uncertain
	Pre-existing eye disease require full opthalmological assessment	Macular degeneration, retinitis pigmentosa, retinal detachment, cataract, may be a contraindication to light therapy
	Concurrent drug therapy (photosensitizer)	Phenothiazine, amiodarone, lithium, tetracycline, chloroquine, St John's wort, methoxypsoralens (psoriasis treatment)

(from Partonen and Rosenthal, 2001; Remé *et al*, 2001)

Patients with a similar presentation to the above case are not uncommon but are not usually seen in the sleep unit. Many patients end up with the diagnosis of chronic fatigue syndrome and undergo a long litany of orthodox and unorthodox treatments. This patient was referred to the sleep unit predominantly for exclusion of sleep apnea, one of the sleep disorders to be excluded in the investigation of chronic fatigue syndrome.

Although attempts to identify positively 'chronic fatigue syndrome' by specific criteria have been made (Fukuda *et al*, 1994; Royal Australasian College of Physicians, 1997) in practice, chronic fatigue syndrome is an umbrella for a variety of conditions, ranging from post-infectious fatigue state, abnormal illness behavior, mood disorders, compensation neurosis, and frequently unrecognized sleep disorders. Patients with narcolepsy or idiopathic hypersomnolence are not uncommonly misdiagnosed as chronic fatigue syndrome (Ambrogetti *et al*, 1998; Ambrogetti and Olson, 1994; Morriss *et al*, 1993).

Unquestionably, there is a group of patients in whom, after a thorough evaluation, fatigue/sleepiness remains a major component of their illness and a diagnostic dilemma. The possibility that patients with subjective sleepiness but without objective evidence, may actually represent a sub-group of patients with an arousal disorder (*Table 8.7*), as distinct to increased sleepiness, has been put forward for many years (Guilleminault and Dement, 1977; Roth, 1980). In these patients, sleepiness/tiredness has also been considered to be of functional origin (Darchia *et al*, 2002). However, awareness of this category is important because, as indicated above, some patients may well benefit from treatment. In some of these patients, the use of stimulant medication may be beneficial (Olson *et al*, 2003).

Table 8.7: Criteria for sub-wakefulness syndrome

❖ Complaint of drowsiness or sleepiness for more than 6 months

❖ Sleepiness is mild and not irresistible (eg. sleep attacks are not present)

 • normal light sleep
 • mean sleep latency during the day >5 min on MSLT

❖ No other medical or mental disorders which may account for the symptoms

❖ No other sleep disorders which may cause sleepiness are present (narcolepsy, idiopathic hypersomnolence, post-traumatic hypersomnia, sleep apnea)

❖ 24-hour EEG monitoring, when available, shows microsleep (brief episodes of stage I sleep (drowsy state) during wakefulness)

Management of hypersomnia and cataplexy

The most important step in the management of sleepiness is to exclude reversible causes which are, in order of importance: chronic sleep deprivation, depression and substance abuse. If there is a suspicion of insufficient resting time of any cause, the patient may have to be taken off work (if possible) for 3–4 weeks and then reassessed. When reversible causes of hypersomnia are excluded, the treatment is symptomatic and includes adjustment to work and lifestyle, naps, and the use of medications (Thackrey, 1989).

Naps

Naps are a useful way to reduce sleepiness in some patients, predominantly in the case of narcolepsy (Roehrs *et al*, 1986). Short naps of 15–20 minutes are restorative and provide temporary relief from sleepiness for 2–3 hours. Naps are usually not refreshing in idiopathic hypersomnolence. Work schedules which increases sleepiness, such as shift working, should be avoided. In children and young adults at school, teachers should be notified in order to minimize learning difficulty. Special consideration should be given during exams, for example, allowing more time.

Use of stimulant medications

It should be stressed that stimulant medications do not restore a normal level of alertness. Narcoleptic patients on treatment remain sleepier than normal controls (Mitler and Hajdukovic, 1991), even though their alertness is improved. Therefore, there may be a subjective improvement even when the patient appears sleepy by multiple sleep latency testing (Sangal *et al*, 1992). It should also be noted that stimulants have a non-specific alerting effect, irrespective of the cause of sleepiness, and so, are not useful in the diagnostic process. An accurate diagnosis needs to precede their use.

The most common medications used are dextroamphetamine, methylphenidate and modafinil (*Table 8.8* and *Chapter 12*). Other agents, methamphetamine, pemoline, mazindol, codeine and beta-blockers (propanolol) have been used (ASDA Standard of Practice, 1994; Banerjee *et al*, 2004; Mitler *et al*, 1994; 1993; Mignot and Nishino, 2005).

Treatment should be started with a small dose (eg. half a tablet of dexamphetamine, 2.5 mg) two or three times a day. The dose is then adjusted every two to three days until a therapeutic effect is obtained. In this stage of dose adjustment, close contact with the patient is essential for treatment success, usually in the form of telephone advice.

Doses late in the afternoon, after 4.00PM or 5.00PM, are best avoided to minimize interference with night sleep. However, an evening dose may be necessary in patients who have to drive late at night. The final dose is different in each individual as there is no direct relationship between blood level of stimulant and alertness response. The time of administration is variable and depends on the individual. More commonly, the medication is spread through the day, but in some patients, one morning dose seems to provide the best result with no significant side effects.

Once a stable and effective dose is achieved, the use of the medication can be flexible. However, the need for a 'drug holiday', ie. omitting the medication on weekends, has no scientific basis (Piscopo, 1992). Stimulants can be daily or intermittent depending on each individual's requirement, the end point being the quality of life and functioning of the patient with no side-effects. During certain activities, such as driving or working with dangerous materials, patients should be advised to use their medication regularly.

The prescriber should be familiar with the potential side-effects and interaction of the stimulant used (*Chapter 12*). Frequent patient concerns include addiction and tolerance (*Chapter 12*). Side-effects, including stomach upset, headache, palpitations, dry mouth, metallic taste, insomnia, tremor and muscle twitching, can be minimized by starting with a low dose. Modafinil appears to have an alerting effect equivalent to amphetamine, but with fewer side-effects except for headache. The risk of reduction in efficacy of contraceptive pills should be explained when modafinil is used in women of childbearing age.

In pregnancy and breast feeding, stimulants should be avoided as safety data is not available (*Chapter 12*). However, the risk to the fetus seems low (Briggs *et al*, 1975; Eriksson *et al*, 1978; Little *et al*, 1988).

Table 8.8 Stimulants used in the treatment of hypersomnolence

Medication	Dose (mgr)	Comments
Methylphenidate	10–60	On occasion, higher doses are necessary, reported up to 240 mg
Dextroamphetamine	5–60	On occasion higher doses are needed
Modafinil	200–400	Usually given twice a day, doses up to 600 mg have been used, but benefit seems maximum at 400 mg. Side-effects are uncommon, except for headache. Contraceptive pill efficacy is reduced
Caffeine	100–200	Mild alerting effect with onset of action within 20 minutes and lasting 3–5 hours. One cup of coffee has 100 mg of caffeine and 5 cups of coffee an alerting effect similar to 5 mg of dextroamphetamine
Mazindol*	2–6	Gastrointestinal side-effects, potential risk of pulmonary hypertension; not a first choice agent. It does have some anti-cataplexy activity
Pemoline*	18.75–112.5 (USA) 20–120 (UK)	Risk of hepatic toxicity; not a first choice agent

* Note that pemoline and mazindol have been withdrawn in most countries (including Australia) because of serious side-effects.

Treatment of cataplexy

Amphetamine stimulants (dextroamphetamine and methylphenidate) have mild anticataplectic activity and are sufficient for some patients. When cataplexy is a prominent symptom, specific treatment is needed with either non-sedating tricyclic antidepressants or serotonin reuptake inhibitors (*Table 8.9*). The combination of amphetamine and tricyclic antidepressants or SSRIs is usually safe, even though there is potential for toxicity, tachycardia, dry mouth and confusion, including serotoninergic syndrome (Prior *et al*, 2002; Thirumalai *et al*, 2000).

The enhancement of monoaminergic transmission by tricyclic antidepressants and SSRIs, together with anticholinergic action, is the likely mechanism in the control of cataplexy. All these agents have REM suppressant activity (*Chapter 1*).

The same medications are also useful in the treatment of sleep paralysis and hypnagogic/hypnopompic hallucinations when these symptoms are bothersome.

Treatment of nocturnal sleep disruption is usually not needed once daytime alertness has improved. However, it has been suggested that short-acting benzodiazepines may improve sleep quality in narcolepsy (Thorpy and Goswami, 1990). GHB, gamma-hydroxy-butyrate, is a compound with complex properties found to improve sleep quality in narcoleptic patients as well as to reduce cataplexy during the day (Lammers *et al*, 1993; Mamelak *et al*, 1986). However, it is not routinely available for use and is subject to strict regulation because of its abuse potential (see also *Chapter 12*).

Table 8.9: Anti-cataplexy medications	
Medication	**Dose (mg)**
Imipramine (Tofranil™)	10–50
Clomipramine (Anafranil™)	25–50
Citalopram (Cipramil™)	20
Fluoxetine (Prozac™)	20–40
Paroxetine (Aropax™)	2–40
Selegiline* (Eldepryl™)	2.5–5
GHB	3–9 (grams)

*Selegiline is a monoaminoxidase type-B inhibitor (MAO-B inhibitor) which increases dopamine transmission, is metabolized to amphetamine with alerting effect as well as anticataplexy action (Reinish *et al*, 1995).
GHB = gamma-hydroxybutyrate.

References

Ambrogetti A, Olson LG (1994) Consideration of narcolepsy in the differential diagnosis of chronic fatigue syndrome. *Med J Aust* 160: 426–8

Ambrogetti A, Olson LG, Sutherland DC, Malcolm JA, Bliss D, Gyulay SG (1998) Daytime sleepiness and REM sleep abnormalities in chronic fatigue: a case series. *J Chron Fatig Syndr* **4**(1): 23

American Academy of Sleep Medicine (2005) *The International Classification of Sleep Disorders. Diagnostic & Coding Manual*. 2nd edn. American Academy of Sleep Medicine, Westchester, IL

American Sleep Disorders Association (1997) *ICSD — International Classification of Sleep Disorders, revised: Diagnostic and Coding Manual*. ASDA, Rochester, Minnesota

American Sleep Disorders Association Standards of Practice (1994) Practice parameters for the use of stimulants in the treatment of narcolepsy. *Sleep* **17**(4): 348–51

Arroyo S, Lesser RP, Gordon B, Uematsu S, Hart J, Schwerdt P *et al* (1993) Mirth, laughter and gelastic seizures. *Brain* **116**: 757–80

Banerjee D, Vitiello MV, Grunstein RR (2004) Pharmacotherapy for excessive daytime sleepiness. *Sleep Med Rev* **8**(5): 339–54

Bassetti C, Aldrich MS (1997) Idiopathic hypersomnia. A series of 42 patients. *Brain* **120**: 1423–35

Billiard M (1996) Idiopathic hypersomnia. *Sleep Disorders* **14**(3): 573–82

Billiard M, Dolenc L, Aldaz C, Ondze B, A Besset (1994) Hypersomnia associated with mood disorders: a new perspective. *J Psychosom Res* **38**(supp 1): 41–7

Bishop C, Rosenthal L, Helmus T, Roehrs T, Roth T (1996) The frequency of multiple onset REM periods among subjects with no excessive daytime sleepiness. *Sleep* **19**(9): 727–30

Broughton RJ (1992) Psychosocial impact of narcolepsy-cataplexy with comparisons to idiopathic hypersomnia and epilepsy. In: Goswami M, Pollak CP, Cohen FL, Thorpy MJ, Kavey NB, eds. *Psychosocial Aspects of Narcolepsy*. The Haworth Press, New York

Brown P, Rothwell JC, Thompson D, Britton TC, Day BL, Marsden CD (1991) The hyperekplexias and their relationship to the normal startle reflex. *Brain* **114**: 1903–28

Briggs GG, Samson J, Crawford DJ (1975) Lack of abnormalities in a newborn exposed to amphetamine during gestation. *Am J Dis Child* **29**: 249–50

Buzzi G, Cirignotta F (2000) Isolated sleep paralysis: a web survey. S*leep Research Online* **3**(2): 61–6

Carskadon MA, Dement WC (1982) Nocturnal determinants of daytime sleepiness. *Sleep* **5**: 573–81

Clinchop DM, Bogner J, Mysiw WJ, Fugate L, Corrigan J (1998) Defining sleep disturbance after brain injury. *Am J Phys Med Rehabil* **77**: 291–5

Dagan Y (2002) Circadian rhythm sleep disorders (CRSD). *Sleep Med Rev* **6**(1): 45–55

Daniels LE (1934) Narcolepsy. *Medicine (Balt)*, **13**: 1–12

Darchia N, Bastawros M, Carlander B, Dauvilliers Y, Espa F, Ondze B *et al* (2002) Pseudo-hypersomnia or a type of hypersomnia not documented by current tests of sleepiness. *ERSR JSR* **11**(Suppl 1): 46

Detre T, Himmelhoch J, Swartzburg M, Anderson CM, Byck R, Kupfer DJ (1972) Hypersomnia and manic-depressive disease. *Am J Psychiat* **128**(10): 1303–5

Douglass AB, Hays P, Pazderka F, Russell JM (1991) Florid refractory schizophrenias that turn out to be treatable variants of HLA-associated narcolepsy. *N Nerv Ment Dis* **179**: 012–017

Duffy JP, Davison K (1968) A female case of Kleine–Levin syndrome. *Br J Psychiat* **114**(506): 77–84

Eagles JM (2001) Sociodemographic aspects. In: Partonen T, Magnusson A eds. *Seasonal Affective Disorder. Practice and Research*. Oxford University Press, New York

Eriksson M, Larsson G, Winbladh B, Zetterström R (1978) The influence of amphetamine addiction on pregnancy and the newborn infant. *Acta Paediatr Scand* **67**: 95–9

Fernandez J-M, Lara I, Gila L, O'Neill OF, Tyrone A, Gimeno A (1990) Disturbed hypothalamic-pituitary axis in idiopathic recurring hypersomnia syndrome. *Acta Neurol Scand* **82**: 361–3

Ferrans CE, Cohen FL, Smith KM (1992) The quality of life of persons with narcolepsy. In: Goswami M, Pollak CP, Cohen FL, Thorpy MJ, Kavey NB, eds. *Psychosocial Aspects of Narcolepsy*.The Haworth Press, New York

Fukuda K, Ogilvie RD, Chilcott L, Vendittelli AM, Takeuchi T (1998) The prevalence of sleep paralysis among Canadian and Japanese college students. *Dreaming* **8**(2): 59–66

Fukuda K, Strauss ES, Hickie I, Sharpe CM, Dobbins GJ, Komaroff A *et al* (1994) The chronic fatigue syndrome: a comprehensive approach to its definition and study. *Ann Int Med* **121**: 953–9

Gelb M, Guilleminault C, Kraemer H, Lin S, Moon S, Dement WC, Mignot E (1994) Stability of cataplexy over several months — information for the design of therapeutic trials. *Sleep* **17**(3): 265–73

Granot R, Berkovic SF, Patterson S, Hopwood M, Drummer OH, Mackenzie R (2004) Endozepine stupor: disease or deception? A critical review. *Sleep* **27**(8): 1597–9

Guilleminault C, Dement WC (1977) 235 cases of excessive daytime sleepiness. *J Neurol Sci* **31**: 13–27

Guilleminault C, Faull KF (1982) Sleepiness in non-narcoleptic, non-sleep apneic EDS patients: The idiopathic CNS hypersomnolence. *Sleep* **5**: S175–S181

Guilleminault C, Faull KF, Miles L, van den Hoed J (1983) Post-traumatic excessive daytime sleepiness: A review of 20 patients. *Neurology* **33**: 1584–9

Guilleminault C, Mondini S (1986) Mononucleosis and chronic daytime sleepiness. A long-term follow-up study. *Arch Inter Med* **146**: 1333–5

Hochman MS, Chediak AD, Ziffer JA (1994) Hyperekplexia: Report of a nonfamilial adult onset case associated with obstructive sleep apnea and abnormal brain nuclear tomography. *Sleep* **17**(3): 280–3

Hublin C, Partinen M, Kaprio J, Koskenvuo M, Guilleminault C (1994) Epidemiology of narcolepsy. *Sleep* **17**: S7–S12

Iranzo A, Santamaria J (1999) Hyperkalemic periodic paralysis association with multiple sleep onset REM periods. *Sleep* **22**(8): 1123–4

Kanbayashi T, Inoue Y *et al* (2003) CSF hypocretin measures in patients with obstructive sleep apnea. *J Sleep Res* **12**(4)

Karacan I, Gokcebay N, Hirshkowitz M, Ozmen M, Ozmen E, Williams RL (1992) Sexual dysfunction in men with narcolepsy. In: Goswami M, Pollak CP, Cohen FL, Thorpy MJ, Kavey NB, eds. *Psychosocial Aspects of Narcolepsy*. The Haworth Press, New York

Kasper S, Hilger E, Willeit M, Neumeister A, Praschak-Rieder N *et al* (2001) Drug therapy. In: Partonen T, Magnusson A, eds. *Seasonal Affective Disorder. Practice and Research*. Oxford University Press, New York

Kesler A, Gadoth N, Vainstein G, Peled R, Lavie P (2000) Klein Levin syndrome in young females. *Sleep* **23**(4): 563–7

Lammers GJ, Arneds J, Declerck AC, Ferrari MD, Schouwink G, Troost J (1993) Gamma-hydroxybutyrate and narcolepsy: a double-blind placebo-controlled study. *Sleep* **16**(3): 216–20

Lankford DA, Wellman JJ, O'Hara C (1994) Post-traumatic narcolepsy in mild to moderate closed head injury. *Sleep* **17**: S25–S28

Little BB, Snell LM, Gilstrap III LC (1988) Methamphetamine abuse during pregnancy: outcome and fetal effects. *Obstet Gynecol* **72**(4): 541–4

Lugaresi E, Montagna P, Tinuper P, Plazzi G, Gallassi R (1998b) Suspected covert lorazepam administration misdiagnosed as recurrent endozepine stupor. *Brain* **121**(pt 11): 2201

Lugaresi E, Montagna P, Tinuper P, Plazzi G, Gallassi R, Wang TC *et al* (1998a) Endozepine stupor. Recurring stupor linked to endozepine-4 accumulation. *Brain* **121**(pt 1): 127–33

Magnusson A, Boivin D (2003) Seasonal affective disorder: an overview. *Chronobiol Int* **20**: 189–207

Mamelak M, Scharf MB, Woods M (1986) Treatment of narcolepsy with gamma-hydroxybutyrate. A review of clinical and sleep laboratory findings. *Sleep* **9**(1 pt 2): 285–9

McIntyre IM, Armstrong SM, Norman TF, Burrows GD (1989) Treatment of seasonal affective disorder with light: preliminary Australian experience. *Aus NZ J Psychiatry* **23**(3): 369–72

Mignot E (1998) Genetic and familial aspects of narcolepsy. *Neurology* **50**(suppl 1): S16–S22

Mignot E, Nishino S (2005) Emerging therapies in narcolepsy-cataplexy. *Sleep* **28**(6): 754–63

Mitler MM, Aldrich MS, Koob GF, Zarcone VP (1994) Narcolepsy and its treatment with stimulants. *Sleep* **17**(4): 352–71

Mitler MM, Hajdukovic R (1991) Relative efficacy of drugs for the treatment of sleepiness in narcolepsy. *Sleep* **14**(3): 218–20

Mitler MM, Hajdukovic R, Erman MK (1993) Treatment of narcolepsy with metamphetamine. *Sleep* **16**(4): 306–17

Mitler MM, van den Hoed J, Carskadon MA, Richardson G, Park R, Guilleminault C, Dement WC (1979) REM sleep episodes during the Multiple Sleep Latency Test in narcoleptic patients. *Electroencephalography Clin Neurophysiol* **46**(4): 479–81

Morriss R, Sharpe M, Sharpley AL, Cowen PJ, Hawton K, Morris J (1993) Abnormalities of sleep in patients with the chronic fatigue syndrome. *Br Med J* **306**: 1161–4

Morrissey SA, Raggatt PT, James B, Rogers J (1996) Seasonal affective disorder: some epidemiological findings from a tropical climate. *Aus NZ J Psychiat* **30**(5): 579–86

Nishino S, Okura M, Mignot E (2000) Narcolepsy: genetic predisposition and neuropharmacological mechanisms. *Sleep Med Rev* **4**(1): 57–99

Nofzinger EA, Thase ME, Reynolds CF III, Himmelhoch JM, Mallinger A, Houck P, Kupfer DJ (1991) Hypersomnia in bipolar depression: a comparison with narcolepsy using the multiple sleep latency test. *Am J Psychiat* **148**: 1177–81

Olson LG, Ambrogetti A *et al* (2003) A pilot randomized trial of dexamphetamine in patients with chronic fatigue syndrome. *Psychosomatics* **44**(1): 38–43

Overeem S, Mignot E, van Dijk G, Lammers GJ (2001) Narcolepsy: clinical features, new pathophysiologic insights, and future perspectives. *J Clin Neurophysiol* **18**(2): 78–105

Parks JD, Chen SY, Clift SJ, Dahlitz MJ, Dunn G (1998) The clinical diagnosis of narcolepsy syndrome. *J Sleep Res* **7**: 41–52

Partonen T, Rosental NE (2001) Symptoms and course of illness. In: Partonen T, Magnusson A, eds. *Seasonal Affective Disorder. Practice and Research*. Oxford University Press, New York

Piscopo JA (1992) A narcolepsy patient role model. In: Goswami M, Pollak CP, Cohen FL, Thorpy MJ, Kavey NB, eds. *Psychosocial Aspects of Narcolepsy*. The Haworth Press, New York

Poirier G, Montplaisir J, Décary F, Momè D, Lebrun A (1986) HLA antigens in narcolepsy and idiopathic central nervous system hypersomnolence. *Sleep* **9**(1): 153–8

Prior FH, Isbister GK, Dawson AH, Whyte IM (2002) Serotonin toxicity with therapeutic doses of dexamphetamines and venlafaxine. *Med J Austral* **176**: 240

Quinto C, Gellido C, Chokroverty S, Masdeu J (2000) Post-traumatic delayed sleep phase syndrome. *Neurology* **54**: 250–2

Rechtschaffen A, Wolpert E, Dement W, Mitchell S, Fisher C (1963) Nocturnal sleep of narcoleptics. *Electroencephalog Clin Neurophysiol* **15**: 599–609

Reinish LW, MacFarlane JG, Sandor P, Shapiro CM (1995) REM changes in narcolepsy with selegiline. *Sleep* **18**(5): 362–7

Reme CE, Grimm C, Hafezi F, Wenzel A (2001) Lamp standards and ocular safety. In: Partonen T, Magnusson A, eds. *Seasonal Affective Disorder. Practice and Research*. Oxford University Press, New York

Reynolds CF III, Black RS, Coble P, Holzer B, Kupfer DJ (1980) Similarities in EEG sleep findings for Kleine-Levin syndrome and unipolar depression. *Am J Psychiat* **137**(1): 116–8

Roehrs T, Zorick F, Wittig R, Sicklesteel J, Roth T (1986) Alerting effect sof naps in patients with narcolepsy *Sleep* **9**(1Pt 2): 194–9

Rosenthal L, Folkerts M, Roehrs T, Zorick F, Roth T (1994) Sleepiness and sleep onset REM periods in the absence of clinical symptomatology. *Biol Psychiat* **36**: 341–3

Roth B (1980) *Narcolepsy and Hypersomnia*. Basel, New York

Royal Australasian College of Physicians Working Group (1997) Chronic fatigue syndrome Online at: http://www.mja.com.au/public/guides/cfs/cfs1.htm

Rye DB, Dihenia B, Weissman JD, Epstein CM, Bliwise DL (1998) Presentation of narcolepsy after 40. *Neurology* **50**: 459–65

Sangal RB, Thomas L, Mitler MM (1992) Disorders of excessive sleepiness. Treatment improves ability to stay awake but does not reduce sleepiness. *Chest* **102**(3): 699–703

Shen J, Shapiro CM (2001). Sleep. In: Partonen T, Magnusson A, eds. *Seasonal Affective Disorder. Practice and Research*. Oxford University Press, New York

Thackrey M (1989) Behavioral management of narcoleptic sleep attacks: a case report. *Med Psychother* **2**: 177–81

Thirumalai SS, Shubin RA (2000) The use of citalopram in resistant cataplexy. *Sleep Med* **1**: 313–6

Thorpy MJ (2005) Which clinical conditions are responsible for impaired alertness? *Sleep Med* **6**(suppl 1): S13–S20

Thorpy MJ, Goswami M (1990) Treatment of narcolepsy. In: Thorpy MJ, ed. *Handbook of Sleep Disorders*. Marcel Dekker, New York

Totah AR, Benbadis SR (2002) Gelastic syncope mistaken for cataplexy. *Sleep Med* **3**: 77–8

van Dijk JG, Lammers GJ, Blansjaar BA (1991) Isolated cataplexy of more than 40 years' duration. *J Psychiat* **159**: 719–21

Vogel G (1960) Studies in the psychophysiology of dreams III. The dream of narcolepsy. *Arch Gen Psychiatry* **3**: 421–8

Yoss RE, Daly DD (1957) Criteria for the diagnosis of narcoleptic syndrome. *Proc Mayo Clin* **32**: 320–8

Zorick F, Roehrs T, Wittig R, Lamphere J, Sicklesteel J, Roth T (1986) Sleep–wake abnormalities in narcolepsy. *Sleep* **9**(1): 189–93

CHAPTER 9

Sleep and other medical conditions

Antonio Ambrogetti

Introduction

There is a close relationship between sleep and wake and neuroendocrine, immunological and cardiorespiratory functions, with the pathology of each system impacting on the others to various degrees. This chapter reviews the associations between sleep and other medical conditions including those that are:

- neurological
- psychiatric
- respiratory
- physiological (eg. pregnancy, menopause).

Neurological syndromes

The syndromes currently most frequently diagnosed as affecting sleep are the chronic neurodegenerative diseases, Parkinson's disease (PD) and its variants, Alzheimer's disease and other dementias. It was the dramatic impact on sleep and wakefulness by acute encephalitis in 1917–1920 (*encephalitis lethargica*) that initiated the first research into the functional anatomy of sleep and wakefulness.

Chronic neurodegenerative diseases result from pathology affecting the anatomical structures common to, or associated with, sleep and wake function (*Tables 9.1* and *9.2*).

Case study 1 – Insomnia, Parkinson's disease, REM-behavior disorder

Mrs Elaine Dwyer is a 64-year-old retired hairdresser with a 12-year history of PD treated with L-dopa/benserizide (Madopar™), a combination of rapid and slow-release formulation, bromocriptine (Parlodel™), and trihexyphenidyl (benzhexol) (Artane™). She has been referred for evaluation because of increased daytime sleepiness and insomnia. Mrs Dwyer is quite healthy apart from PD and a sacroileitis causing chronic hip pain, which was partially controlled with celecoxib (Celebrex™).

Table 9.1: Anatomical structures involved in neurodegenerative disorders

Disease	Pathology
PD and associated syndromes (eg. progressive supranuclear palsy, multiple system atrophy)	Pons, midbrain, basal ganglia with dopaminergic, cholinergic and serotonergic neurones involvement
Dementia syndromes (Alzheimer's disease, Lewy body dementia, frontotemporal and vascular dementia)	Forebrain including suprachiasmatic nuclei, subthalamic nuclei, with predominant acetylcholine and noradrenergic neuron involvement.
Multiple sclerosis	Variable involvement of subcortical, brainstem pathways
Myotonic distrophy	Thalamic dorsomedial nuclei
Motor neuron disease	Involvement of variable areas of the brainstem

Table 9.2: Neuroanatomy and sleep-related symptoms

Degenerative changes	Symptom
Anterior hypothalamus	Insomnia
Basal frontal lobes	Insomnia
Dorsomedial thalamus	Insomnia
Ventral pons	Insomnia
Posterior hypothalalmus	Hypersomnolence
Midbrain reticular formation	Hypersomnolence
Rostral pontine reticular formation	Hypersomnolence
Paramedian thalamic regions	Hypersomnolence
Suprachiasmatic nucleus	Circadian rhythm disorder
Retinohypothalamic tract	Circadian rhythm disorder
Retinal degeneration	Circadian rhythm disorder
Pons and medulla	Sleep behavior disorder

(Aldrich, 1993)

Mrs Dwyer goes to bed after midnight usually around 1.00AM after watching television or using the internet. She sleeps for 3–4 hours before being woken up by her hip pain and is unable to go back to sleep. She had been taking temazepam (Normison™) or nitrazepam (Mogadon™) three to four times a week to try to sleep longer. Mrs Dwyer takes a daily nap in the afternoon for 10–15 minutes but wakes without feeling refreshed. She feels drowsy socially, at the table, talking to people and watching television. She is a heavy snorer, but apneas are not reported by her husband who does, however, describe his wife's abnormal behavior during sleep, with loud vocalization, fist clenching and violent lower and upper limb movements.

On examination, Mrs Dwyer is an overweight lady with dyskinetic movements of the head and upper limbs secondary to L-dopa treatment. Oropharyngeal examination is normal.

The initial diagnosis includes:
- delayed sleep phase syndrome
- REM-behavior disorder
- sleep fragmentation due to PD
- sleep fragmentation due to chronic hip pain
- possible sleep apnea.

A sleep study shows snoring but no evidence of disturbed breathing. Sleep efficiency is markedly reduced at 59% (normal value above 85%). There are no leg movements recorded but the patient is restless, thrashing around in bed. Multiple sleep latency test shows a mean sleep latency of 10.5 minutes (normal is above 10 minutes), with an Epworth sleepiness scale (ESS) of 23 out of 24, in keeping with severe subjective sleepiness.

The above combination of factors is explained to the patient and her husband. Mrs Dwyer is started on a more regular sleep schedule requiring a bedtime of 11.30PM and waking at 6.30AM. Computer activity is not permitted after 9.00PM. She is prescribed melatonin 3 mg to be taken at 9.00PM together with slow-release morphine to control her hip pain at 11.00PM. No changes are made to her anti-Parkinson medications.

Sleep quality improves with Mrs Dwyer sleeping 5–6 hours at night. Her husband reports that the abnormal movements have stopped. Mrs Dwyer wakes feeling more refreshed and her daytime sleepiness improves, although it is not completely alleviated. Stopping the melatonin 4 weeks after the initial treatment causes her sleep to deteriorate and 3 mg of melatonin is continued long term.

Case study 2 — *Severe daytime sleepiness, Parkinson's disease*

Mr Jacob Gardener is a 72-year-old man with an eleven-year history of moderately severe PD for which he takes L-dopa (Madopar™), both normal and slow-release formulations, as well as bromocriptine (Parlodel™) 10 mg three times daily. He had bowel cancer in 1982 but no other medical problems.

Mr Gardener was referred predominantly for investigation of severe daytime sleepiness as reported by his wife. He does not perceive that he has a problem and says he functions satisfactorily during the day. However, his wife says that he falls asleep while talking to her and even at the table while having breakfast. It is also common for him to fall asleep while reading the paper. Sleepiness of the degree described by his wife has been present for about 2 years. There are no symptoms suggestive of narcolepsy.

Mr Gardener goes to bed between midnight and 1.00AM with a short sleep latency. He sleeps undisturbed through the night with no awakening and has denied choking arousals. Snoring is only occasionally present and apneas have never been reported by the family. He gets up at 6.30AM usually feeling refreshed. As the day passes, he feels somewhat sleepier and tends to take a nap on purpose during the afternoon.

The diagnosis includes:
- delayed sleep phase syndrome
- sleep fragmentation due to PD and/or his medications
- hypersomnia associated with PD.

A sleep study shows snoring but no disturbed breathing. Oxygen saturation is well maintained throughout. There are no leg movements and only five arousals per hour. Sleep efficiency is 79% with a marked reduction of 8% of slow-wave sleep (normal is 20–24%) and reduction of 6% REM (normal value ~ 20%). A multiple sleep latency test performed the day after the sleep study shows pathological daytime sleepiness with a mean sleep latency of 1.6 minutes (normal is above 10 minutes). No REM sleep abnormality is noted.

The findings are explained to Mr Gardener and his wife and they are warned that driving is contraindicated given Mr Gardener's increased risk of having a motor vehicle accident. There is no evidence of a reversible cause for Mr Gardener's daytime sleepiness, except a somewhat curtailed amount of sleep given the delayed sleep onset at night. A trial of stimulant medication, dexamphetamine, starting with 5 mg twice daily at breakfast and midday is commenced, and this sees some improvement in his daytime sleepiness. However given the fact that Mr Gardener does not perceive that the sleepiness is interfering with his quality of life and he is happy to stop driving, the medication is stopped.

Sleep disturbances in PD are self-reported in approximately 75% of patients (Larson and Tandberg, 2001). The sleep of the PD patient's spouse is also significantly disrupted (48% of female spouses and 27% of male spouses) (Smith *et al*, 1997). Sleep disturbance in PD has a variety of presentations (*Table 9.3*), often with more than one component. Although there is a different mechanism leading to sleep disruption, the more severe the PD, the more disturbed the patient's sleep and daytime function. Progressive deterioration of sleep structure seems to be part of the degenerative process in Parkinson's disease (Diederich *et al*, 2005).

Difficulty initiating and maintaining sleep (insomnia) is probably the most frequent complaint (60% of patients) (Larson and Tandberg, 2001). Difficulty initiating and maintaining sleep can be related to severe tremor, L-dopa dyskinetic movements, direct alerting effect of the aminergic medications and depression. In more advanced PD, reversal of the sleep cycle may be associated with a highly fragmented night sleep and multiple sleep episodes through the day. Increased stiffness and akinesia can lead to added fragmentation of sleep. Although tremor tends to decrease in stage 1 and stage 3 and 4 sleep, it may increase during periods of arousals and during stage 2. Repetitive muscle contraction may occur during non-REM sleep (Garcia-Borreguero *et al*, 2003).

Dopaminergic medications, including L-dopa and other dopamine agonists, have multiple effects on sleep depending on the dose and time of administration. Doses that improve motility and stiffness are likely to have a beneficial effect on sleep continuity. However, high doses and administration late in the evening (eg. L-dopa night dose, selegiline after midday) can cause insomnia due to the alerting effect, increased fragmentation of sleep and alteration in sleep structure (eg. REM suppression). Paradoxically, dopaminergic agents can be associated with increased somnolence 30–60 minutes after administration (Rodnitzky, 2000) and acute sudden sleep episodes. After prolonged use of L-dopa, dyskinetic movements may be prominent enough to interfere with sleep onset. Hallucinations and vivid dreams are also associated with long term use of anti-Parkinson agents.

Table 9.3: Sleep disturbances in Parkinson's disease and Parkinsonian syndromes	
Clinical presentation	**Mechanisms**
Difficulty initiating sleep	Circadian rhythm sleep disorders (delayed or advanced sleep phase), alerting effect of L-dopa, dyskinesias
Difficulty maintaining sleep	Fragmentation of sleep due to PD stiffness, L-dopa, depression, restless leg, syndrome sleep apnea, low melatonin
Abnormal movements and violent behavior during sleep	REM sleep behavior disorder, L-dopa induced myoclonus, end-of-dose dyskinesias
Nocturnal cramp	Focal dystonia
Nightmares and hallucinations	Dopaminergic medications, disturbance of REM sleep mechanisms
Excessive daytime sleepiness	Fragmentation of sleep due to PD, restless leg syndrome, sleep apnea Direct effect of dopaminergic agents, eg. pramipexole, ropinirole, pergolide Degeneration of wakefulness-related systems

Abnormal movement during sleep are common in PD. REM sleep behavior disorder (RSBD), (*Chapter 6*) is related to degeneration of the pontine–medulla pathways, which stop the physiological muscle atonia that should occur during REM. As a result, the patients tend to act out their dreams often injuring themselves or the bed partner. This phenomena is reported in up to 21% of unselected PD patients. Other parasomnias, such as sleep terrors and sleep-walking often coexist (Comella *et al*, 1998).

Dystonic dyskinesias (leg cramps) in the form of painful plantar flexion of the foot and sometimes extension of the big toes can occur at the time of waking when the effect of L-dopa is wearing off. L-dopa-induced myoclonus and akathisia are also related to long-term use. In akathisia, the patient has a compulsive need to move which can interfere with sleep onset and maintenance of sleep (Linazasoro *et al*, 1993). Contrary to restless leg syndrome, also frequent in PD, there is no associated paraesthesia.

Symptoms of depression are common and are reported by 40–50% of PD (Larson and Tandberg, 2001) and need treatment in their own right.

Excessive daytime sleepiness is a common complaint reported in 15–50% of patients (Garcia-Borregnero *et al*, 2003). It has a multifactorial origin. In *Case studies 1* and *2*, significant delayed sleep onset was a contributing factor. Other circadian rhythm sleep disorders are also common in PD, including advanced sleep phase syndrome and reversal of the sleep and wake cycle. Fragmentation of sleep due to PD and anti-Parkinson medications can contribute to unrefreshed sleep and daytime sleepiness.

Obstructive and central sleep apneas are also said to be common in PD patients, even though they may be the reflection of changes associated with age rather than with PD *per se*. Acute sleep attacks have been reported in patients using dopamine agonists, pramipexole and ropinirole (Frucht *et al*, 1999), but also with other dopamine agonist compounds such as pergolide (Pal *et al*, 2001).

Management of sleep disturbance in Parkinson's disease

The same general rules of sleep hygiene apply to PD patients as to any other individual, but specific issues are important in this group of patients.

Optimization of anti-Parkinson therapy

As described above, L-dopa and dopa agonists have the potential to improve sleep by improving the mobility and hypokinesia but there is also the potential for disturbing sleep. Insufficient doses can be responsible for end-of-dose dystonia. Dose and time of medication need to be adjusted individually on a trial-and-error basis.

Abnormal movements during sleep (see *Case study 1*) are treated along the same lines as in a non-Parkinson patient. Periodic limb movement disorder (PLMD), and REM-sleep behavior disorder (RSBD) respond well to a small dose of benzodiazepine, such as clonazepam 0.5–1 mg, temazepam 10–20 mg, and slow-release opioids (see *Case study 1*).

Daytime sleepiness requires optimization of any potential cause of sleep fragmentation. The use of stimulant medications, such as dexamphetamine or methylphenidate can be tried (*Case study 2*), but the response is not usually as rewarding as in other hypersomnolent states (eg. narcolepsy). Modafinil may be a better choice as an alerting medication, given the lack of dopaminergic activity of this compound.

Vivid dreams and hallucinations, associated with increased dose of dopaminergic agents, can be controlled with a small dose of olanzapine (Zyprexa™) at a dose of 2.5–5 mg at night and rispiridone (Risperdal™) at 0.5–1 mg at night. Both these antipsychotic medications are less likely to impact on PD symptoms.

Depression requires management similar to that of non-PD patients. Concerns have been raised over the potential of SSRIs (eg. fluoxetine) to exacerbate PD motor symptoms in some patients. However, it is suggested (Larsen and Tandberg, 2001) that citolapram (Cipramil™) 20–40 mg in the morning, is safe in PD. The occurrence of serotonin syndrome (confusion, incoordination, fever, hyperreflexia, and diarrhea) has been reported with the concurrent use of selegiline and SSRIs, but it is a rare complication (Zesiewicz and Hauser, 2000).

The management of circadian rhythm sleep disorders (*Case studies 1* and *2*) follow the same principal as non-PD patients. Based on individual experiences, bright-light exposure in the morning and the use of melatonin are worthwhile strategies. The above therapeutic considerations apply to other neurodegenerative syndromes (*Table 9.4*), such as multiple system atrophy (MSA), progressive supranuclear palsy and vascular Parkinsonism.

Table 9.4: Sleep disturbance in degenerative neurological diseases

	Sleep architecture and EEG features	Respiration	Parasomnias
Parkinson's disease	30–50% awake	Obstructive sleep apnea (mild) more severe when dysautonomia	Hallucinations, vocalizations, PLMs, tremor, Fragmentary myoclonus, REM sleep behavior disorder
Olivopontocerebellar degeneration	10–30% awake Reduced or absent REM sleep Loss of REM/NREM differentiation	Obstructive and central sleep apnea, Stridor and irregular breathing Increased risk of sudden death	REM sleep behavior disorder
Huntington's disease	15–40% awake Low voltage EEG	Normal	Choreiform movements in stage 1–2 sleep
Progressive supranuclear palsy	30–70% awake Alpha during sleep Loss of EEG features of NREM sleep Reduced amounts of REM sleep	Normal	REM sleep behavior disorder (occasional)
Alzheimer's disease	20–70% awake Reduced amounts of REM sleep	Probably some increase In obstructive sleep apnea. Usually mild	Sundowning 20% or more Nocturnal wandering
Fatal familial insomnia	80–100% awake Loss of EEG features of NREM sleep		REM sleep behavior disorder

(Aldrich, 1993)

Case study 3 — dementia, Alzheimer's disease

Barry McEwan is a 65-year-old man with a diagnosis of dementia, with moderate to severe cognitive impairment. He was referred by his neurologist because of a history of snoring and apnea reported by the family. The patient does not perceive he has any problems and his wife and children initiated the referral.

Mr McEwan had a coronary artery bypass graft 2 years ago and his daytime functioning appears to have deteriorated markedly since the surgery. He is able to look after himself for the activities of daily living but his memory has deteriorated. He can become confused in place and time and he is agitated and restless at night. The question as to whether sleep apnea is a contributing factor to his cognitive impairment and night-time disturbance has been raised.

An overnight sleep study shows poor sleep quality with no slow-wave sleep (stages 3 and 4), intermittent snoring and apnea/hypopnea (disturbed breathing) of 25 times per hour, with fifteen arousals per hour (normal is less than ten). He also has seven leg movements per hour but only one associated with arousal. Oxygen saturation was maintained above 90% all through the recording.

A diagnosis of mild sleep apnea and dementia (Alzheimer's disease), is made. The findings are discussed with Mr McEwan and his wife. It is pointed out that the condition is mild and may not be the reason for his disturbed sleep or for his cognitive impairment. However, a trial of nasal continuuous positive airways pressure (CPAP) is undertaken. During the titration night the disturbed breathing is abolished but sleep quality does not improve. A trial at home is unsuccessful as the patient becomes agitated and his sleep is more disturbed than before. A second trial is undertaken a few weeks later after further education on the use of nasal CPAP, but is again unsuccessful.

With the world population aging in numbers greater than any other time in history, there is an increase in the number of elderly with dementia. Alzheimer's dementia is the most common type with others including frontal lobe dementia, vascular dementia and other neurodegenerative syndromes. Sleep and wake function disturbance is common in Alzheimer's disease with a prevalence estimated between 29% and 45% (McCurry *et al*, 2000; Vitiello and Borson, 2001). The disruption of sleep and wake is proportional to functional derangement in terms of cognitive deficit, as well as the ability to manage daily living tasks, even though a U-shaped distribution has been described, with a higher prevalence in moderate Alzheimer's disease than in mild or severe disease.

Dementia syndromes involve not only the sufferer, but also the caregivers whose sleep may be affected. When considering management, an important issue to clarify (McCurry *et al*, 2000) is how much of the treatment is for the benefit of the patient and how much is for the benefit, and sometimes the convenience, of the caregivers, be it the family or the health workers.

The pathophysiology of sleep and wake derangement in dementia is multifactorial (*Table 9.5* and *Figure 9.1*) and the management should, in response, be multimodal. It involves intervention during the day as well as at bedtime and night-time. Therefore, the debate which often focuses on the use of pharmacological agents, eg. which medication should or should not be used is, in reality, a non-issue. Medications are a useful adjunct to management (see below), but are insufficient on their own. Their use in isolation may be more harmful than beneficial.

Table 9.5: Factors responsible for sleep-wake disturbances in dementia
• Increased fragmentation of sleep and decreased slow-wave sleep similar to, but more severe than changes associated with healthy elderly
• Neuron loss associated with neurodegeneration of dementia (mostly cholinergic and adrenergic neurons)
• Degeneration of the suprachiasmatic nuclei and hypothalamic pathways (prominent in Alzheimer's disease)
• Depression
• Associated medical conditions
• Medications (often polypharmacy)
• Sundowning
• Poor environmental conditions (particularly nursing homes)

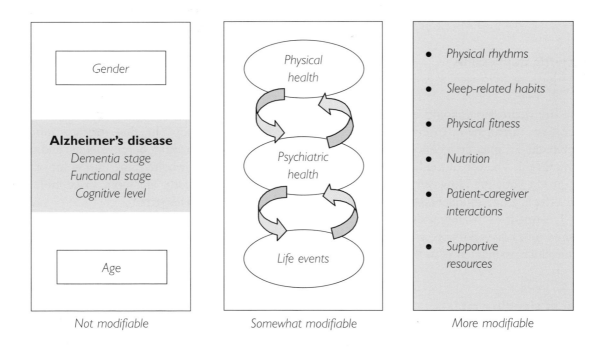

Figure 9.1: Factors contributing to sleep disturbances in Alzheimer's disease (McCurry et al, 2000).

Environmental factor modification

Due to poor mobility and an increased dependence on others for daily care, many of the environmental clues which synchronize the body's functions become weak in dementia patients. Light exposure is often reduced or even absent, especially in institutionalized care facilities (Alessi and Schnelle, 2000; Shochat *et al*, 2000). Meal times can be irregular, and exercise and physical activity is reduced for safety reasons, or because of concurrent medical problems. Social interactions are diminished because of social isolation or the severity of cognitive impairment.

There is evidence that when patients with dementia can engage in daytime activities such as exposure to light, physical activity, regular routine and social interaction, night-time sleep is improved in terms of continuity and quality, when examined objectively (by actigraphy) or as reported by the caregiver (McCurry *et al*, 2000; Alessi and Schnelle, 2000).

Management of medical and psychiatric comorbidity

In the dementia age group, other medical problems are prevalent and can be contributing factors to poor day and night function and daytime disruption. Ischemic heart disease, left ventricular failure from any cause, asthma, gastroesophageal reflux and chronic painful rheumatological conditions, nocturia due to prostatism or diuretic treatment should all be looked at when a dementia patient has sleep disorders, as these are conditions which can be improved.

Late-life depression

Late-life depression should always be considered in this age group, because it can exacerbate cognitive impairment (pseudo-dementia), as well as affect sleep. In this setting, family circumstances may be a contributing factor to depression (social isolation, bereavement) and can be modified. The use of medication for treatment of depression follows the same line as for other age group patients. However, it should be remembered that the elderly are more susceptible to side-effects from antidepressants, both of the tricyclic type as well as SSRIs.

Treatment of Alzheimer's disease with cholinergic agents (eg. donepezil and rivastigmine, galantamine) does not appear to improve sleep. However, there is no evidence of significant sleep disturbance associated with this treatment.

Use of sleeping tablets

The use of hypnotics such as benzodiazepines or even non-benzodiazepine hypnotics (zolpidem, zoplicone and zaleplon) are best avoided. They are often unhelpful and may add to confusion and the risk of night-time injury in this group of patients.

Sundowning and nocturnal agitation

Sundowning is a syndrome seen in patients with moderate to severe dementia and is characterized by agitated behavior in the evening, between 7.00PM and 10.00PM. The patient may appear restless, fearful, angry and confused (Morley, 1993). It has been suggested that post-prandial hypotension, concomitant chronic obstructive airway disease with oxygen level fluctuation following a large meal and large fluctuation in glucose levels following a meal rich in carbohydrates are associated with sundowning (Morley, 1993). Attention to these factors can reduce the occurrence of nocturnal agitated behavior which can spill over from the evening into the night-time or may occur only during the sleep period.

Other factors such as sensory deprivation, both visual and auditory due to sensory deficit, poor environmental setting (poorly lit environment), and intermittent febrile illnesses can trigger sundowning. This is particularly evident in patients who are hospitalized.

Management of nocturnal agitation includes attention to any modifiable factors and at times, pharmacological treatment. These include:

- minimizing sensory deprivation by the use of a dimmed night light as well as reassurance from hospital or nursing home staff
- light exposure during the day and physical activity when possible
- adapting bedtime to the patient's needs rather than for the convenience of others. In particular, nursing homes and hospitals should avoid enforcing unrealistic bed times (7.00PM–8.00PM) and expecting the patient to stay in bed until 6.00AM–7.00AM
- relief of physical discomfort due to painful conditions.

Physical restraint to avoid nocturnal wandering is not acceptable and adds to the patient's agitation.

If conservative approaches fail, the use of medication may be necessary. A small dose of pericyazine (Neulactil™) 2.5–5mg, olanzapine (Zyprexa™) 5mg or rispiridone (Respirdel™) 1mg may reduce agitated behavior. These new, atypical anti-psychotic agents should be the first line of choice as their use is less likely to disrupt the circadian rest–activity cycle (Wirz-Justice *et al*, 2000). However, it cannot be emphasized enough that the use of medications as a form of 'pharmacological restraint' is not appropriate.

Management of specific sleep disturbances

Obstructive sleep apnea, with its associated hypoxemia and fragmentation of sleep, is often blamed for worsening dementia (*Case study 3*). Patients with dementia have a higher number of apneas and hypopneas than aged-matched controls; female more than male (Mant *et al*, 1988; Pond *et al*, 1990). This is a difficult problem because the current criteria for the diagnosis of obstructive sleep apnea (apnea/hypopnea index more than five per hour) are based on a younger population (less than 60 years of age), and criteria for clinical significance in the elderly is not established (*Chapter 4*). Although the presence of unequivocal severe obstructive sleep apnea (eg. apnea/hypopnea more than thirty events per hour with oxygen desaturation) is likely to affect cognitive function and aggravate dementia, a low level of apnea/hypopnoea index (less than thirty events per hour), particularly in the absence of hypoxemia, is of questionable relevance and probably not significant (*Case study 3*). Attempted treatment with nasal CPAP often results in failure and may add to the distress of the patient, disturbed sleep and agitation.

Other sleep-related conditions, such as periodic limb movement disorder, restless leg syndrome and REM sleep behavior disorder, are also common in dementia and are treated as in any other patient if it is clinically significant. The medications of choice are short-acting benzodiazepines or opioids (*Chapter 6*).

In patients who are lethargic and apathetic during the day, the use of stimulant medication (eg. methylphenidate) has been reported to improve daytime alertness and sleep quality (Kittur and Hauser, 1999).

Low melatonin syndrome

The circadian rhythm of melatonin is maintained in the elderly but the amplitude is reduced. A further reduction in melatonin level is seen in patients with Alzheimer's disease when compared to age controls. This is in keeping with the notion that circadian rhythms decline with age.

Allowing for the methodological problems inherent in studying biological rhythms in dementia patients (Bliwise, 1997), the decline in the neuron population in the suprachiasmatic nuclei (SCN) in dementia patients seems to support the idea that some of the sleep–wake abnormalities seen in Alzheimer's disease could benefit from chronobiotic agents, such as melatonin.

Anecdotal reports suggest that melatonin 3–9 mg at bedtime improves sleep quality and continuity (McCurry and Arendt, 2000).

Sleep and stroke

Case study 4

Mr Michael Conrad is a 71-year-old man with a history of polymyalgia rheumatica for which he takes 12.5 mg of prednisone, and hypertension which is treated with a calcium-channel blocker and diuretic. He has been referred for investigation of snoring and daytime sleepiness on a background of a brainstem infarct 4 months previously. He has had a good functional recovery and he is living independently with his wife.

Mr Conrad's family feels his snoring and apnea have become more obvious since the stroke. However, while on prednisone over a period of 6 months he has put on about 9 kg in weight. He feels tired on awakening and he becomes sleepy during the day.

Overnight polysomnography reveals a sleep efficiency of 75% with severe sleep apnea (85 apneas/

hypopneas per hour), and an oxygen saturation below 90% for 95% of the time and 50% for below 80% of the time. Mr Gardener is started on nasal CPAP with marked improvement in his daytime level of energy and improved sleep quality.

Case study 5

Mr Peter Mercurio is a 50-year-old retired truck driver referred because of daytime fatigue and sleepiness, on a background of snoring and multiple infarcts involving the pons and right temporal lobe 4 months ago. He has made a very slow recovery needing assistance for walking as well as prolonged difficulty with swallowing. He has a background history of maturity onset diabetes, hypothyroidism, and depression.

Due to his occupation as a truck driver he was seen and studied with a polysomnography 4 years before this presentation. At the time, he was found to be a snorer but sleep apnea was not present.

Overnight polysomnography is performed which shows sleep efficiency of 88% with absent slow-wave sleep and 20% stage REM. There is minimal snoring and no disturbed breathing. Oxygen is maintained around 90% through the recording. A multiple sleep latency test is performed during the day which shows a mean sleep latency of 17.3 minutes (normal > 10 minutes).

As in the examination 4 years previously, Mr Mercurio shows no evidence of sleep apnea. His limited function and daytime tiredness are more likely to be related to the significant functional impairment due to the embolic stroke, his diabetes, and possibly depression.

These two cases highlight the complexity of the potential relationship between obstructive sleep apnea and cerebrovascular events. In both cases there are significant risk factors for stroke including diabetes, hypertension and obesity.

In the first case, although the family perceived the relationship between the stroke and the increase in snoring and apnea, a strong case could be made for the increase of 9 kg in weight as being a stronger risk factor and one which occurred at the same time as the cerebrovascular event. In the second case, there was significant functional impairment but no evidence of disturbed breathing.

The occurrence of stroke follows a circadian incidence pattern with the peak in the morning between 6.00AM and 10.00AM (Elliot, 2001) with around 18% of strokes occurring during sleep (Bornstein *et al*, 1999). During the acute phase of a stroke and the recovery period, which can last months, sleep disturbances are frequent (*Table 9.6*).

Studies of patients with acute cerebrovascular events are difficult to undertake, but the available evidence suggests that derangement in sleep and wake function is proportional to the neurological deficit and the location of the lesion. Thalamic and subcortical stroke can be associated with significant daytime sleepiness, sometimes with no significant derangement in nocturnal sleep structure, presumably due to damage to the arousal system. Brainstem vascular lesions, given the close association with the autonomic nervous system, in particular respiratory control, are often associated with disturbed REM and slow-wave sleep regulation (Landau *et al*, 2005).

An unusual, although possibly under-recognized syndrome is Ondine's curse: primary failure of automatic respiration. In this condition, which has been described in both bilateral as well as unilateral brainstem lesions, there is failure of the autonomic drive to breathe, whereby the person can breathe on command but becomes apneic during sleep (Kuhn *et al*, 1999; Severinghaus and Mitchell, 1962). Similar presentation occurs not only in vascular lesions of the brainstem, but also in the presence of trauma and tumors in the brainstem region.

Disturbed breathing during sleep is common and can present with either central

Table 9.6: Sleep disturbances following stroke
• Decrease in REM sleep
• Reduction in slow-wave sleep (stages 3 and 4)
• Reduction in slow-wave sleep — REM sleep cycles
• Respiratory disturbances (central and obstructive sleep apnea)
• Depression
• Daytime sleepiness

apnea (periodic breathing of Cheyne–Stokes pattern) or obstructive sleep apnea. The relationship between sleep apnea and stroke is bidirectional and still to be clearly defined (*Chapter 5*). As for patients with dementia, the issue is confounded by the lack of a clinically meaningful definition of sleep apnea. This is particularly relevant given the fact that a disturbed breathing of 15–20 events/hour is frequently found in healthy, asymptomatic elderly subjects (*Chapter 5, Figure 5.13*).

For the clinician there are two practical questions:

1. Should elderly patients with sleep apnea be treated (and how) to prevent cerebrovascular accident? More precisely, what clinical and polysomnographic features of disturbed breathing (eg. number of apneas/hypopneas per hour, oxygen desaturation), identify patients who would need treatment.
2. After a stroke, does a patient with disturbed breathing need treatment (and how)? As above, the issue is one of defining a combination of clinical and polysomnographic parameters associated with worse post-stroke outcome and demonstrating that treatment improves prognosis and quality of life.

So far, there is no answer to either of these questions.

It seems reasonable that sleep apnea syndrome, if present post-stroke, should be treated along the same lines as in non-stroke patients (*Chapter 5*). In the first days after a stroke, assisted ventilation may need to be considered if there is evidence of respiratory failure (hypoxemia with or without hypercapnia).

Headache and sleep

Case study 6

Mr Ernest Christie is a 57-year-old retired power station operator, non-smoker, occasional drinker on a calcium-channel blocker for hypertension, who presents with recurrent nocturnal headache which wakes him through the night.

He described a 10-year history of recurrent (three to four times/week) headache which wakes him between 2.00AM and 3.00AM lasting between 30 and 60 minutes. The headache is dull, not throbbing, not associated with nausea or vomiting or with lacrimation. There is no history of migraine in the patient or in the family. He did not appear anxious or depressed. He has a history of snoring but apneas are not reported by his wife.

Overnight polysomnography shows a sleep efficiency of 88% and reduction in REM sleep. No headache occurs during the night's recording.

The diagnosis includes:
- hypnic headache
- tension headache (less likely).

Case study 7

Mrs Emily Miller is a 51-year-old retired public servant presenting with severe, sudden shock-like headache. She has a background of gastroesophageal reflux, hypertension, fibromyalgia, depression and anxiety. She is a non-smoker, occasional drinker. Her only medications at the time of presentation include hormone replacement and antacids.

Mrs Miller describes a sensation like an electrical shock going through her head, a 'buzzing and zapping' lasting a few seconds at the time of falling asleep. This occurs once or twice per week. Each episode is followed by an overwhelming need to fall asleep. Sleep lasts from thirty minutes to 3 hours. She wakes feeling 'washed out'.

She has attended the local casualty department but, by the time she was seen, no abnormalities were found. The CT of the head was normal.

On examination, she presents with a three-page spreadsheet detailing a medical history including doctor encounters at the age of 8. The past history is relevant for recurrent episodes of depression and anxiety associated with work and family stresses. She has fibromyalgia symptoms and daytime tiredness.

An overnight polysomnography shows a sleep efficiency of 75% with reduction in REM sleep, no disturbed breathing and alpha intrusion in < 10% of slow-wave sleep. Multiple sleep latency test shows a mean sleep latency of 17 minutes (normal value > 10).

Patients with nocturnal headache and headache on waking are often referred to sleep clinics for evaluation of possible sleep apnea, because a dull frontal headache is reported as one of the symptoms typical of obstructive sleep apnea syndrome. However, in the general population self-reported headache is more common in patients without disturbed breathing than in patients with evidence of sleep apnea (Olson *et al*, 1995).

In a sleep clinic setting, headache is uncommon even in patients with severe hypoxemia. The dull, frontal headache associated with obstructive sleep apnea, when present, is related to hypercapnia and is resolved within 30–60 minutes of awakening.

The association between headache and sleep is well established but complex (*Table 9.7*). The neural pathways putatively involved in migraine, serotonergic and noradrenergic pathways are also intimately linked with wake and sleep function. Often, migraine ends up with episodes of sleep which release the migraine, but the migraine is also known to be triggered during sleep particularly during REM sleep (Culebras, 2000; Mathew, 1992).

Table 9.7: Headache and sleep

Time of onset	Type	Comment
Only during sleep	Hypnic headache	Usually bilateral headache, waking the patient at approximately the same time each night
	Exploding head syndrome	Very brief, usually when falling asleep or during brief arousals
Day and night	Migraine (common) Cluster headache Paroxysmal hemicrania (REM sleep lock headache)	Usually or exclusively unilateral headache Associated with aura and autonomic symptoms (lacrimation, face flushing, nausea, vomiting)
On awakening	Obstructive sleep apnea Bruxism Tension headache (psychogenic) Poorly controlled hypertension Depression Alcohol abuse	Specific history and/or physical findings should suggest the diagnosis

NB: More than one type of headache may be present

Cluster headache and paroxysmal hemicrania are common at night. Both forms of migraine are characterized by episodes of unilateral, peri-orbital–temporal, frontal headache, associated with autonomic activations, such as lacrimation (epiphora), nasal congestion, injection of the conjunctiva and a sensation of flushing in the face. However contrary to migraine, aura is not present. Cluster headaches occur in multiple episodes (two to three a day on average) lasting 1–2 hours, occurring through the day as well as at night (in cluster headache, 75% of the episodes occur at night). The cluster periods last 2–3 months at a time (Sahota and Dexter, 1993). It is more common in men between the ages of 20 and 50 years, heavy smokers and often in those with increased alcohol intake.

Paroxysmal hemicrania has a similar presentation with unilateral headache which, however, is more severe, lasting 5–10 minutes, but recurring five to twenty times per day (Kayed *et al*, 1978). It is more common in women than men. Paroxysmal hemicrania characteristically responds to indomethacin 25–50 mg at night.

Cluster headache responds to inhalation of a high concentration of oxygen in the acute phase, which is feasible in hospital, but impractical as an outpatient. The episode of cluster headache can be aborted by the use of methysergide (Deseril™) 6–8 mg daily, ergotamine derivative either orally or parenterally, prednisone 25–50 mg daily, sumatriptan 50 mg orally or 10–20 mg by nasal spray.

Case studies 6 and *7* are examples of two conditions, which are neither common nor widely reported: hypnic headache and exploding head syndrome. They are both characterized by occurring exclusively during sleep.

Hypnic headache is more commonly reported in people over 50 years, even though cases in the younger population are described. It is thought to be more common in women (Dodick *et al*, 1998; Dodick 2000). The headache is usually bilateral (contrary to the unilateral pain in cluster migraine and paroxysmal hemicrania) and autonomic activation symptoms are not present. Because it seems to occur at a particular time of the night in each individual it is also referred to as 'alarm clock' headache. When polysomnography documentation is available it seems that it is triggered during REM sleep. In the elderly, other organic pathology needs to be considered and excluded by appropriate investigation (eg. head CT scan). Spontaneous remissions do occur, but when treatment is needed, hypnic headache seems to respond to the use of lithium 250–500 mg at night, indomethacin 25 mg at night (Ivafiez *et al*, 1998). Melatonin 3 mg at night has also been effective in some patients as well as the use of coffee, such as one to two cups of coffee before going to bed.

Exploding head syndrome, as in *Case study 7*, is an uncommon, benign condition which is usually self-limiting. When polysomnography documentation is available, the attacks occur during periods of arousals or when the patient is in a relaxed, drowsy state. No epileptic activity is documented. It is described as a sudden, brief (seconds) abnormal sensations of banging, lightening, electric shock, and zapping, rather than as pain (Pearce, 1989; Sachs and Svanborg, 1991). It can occur once or more through the night and persists for weeks. There is a firm association with a fairly anxious personality and it often occurs during periods of stress at work or in the family. The condition's dramatic nature leads to significant concern and sleep disturbance.

Investigations to exclude more sinister pathology, such as subarachnoid hemorrhage or brain tumour, by CT or MRI of the head, are normal. Management may simply be by reassurance of the benign nature of the episodes but when treatment is needed, clomipramine (Anafranil™) 50 mg at night has been reported to be effective (Sachs and Svanborg, 1991).

When headache is symptomatic of other sleep disorders, such as obstructive sleep apnea or bruxism, specific treatment needs to be undertaken.

Sleep and multiple sclerosis

Case study 8

Mrs Lucy Chandler is a 46-year-old woman with a history of chronic tiredness on a background of multiple sclerosis (MS). She does not smoke or drink. She was diagnosed with MS 2 years prior to this referral, even though symptoms were present for a few years prior to the final diagnosis. She had been taking beta-interferon, but ceased this because of side-effects and now she is on glatiramer (Copaxone™).

She describes her fatigue as a combination of lack of energy and sleepiness. This has been continuous, of subacute onset, and present for the last 2–3 years. She has two children aged 8 and 11, works part-time as a clerk, and attends university six hours/week, usually in the evening.

Mrs Chandler goes to bed between 8.00PM and 9.30PM, falling asleep within 5 minutes. Snoring is not reported by her husband. There is no history of leg movement. She wakes at 7.00AM feeling unrefreshed. She sleeps in the afternoon for a couple of hours, but not every day, and feels refreshed after the nap. She has no REM-related symptoms (hypnagogic hallucinations, sleep paralysis or cataplexy). A sleep diary kept for a week seems to confirm her sleep history.

On examination she is an overweight lady with a body mass index (BMI) of 30, with normal cardiorespiratory findings including normal oropharyngeal exam. She does not appear to be anxious or depressed. Polysomnography shows loud snoring with no disturbed breathing. Sleep stages and sleep structure are within normal limits. Arousals were six per hour (normal value up to 10). A multiple sleep latency test shows a mean sleep latency of 6.3 minutes (normal value > ten minutes) in keeping with severe daytime sleepiness, but no early onset REM sleep (usually found in narcolepsy). Thyroid function tests had been done in the past and were normal.

The diagnosis includes:
- hypersomnolence and fatigue associated with multiple sclerosis (MS)
- insufficient sleep syndrome.

In a person with a part-time job, studying commitments, and looking after two young children, the possibility of insufficient resting time should always be considered. With Mrs Chandler, this possibility does not seem to be a major contributing factor. Given the significant daytime sleepiness documented on MSLT, which is likely to be contributing to her tiredness, treatment with stimulant medication, dexamphetamine or modafinil, is offered and discussed with the patient. However she feels that the tiredness is not significant enough to interfere with her activity and pharmacological treatment is not undertaken.

Chronic tiredness, both in terms of lack of energy and increased sleepiness are common symptoms in MS patients. Similarly sleep disturbances with difficulty initiating and maintaining sleep are commonly reported (Culebras, 2000; Saunders *et al*, 1991; Taphoorn *et al*, 1993). The origin of sleep disturbances in an MS patient is multifactorial, including:

- disability and functional status (bladder problems, muscle spasms, chronic muscular skeletal pain)
- hypersomnolence (narcoleptic-like) or secondary to other sleep disturbances, such as periodic limb movement disorder, obstructive sleep apnea, delayed sleep phase syndrome
- depression.

Depending on the extent and location of the demyelinating process, sleep and wake disturbances can have a variable presentation. Cases indistinguishable from narcolepsy (secondary narcolepsy or symptomatic narcolepsy, see *Chapter 8*) have been reported in MS patients (Schrader *et al*, 1980). Cataplexy (episodes of partial or complete loss of muscle power) can occur in multiple sclerosis and could be the underlying mechanism for symptoms such as knee weakness, unexpected falls, slurring of speech and blurring of vision. Similar to narcolepsy, the symptoms can be exacerbated by stress or emotions. The use of anti-cataplectic agents, such as SSRIs, could be beneficial (Sandyk, 1995).

Patients with MS can have disturbed breathing, including Ondine's curse (Auer *et al*, 1996), characterized by an inability to breathe while asleep due to failure of the automatic regulation of breathing, restless leg syndrome and periodic limb movement disorder (Yokota *et al*, 1991). Proper investigation of sleep disorders, including polysomnography, should be undertaken in MS patients who are symptomatic of sleep and wake disturbances because treatment can be undertaken to alleviate these conditions (Poirier *et al*, 1987).

Sleep and myotonic muscular dystrophy

Case study 9

Mr Andrew Williams is a 40-year-old male, with known myotonic dystrophy, referred for investigation of snoring, apnea and daytime sleepiness, reported by his wife over a period of 7 years. He is one of three members of his family with myotonic dystrophy, he is employed as a clerk in a government agency, a non-smoker and occasional drinker. His only medication is a statin for hypercholesterolemia.

His bedtime is between 10.00PM and 11.00PM with a sleep latency of 30 minutes. He denies waking through the night. According to his wife, he would snore in all body positions and she reported apnea. He wakes at 7.00AM feeling unrefreshed and takes a nap in the afternoon if not busy. He becomes drowsy while talking to people.

On examination, he appears to be quite apathetic, almost disinterested in the investigation. He has typical facial features of myotonic dystrophy (elongated face with nasal speech and frontal baldness) and high-arched palate with soft palate slightly edematous and inflamed.

Mr Williams' respiratory function shows restrictive lung disease with 50% reduction in maximal inspiratory and maximal expiratory pressures, in keeping with respiratory muscle weakness (predominantly diaphragm muscle). He has no symptoms of heart failure but an echocardiogram shows hypertrophy of the myocardium with normal function. There is no evidence of arrhythmia on ECG.

An overnight polysomnography (*Figure 9.2*) shows evidence of severe sleep apnea, with marked hypoxemia during REM sleep, even though the average apnea/hypopnea index is thirteen events per hour. An MSLT shows daytime sleepiness with a mean sleep latency of 7 minutes and three out of four naps with early onset REM. Nasal CPAP is undertaken but the patient does not find it useful and does not continue with treatment. The patient perceives that he has no problem and is not willing to consider any intervention.

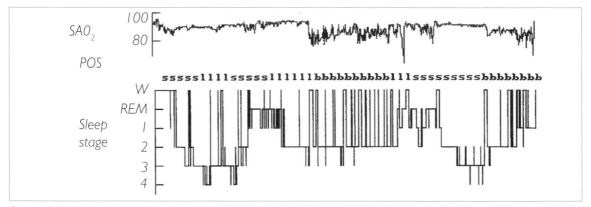

Figure 9.2: Severe sleep apnoea, with marked oxygen desaturation during REM-sleep, in a 41-year-old patient with myotonic dystrophy. Sleep stages: W = wake; REM = rapid eye movement sleep; S1 = stage 1 sleep; S2 = stage 2 sleep; S3 = stage 3 sleep; S4 = stage 4 sleep; MT = movement time; SaO_2 = oxygen saturation; POS = sleeping position: s = supine, l = left side.

Mr Williams is followed-up yearly and about 5 years later a bi-level CPAP trial is undertaken. This is better tolerated even though daytime sleepiness continues despite improvement in apnea/ hypopnea. He is given methylphenidate up to three tablets per day to improve excessive daytime sleepiness. Mr Williams however, remains poorly compliant until about 5 years after the initial presentation, when he is unable to hold his job due to significant muscle weakness, particularly in the upper limbs. He remains on nasal bi-level CPAP.

Central to neuromuscular disorders and sleep is the development of disturbed breathing, particularly during REM sleep, when hypotonia (loss of muscle power) compounds the already weakened muscles. Hypoxemia and hypercarbia result from hypoventilation due to muscle weakness (particularly the diaphragm), from central and obstructive sleep apnea. Myotonic dystrophy patients are of particular interest because on top of the respiratory disturbance, like other neuromuscular disorders, they often have an increased sleepiness tendency with narcoleptic-type features. These patients, as in narcolepsy, benefit from treatment with stimulant medications (Coccagna *et al*, 1975; Van der Meche *et al*, 1986).

Myotonic muscular dystrophy is a genetic autosomal dominant disease, which affects skeletal muscles and other systems including the cardiac, endocrine and central nervous systems. Hypersomnia often persists despite ventilatory assistance with nasal CPAP or bi-level CPAP, and requires stimulant treatment as described in *Case study 9*. However, in practice, treatment can be difficult because of cognitive decline in myotonic dystrophy patients who often appear apathetic and disinterested in their condition, making treatment compliance difficult to achieve.

Neuropathological examination in patients with myotonic dystrophy has shown an area of degeneration in the lateral thalamus, which may be one of the reasons for their increased sleepiness. Polysomnography examination often reveals fragmentation of sleep, including early onset REM, both in overnight polysomnography and the multiple sleep latency test during the day, with a pattern similar to narcolepsy.

Other neuromuscular conditions, such as post-polio syndrome, *myasthenia gravis* and motor neuron disease also present with derangement of sleep structure usually associated with respiratory failure.

Psychiatric and other medical conditions

Sleep and schizophrenia

Case study 10

Mr Tim Paxton is 26 years old with a history of developmental disability and schizophrenia, for which he takes olanzapine (Zyprexa™) 10 mg at night, fluvoxamine (Luvox™) 50 mg in the morning and pericyazine (Neulactil™) 10 mg at night. He is a competitive swimmer and goes to bed between 7.00PM–8.00PM rising at 8.00AM. However, if he is training he gets up at 4.00AM and trains until 7.30AM, naps in the afternoon and then trains again in the late afternoon.

Tim is a known snorer and apneas have been reported by his family. He describes a choking sensation, occurring just as he is falling asleep, associated with dry mouth, but it is felt that this is more likely to be due to his current medications. On examination he is a quiet, shy young man who lets his mother answer most of the questions. Physical examination is unremarkable, but for his nose which is partially blocked bilaterally, but his pharynx is of normal size and not inflamed. The diagnosis to be considered to explain his presentation with tiredness would include the following:

- irregular sleep and wake pattern
- schizophrenia
- effect of medications on sleep structure
- obstructive sleep apnea, even though clinically this is less likely.

Tim undergoes a sleep study (*Figure 9.3, bottom part*) which shows high sleep efficiency of 95% with only three apnea/hypopneas per hour (normal is up to five events per hour). There is marked reduction in slow-wave sleep but no other abnormalities and mild to moderate snoring.

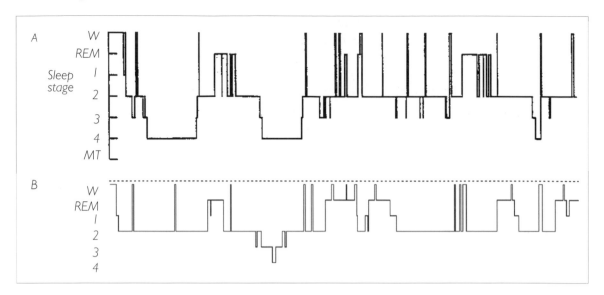

Figure 9.3: Panel B: minimal amount of stage 3 & 4 , normal oxygen saturation in the patient described above. Panel A: Example of 'normal' sleep stage distribution. Sleep stage: W = wake; REM = rapid eye movement sleep; S1 = stage 1 sleep; S2 = stage 2 sleep; S3 = stage 3 sleep; S4 = stage 4 sleep; MT = movement time.

In patients with schizophrenia, the presence of positive psychotic symptoms of hallucinations and delusions, with similarities to dreaming state and to narcolepsy, led to the hypothesis that derangement of the REM-system has a role in its pathogenesis (Douglass *et al*, 1991). Studies in patients with schizophrenia free of medication, suggest a pattern characterized by decrease in stage 4 and decreased latency to onset of REM sleep even though the total amount of REM sleep is not increased (*Table 9.8*) (Feinberg and Hiott, 1978; Keshavan and Tandon, 1993).

REM sleep changes are thought to be related to hyperactivity of the pontine tegmental cholinergic system, peduncular pontine tegmental nuclei (PPT) and lateral dorsal tegmental nuclei (LDT), which increase dopaminergic neurons in the thalamic area (see *Chapter 1* for the anatomy). The clinical observation that anticholinergic agents (atropine, scopolamine) can induce visual tactile and auditory hallucinations together with confusion and disruption of thinking (antimuscarinic psychosis) seems to support this theory. It is hypothesized that the anticholinergic agents act on the autoreceptors in the mesopontine area (autoreceptors usually have an autoinhibitory action on the cells), therefore increasing cholinergic drive by reducing self-inhibition (Yeomans 1995). Treatment with antipsychotic improves sleep parameters (*Table 9.8*).

The new antipsychotics rispiridone and olanzapine seem to have a better profile than the more traditional antipsychotic agents (chlorpromazine, pericyazine, fluphenazine and haloperidol) (Dursum *et al*, 1999; Maixner *et al*, 1998; Salin-Pascual *et al*, 1999). It is also suggested that melatonin (2 mg slow-release) improves sleep efficiency in some patients with schizophrenia (Shamir *et al*, 2000).

Treatment of schizophrenia can be complicated by circadian rhythm sleep disorders. The patient in *Case study 10* was on fluvoxamine, which has been reported to be associated with delayed sleep phase syndrome (Dagan, 2002). Similarly, haloperidol may cause significant disruption of the sleep and wake cycle (Wirz-Justice *et al*, 1997).

Table 9.8: Sleep changes in patients with schizophrenia	
Sleep changes in schizophrenia	**Comments**
Reduced slow-wave sleep, stage 4	Consistent finding
Reduced REM-sleep onset latency	Observed, but not in all subjects
Impaired sleep continuity	Possibly confounded by coexisting psychiatric morbidity, eg. depression
The total amount of REM sleep as a percentage of total sleep is not increased	A finding which weakens REM sleep theory of schizophrenia
Sleep continuity and slow-wave sleep improved by medications	Olanzapine, rispiridone, clozapine and melatonin

Circadian rhythm sleep disorders associated with SSRI and antipsychotic medications are important as they can lead to increased sleep fragmentation, a side-effect which has only recently been reported and is little known.

Reduced REM sleep latency, reduction in stage 4 and fragmentation of sleep are not exclusive to schizophrenia. These changes in the macrostructure of sleep are described in other psychiatric syndromes, specifically depression and anxiety disorders. Major depression disorders have received the most attention. In particular, the role of REM sleep in the pathogenesis of major depression and its role as a prognostic parameter and as an index of response to therapy has been subject to debate (*Table 9.9*).

However, not all patients with depression seem to show sleep abnormalities and, it has been argued, that some of the changes may be confounded by age (REM onset latency and slow-wave sleep decrease with age), gender (slow-wave sleep is reduced in males) severity of depression (the more symptomatic the greater the disruption) (Armitage and Hoffman, 2001; Berger and Rieman, 1993). The fact that antidepressants and electric convulsive therapy (ECT) suppress REM sleep would support its pathogenic role in depression, except that some antidepressants, trimipramine, trazodone and nefazodone, as well as psychotherapy, do not suppress REM significantly but they are still effective treatments.

Other agents used in depressive illness treatment, such as carbamazepine, lithium and epilim, have minimal impact on REM sleep and tend to increase slow-wave sleep.

Sleep and post-traumatic stress disorder (PTSD)

Case study 11

George Lidwinski is a 49-year-old man, a leading hand in a coal mine who is referred for assessment of daytime sleepiness/fatigue, mood changes and aggressive behavior. He is on testosterone replacement because of hypogonadism but takes no other medication. He has a history of heartburn. He is a non-smoker and admits drinking up to a bottle of scotch per week, usually over a period of 2–3 days. He describes tiredness going back to the Vietnam War years, some 25 years prior to this presentation, when he was engaged as a marine engineer on a landing craft transporting damaged goods.

Mr Lidwinski complains of poor sleep, aggression towards his family, which he describes as being violent to his sons, reluctance to attend work where he attacked a man after a minor argument, tiredness and tearfulness. He seems very depressed and describes feeling like 'sitting in a gutter' after becoming overwhelmed with emotions and like 'being in a black tunnel'.

In the Vietnam War he remembers percussion grenades being thrown around him and seeing a serviceman have his leg blown off by a mine. He also recalls a distressing experience where another soldier held a child against a wall with a revolver to the child's head.

Mr Lidwinski says he sleeps badly, feels chronically tired and falls asleep during the day. He is irritable and intolerant of crowds. He describes himself as having no friends, his closest friend being his wife. He says he has poor concentration and memory, decreased libido, low self-esteem and a diminished sense of optimism. He is troubled by feelings of guilt and talks about death. He has suicidal thoughts but no plan to take his life.

He goes to bed between 7.00PM and 7.30PM with a variable sleep latency. He snores every night but his wife does not report apnea. He sometimes wakes up through the night with deep breathing but no choking sensation. He has violent jerks at night and he is a restless sleeper with a history of leg movement. He has nightmares about military experiences, reliving military events as if they were a 'videotape'. The nightmares are worse if he is exposed to anything which reminds him of his military experiences. He wakes between 5.00AM and 6.30AM, usually feeling unrefreshed. He takes a regular nap in the afternoon of ½–1 hour. He feels drowsy when driving, visiting or talking to people. There is no history suggestive of REM-related symptoms, such as hypnagogic (at the beginning of sleep) hallucinations, sleep paralysis, cataplexy or automatic behavior.

The diagnosis would include the following:
- post-traumatic stress disorder
- major depression
- advanced sleep phase syndrome
- alcohol-induced sleep disturbance
- restless leg syndrome and periodic limb movement disorder
- nightmares
- sleep apnea (less likely).

Mr Lidwinski has a sleep study and multiple sleep latency test, as well as formal psychiatric assessment. Overnight sleep study shows a reduction in sleep efficiency to 77%, an average of ten arousals per hour, reduction in slow-wave sleep and early onset REM at 52 minutes, with an overall reduction in REM sleep of 12% (normal value 20–24%). There is mild snoring but no disturbed breathing. The daytime test shows a mean sleep latency of 10.5 minutes, which is increased sleepiness for a man of his age but not pathologically sleepy. There is no early onset stage REM in any of the daytime naps. A detailed psychiatric interview confirms major depressive illness, as well as moderately severe post-traumatic stress disorder (PTSD).

The above findings are discussed with the patient, including the disruptive effect of alcohol on sleep, particularly in high doses. A more regular sleep and wake pattern is instituted and Mr Lidwinski is encouraged to reduce his alcohol intake. He is started on paroxetine with good symptomatic response in terms of his mood and reduced frequency of nightmares. He continues ongoing psychiatric counselling.

PTSD refers to long-lasting psychological, personal, social and occupational consequences of exposure to traumatic events. These are not only war-related but can include threats to personal integrity (eg. hold-ups, being the victim of aggression), or witnessing tragic events. The effects of psychological trauma on sleep can be considered in terms of immediate effects (6–12 months) and long-term (more than 12 months) (*Table 9.10*) (Hefez *et al*, 1987).

PTSD may coexist with other psychiatric morbidities, such as major depression, phobia and substance/alcohol abuse (O'Toole *et al*, 1996). Sleep disorders are more common in PTSD patients than in comparable subjects without PTSD (*Table 9.11*) (Mellman *et al*, 1995; Ross *et al*, 1989). In particular PTSD patients have an increased hyperarousal state which causes difficulty in initiating and maintaining sleep and fragmentation of sleep. This alteration may be mediated by dis-regulation of catecholamine and serotonin pathways (Southwick *et al*, 1999).

Patients with PTSD are also found to have increased upper limb movements during sleep, with similarity to REM behavior disorder, suggesting REM sleep deregulation in this group of patients (Ross *et al* 1994).

The presence of repetitive anxiety dreams (nightmares) is prevalent in PTSD (*Table 9.9*). While 20–24% of healthy students report nightmares once a year, 50–70% of combat patients report nightmares at least once a month (Ross *et al*, 1989). Coexisting psychiatric morbidity makes it difficult to interpret polysomnographic studies in this group of patients, but the available evidence suggests significant sleep disruption (*Table 9.12*) (Mellman *et al*, 1997).

Table 9.9: Predictors of antidepressant response to amitryptiline, which apply to other tricyclic antidepressants

Polysomnography predictors of poor response	Polysomnography predictors of favorable response
Very short REM sleep onset latency (<20 min)	Moderately shortened REM sleep onset latency (20–30 mins)
Poor suppression of REM in the first two nights on amitriptyline	Prolongation of REM onset latency (>150% of initial latency) while on amitriptyline
Lack of initial sedative response to amitriptyline	Suppression of total amount of REM while on amitriptyline

(Kupfer and Thase, 1987)

Table 9.10: Effects of trauma on sleep	
Immediate response (6–12 months)	**Long-term response (>12 months)**
Multiple awakenings	Less REM sleep and less dream recall
Increased motor activity	Persistent nightmares both in REM and slow-wave sleep (non-REM sleep)
Increase in nightmare	The nightmares incorporate elements of the trauma

(Hefez *et al*, 1987)

Management

Management of sleep disturbances in PTSD needs to be integrated with the treatment of the syndrome itself and other coexisting medical problems. In *Case study 11*, depression and alcohol abuse need to be addressed as they are an integral part of the sleep disruption.

In this instance, sleep management requires a co-operative patient who understands the multifactorial origin of the poor sense of well-being and poor sleep quality. The patient must be willing to take an active part in the treatment. A passive patient who expects a pharmacological treatment to solve all problems will lead to failure. Response to treatment is better if the patient has a supportive spouse or a friend. Maintaining a regular sleep and wake pattern, and respecting sleep hygiene, including avoiding excessive alcohol intake, are important elements in the management.

Selective serotonin reuptake inhibitors (SSRIs) are useful in post-traumatic stress disorder as some of the symptoms, aggression, impulsivity and sleep disturbance, may be related to low serotonin level (Southwick *et al*, 1999). Monoamino oxidase inhibitors (meclobomide and fluphenazine) have been reported to be useful in controlling nightmares as well. Tricyclic antidepressants (amitriptyline) and lithium have also been reported to be effective. Clonidine, an alpha-2 receptor antagonist, has also been used successfully.

Table 9.11: Sleep disturbances in Vietnam veterans with and without post-traumatic stress disorder (PTSD)		
Sleep	**PTSD (%)**	**Non-PTSD (%)**
Non-refreshing	73	38
Insomnia	68	24
Nightmares	65	5
Thrashing	59	19
Startle awakenings	51	5
Hallucinations	41	0
Night terrors	38	10
Sleep paralysis*	24	0
Sleep-walking	3	0

* Sleep paralysis refers to a sensation of being paralysed on waking up. The person is able to breathe and move his eyes, but no other movements. Sleep paralysis is usually associated with feeling frightened.

(Mellman *et al*, 1995)

Effect of chronic alcohol abuse on sleep pattern

Alcohol has pervasive effects on sleep and wake and, in cases of alcohol abuse, the effects are severe and long-lasting, even after withdrawal.

Alcohol has consistent effect on sleep of normal volunteers, with euphoria as the alcohol level rises in the blood within the first hour or so, followed by sedation, shortening of sleep onset latency and REM suppression in the first 2–4 hours as blood alcohol levels increase. A slight increase in stages 3 and 4 is also reported.

Ethanol is metabolized within 4–6 hours, with withdrawal occurring in the second half of the night causing increased fragmentation of sleep and REM rebound. If alcohol is taken over several continuous nights some of these changes, including the sedative effects, tend to decrease and an increased dose is needed to maintain sedation, increasing the severity of disturbance in the second part of the night (Landolt and Gillin, 2001; Roehrs and Roth, 2001). Importantly, sleep disruption and subjective reports of poor sleep occur in non-alcohol dependent individuals after the consumption of high alcohol (three to four standard drinks) early in the evening, around 5.00PM, even when bedtime is around 11.00PM and alcohol levels in the blood are undetectable (Landolt and Gillin, 2001).

In patients with alcohol dependence, sleep and wake disturbances are even more severe and longer lasting, possibly due to permanent neuronal damage. Often patients with alcohol dependency state that alcohol is needed for them to fall asleep. They have short periods of sleep, followed by arousals, which require further drinking to fall asleep, creating a pattern known as 'polyphasic sleep–wake behavior'.

Following alcohol abstinence, the clinical pattern is complicated by hyperarousal, intense REM rebound with intrusion of REM during the day, leading to visual and auditory hallucinations with gross sleep fragmentation, which reaches its most dramatic presentation in delirium tremens (DT). EEG recording is characterized by reduction or absence of slow-wave sleep, with predominant stage 1 with REM intrusion. REM is often atypical with no atonia (Lugaresi and Provini, 2001). Depression in the first few weeks of withdrawal can complicate the sleep and wake disturbance. It should be noted that the disruption of sleep and difficulty falling asleep can persist for a few years after alcohol abstinence, and this is a contributing factor to drinking relapse.

Daytime function is impaired as a consequence of disturbed sleep and the direct effect of alcohol consumption. It should be emphasized that the effect of alcohol is more pronounced in subjects who are sleep-deprived, either because of voluntary sleep restriction or due to other sleep disorders. Therefore, alcohol in the presence of sleep apnea, periodic limb movement disorder or narcolepsy can increase daytime impairment, and patients should be warned of this risk. The underlying neuromechanism of alcohol effects is likely to be complex, and is due to the interaction of ethanol with important neurotransmitters (*Table 9.13*).

Table 9.12: Overnight sleep studies in PTSD patients compared to normal controls

- Sleep efficiency is reduced
- Reduction in REM sleep
- Reduction in slow-wave sleep
- Increased in REM density*
- Increased limb movement (upper limbs in particular)

* REM density is the number of eye movements per unit of time

(Mellman *et al*, 1995; Ross *et al*, 1994)

The clinical manifestations of alcohol abuse are varied and include:

- difficulty initiating and maintaining sleep
- increased risk of sleep apnea
- delayed and advanced sleep phase syndrome
- nightmares
- REM behavior disorder.

Patients with chronic alcohol dependency have an increased prevalence of both obstructive and central sleep apnea, in both men and women independent of age and body mass index (BMI). During abstinence, men are at increased risk of nocturnal hypoxemia (Vitiello *et al*, 1990). The effect of alcohol and alcohol abstinence on sleep in patients with ethanol dependence should be considered in the management of alcohol detoxification.

Sleep in chronic renal disease

Case study 12

Mr Matthew Jones is a 45-year-old miner with a background of end-stage renal failure on home haemodialysis. He works as a shift worker on permanent night shift 5 days a week. He presents with profound tiredness and sleepiness. He is a non-smoker and non-drinker. He is on a waiting list for a kidney transplant.

Mr Jones goes to bed between 8.30AM and 9.00PM and wakes at 3.00PM, getting up once to go to the toilet. He has home hemodialysis three times a week between 8.30AM and 1.30PM. His wife reports habitual snoring and apneas, as well as limb movement. Mr Jones says he experiences restless legs before going to bed.

Mr Jones has overnight polysomnography which shows severe obstructive sleep apnea with an apnea/hypopnea of ninety-five events per hour with minimal oxygen desaturation, which is below 90% for 1% of the time. He is restless but periodic limb movements only occur seven times an hour on the night of recording.

The diagnosis with regard to his symptoms of tiredness and sleepiness includes the following:
- severe sleep apnea
- restless leg syndrome and periodic limb movement disorder
- shift working
- chronic renal failure and hemodialysis.

Home dialysis three mornings a week between 8.30AM and 1.30PM would cause a reduction in resting time, coming on top of permanent nightshift working. Severe sleep apnea would be a major contributor to this man's unrefreshing sleep and feelings of tiredness.

Mr Jones starts nasal CPAP which greatly improves his sleep quality and sense of well-being. Interestingly, on the night of nasal CPAP titration, the number of periodic limb movements increases to twenty-five events per hour.

Table 9.13: Neurochemical effects of alcohol	
GABA (gamma-aminobutyric acid)	GABA is the major inhibitory neurotransmitter and it is activated by ethanol, increasing chloride flux, in similar fashion to other CNS depressants such benzodiazepines, barbiturates and the newer non-benzodiazepine hypnotics. Tolerance to this action occurs by down-regulation of $GABA_A$ receptors
Direct increase of chloride flux (GABA independent)	This CNS depressant activity is not subject to tolerance
Adenosine	Ethanol seems to facilitate adenosine action by stimulation of Adenosine type 2 receptors. Adenosine is considered one of the mediators of sleep propensity
Acetylcholine	Increased synthesis, and release of acetylcholine after chronic alcohol intake. Acetylcholine mediates REM sleep regulation and its increased activity may explain the abnormalities of REM in patients with chronic alcohol abuse and during withdrawal
Glutamate (central nervous system excitatory neurotransmitter, promoting wakefulness)	Ethanol acutely inhibits glutamate receptors, reducing wakefulness, therefore mediating the sedative effects of alcohol

(Roehrs and Roth, 2001; Brust, 1993)

Sleep disorders in advanced chronic renal failure are common. The metabolic derangement associated with renal failure of any cause, affects many body functions including sleep and wake, with disturbed nocturnal sleep, daytime sleepiness and tiredness. The following factors are relevant to patients with end-stage renal failure:

- increased risk of sleep apnea
- increased prevalence of restless leg and periodic limb movement disorder
- effect of uremia on sleep structure
- effect of different type of dialysis on sleep.

The effects of uraemia on sleep EEG is reflected in the reduction of total sleep time and fragmentation of sleep (Reichenmiller *et al*, 1971). The prevalence of sleep apnea syndrome (daytime sleepiness associated with snoring and disturbed breathing) is increased compared to the normal population, being estimated as being between 31% and 63% (although studies usually include small numbers and different criteria for sleep apnea) (Fletcher, 1993; Kraus and Hamburger, 1997; Kuhlmann *et al*, 2000; Stepanski and Zorick, 1995).

The reasons for the increased prevalence of disturbed breathing in chronic renal failure are not fully understood, but it is thought that the metabolic abnormalities due to metabolic acidosis and compensatory hypocapnia may affect central nervous system regulation of respiration during sleep, as well as the direct effect of uraemia.

The observation that intense dialysis (Mendelson *et al*, 1990) and kidney transplant (Langevin *et al*, 1993; Auckley, 1999) improves disturbed breathing seems to support this hypothesis. Similarly, restless leg syndrome improves with better metabolic control (Winkelmann *et al*, 2002).

In patients with end-stage renal disease complicated by heart failure, central sleep apnea can be a more prominent component than obstructive sleep apnea. Treatment follows the same line as in the general population, with nasal CPAP being effective treatment, particularly in more severe cases like that described in *Case study 12* (Pressman *et al*, 1993).

The association of obstructive sleep apnea and kidney dysfunction is probably bidirectional: the hypoxemia, pulmonary hypertension and systemic hypertension of sleep apnea syndrome may affect glomerular function, causing glomerular hypertrophy and increasing the risk of proteinuria (Fletcher, 1993). Treating disturbed breathing may not only improve the patient's sleep quality and sense of well-being, but also reduce the risk of further deterioration of kidney function.

A diagnosis of obstructive sleep apnea should be suspected in patients with end-stage renal disease complaining of loud snoring, a body mass index above 25 and hypertension. An overnight oximetry is an effective, minimally intrusive, and inexpensive way to screen patients on dialysis (Pfister *et al*, 1999).

Restless leg and periodic limb movement disorder are common in patients with end-stage renal disease (62%) (Hui *et al*, 2000), and can be an important contributor to fragmentation of sleep and insomnia. Treatment is along the same lines as in the general population, as well as pursuing metabolic control by dialysis and kidney transplant.

The effect of dialysis on sleep depends on the type (peritoneal versus hemodialysis, versus nocturnal continuous hemodialysis) as well as time and effectiveness of treatment. Good metabolic control, including ideal weight, is likely to result in an improvement in sleep quality. Concern has been raised about the possible effect on respiration of the mechanical effect of peritoneal dialysis (Wadhwa *et al*, 1992), even though the prevalence of obstructive sleep apnea is similarly increased in hemodialysis and peritoneal dialysis patients (Wadhwa and Mendelson, 1992). A new form of hemodialysis, nocturnal hemodialysis, seems to be much more effective than conventional hemodialysis in improving disturbed breathing during sleep, even though periodic limb movement disorder does not improve as well as disturbed breathing (Hanly *et al*, 2002).

Obstructive airway disease and sleep

Case study 13

Mr Warwick Carr is a retired, 65-year-old steel industry supervisor referred because of difficulty maintaining sleep, waking unrefreshed and daytime sleepiness. He smoked for fifty years but stopped 5 years ago. He is an habitual snorer but whether he has apnea is uncertain as he has been sleeping separately from his wife for several years. He has no orthopnea and can walk at his own pace up to 100 meters before being breathless.

Spirometry shows a forced expiratory volume, (FEV_1) of 0.8 (predicted 2.9 litres), a forced vital capacity (FVC) of 1.5 (predicted 3.7), a finding in keeping with moderate to severe obstructive airway disease. His body mass index was 30.4, in keeping with obesity. Mr Carr uses bronchodilators and inhaled steroids even though asthma, as such, is not present. He has been using temazepam intermittently because of his sleep problem.

Overnight polysomnography shows low baseline oxygen saturation (mean value of 89%), with oxygen below 90% for 45% of the time. There are twenty apnea/hypopnea events per hour and marked oxygen desaturation during sleep (*Figure 9.4*).

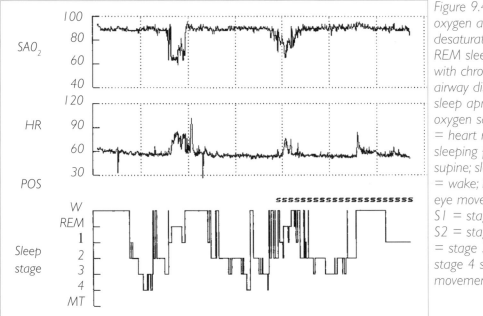

Figure 9.4: Low baseline oxygen and marked desaturation during REM sleep in a patient with chronic obstructive airway disease and sleep apnea. SaO_2 = oxygen saturation; HR = heart rate; POS = sleeping position: s = supine; sleep stage: W = wake; REM = rapid eye movement sleep; S1 = stage 1 sleep; S2 = stage 2 sleep; S3 = stage 3 sleep; S4 = stage 4 sleep; MT = movement time.

The history suggests a diagnosis overlap syndrome (COAD with hypoventilation and obstructive sleep apnea). He is started on nasal CPAP, which corrects the respiratory disturbance. No oxygen needs to be added. He is enrolled in a rehabilitation programme to improve his lung function and reduce his weight .

A high index of suspicion needs to be maintained for respiratory disturbance in patients with moderate to severe COAD, especially in the presence of snoring, obesity, unrefreshed sleep and daytime hypoxemia. The majority of patients with symptomatic obstructive airway disease have an increased risk of sleep-related disturbed breathing related to the following:

- decreased respiratory reserve

- reduction in upper airway cross-section, causing increased upper airway resistance during sleep
- a decrease in ventilation associated with sleep
- decreased response to hypoxia and hypercapnia
- circadian variation in respiratory function (decrease during sleep at night-time, independent of sleep itself).

Changes in ventilation with associated reduced PO_2 and increased PCO_2 at alveolar level occur in slow-wave sleep as well as in REM. However, in REM sleep the effect of marked hypotonia increases the possibility of hypoventilation and obstructive events, as described in *Case study 13* (Cormick *et al*, 1986; Stradling *et al*, 1985). Polysomnography in patients with COAD shows significant disturbance in sleep quality and structure (*Table 9.14*). The lower the patient's arterial oxygenation, the more disturbed the breathing (Cormick *et al*, 1986; Weitzenblum and Chaouat, 2004).

The level of PO_2 and PCO_2 during the day, when the patient is awake, are the best predictors of sleep-related hypoventilation. Clinicians should suspect significant sleep disturbance in patients with low oxygen during the day (eg. oxygen saturation of less than 92%) and more so if hypercapnea is present.

Table 9.14: Sleep in chronic obstructive airway disease (COAD)
- Increased difficulty falling asleep and staying asleep
- Increased daytime sleepiness
- Increased use of hypnotics
- Arterial hypoxaemia common, and often severe in REM sleep
- Increased number of arousals related to hypoventilation

A simple and effective way to screen at-risk patients is an overnight oximetry. Most oximetry software allow quantification of a variety of oxygen saturation indices, which can be used to quantify the severity of hypoxemia, usually expressed as a percentage of oxygen saturation (SaO_2) below 90%, or mean nocturnal $SaO_2 < 90$. *Figure 9.5* shows the overnight oximetry of a patient with COAD and hypoventilation.

Management requires optimization of the lung condition, including treatment of pulmonary hypertension, a common coexisting problem contributing to hypoxemia. Nasal CPAP or non-invasive nasal ventilation (NIV), with or without oxygen, should be considered in this group of patients (*Chapter 14*). Low flow (1–2 L/min) oxygen is usually sufficient, and the risk of worsening hypercapnea is small.

Use of sleeping tablets in obstructive airway disease

Patients with COAD often complain of difficulty falling asleep and request the prescription of hypnotic agents. Prescription should follow the same guidelines as for any other patient presenting with symptoms of insomnia. However special precaution is needed in COAD patients, as most sleeping tablets have a muscle relaxant effect and tend to decrease the breathing drive, therefore worsening sleep-related hypoventilation. This is particularly relevant in patients with severe lung function impairment, such as $FEV_1 < 40\%$, awake oxygen saturation <92%, and hypercapnia.

There is some evidence that the new non-benzodiazepine hypnotics (zolpidem, zoplicone, zaleplon), because of their lack of muscle relaxant activity, may have a safer profile in this group of patients (Girault *et al*, 1996).

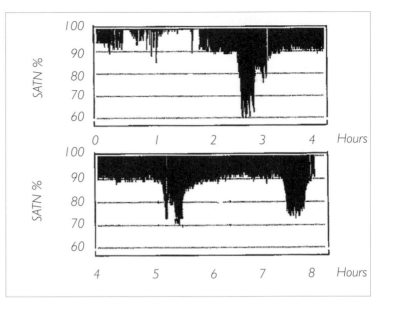

Asthma

Patients with moderate to severe symptomatic asthma often have disturbed sleep with increased sleep fragmentation, unrefreshing sleep and poor daytime function. Medications used in asthma such as beta-agonists, theophylline and oral steroids, can affect sleep by increasing wakefulness.

Figure 9.5: Oximetry in patient with COAD and marked hypoventilation episodes, with a recurrent pattern suggestive of REM-related hypoventilation. SATN = oxygen saturation

Gastroesophageal reflux is often a concomitant factor contributing to sleep fragmentation. However, patients with asthma are rarely referred to a sleep unit.

The relationship between asthma and sleep is complex and bi-directional. Asthma gets worse at night (*Figure 9.6*) due to two factors:

- circadian effect
- sleep effects.

Evidence of worsening broncho-constriction, using peak respiratory flow, is present at night time when the patient is kept awake (independent from sleep) with a nadir at about 4.00AM. However, it is worse if the person is allowed to sleep (*Figure 9.6*), pointing to two independent mechanisms, one related to circadian variation of bronchoconstriction and the other, the direct effect of sleep itself.

Management should seek to optimize:

- asthma treatment
- co-morbidities such as esophageal reflux.

In asthma, attention to current chronopharmacology knowledge is important (*Chapter 2*). A simple but important example is the timing of steroid administration (Gibson, 1990; Smolensky and D'Alonzo, 1997). During an acute asthma attack, steroids should be administered in a split dose, morning and afternoon, so that night-time inflammation is properly treated. If steroids are administered only in the morning, there is insufficient antiinflammatory activity after midnight when bronchoconstriction is actually more intense.

Interstitial lung disease and cystic fibrosis

Sleep in patients with interstitial lung disease is fragmented, with hypoxemia more likely to occur in REM sleep. These patients have an increased number of arousals associated with bouts of coughing, and unrefreshed sleep with daytime tiredness (Ambrogetti *et al*, 1994). When hypoxemia is documented, oxygen therapy should be considered, particularly if there is clinical evidence of pulmonary hypertension.

The use of assisted ventilation is not well tolerated in patients with interstitial lung disease, unless there is coexisting obstructive sleep apnea. In patients with cystic fibrosis, sleep quality deteriorates with increasing severity of the lung disease. There is an increase in fragmentation of sleep and development of sleep-related hypoxemia and hypercapnia, due to nocturnal hypoventilation. These sleep-related changes can lead to deterioration in daily functioning and contribute to pulmonary hypertension and cor pulmonale.

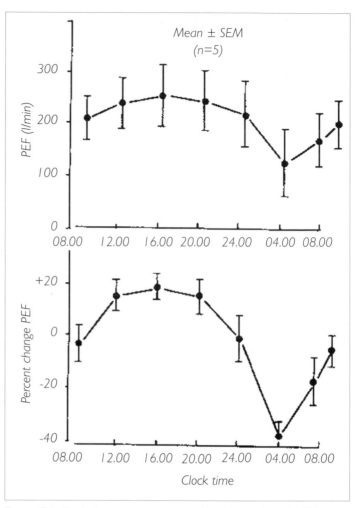

Figure 9.6: *Peak flow drops in the middle of the night (4.00AM) both in absolute value and as a percentage in all subjects, but it is more marked in asthma patients. PEF = peak expiratory flow.*

The risk of sleep disorder breathing and nocturnal hypoventilation is increased when the resting oxygen saturation is <94%, and with moderate to severe obstructive airway disease (FEV_1 <65% of predicted value) (Milross *et al*, 2004). As the lung disease progresses, the use of oxygen therapy and non-invasive ventilation are useful strategies to improve sleep quality and daytime function, and as supportive patient care while waiting for lung transplant.

Sleep and wake function in human immunodeficiency virus (HIV) patients

Given the neurotropism of HIV and the neuropsychiatric complications of acquired immune deficiency syndrome (AIDS), it is not surprising that derangement of sleep and wake function is common in this group of patients. The subjective complaint varies from difficulty initiating and maintaining sleep (insomnia with prolonged latency to sleep onset and early morning arousals), to lethargy and excessive daytime sleepiness during the day (Nokes and Kendrew, 1996). Sleep disturbance can precede the diagnosis of HIV infection (Phillips, 1999).

Sleep abnormalities are reported in asymptomatic HIV-infected patients (Norman *et al*, 1992) and seems to worsen with progression of the infection (Darko *et al*, 1992; Moeller *et al*, 1991).

In HIV-positive patients with daytime somnolence, the possibility of obstructive sleep apnea (OSA) should be considered, even when the patient is young and with a normal body mass index (BMI). Adenotonsillar hypertrophy is often present in HIV-infected patients, and it is thought to be a potential reason for increased risk of OSA Epstein *et al*, 1995)

The structure of sleep also seems to be affected in HIV infection. An increase in total amount and percentage of slow-wave sleep (SWS) is reported with an increase in slow-wave sleep in the second part of the night (Norman *et al*, 1990), even though this finding is not always confirmed (Ferini-Strambi *et al*, 1995). Alpha-delta sleep has also been reported to be more common in these patients. Alpha-delta is an EEG finding characterized by the presence of alpha rhythm (8–12 Hz) overriding a slow-wave rhythm (2–4 Hz). It is a non-specific finding associated with other conditions, characterized by poor sleep quality and sleep fragmentation, such as fibromyalgia, rheumatoid arthritis, anxiety, depression and schizophrenia.

Analysis of cyclic alternating pattern (CAP, *Chapter 4*), a measure of arousal levels, in HIV-infected patients suggests an increase in CAP rate (percentage of CAP over sleep time), which is considered a marker of poor subjective sleep quality (Ferini-Strambi *et al*, 1995).

There are many factors which may contribute to sleep and wake abnormality in HIV patients. These include: HIV encephalopathy, variation in cytokines level (interleukins-1 and 2, IL-1 and IL-2, and tumor necrosis factor (TNF). Coexistent anxiety and depression are often contributing factors. The use of prescribed and non-prescribed medication/substances is also likely to be important (*Table 9.15*). Treatment with zidovudine has been reported to be associated with insomnia (Moeller *et al*, 1991, 1992).

Treatment of sleep and wake disturbances in HIV patients will need to take into consideration the likely multifactorial etiology summarized above.

Physiological states

Pregnancy associated sleep disorders

Case study 14

Naomi Thompson is a 31-year-old woman who is referred 10 days after delivery of her second son, 1 day after discharge from hospital. The nursing staff noticed recurrent apneas in her sleep and oxygen desaturation. Retrospectively, she was tired and somnolent before becoming pregnant and this became more pronounced during pregnancy. She recalls having to pull off the road while driving to work due to sleepiness. She left her job after 7 months of pregnancy as she was profoundly tired and unable to keep up with the work. Her confinement, however, was uncomplicated with delivery of a healthy infant of normal weight.

Examination reveals evidence of rhinitis with grossly enlarged adenoids and tonsils. A sleep study reveals severe obstructive sleep apnea (*Figure 9.7*). Ms Thompson is started on nasal CPAP with immediate benefit. She is also prescribed an inhaled steroid.

Two months later, and 4 weeks after adeno-tonsillectomy, there is no further snoring and Ms Thompson has good quality sleep without nasal CPAP. A follow-up study shows complete resolution of disturbed breathing (*Figure 9.8*). Her body mass index is 33 and this remains unchanged between the two studies.

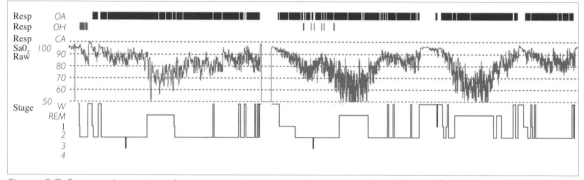

Figure 9.7: Severe obstructive sleep apnea in postnatal patient with evidence of rhinitis and grossly enlarged adenoids and tonsils. Resp = respiratory event: OA = obstructive apnea, OH = obstructive hypopnea, CA = central apnea; SaO₂ Raw = oxygen saturation; Stage = sleep stage: W = wake; REM = rapid eye movement sleep; 1 = stage 1 sleep; 2 = stage 2 sleep; 3 = stage 3 sleep; 4 = stage 4.

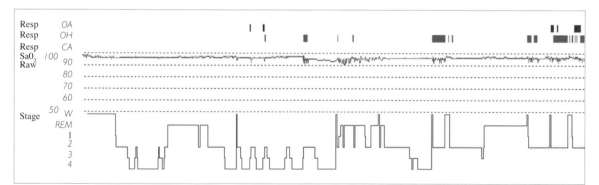

Figure 9.8: Normal sleep study following adenotonsillectomy. Resp = respiratory event: OA = obstructive apnea, OH = obstructive hypopnea, CA = central apnoea; SaO₂ Raw = oxygen saturation; W = wake; REM = Rapid eye movement sleep; 1 = stage 1 sleep; 2 = stage 2 sleep; 3 = Stage 3 sleep; 4 = stage 4 sleep.

Table 9.15: Medications and sleep in HIV disease

Organisms targeted	Drug	Effect on sleep
HIV	Didanosine (ddI)	Insomnia
	Lamivudine	Insomnia
	Stavudine (d4T)	Sleep disorder
	Zalcitabine (ddC)	Insomnia
	Zidovudine (AZT, ZDV)	Insomnia
	Delavirdine	Insomnia
	Nevirapine	Somnolence
	Indinavir	Insomnia
	Nelfinavir mesylate	None reported
	Ritonavir	Insomnia
	Saquinavir	Somnolence
		Insomnia
		Sleep disorders
		Somnolence
		Insomnia
		Somnolence
		None reported
Viruses	Aciclovir	None reported
	Foscarnet	Insomnia
	Ganciclovir	Somnolence
		Somnolence
Pneumocystis carinii	Atovaquone	Insomnia
	Clindamycin	None reported
	Dapsone	Insomnia
	Pentamidine	None reported
	Primaquine	None reported
	Trimethoprim-sulfamethoxazole	None reported
	Trimetrexate	None reported
Mycobacterium tuberculosis	Ethambutol	None reported
	Isoniazide	None reported
	Pyrazinamide	None reported
	Rifampin	Drowsiness
Mycobacterium avium	Azithromycin	Somnolence
	Ciprofloxacin	Insomnia
	Clarithromycin	Somnolence
	Clofazimine	None reported
	Ofloxacin	None reported
	Rifabutin	Insomnia
		Sleep disorders
		None reported
Fungi	Amphotericin B	None reported
	Fluconazole	None reported
	Flucytosine	Sedation
	Itraconazole	Somnolence
	Ketoconazole	Somnolence

This case is remarkable for a series of reasons. One can only speculate that the degree of hypoxemia present before delivery was likely to be much worse than when the patient presented post-delivery. Despite this, there were no pregnancy associated complications, in particular, there was no hypertension or pre-eclampsia. The infant was born with no apparent distress and of normal weight.

Sleep-disordered breathing during pregnancy is a topic of increasing attention because of a possible link with pregnancy-related hypertension, eclampsia and fetal growth retardation (Santiago *et al*, 2001). Hypoxemia of whatever cause — poorly controlled asthma, cardiac malformations or high altitude — increases the risk of fetal growth retardation. There are well-documented cases of fetal distress in mothers with obstructive sleep apnea and hypoxia (Joel-Cohen and Schoenfield, 1978; Kowall *et al*, 1989).

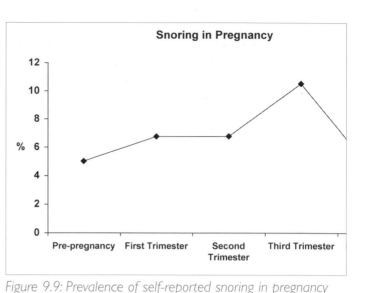

Figure 9.9: Prevalence of self-reported snoring in pregnancy (from Hedman et al, 2002).

Snoring is increased in pregnant women compared to matched non-pregnant subjects. It increases in prevalence from the first to the third trimester (Hedman *et al*, 2002; Loube *et al*, 1996) and it is reduced to pre-pregnancy level 3 months after delivery (*Figure 9.9*).

While in an unselected group of pregnant women there appears to be no adverse fetal outcome, obstructive sleep apnea syndrome is well documented in pregnancy and a high index of suspicion should trigger full evaluation, including polysomnography or at least overnight oximetry in an at-risk group (*Table 9.16*).

Some of the physiological changes occurring during pregnancy may favor upper airway narrowing. The increase in estrogen, for example, can cause fluid retention and edema of the upper airway, increasing the likelihood of obstruction. To some degree, these changes are counterbalanced by progesterone which increases the frequency and depth of breathing.

Management of obstructive sleep apnea in pregnancy follows the same line as in a non-pregnant subject. Weight control, avoiding alcohol and optimization of nasal obstruction are important conservative measures. Nasal CPAP is both safe and effective in pregnancy, as seen in

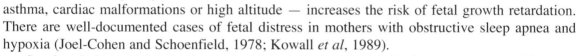

Table 9.16: At risk subjects for OSA in pregnancy
Obese patients with a history of snoring
• Habitual snoring • Apnea reported by the family • Daytime sleepiness
Known disturbed breathing before becoming pregnant (even if mild)
History of hypertension or pre-eclampsia
Coexisting medical conditions which increase the risk of disturbed breathing:
• Diabetes • Thyroid dysfunction • Asthma
Fetal growth delay

Case study 14. Mandibular advancing devices (mouthguards) are also appropriate in cases where disturbed breathing is mild, or in patients who are unable to use nasal CPAP. Documentation of resolution of disturbed breathing and normalization of oxygen levels should be obtained by objective measures such as polysomnography or oximetry.

Sleep during pregnancy goes through a series of changes related to the effect of hormones and other physiological variables on sleep and wake (*Table 9.17* and *Figure 9.10*). As the pregnancy progresses other factors influence fragmentation of sleep, including discomfort related to the enlarged uterus, backache, esophageal reflux, leg cramps and increased need to urinate. Nocturnal backache, particularly after the twentieth week of gestation, disturbs sleep in 18–36% of pregnant women (Fast and Hertz, 1992; Schweiger, 1972).

When symptoms of sleepiness (more common in early pregnancy) and/or insomnia (more common in the second part of pregnancy) become prominent they are referred to as pregnancy-associated sleep disorder, which is defined by the international classification of sleep disorders (American Sleep Disorders Association, 1997) as, '... the occurrence of either insomnia or excessive daytime sleepiness that develops in the course of pregnancy'.

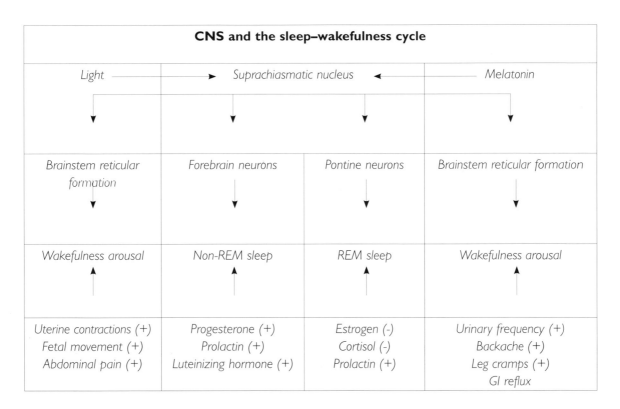

Figure 9.10: Pregnancy influences on sleep (Santiago et al, 2001). CNS = central nervous system.

Table 9.17: Subjective and objective sleep changes in pregnancy

Stage of pregnancy	Subjective (surveys and sleep logs)	Objective (polysomnography)
First trimester	Increased total sleep time due to naps Increased daytime sleepiness Increased nocturnal insomnia	Increased total sleep time Decreased stage 3 and 4 non-REM sleep
Second trimester	Normalization of total sleep time Increased awakening	Normal total sleep time Decreased stage 3 and 4 non-REM sleep Decreased REM sleep
Third trimester	Decreased total sleep time Increased insomnia Increased nocturnal awakening Increased daytime sleepiness	Decreased total sleep time Increased waking after sleep onset Increased stage 1 non-REM sleep Decreased stage 3 and 4 non-REM sleep Decreased REM sleep

(Santiago *et al*, 2001)

The prevalence of primary sleep disturbances (snoring, restless leg syndrome with periodic limb movement disorder, sleep walking, narcoleptic syndrome) shows a variable increase in pregnant women (Santiago *et al*, 2001). The change in sleep pattern results in more fragmentation of sleep, symptoms of insomnia and increased daytime sleepiness, as distinct from alteration of sleep due to pregnancy itself. Restless leg syndrome and periodic limb movement disorder are more common in the third trimester and improve to pre-pregnancy level after delivery (*Figure 9.11*) and does not seem to vary with age group (Hedman *et al*, 2002).

Management of primary sleep disorders during pregnancy is complicated by the possible adverse affects of medications on the fetus, and non-pharmacological intervention should be tried first. Predisposing factors, such as iron and folate deficiencies, should be ascertained and corrected if present. Avoidance of caffeinated beverages is also recommended and can be beneficial. The use of medications, such as benzodiazepines, opioids or dopa-agonists is preferably omitted because they fall into category C and are considered unsafe in pregnancy (*Table 9.18*).

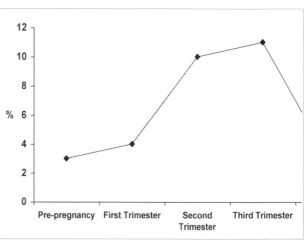

Figure 9.11: Restless leg incidence in pregnancy (from Hedman et al, 2002).

Table 9.18: The US Food and Drug Administration assigned five categories of labeling for drug use in pregnancy:

A: Controlled studies in women have failed to demonstrate a risk to the fetus in the first trimester, and the possibility of fetal harm seems remote.

B: Animal studies do not indicate a risk to the fetus; no controlled human studies have been published, or animal studies show an adverse effect on the fetus but well-controlled studies in pregnant women have failed to demonstrate a risk to the fetus.

C: Studies have shown teratogenic or embryocidal effects in animals, but no controlled studies are available in women or no studies are available in either women or animals.

D: Positive evidence of human fetal risk exists, but benefits from use in pregnant women may be acceptable despite this risk (for example, when the life of the mother is in danger or she risks serious disease for which safer drugs are ineffective or cannot be used).

X: Studies in animals or humans have demonstrated fetal abnormalities or evidence of fetal risk exists on the basis of experience in humans (or both) and the risk of use clearly outweighs any possible benefit. The drug is contraindicated in women who are or may become pregnant.

Drug	Pregnancy category
Sedatives and hypnotics	
Alprazolam	D
Diazepam	D
Lorazepam	D
Midazolam	D
Temazepam	X
Clonazepam	C
Diphenhydramine	B
Secobarbital	D
Zolpidem	B
Zaleplon	C
Stimulants	
Dextroamphetamine	C
Methamphetamine	C
Pemoline	B
Mazindol	C
Methylphenidate	C
Modafinil	C
Antidepressants	
Fluoxetine	B
Paroxetine	B
Amitriptyline	D
Other	
Carbamazepine	C
Carbidopa	C
Levodopa	C
Codeine	C

Daytime tiredness and fatigue are common in pregnancy, possibly related to the increase in progesterone. On occasion, pathological sleepiness manifests itself in pregnancy. However before a firm diagnosis of narcolepsy, or non-REM narcolepsy is made, other causes of sleepiness such as insufficient sleep or sleep fragmentation due to pregnancy need to be considered. A final diagnosis should be delayed until well after confinement.

More important is the management of the patient known to have narcolepsy or idiopathic hypersomnolence syndromes during pregnancy. All patients treated with stimulant medications, such as dexamphetamine methylphenidate, modafinil and pemoline, should be counselled to stop treatment when they are planning to conceive and should not take these medications during pregnancy. This is particularly important in the first trimester. It is suggested that pemoline (Santiago et al, 2001) which is not available in Australia, is the safer of the stimulants available.

In practice, the potential risks of using stimulant medications in the second and third trimester must be weighed against the deleterious effect of stopping treatment on the patient's function and well-being. Evidence based on small groups of patients who have used stimulants throughout pregnancy shows little indication of toxicity (Briggs et al, 1975; Eriksson et al, 1978; Little et al, 1988; Milkovich and Van den Berg, 1977).

Other primary sleep disturbances said to be common in pregnancy include sleep-walking and sleep terrors. These disturbances may be explained by the increased number of arousals, as parasomnias often occur during the transition between slow-wave sleep and awake state (American Sleep Disorders Association, 1997).

Pre-eclampsia and sleep

Pre-eclampsia is an important cause of perinatal morbidity associated with sleep disturbances. Indirect measures of sleep quality (Ekholm et al, 1992) and polysomnography studies (Edwards et al, 2000) suggest that there is increased restless sleep, reduced latency to REM sleep, reduction of total REM and an increase in slow-wave sleep with pre-eclampsia, although some of these findings may be confounded by the medications used to treat this condition.

Of particular interest is the relation of sleep and disturbed breathing with pregnancy-induced hypertension and pre-eclampsia (Franklin et al, 2000). There is difficulty in predicting early on which subjects will progress to a full pre-eclampsia/eclampsia syndrome. Studies which consider circadian variability of blood pressure recorded throughout pregnancy (Hermida et al, 1997) have shown that the blood pressure profile in patients who go on to develop gestational hypertension of pre-eclampsia is recognizable after a few weeks of gestation. Specifically in uncomplicated pregnancy, both systolic and diastolic blood pressure progressively decrease from the beginning of pregnancy up to 20 weeks of gestation, and then increase steadily up to confinement. In complicated pregnancy, although the initial blood pressure is similar to that recorded in uncomplicated patients, the blood pressure profile shows a linear increase throughout pregnancy.

Unfortunately, conventional blood pressure monitoring, including mean value of 24-hour monitoring, does not have enough sensitivity and specificity to be useful in individual patients (Brown et al 2001). However, by reevaluation of the definition of what constitutes systolic and diastolic hypertension in pregnancy, it is possible to provide a clinically useful instrument which can be used to identify at-risk patients early on in pregnancy (Hermida et al, 1997).

Given the reported association between snoring and hypertension, current lines of investigation are looking at the potential benefit of nasal CPAP in the third trimester of pregnancy in pre-eclamptic patients (Edwards *et al*, 2000). However, the value of this approach is not proven and requires further study.

The menopause and sleep

Subjective report of poor sleep quality is linked to physiological changes in the gonadal hormones associated with the menopause. The decrease in estrogen and progesterone seems to affect a variety of functions apart from the reproductive one. Autonomic instability with hot flushes, dryness of sexual organs, mood and cognitive changes, and sleep disturbances are common complaints.

When symptoms become clinically significant, the clinician is faced with the following two questions:

1. Are the symptoms only related to menopausal changes, or are they related to age and psychiatric comorbidity?
2. Is hormone replacement therapy (HRT) effective and indicated in patients with menopause-associated sleep disorders?

Menopause, insomnia and hormone replacement therapy (HRT)

Women at menopause present with a complex array of symptoms, including hot flushes, sweating, declining libido, headache, anxiety and depression, tiredness, palpitations, weight increase, lack of concentration, as well as sleep disturbances. At least some of these symptoms reach levels which interfere with normal functions (Polo-Kantola *et al*, 2001).

Insomnia is self-reported by twice as many women in the 5 years post-menopause then pre-menopausal subjects (Ballinger, 1976). The insomnia predominantly appears to be difficulty in initiating and maintaining sleep, rather than early waking (Ballinger, 1976), and seems independent from psychiatric symptoms which are more prominent in pre-menopausal women (aged 45–50), than postmenopausal.

A widely held theory that hot flushes occurring at night are a major contributing factor to disturbed sleep in this group of patients is not supported by studies where objective measurement of hot flushes (skin temperature and increase in heart rate) were monitored (Purdie *et al*, 1995).

Treatment with HRT is reported to improve *subjective* sleep quality, reducing sleep onset latency, increasing the total amount of REM as well as improving psychological well-being (Polo-Kantola, 2001; Schiff *et al*, 1979; Thompson and Oswald, 1997). The impact of menopausal changes and the benefit of HRT are probably more obvious in the more severely affected patients (Schiff *et al*, 1979).

There are, however, discrepancies between subjective reported improvement and a lack of significant polysomnography (objective) changes when sleep is recorded overnight (Purdie *et al*, 1995). Subjective versus objective sleep perception differences apply in both directions. While one in four subjects who complain of insomnia may have no objective evidence (such as sleep onset latency of more than thirty minutes and increased number of arousals), one in five who report good sleep quality have objective evidence of disturbed sleep.

Management of menopausal-related sleep disturbances

Perimenopausal women presenting with sleep disturbances, unrefreshing sleep and daytime tiredness require a full assessment before the symptoms can be ascribed to menopause. Specifically, the following points should be considered:

❖ Is there clinical depression?
❖ Is there anxiety and psychophysiological insomnia? (*Chapter 7*)
❖ Is there obstructive sleep apnea? (more common after the menopause)
❖ Is there restless leg and periodic limb movement disorder and the often associated iron deficiency?

When the above issues are clarified, a trial of HRT for a few months can be undertaken. Another approach is to prescribe a 3–6-month HRT replacement as the first line of treatment (Polo-Kantola *et al*, 2001). However in view of the evidence of the increased risk of breast malignancy with hormone replacement therapy, caution is needed together with well-informed patients.

Perimenstrual sleep disorders

During the perimenstrual period, some women suffer disturbed sleep similar to the menopausal sleep disturbances, but on a smaller scale. These women have increased sleep fragmentation, difficulty initiating sleep, increased arousals, as well as a clinical picture characterized by increased sleepiness tendency (hypersomnolence) (American Sleep Disorders Association, 1997). A subjective increase in sleepiness is also reported around ovulation. However objective assessment of sleep structure across the menstrual cycle fails to reveal significant differences (Moline *et al*, 2003).

Sleep disorders in hospitalized patients

Sleep and wake disturbances in hospitalized patients are common and despite the significant impact on patient care and well being, have received little attention. A brief round on a medical ward at 10.00AM often reveals that up to 30–40% of patients are either soundly asleep or dozing. In fact, in a questionnaire survey 51% of patients report poor sleep in hospital with difficulty falling and staying asleep (Yinnon *et al*, 1992). The sleep and wake problems vary among different groups of patients and settings, such as medical, surgical and ICU environments. Often patients request hypnotic medications and one in three patients has their first exposure to sleeping tablets while in hospital.

For the clinician there are a series of important questions:

- What is the impact of sleep disturbances on patient care?
- Is there long-term effect after the patient has been discharged from hospital?
- What are the determinants of sleep and wake disturbances in hospital?
- How should this problem be dealt with?
- What is the role of sleeping tablets in hospitalized patients?

The impact of sleep disturbances on patient care will depend on the patient's age, morbidity and the hospital setting. For example, in a geriatric hospital (Manabe *et al*, 2000), the patients with insomnia, sleep onset delay and daytime sleepiness have increased mortality at 2 years follow-up after adjusting for other variables (age, gender, functional status).

In surgical units (Rosenberg, 2001), a patient's sleep is altered in the first few days post-operatively as a consequence of the surgical procedure itself, post-operative pain and ward routine, including noise (*Table 9.19*). There is often a reduction of total night-time sleep, even though how much sleep the patient may actually get in 24 hours is not known as daytime sleep is not usually accounted for (Kavey and Altshuler, 1979). It is common for patients to be referred to a sleep unit for an evaluation of sleep apnea that has been first identified after a surgical admission.

Table 9.19: Factors affecting sleep in surgical patients	
Extent and length of surgery	Presumably related to prolonged stress and tissue damage
Stress response	Increase in cortisol, norepinephrine and dopamine, which favor arousal
Inflammatory response IL-1 (interleukin-1) IL-6 (interleukin-6) TNF (tumour necrosis factor) GCSF (granulocyte colony stimulating factor)	The cytokines mediating the inflammatory response are known to affect sleep stage distribution, reducing REM sleep, and variable effect on slow-wave sleep
Post-operative pain, and reduced mobility	These factors are important in the first few days
Ward routine and noise	The noise can be as high as 80 dB (traffic noise)
Circadian rhythm disturbances	Poorly lit environment, loss of daily routine favor derangement of biological rhythms, including sleep and wake

Constant findings on EEG monitoring are the reduction of slow-wave sleep (SWS) and REM sleep, with rebound towards the end of the first week after surgery. In particular REM rebound may be responsible for postoperative nightmares, increased risk of obstructive sleep apnea (because of the increased hypotonia during REM), periods of hypoxemia which may lead, in predisposing individuals to increased risk of myocardial and brain ischemia, resulting in cardiac arrhythmia as well as a confusional state (ICU psychosis) (Gill *et al*, 1992; Rosenberg, 1991; Reeder *et al*, 1991).

ICU psychosis is seen in some patients after a few days in intensive care, characterized by confusion, agitation, hallucinations and paranoid ideation. Apart from the effect of the illness or surgical intervention which led to the ICU admission, sleep deprivation is considered to be a contributing factor to the syndrome (Helton *et al*, 1980). ICU psychosis appears to resolve spontaneously after the patient is discharged to more routine care.

The type of anesthesia does not appear to be a major determinant of sleep disturbance, but the extent and duration of surgery are related to sleep derangement, with some evidence that minimally intrusive techniques, such as laparoscopic surgery, lead to a more preserved sleep structure (Rosenberg, 2001). General anesthesia itself however, is associated with significant disruption in sleep length and structure in the first 24 hours with reduction of REM, stages 2, 3 and 4. These changes are more marked in the elderly (Lehmkuhl *et al*, 1987).

Postoperative pain is reported by the surgical patient to be perhaps the most important factor in disturbing their sleep. However, the best way to relieve postoperative discomfort is a subject of debate. Concern has been raised over the use of opioids, as morphine in healthy individuals is reported to reduce slow-wave and REM sleep. However, this data should not be extrapolated to medical or surgical patients, because a decrease in REM sleep and slow-wave sleep occur post-operatively independent from the use of opioids (Cronin *et al*, 2001). Clinical experience suggests that morphine is a very effective agent, at least subjectively, in patients with chronic, painful conditions and other medical syndromes, such as heart failure.

Surgical patients often report nightmares in the first week postoperatively, with highest incidence following cardiac surgery (27.9%) (Brimacombe, 1993). The sleep changes described in surgical patients also apply to the medical ward, particularly in subjects who have undergone acute events, such as ischemic stroke, myocardial infarct or trauma (Rosenberg, 2001).

The underlying pathophysiology of sleep and wake deregulation in hospital is multifactorial (*Table 9.18*). Despite being underestimated, circadian rhythm disorders are likely to be important. The amount of light exposure in hospital is variable and a clear distinction between day and night is sometimes completely lost. Other time givers, such as meal times and attendance to daily functions are usually dictated by rigid and patient-unfriendly routines, contributing to the alteration of circadian rhythms. Patients often experience either an advanced sleep phase or, more commonly, a delayed sleep phase, which would explain the common finding of patients sleeping late into the morning.

The fact that melatonin secretion is deranged in hospitalized patients (Baskett *et al*, 1991) and the recent observation that melatonin treatment improves the sleep quality of patients with exacerbations of chronic obstructive airway disease admitted to ICU (Shilo *et al*, 2000), would suggest that biological rhythm disturbances are important factors.

Management requires attention to the following points:

* medical and nursing education regarding sleep and wake in hospitalized patients
* adapting ward activities to benefit the patient, such as avoiding any routine activity before 7.00AM–8.00AM. For example, there is no reason to collect blood at 5.00AM to have the result

by 8.00AM–9.00AM for the convenience of the doctors, as happens in many ICUs. There is also no reason to start showering and taking routine measurements at 6.00AM when these could be done at 8.00AM

* proper lighting during the day and minimizing light and noise at night
* use of appropriate analgesia and hypnotic medications.

The use of sleeping tablets is prevalent in hospitalized patients either on a prn (as required) or on a regular basis (Berlin, 1984; Perry, 1984). It is important to note that the use of benzodiazepines is not associated with reports of improved sleep (Freter and Becker, 1999). The new group of non-benzodiazepines (zolpidem, zoplicone, and zaleplon) are less likely to impact on sleep structure, but they are not widely available in hospital because of cost. It is important to educate the patient to avoid hypnotic medications being continued at home as appears to be the case in 15–21% of patients discharged from hospital (Clift, 1975; Halfens *et al*, 1994).

References

Aldrich MS (1993) Insomnia in neurological diseases. *J Psychosom Res* **37**(suppl 1): 3–11

Alessi CA, Schnelle JFF (2000) Approach to sleep disorders in the nursing home setting. *Sleep Med Rev* **4**(1): 45–56

Ambrogetti A, Olson LG, Hensley MJ (1994) Sleep and breathing in asthma, cystic fibrosis and interstitial lung disease. In: Saunders, Sullivan, eds. Sleep and Breathing, 2nd edn. Marcel Dekker, New York

American Sleep Disorders Association (1997) *International Classification of Sleep Disorders revisited: Diagnostic and Coding manual.*ASDA, Rochester, Minnesota

Armitage R, Hoffman RF (2001) Sleep EEG, depression and gender. *Sleep Med Rev* **5**(3): 237–46

Auckley DH, Schmidt-Nowara W, Brown LK (1999) Reversal of sleep apnea hypopnea syndrome in end-stage renal disease after kidney transplantation. *Am J Kidney Dis* **34**(4): 739–44

Auer RN, Rowands CG, Perry SF, Remmers TF (1996) Multiple sclerosis with medullary plaques and fatal sleep apnea (Ondine's curse). *Clin Neuropath* **15**(2): 101–5

Ballinger CB (1976) Subjective sleep disturbance at the menopause. *J Psychosom Res* **20**: 509–13

Baskett JJ, Cockrem JF, Todd MA (1991) Melatonin levels in hospitalized elderly patients: A comparison with community based volunteers. *Age Ageing* **20**: 430–4

Berger M, Rieman D (1993) REM sleep in depression — an overview. *J Sleep Res* **2**: 211–23

Berlin RM (1984) Management of insomnia in hospitalized patients. *Ann Intern Med* **100**: 398–404

Bliwise DL (1997) Sleep and circadian rhythm disorders.In: Turek FW, Zee PC, eds. *Aging and Dementia in Regulation of Sleep and Circadian Rhythm*. Marcel Dekker, New York.

Bornstein N, Gur AY, Fainshtein P, Korczyn AD (1999) Stroke during sleep: Epidemiological and clinical features. *Cerebrovascular Dis* **9**: 320–2

Briggs GG, Samson JH, Crawford DJ (1975) Lack of abnormalities in a newborn exposed to amphetamine during gestation. *Am J Dis Child* **129**: 249–50

Brimacombe MB, Macfie AG (1993) Perioperative nightmares in surgical patients. *Anaesthesia* **48**: 527–9

Broughton R, Baron R (1978) Sleep patterns in the intensive care unit and on the ward after acute myocardial infarction. *Electroencephalogr Clin Neurophysiol* **45**: 348–60

Brown MA, Bowyer L, McHugh L, David GK, Mangos GJ, Jones M (2001) Twenty-four-hour automated blood pressure monitoring as a predictor of preeclampsia. *Am J Obstet Gynecol* **185**(3): 618–22

Brust JCM (1993) *Neurological Aspects of Substance Abuse*. Butterworth-Heineman, Boston

Clift AD (1975) Dependence of hypnotic drugs in general practice. In: Clift AD, ed. *Sleep Disturbance and Hypnotic Dependence*. Excerpt Medica, Amsterdam: 71–95

Coccagna G, Mantovani M, Parchi C, Mironi F, Lugaresi E (1975) Alveolar hypoventilation and hypersomnia in myotonic dystrophy. *J Neurol Neurosurg Psychiat* **3**: 977–84

Comella CL, Nardeine TM, Diedrich WJ, Stebbins GT (1998) Sleep-related violence, injury, and REM sleep behavior disorder in PD. *Neurology* **51**: 516–28

Cormick W, Olson GL, Hensley MJ, Saunders NA (1986) Nocturnal hypoxaemia and ability of sleep in patients with chronic obstructive lung disease. *Thorax* **41**: 846–54

Cronin AJ, Keifer JC, Davies MF, King TS, Bixler EO (2001) Postoperative sleep disturbance: influences of opioids and pain in humans. *Sleep* **24**(1): 39–44

Culebras A, ed (2000) *Sleep Disorders and Neurological Disease*. Marcel Dekker, New York

Dagan Y (2002) Circadian rhythm sleep disorders (CRSD). *Sleep Med Rev* **6**(1): 45–55

Darko DF, McCutchan JA, Kripke DF, Gillin JC, Golshan S (1992) Fatigue, sleep disturbance, disability, and indices of progression of HIV infection. *Am J Psychiatry* **149**(4): 514–20

Diederich NJ, Vaillant M, Mancuso G, Lyen P, Tiete J (2005) Progressive sleep 'destructuring' in Parkinson's disease. A polysomnographic study in 46 patients. *Sleep Med* **6**(4): 313–8

Dodick DW (2000) Polysomnography in hypnic headache syndrome. *Headache* **40**: 748–52

Dodick DW, Mosek AC, Campbell JK (1998) The hypnic ('alarm clock') headache syndrome. *Cephalalgia* **18**: 152–6

Douglass AB, Hays P, Pazderka F, Russell JM (1991) Floris refractory schizophrenias that turn out to be treatable variants of HLA-associated narcolepsy. *J Neur Ment Dis* **179**: 12–17

Dursum SM, Patel JK, Burke JG, Reveley MA (1999) Effects of typical antipsychotic drugs and risperidone on the quality of sleep in patients with schizophrenia: a pilot study. *J Psychiat Neurosci* **24**(4): 333–7

Edwards N, Blyton DM, Kirjavainen T, Kesby GJ, Sullivan CE (2000) Nasal continuous positive airway pressure reduces sleep-induced blood pressure increments in preeclampsia. *Am J Respir Crit Care Med* **162**(1): 252–7

Ekholm EMK, Polo O, Rauhala ER, Ekblad UU (1992) Sleep quality in pre-eclampsia. *Am J Obstet Gynecol* **167**: 1262–6

Elliott WJ (2001) Cyclic and circadian variations in cardiovascular events. *Am J Hypertens* **14**(9, supple 1): S291–S295

Eriksson M, Larsson G, Winbladh B, Zetterstrom R (1978) The influence of amphetamine addiction on pregnancy and the newborn infant. *Acta Paediatr Scand* **67**: 95–9

Epstein LJ, Strollo PJ, Donegan RB, Jr, Delmar J, Hendrix C, Westbrook PR *et al* (1995) Obstructive sleep apnea in patients with human immunodeficiency virus (IV) disease. *Sleep* **18**(5): 368–76

Fast A, Hertz G (1992) Nocturnal low back pain in pregnancy: polysomnographic correlates. *Am J Reprod Immunol* **28**: 251–53

Feinberg I, Hiott JF (1978) *Sleep Patterns in Schizophrenia: A Selective Review in Sleep Disorders, Diagnosis and Treatment.* Williams RL, Daracan I, eds. John Wiley and Sons, New York

Ferini-Strambi L, Oldani A *et al* (1995) Slow-wave sleep and cyclic alternating pattern (CAP) in HIV-infected asymptomatic men. *Sleep* **18**(6): 446–50

Fletcher EC (1993) Obstructive sleep apnea and the kidney. *J Am Soc Nephrol* **4**: 1111–21

Franklin KA, Holmgren PA, Jonsson F, Poromaa N, Stenlund H, Svanborg E (2000) Snoring, pregnancy-induced hypertension, and growth retardation of the fetus. *Chest* **117**(1): 137–41

Freter SH, Becker MR (1999) Predictors of restful sleep in a rehabilitation hospital. *Am J Phys Med Rehabil* **78**(6): 552–6

Frucht S, Rogers JD, Greene JD Gordon PE, Fahn S (1999) Falling asleep at the wheel: Motor vehicle mishaps in persons taking pramipexole and ropinirole. *Neurology* **52**: 1908–10

Garcia-Borreguero DC, Schwarz *et al* (2003) L-DOPA-induced excessive daytime sleepiness in PD: a placebo-controlled case with MSLT assessment. *Neurology* **61**(7): 1008–10

Gibson PG (1990) Corticosteroids — clinical applications: exacerbations of asthma in adults. *Austral Prescrib* **19**(2):44–7

Gill NP, Wright B, Reilly CS (1992) Relationship between hypoxaemic and cardiac ischaemic events in the perioperative period. *Br J Anaesth* **68**: 471–3

Girault C, Muir JF, Mihaltan F, Borderies P, de la Gicleis B, Verdure A *et al* (1996) Effects of repeated administration of zolpidem on sleep, diurnal and nocturnal respiratory function, vigilance and physical performance in patients with COPD. *Chest* **119**: 1203–11

Halfens R, Cox K, Kuppen-Van Merwijk A (1994) Effect of use of sleep medication in Dutch hospitals on the use of sleep medication at home. *J Adv Nurs* **19**(1): 66–70

Hanly P, Gabor J, Pierratos A (2002) Daytime sleepiness in patients with end-stage renal disease — impact of nocturnal hemodialysis. 8th International Symposium on Sleep and Breathing, Reykjavik, Iceland

Hedman C, Pohjasvaara T, Tolonen U, Suhonen-Malm AS, Myllyla VV (2002) Effects of pregnancy on mothers' sleep. *Sleep Med* **3**: 37–42

Hefez A, Metz L, Lavie P (1987) Long-term effects of extreme situational stress on sleep and dreaming. *Am J Psychiat* **144**: 344–7

Helton MC, Gordon SH, Nunnery SL (1980) The correlation between sleep deprivation and the intensive care syndrome. *Heart and Lung* **9**: 464–8

Hermida RC, Ayala DE, Mojon A, Fernandez JR, Silva I, Ucieda R, Iglesias M (1977) High sensitivity test for the early diagnosis of gestational hypertension and preeclampsia. I. Predictable variability of cardiovascular characteristics during gestation in healthy and hypertensive women. *J Perinat Med* **25**: 101–9

Hermida RD, Ayala DE, Mojon A, Iglesias M (1997) High sensitivity test for the early diagnosis of gestational hypertension and preeclampsia. II. Circadian blood pressure variability in healthy and hypertensive pregnancy women. *J Perinat Med* **25**: 153–67

Hui DS, Wong TY, Ko FW, Li TS, Choy DK, Wong KK *et al* (2000) Prevalence of sleep disturbances in Chinese patients with end-stage renal failure on continuous ambulatory peritoneal dialysis. *Am Kidney Dis* **36**(4): 783–8

Ivafiez V, Soler R, Barriers P (1998) Hypnic headache syndrome; a case with good response to indomethacin. *Cephalalgia* **18**: 225–6

Joel-Cohen SJ, Schoenfeld A (1978) Fetal response to periodic sleep apnea: a new syndrome in obstetrics. *J Obstet, Gynec Reprod Biol*, 8(2): 77–81

Johns MW, Egan P, Gay TJA, Masterton JP (1970) Sleep habits and symptoms in male medical and surgical patients. *Br Med J* **2**: 509–12

Kavey NB, Altshuler KZ (1979) Sleep in herniorrhaphy patients. *Am J Surg* **138**(5): 682–7

Kayed K, Godtlibsen OB, Sjaastad O (1978) Chronic paroxysmal hemicrania IV: 'REM sleep locked' nocturnal headache attacks. *Sleep* **1**: 91–5

Keshavan MS, Tandon R (1993) Sleep abnormalities in schizophrenia: pathophysiological significance. *Psycholog Med* **23**: 831–5

Kittur S, Hauser P (1999) Improvement of sleep and behavior by methylphenidate in Alzheimer's disease. *Am J Psychiat* **156**: 7

Kowall J, Clark, G, Non-Murcia G, Powell N (1989) Precipitation of obstructive sleep apnea in pregnancy. *Obstet Gynecol* **74**: 543

Kraus M, Hambuger RJ (1997) Sleep apnea in renal failure. *Adv Peritoneal Dialysis* **13**: 88–92

Kuhlmann U, Becker HG, Birkhahn M *et al* (2000) Sleep-apnea in patients with end-stage renal disease and objective results. *Clin Nephrol* **53**(6): 460–6

Kuhn M, Lutolf M, Reinhart WH (1999) The eye catecher: Ondine's curse. *Respiration* **66**: 265

Kupfer DJ, Thase ME (1987) The use of sleep laboratory in the diagnosis of affective disorders diagnosis and treatment of affective sleep disorders. *Psychiatr Clin N Am* **10**(4): 3–250

Landau ME, Maldonado JY, Jabbari B (2005). The effects of isolated brainstem lesions on human REM sleep. *Sleep Med* **6**(1): 37–40

Landolt HP, Gillin JC (2001) Sleep abnormalities during abstinence in alcohol-dependent patients. *CNS Drugs* **15**(5):413–25

Langevin B, Fouque D, Leger P, Robert D(1993) Sleep apnea syndrome and end-stage renal disease. Cure after renal transplantation. *Chest* **103**(5): 1330–5

Larson JP, Tandberg E (2001) Sleep disorders in patient with PD epidemiology and management. *CNS Drugs* **15**(4): 267–75

Lehmkuhl P, Prass D, Pichlmayr I (1987) General anesthesia and postnarcotic sleep disorders. *Neuropsychobiology* **18**: 37–42

Linazasoro G, Martí Massó JF, Suárez JA (1993) Nocturnal akathisia in Parkinson's disease: Treatment with clozapine. *Movement Disorders* **8**(2): 171–4

Little BB, Snell LM, Gilstrap LC III (1988) Methamphetamine abuse during pregnancy: outcome and fetal Effects. *Obstet Gynecol* **72**(4): 541–4

Loube D, Poceta JS, Morales MC, Peacock MD, Mitler MM (1996) Self-reported snoring in pregnancy association with fetal outcome. *Chest* **109**(4): 885–9

Lugaresi E, Provini F (2001) Agrypnia exitata: clinical features and pathophysiological implications. *Sleep Med Rev* **5**(4): 313–22

Maixner S, Tendon R, Eiser A, Taylor S, DeQuardo JR, Shipley J (1998) Effects of antipsychotic treatment on polysomnographic measures in schizophrenia; a replication and extension. *Am J Psychiat* **155**(11): 1600–2

Manabe K, Matsui T, Yamada M, Sato-Nakagawa T, Okamura N, Arai H, Sasaki H (2000) Sleep patterns and mortality among elderly patients in a geriatric hospital. *Gerontology* **46**(6): 318–22

Mant A, Saunders NA, Eland AE, Pond CD, Chancellor AH, Webster IW (1988) Sleep-related respiratory disturbance and dementia in elderly female. *J Gerontol* **43**: 140–4

Mathew NT (1992) Cluster headache. *Neurology* **42**(suppl 2): 22–31

Mellman TA, Kulick-Bell R, Aslock LE, Nolan B (1995) Sleep events among veterans with combat-related post traumatic stress disorder. *Am J Psychiat* **152**(1): 110–15

Mellman TA, Nolan B, Hebding J, Kulick-Bell R, Dominguez R (1997) A polysomnographic comparison of veterans with combat-related PTSD, depressed men and non-ill controls. *Sleep* **20**(1): 46–51

Mendelson WB, Wadhwa NK, Greenberg HE, Gujavarty K, Bergofsky E (1990) Effects of hemodialysis of sleep apnea syndrome in end-stage renal disease. *Clin Nephrol* **33**(5): 247–51

McCurry, Arendt J (2000) In what circumstances is melatonin a useful sleep therapy? Consensus statement, WFSRS Focus Group, Dresden, November 1999. *J Sleep Res* **9**: 397–8

Milkovich L, van den Berg BJ (1977) Effects of antenatal exposure to anorectic drugs. *Am J Obstet Gynecol* **129**: 637

Milross MA, Piper AJ, Dobbin CJ, Bye PTP, Grunstein RR (2004) Sleep disorder breathing in cystic fibrosis. *Sleep Med Rev* **8**(4): 295–308

Moeller AA, Oechsner M *et al* (1991) Self-reported sleep quality in HIV infection: corrlation to the stage of infection and zidovudine therapy. *J Acq Immune Defic Syndr* **4**(10): 1000–3

Moline ML, Broch L *et al* (2003) Sleep in women across the life cycle from adulthood through menopause. *Sleep Med Rev* **7**(2): 155–77

Morley JE (1993) Nocturnal agitation in sleep disorders and insomnia in the elderly. In: Roth T, Morley JH, eds. *Facts and Research in Gerontology Vol 7*. Serdi Publishers, Paris

Norman SE, Chediak AD, Kiel M, Cohn MA (1990) Sleep disturbances in HIV-infected homosexual men. *Aids* **4**(8): 775–81

Norman SE, Chediak AD, Freeman C, Kiel M, Mendez A, Duncan R *et al* (1992) Sleep disturbances in men with asymptomatic human immunodeficiency (HIV) infection. *Sleep.* **15**(2): 150–5

Olson LG, King MT, Hensley MJ, Saunders NA (1995) A community study of snoring and sleep-disordered breathing: symptoms. *Am J Respir Crit Care Med* **152**: 707–10

O'Toole BI, Marshall RP, Grayson DA, Schureck RI, Dobson M, French M *et al* (1996) The Australian Vietnam Veterans Health Study: III. Psychological Health of Australian Vietnam Veterans and its Relationship to Combat International. *J Epidemiol* **25**(2): 331–9

Nokes KM, Kendrew J (1996) Sleep quality in people with HIV disease. *J Assoc Nurses AIDS Care* **7**(3): 43–50

Pal S, Bhattacharya F, Agapito C. Chandhuri KR (2001) A study of excessive daytime sleepiness and its clinical significance in these groups of PD patients taking pramipexole, carbergoline and levodopa mono and combination therapy. *J Neurol Trans* **108**: 71–7

Pearce JM (1989) Clinical features of the exploding head syndrome. *J Neurol Neurosurg Psychiat* **52**: 907–10

Perry SW, Wu A (1984) Rationale for the use of hypnotic agents in a general hospital. *Ann Intern Med* **100**: 441–6

Pfister M, Jakob SM, Marti HP, Frey FJ, Gugger M (1999) Ambulatory nocturnal oximetry and sleep questionnaire-based findings in 38 patients with end-stage renal disease. *Nephrol Dial Transplant* **14**: 1496–1502

Phillips KD (1999)Physiological and pharmacological factors of insomnia in HIV disease. *J Assoc Nurses AIDS Care* **10**(5): 93–7

Poirier G, Montplaisir J, Dumont M, Duquette P, Decary R, Pleines J, Lamoureux G (1987) Clinical and sleep laboratory study of narcoleptic symptoms in multiple sclerosis. *Neurology* **37**: 693–5

Polo-Kantola P, Saaresranta T, Polo O (2001) Aetiology and treatment of sleep disturbances during perimenopause and postmenopause. *CNS Drugs* **15**(6): 445–52

Pond CD, Mant A, Eyland EA, Saunders NA (1990) Dementia and abnormal breathing during sleep. *Age Ageing* **19**(4): 247–52

Pressman MR, Benz RL, Schleifer CR, Peterson DD (1993) Sleep disordered breathing in ESRD: Acute beneficial effects of treatment with nasal continuous positive airway pressure. *Kidney Int* **43**: 1134–9

Purdie DW, Empson JA, Crichton C, Macdonald L (1995) Hormone replacement therapy, sleep quality and psychological wellbeing. *Br J Obstet Gynaecol* **22**: 735–9

Reeder MK, Muir AD, Foex P, Goldman MD, Loh L, Smart D (1991) Postoperative myocardial ischaemia: temporal association with nocturnal hypoxaemia. *Br J Anaesth* **67**: 626–31

Reichenmiller HE, Reinhard U, Durr F (1971) Electroenceph. *Clin Neurophysiol* **30**: 255–74

Rodnitzky RL (2000) Parkinson's disease and extrapyramidal disorders in sleep disorders and neurological disease. In: Culebras A, ed. *Sleep Disorders and Neurological Disease*. Marcel Dekker, New York

Roehrs T, Roth T (2001) Sleep, sleepiness, sleep disorders and alcohol use and abuse. *Sleep Med Rev* **5**(4): 287–97

Rosenberg J (2001) Sleep disturbances after non-cardiac surgery. *Sleep Med Rev* **5**(2): 129–37

Ross RJ, Ball WA, Sullivan KA, Caroff SN (1989) Sleep disturbances as the hallmark of post-traumatic stress disorder. *Am J Psychiat* **146**: 697–707

Ross JR, Ball AW, Dinges DF, Kribbs NB, Morrison AR, Silver SM, Mulvaney FD (1994) Motor dysfunction during sleep in post-traumatic stress disorder. *Sleep* **17**(8): 723–32

Sachs C, Svanborg E (1991) The exploding head syndrome: polysomnographic recordings and therapeutic suggestions. *Sleep* **14**(3): 263–6

Sahota DP, Dexter JD (1993) Transient recurrent situational insomnia associated with cluster headache. *Sleep* **16**(3): 255–7

Salin-Pascual RJ, Herrera-Estrella M, Galicia-Polo L, Lanrrabaquio MR (1999) Olanzapine acute administration in schizophrenic patients increases delta sleep and sleep efficiency. *Biol Psychiat* **46**(1): 141–3

Sandyk R (1995) The pineal gland, cataplexy and multiple sclerosis. *Int J Neurosci* **83**(3–4): 153–63

Santiago JR, Nolledo MS, Kinzler W, Santiago TV (2001) Sleep and sleep disorders in pregnancy. *Ann Intern Med* **134**: 396–408

Saunders J, Whitham R, Schanmann B, Portland OR (1991) Sleep disturbance, fatigue and depression in multiple sclerosis. *Neurology* **41**(suppl 1): 320

Schiff I, Regestein Q, Tulchinsky D, Tyan KJ (1979) Effects of estrogens on sleep and psychological state of hypogonadal women. *JAMA* **242**: 2305–407

Schrader H, Godlibsen OB, Skomedal GN (1980) Multiple sclerosis and narcolepsy–cataplexy in monozygotic twin. *Neurology* **30**: 105–8

Schweiger MS (1972) Sleep disturbance in pregnancy. A subjective survey. *Am J Obstet Gynecol* **114**(7): 879–82

Severinghaus JW, Mitchell RA (1962) Ondine's curse-failure of respiratory centre automaticity while awake. *Clin Res* **10**: 122

Shamir E, Landon M, Barek Y, Anis Y, Rotemberg V, Elizur A, Zisapel N (2000) Melatonin improves sleep quality of patients with chronic schizophrenia. *J Clin Psychiat* **61**(5): 373–7

Shilo L, Dagan Y, Smorjik Y, Weinberg U, Dolev S, Komptel B, Shenkman L (2000) Effect of melatonin on sleep quality of COPD intensive care patients: a pilot study. *Chronobiol Int* **17**(1): 71–6

Shochat T, Martin J, Marler M, Ancoli-Israel S (2000) Illumination levels in nursing home patients: effects on sleep and activity rhythms. *J Sleep Res* **9**: 373–9

Smith MC, Ellgring H, Oertel WH (1997) Sleep disturbances in PD and spouses. *J Am Geriatr Soc* **45**: 194–9

Smolensky MH, D'Alonzo GE (1997) Progress in the chronotherapy of nocturnal asthma. In: Redfern PH, Lemmer B, eds. *Physiology and Pharmacology of Biolotical Rhythms.* Springer, Berlin

Southwick MS, Paige S, Morgan III CA, Bremmer JD, Krystal JH, Charney DS (1999) Neurotransmitter alterations in PTSD: catecholamines and serotonin. *Semin Clin Neuropsychiat* **4**(4): 242–8

Spath-Schwalbe E, Hansen K, Schmidt F, Schrezenmeier H, Marshall L, Burger K *et al* (1998) Acute effects of recombinant human interleukin-6 on endocrine and central nervous sleep functions in healthy men. *J Clin Endorinol Metab* **83**: 1573–9

Stepanski E, Basner R, Faber M, Zorick F, Roth T (1995) Sleep disorders in patients on continuous ambulatory peritoneal dialysis. *J Am Soc Nephrol* **6**: 192–7

Stradling JR, Chadwick GA, Frew AJ (1985) Changes in ventilation and its components in normal subjects during sleep. *Thorax* **40**: 364–70

Taphoorn MJ, van Someren E, Snoek FJ, Stijers RL, Swaab DF, Visscher F, de Vaal CP *et al* (1993) Fatigue, sleep disturbances and circadian rhythm in multiple sclerosis. *J Neurol* **240**: 446–8

Thomson J, Oswald I (1977) Effect of oestrogen on the sleep, mood, and anxiety of menopausal women. *Br Med J* **2**: 1317–19

Van der Meche FGA, Boogaard JM, van der Berg BV (1986) Treatment of hypersomnolence in myotonic dystrophy with CNS stimulant. *Muscle Nerve* **9**: 341–4

Vitiello VM, Borson S (2001) Sleep disturbances in patients with Alzheimer's disease. Epidemiology, pathophysiology and treatment. *CNS Drugs* **15**(10): 777–96

Vitiello MV, Prinz PN, Personius JP, Nuccio MA, Keorker RM, Scurfield R (1990) Night-time hypoxemia is increased in abstaining chronic alcoholic men. *Alcohol Clin Exp Res* **14**(1): 38–41

Wadhwa NK, Mendelson WB (1992) A comparison of sleep-disordered respiration in ESRD patients receiving hemodialysis and peritoneal dialysis. *Adv Peritoneal Dialysis* **8**: 195–8

Wadhwa NK, Selinger M, Greenberg HE, Bergofsky E, Mendelson WB (1992) Sleep-related respiratory disorders in end-stage renal disease patients on peritoneal dialysis. *Peritoneal Dialysis Int* **12**: 52–6

Weitzenblum E, Chaouat A (2004) Sleep and chronic obstructive airway disease. *Sleep Med Rev* **8**(4): 281–94

White DP, Douglas NJ, Pickett CK, Zwillich CW, Weil JV (1983) Sleep deprivation and the control of ventilation. *Am Rev Respir Dis* **128**: 984–6

Winkelmann J, Stautner A, Samtleben W, Trenkwalder C (2002) Long-term course of restless legs syndrome in dialysis patients after kidney transplantation. *Move Disord* **17**(5): 1072–6

Wirz-Justice A, Cajochen C, Nussbaum P (1997) A schizophrenic patient with an arrhythmic circadian rest-activity cycle. *Psychiatry Res* **73**: 83–90

Wirz-Justice A, Werth E, Savaskan E, Knoblanch V, Fontana Gasio P, Muller-Span F (2000) Haloperidol disrupts, clozapine reinstates the circadian rest–activity cycle in a patient with early-onset Alzheimer's disease. *Alzheim Dis Assoc Disord* **14**(4): 212–15

Yeomans JS (1995) Role of tegmental cholinergic neurons in dopaminergic activation, antimuscarinic psychosis and schizophrenia. *Neuropsychopharmacology* **12**: 3–16

Yinnon AM, Ilan Y, Tadmor B, Altarescu G, Hershko C (1992) Quality of sleep in the medical department. *Br J Clin Pract* **46**(2): 88–91

Yokota T, Hirose K, Tanabe H, Tsukagoshi H (1991) Sleep-related periodic leg movements (nocturnal myoclonus) due to spinal cord lesion. *J Neurol Sci* **104**(1): 13–18

Zesiewicz TA, Hauser RA (2000) Depression in patients with PD. Epidemiology, pathophysiology and treatment options. *CNS Drugs* **13**(4): 253–64

CHAPTER 10

Sleep disorders in children

Karen Waters and Antonio Ambrogetti

Introduction

Sleep-associated disorders may arise through interactions with behavioral or physiological functions. Disorders of sleep, or medical disorders associated with sleep, are common during childhood. Primary clinicians need to recognize and understand the characteristics and appropriate intervention strategies that are now available for most pediatric sleep disorders.

Surveys show that 10–20% of parents believe that their children have sleep problems, yet only half of those parents had discussed these problems with their family doctor (Mindell *et al*, 1999; Stein *et al*, 2001). In addition, sleep-related disorders have not been included in most formal medical education programmes (Owens, 2001).

This chapter provides descriptions and case studies of several common sleep problems, including how physiological or pathophysiological disturbances interact with sleep. The presentations, differential diagnoses and management strategies for common clinical sleep disorders are provided with management guidelines for common sleep-associated disorders.

Clinical evaluation of paediatric sleep problems

Assessment of a child's sleep should include taking a detailed history, examination of the child and, when appropriate, sleep investigations.

Sleep history

Important features of the clinical history for infants and children presenting with sleep-associated problems include, evaluation of the development of the circadian cycle, features of the sleep environment, sleep onset, and characteristics of any arousals that are causing concern. Behavior during wakefulness and surrounding sleep times should be evaluated, along with the medical and family history. A thorough history will generally distinguish problems requiring additional medical investigations or interventions. If medical and psychosocial problems are excluded, sleep problems amenable to simple behavioral management strategies, and the points where management interventions can alleviate them, can usually be diagnosed on history (*Table 10.1*).

Table 10.1: Sleep history

Circadian
Sleep log x 2 weeks (time in bed, sleep onset, wake time) for weekday and weekend
24-hour daily schedule (school, work, meals, play)
Amount of light in room
Seasonal variations

Sleep environment
Describe bedroom (What is in it? Who is there? How much natural light is there? Television? Radio?)

Sleep onset
How does the child fall asleep?
Who is present at sleep onset and what do they do?
Are there curtain calls, fears, hypnagogic hallucinations, sleep-onset paralysis, restless legs?
Head banging? Body rocking?

Arousals
Time of night
Triggers
Description of arousal
Level of agitation/ambulation
Associated with eating/drinking
Level of consciousness
Duration
Associated with injury
How does arousal terminate?
How does child return to sleep?
Frequency
Recall the next day
Age of onset

Other sleep behavior
Seizures, enuresis, diaphoresis, restlessness, snoring, cough, choking, apnea, periodic movements of sleep, vomiting, nightmares, bruxism

Waking behavior
Hypnopompic hallucinations, paralysis, headaches

Daytime sleep
Naps, cataplexy, excessive daytime sleepiness

Table 10.1: Sleep history

Medical

Neurologic: migraine headaches, attention deficit disorder, seizures, tics, mental retardation, narcolepsy, neuromuscular disease

Psychiatric: depression, anxiety, dissociative disorders, conduct disorder, panic disorder, physical/sexual abuse

Ear, nose, throat: ear infections, ear effusions, daytime airway nasal obstruction, sinusitis streptococci infections, swallowing problems

Cardiorespiratory: asthma, cough, heat disease pneumonia

Gastrointestinal: vomiting, diarrhea, constipation, feeding problems

Growth: failure to thrive

Allergies: milk, seasonal, asthma, eczema

Drug: legal/illegal

School behavior: behavioral problems, school/developmental problems

Acute medical illness

Family history

Sleep apnea/snoring

Arousals (sleep-walking, confusional arousals, night terrors, restless legs/periodic movements)

Psychiatric disease (depression)

Social issues (stress at home, divorce, family violence, drug/ETOH use)

Narcolepsy, hypersomnolence

Restless leg syndrome

Additional features of the history relating to sleep problems include documentation of a child's sleep patterns using a sleep diary (sleep log) to evaluate circadian rhythm disturbances. Bedtime rituals are repeated behaviors that preceed sleep onset. Assessing the sleep environment includes establishing how and where the child falls asleep, and the bedtime rituals, including interactions between the child and parents (or primary carer) around sleep onset. Sample questions include: 'Is bedtime preceded by behaviors that encourage relaxation such as bath and story telling?' 'Is the child put to bed asleep or awake?' 'Does the child require the presence of a parent to fall asleep?' 'Do the parents pat, rock, or feed the infant while (s)he is falling asleep?'

After sleep onset, the characteristics of any wakening should clarify whether arousals or behavioral issues surrounding the subsequent sleep onset are causing distress. Parental expectations regarding sleep patterns may underlie the presentation and there may be a need for education rather than intervention. If behavioral problems extend into the daytime, consideration should be given as to whether these represent issues requiring comprehensive psychological review, including other problems within the family.

Examination

General physical and psychomotor development should be assessed in all children, including accurate measurement of growth parameters and exclusion of other physical conditions relevant to the presentation. Sleep disruption may be caused by physical problems, particularly sleep-disordered breathing, so the examination should include attention to upper airway morphology.

An ear, nose and throat (ENT) examination should always be included, seeking evidence of current or past middle ear infections, and signs of airway obstruction when awake or asleep in the consulting room. A small, or compromised upper airway may be caused by soft tissue or bony abnormalities. Soft tissue signs include poor nasal airflow usually due to adenoidal hypertrophy or tonsillar enlargement on direct visualization. Bony abnormalities include a small mid-face, a high-arched palate, or abnormal bite (whether this is due to a small maxilla or small mandible). Other problems that may underlie or compound respiratory and airway abnormalities, include atopic illness, particularly rhinitis and asthma, specific syndromes, and neuromuscular abnormalities.

Sequelae of OSA can include palatal petechiae and/or edema, Harrison's sulci, and signs of insulin resistance, such as acanthosis nigricans. Cardiac and respiratory assessment may reveal concomitant conditions, such as asthma, esophageal reflux or valvular heart disease which may mimic symptoms of sleep apnea or be a complication of it. Blood pressure should also be taken to exclude hypertension.

Normal development of sleep states and the sleep–wake cycle

Sleep state maturation is closely linked to conceptional age (*Figure 10.1*). Biological rhythms are documented in the fetus and by the third trimester of pregnancy two sleep stages are identifiable: active sleep (AS) predominates and is characterized by irregular respiratory effort, motor activity and eye movements; quiet sleep (QS) is characterized by regular breathing and the absence of motor activity (Meirs, 1994).

At birth, a sleep and wake rhythm of 3–4 hours is normal and associated with feeding episodes (Kleitman, 1987; McGraw *et al*, 1999; Meier-Koll *et al*, 1978). At this age, three sleep stages are distinguished using behavioral and/or physiological criteria: active sleep (AS), quiet sleep (QS) and indeterminate sleep (IS) (Anders and Keener, 1985). Behavioral features of AS continue to include irregular respiratory effort, motor activity, and eye movements.

Physiologically, AS is characterized by mixed frequency, low-amplitude electroencephalogram (EEG) and reduced postural muscle tone that is measured under the chin as submental electromyogram (EMG). Behavioral features of QS continue to include regular breathing and absence of both motor activity and eye movements, with physiological monitoring showing low frequency, high-amplitude EEG. Indeterminate sleep is a transition phase that may include behavioral and physiological features of AS and/or QS.

The first 6 months of postnatal life are characterized by rapid maturation of all cerebral functions, reflected in the maturation of sleep-wake cycles (de Veerd and Van den Bossche, 2003). The proportion of time spent in AS decreases, while QS continues to increase. After 6 months of age, rapid eye movement (REM) replaces AS, mature slow-wave sleep (SWS) replaces QS and mature stage 1 and 2 (light non-REM) sleep replace IS (intermediate sleep).

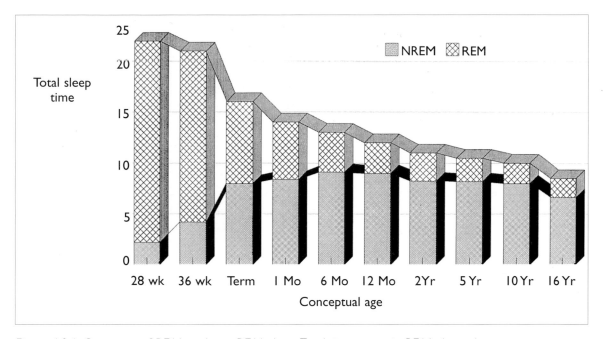

Figure 10.1: Ontogeny of REM and non-REM sleep. Total time spent in REM sleep decreases considerably throughout infancy and early childhood. By 3–5 years of age the adult level of about 25% of the total sleep time is reached (From Sheldon et al, 1992).

During early infancy circadian (24-hour) rhythms mature in a sequential manner. Body temperature rhythms appear first, followed by melatonin secretion, wakefulness, and then sleep rhythms (McGraw *et al*, 1999). Circadian sleep-wake cycles are usually well established by 16 weeks of age but there is large variability between individuals, and a circadian sleep-wake rhythm has been documented as early as 30 days (Kleitman, 1987; McGraw *et al*, 1999; Tomioko and Tomioko, 1991). Social cues, such as regularity of sleep opportunities and feeds contribute to the reinforcement of this 24-hour cycle (Kleitman, 1987) (*Figure 10.2*).

Clinically important features of sleep-wake cycle development include:

❖ The circadian wakefulness rhythm which can be distinguished before the sleep rhythm. This wake rhythm may be essential to establishing a proper sleep pattern, and derangement of this wake (circasemidian) pattern may contribute to sleep disturbances.

❖ Photic (light/dark) stimulation is an important determinant of the sleep–wake cycle (*Chapter 2*).

However wakefulness may be prolonged in response to social cues, such as interaction with family members for infants, or with peers during adolescence.

Night wakenings are normal. Several brief wakenings are normal during night sleep. Most infants re-establish sleep without any parental intervention ('self-soothers') (Anders and Keener, 1985; Anders *et al*, 1992; Wolfson, 1996). By one year of age, 60–70% of children have developed the ability to settle back to sleep spontaneously.

The polyphasic sleep pattern of young children includes a prolonged night period and distinct daytime episodes, so daytime naps are normal during early childhood. Morning naps disappear first, at 15–24 months of age, but approximately 12% of 7-year-olds still have a daytime nap (Weissbluth, 1995).

Common sleep problems

Behavioral sleep problems

The prevalence of difficulty falling asleep, bedtime struggles and night awakenings is variably reported between 6% and 15% in young children of school age, and becomes a persistent problem lasting more than 12 months in approximately 50% (Owens *et al*, 2000; Smedje *et al*, 2001).

Case study 1 — infant

Andrew presents at 6 months of age with a history of night-waking, and difficulty in settling. As he gets older, Andrew's episodes of awakening have become more prolonged and he is increasingly difficult to settle. His mother is physically exhausted because Andrew wakes with bouts of crying 2–3 times every night, and three to four times a week he will only settle after his mother drives him around in the car for about 30 minutes.

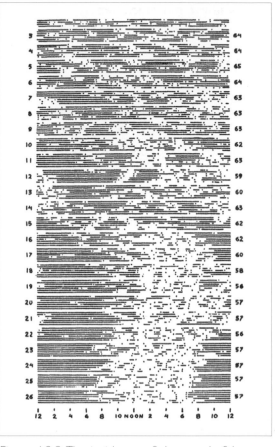

Figure 10.2: The incidence of sleep, wakefulness, and feeding in an infant, from the 11th to the 182nd day of life. Each line represents a 24-hour calendar day. The lines are sleep periods, measured to the nearest 5 minutes; the breaks in the lines, wakefulness; the dots, feedings. Each group of seven lines is separated from adjacent groups by a double space. The weeks are indicated on the left; percentages of time spent in sleep during the successive weeks, on the right; in 2-hourly intervals, at the bottom (from Kleitman, 1987).

Andrew was born at 36 weeks following a normal pregnancy; was breast-fed for 4 weeks and then changed to bottle feeds for maternal (non-medical) reasons. His growth and psychomotor development have been consistently normal. He has woken during the night from early infancy, but would initially settle to sleep with feeding and rocking. When he was 3 months old, the family were told that Andrew was a 'colicky baby' and his behavior would improve as he got older. The parents abandoned attempts to let Andrew cry himself to sleep (controlled crying), because he became so distressed and they were concerned for his well-being. The parents are not happy to use medication.

Case study 2 — older child

Ben was referred at 9 years of age. He has a diagnosis of ADHD and has also been noted to snore, with restless sleep since the age of 7 years. Ben's current sleep history includes bedtime between 9.30PM and 10.30PM, with sleep onset usually 1 hour after that. On school days he is woken between 7.00AM and 7.30AM and is slow to get up. On weekends, or if not disturbed, he sleeps until 8.30AM or 9.00AM. His sleep is restless and he keeps a light on in his room all night. Since he sleeps in his own room, his parents are unsure about his breathing when he is asleep. He has no history of sleep-walking or sleep-talking. He still wets the bed 2–3 times a week. He denies daytime sleepiness and his school performance is borderline.

Ben was born at term with no perinatal problems. However, he suffered viral meningitis at the age of 3, bronchiolitis at the age of 5, and currently has mild asthma requiring no regular medication. He had heavy breathing during sleep as a toddler, and his mother reports witnessing apneas at that time. His current medication is methylphenidate (10 mg), three tablets at breakfast, two at lunch time, and one at 4.00PM.

On examination, Ben's height is 140 cm but he is overweight at 46 kg and his BMI is 2.5 standard deviations above normal. He has no nasal obstruction but does have a high-arched palate and an inverted bite. Blood pressure is 100/65. His pharynx is mildly inflamed, with the tonsils occupying 50% of the oropharyngeal space.

Management of sleep infant disturbance

A useful mnemonic for approaching behavioral problems of infants and children is to address 'fact, tact and then act' (France *et al*, 1996).

❖ *Facts:* includes full elucidation of the problem, including prior advice the family have received, regardless of the source, ie. relatives, magazines, books, or electronic media, such as the Internet. This should be followed by education and explanation of that problem to the parent(s).
❖ *Tact*: is required because children's sleep disturbances can be associated with high emotional loads, guilt, and can sometimes be compounded by, or symptomatic of, other conflicts within the families.
❖ *Act(ion):* is the final process, when parents become involved in altering their behaviors towards the infant or child to achieve and reinforce new patterns. This may include reduced intervention when their child cries, or a more structured approach to sleep onset.

Table 10.2: Facts and beliefs about children and sleep

Belief	Facts
Infant sleep disturbance is normal and inevitable	
Most babies wake at night	Sleep disturbance is related to behavior upon awakening — not awakening *per se*
Infant sleep disturbance is so frequent it cannot be a disorder	Help-seeking is related to severity of infant sleep disturbance Any behavior problem can become maladaptive Relief of infant sleep disturbance may relieve associated problems
Infant sleep disturbance should be accommodated in Western and in non-Western families	
Co-sleeping is natural and adaptive Western expectations about infant behavior are unreasonable	Ethnic differences in sleeping practices have not been well established or explained; true comparisons are difficult to make
Co-sleeping is a way to cope with infant sleep disturbance	Co-sleeping is not a solution to infant sleep disturbance for many families
Infant sleep disturbance reflects a need state	
Human infants share with other mammals a need to wake and feed at night	Night feeding of healthy infants, after 6 months of age, is not a developmental need
Infants who cry at night need more nurturing	Parents of sleep-disturbed infants are at least as nurturing as other parents
Management techniques based on extinction are harmful	
Systematic ignoring may be harmful	Only positive effects have been reported following unmodified systematic ignoring
Systematic ignoring goes against parents 'instincts'	Systematic ignoring is regularly used by parents, regardless of advice, and often incorrectly

Education

The tactful provision of educational information about normal infant sleep aims to achieve:

- reassurance and reduced anxiety in the parents

- reasonable expectations for their child regarding settling, prolonged night sleep periods and factors underlying unsettled behaviors
- the rationale behind treatment interventions. Sleep behavior modification promotes different behavioral responses to wakening, rather than a change in sleep patterns (eg. being able to fall asleep on their own). This includes removal of transitional objects that would require a parent's attendance, such as having a bottle when settling to sleep
- reasonable expectations of the improvements that behavioral intervention can achieve, and the time course over which these will occur
- parental participation in choosing the behavioral programme that they will undertake to manage their infant's sleep problem
- reassurance for the parents that the problem is amenable to intervention.

Interventions (actions)

Strategies for interventions vary from systematically ignoring or controlled crying, to graduated extinction (*Table 10.3*). At one extreme, after confirming that the child is not ill, parents do not attend to them again at all until a pre-defined morning time. This method can produce rapid changes in the child's behavior but it is difficult for most parents. More gradual programmes allow the parents to interact but to set progressive and stepwise increases on their limits for physical and verbal interactions with the infant. For example, the parents may initially attend to the child, including a brief cuddle and then progressively work towards leaving the room once the child is drowsy, returning only if the child fails to settle at pre-defined and progressively longer intervals.

Enhancing successful behavioral interventions:

- consistency of implementation is probably more important than the type of intervention
- support for the parents, for example, by telephone contact with the treating clinical team, especially when their motivation is flagging
- focusing on high impact interventions. This includes consistent intervention at sleep onsets for daytime naps and at the start of the night, when the parents are awake and motivated. Permission to 'do whatever works' during early morning awakenings can often assist the overall success of the intervention
- framing the intervention as a teaching process can enhance parental self-confidence. The parents view the process as teaching their child to settle to sleep independently. This will ensure that the agreed programme is consistent with methods they use for teaching or correcting other behaviors in their child
- anticipating and planning strategies to cope with the phenomenon of a post-extinction response boost (PERB) will limit its impact. The PERB is the tendency for behaviors to revert or even be worse than they originally were, after the intervention has had an initially successful response. It is important that parents persist with their altered strategy at this time, and do not respond with increased anxiety, or by abandoning the programme (*Figure 10.3*).

Table 10.3: Advantages, disadvantages and application of specific behavioral treatments

Techniques	Advantages	Disadvantages	Applications	Contraindications
Unmodified systematic ignoring	Rapid; consistent parental responses promote efficient learning	Parental resistance and noncompliance; duration of crying; spontaneous recovery	First-time interventions; motivated parents	Previous intervention failure; negative conditioned responses
Minimal check with systematic ignoring	Rapid; crying may be of longer duration; parent reassured about infant well-being	Parental presence may trigger intense crying bursts	First-time interventions; parents who wish to check the infant	Previous intervention failure; negative conditioned responses
Parental presence with systematic ignoring	Rapid; less infant crying; less anticipatory parental anxiety; parent reassured about infant well-being	Parental distraction from crying not possible; parental resistance for practical reasons	Flexible parents; parents or infants with separation anxiety	Parents unable to be in close proximity to their infant without intervention
Graduated systematic ignoring	Gradual; parent reassured about infant's well-being	Requires long-term commitment; parent must be well organized; possibility of delayed PERB; settling problems cannot be handled gradually; more risk of disruptions due to illness	Healthy infant; well-organized parents; anxious parents	Infants with settling problems; infants with regular minor illnesses; parents unable to time and carefully reduce interventions; co-sleeping
Trimeprazine with systematic ignoring	Relatively rapid; less infant crying; less anticipatory parental anxiety	Parental resistance to medication	Anxious parents; previous intervention failures; infants with negative conditioned responses	None other than those associated with medication

PERB = post-extinction response burst.

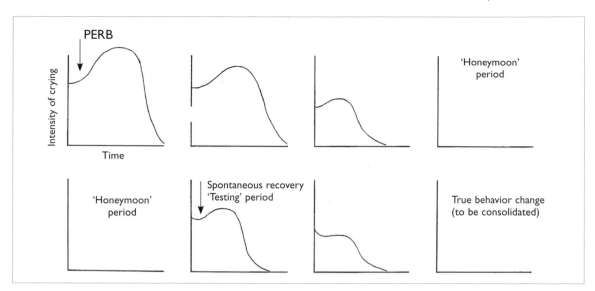

Figure 10.3: *The parent should be made aware that, irrespective of the strategy used (see text), crying may recur after apparent improvement (PERB = post-extinction response boost). This is not a sign of failure and intervention should continue with eventual persistent resolution of the problem (France et al, 1996).*

Medications

Although frequently prescribed the use of medications has not been subjected to rigorous assessment (Ramchandani *et al*, 2000). Currently, it is suggested that the use of medications be:

- intermittent, or short-term only, including use for parental respite
- used with supervision
- used in combination with behavioral interventions, which assure a more prolonged results.

There is no evidence that sedative medications enhance the entrainment of sleep times or new patterns of settling.

Issues raised by *Case study 1* (Andrew)

Behavioral sleep problems are not uncommon when there is a history of prematurity. This is most likely due to the association between prematurity and difficult or traumatic perinatal events, which are associated with an increased prevalence of subsequent sleep disturbance in infants (Wolfson, 1996).

There is no firm evidence that style of feeding (breastfeeding versus bottle feeding, or demand versus schedule) is related to nocturnal awakenings. Night feeds are not usually required after 6 months of age, as long as appropriate daytime feeding ensures hunger and physical discomfort are not present at night.

Colic is the common name given to a pattern of paroxysmal crying occurring in the evening in the first 3–4 months of life, and is a diagnosis made once other causes for distress have been excluded. Crying in the first few months of life may reflect (and be part of) the infants' transition between states of wakefulness and sleep. In either case maneuvers to soothe the infant have variable success and medications are not indicated. Bouts of crying usually terminate with sleep, although sleep episodes that follow crying bouts tend to be fragmented. Once a diagnosis of colic is established, the management is to counsel parents about the nature of the episodes, and reassure regarding the self-limiting nature of the problem.

The circumstances of falling asleep are important, even during infancy. Consistency of bedtime routines facilitates sleep onset. Irregular routines, such as only intermittently allowing the child in the parent's bed, convey confusing messages to the child (Lozoff, 1995). Consistency or disruptive aspects of the physical environment are also relevant and include single versus shared rooms, the presence or absence of a bedroom light and the proximity of the child and parents' bedrooms.

The issue of co-sleeping is controversial. In Western societies, it is often recommended that the child sleeps alone in a separate room from an early age. Some studies suggest that children who share their parent's bed regularly (more than once a week) have more sleep problems. It remains unclear whether co-sleeping causes sleep fragmentation, or if children who have a sleep problem are more likely to co-sleep (Madansky and Edelbrock, 1990). Infants who are put in the crib awake and fall asleep without the presence of the parents are more likely to fall asleep again after spontaneous awakening through the night (Adair *et al*, 1991). These observations can help parents prevent the development of infant sleep disturbances, to identify how they can stop co-sleeping, and retrain an infant who does not settle to sleep independently (see later in this chapter).

It is important to explore social and family circumstances of a child presenting with sleep disturbance, including family structure, social supports available to the parents, and any specific stressors including financial, personal or work-related issues. The issue of early return to work by the mother is controversial with conflicting evidence of the effect on the infant's sleep (Lozoff, 1995). Postnatal depression is diagnosed in up to 30% of mothers whose infants are admitted to in-patient facilities to treat sleep disturbance.

Case study 1 — summary

Andrew was born 4 weeks prematurely; however, there were no perinatal medical problems. The pattern of waking 2–3 times a night in the first 1–2 months is considered normal. The major problem was his persisting requirement for parental attendance to re-establish sleep, and it was the interaction between the infant and the parents that needed to be addressed. This case was compounded by maternal sleep deprivation, although postnatal depression had not been excluded.

Allowing for variations in presentation, Andrew's case represented a problem of sleep onset routines. Initial management would be directed towards educating the parents to facilitate activities that will teach Andrew to settle to sleep independently. Especially in the presence of parental sleep deprivation, the primary focus should be the first sleep onset of the night. A consistent pattern of consoling their baby until he falls asleep means that he associated sleep onset with parental presence and a variety of soothing activities (cuddling, strolling and feeding). It would be relevant to reassure the parents that night waking occurs in all children. They would need to be aware that infants can learn to put themselves back to sleep, and interventions would primarily aim to change the interactions between the parent(s) and infant at sleep onset.

Issues highlighted by *Case study 2* (Ben)

Average sleep requirements across the pediatric age spectrum are illustrated in *Figure 10.4*. Prepubertal, school-age children require an average of 10 hours sleep per day. Appropriate sleep schedules are particularly important for children whose sleep-wake rhythms are easily disrupted. These are often experienced as difficulty initiating or maintaining sleep. The process of implementing changes to bedtime, for example from 10.30PM to 8.30PM, needs to be undertaken gradually. Attempting to make rapid and major shifts in the time of sleep onset are likely to fail. Parents need to understand the difference for a child who cannot fall asleep earlier, rather than attributing the problem to wilfulness or not wanting to fall asleep. The most successful strategy is a gradual progression, 15–20 minutes earlier every 3–4 days.

An important component of the management is a commitment to a fixed wake-up time that suits the child's weekday schedule. This wake-up time should be maintained at the weekends, since 'catch-up' sleep on weekends can exacerbate sleep phase disruptions.

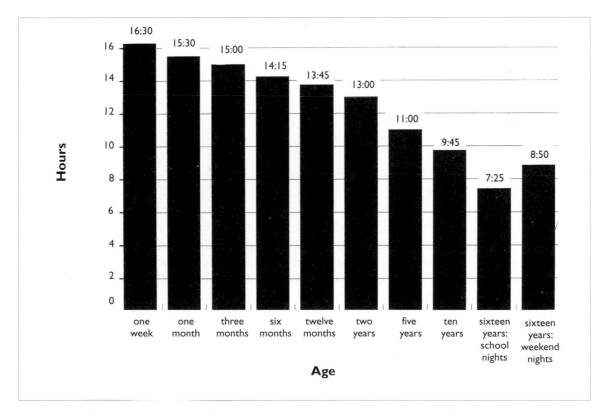

Figure 10.4: Total sleep time (per 24 hours clock time) across age groups. Wolfson, 1996.

Discipline and firmness in setting bedtime and wake-up time limits are essential. Resistance from the child is to be expected, so strategies to enlist their cooperation may require some form of reward system, such as star charts in younger children. A long difference between bedtime and sleep time can present worries and fears being experienced during the delay to sleep onset. If these are due to other reasons such as separation anxiety, the problem will persist despite simple behavioral management, and expert psychological advice may be required to assess further the child's and family's needs. In younger children, the use of security objects and/or the presence of the parents in the room may be beneficial.

Attention deficit/hyperactivity disorder (ADHD) has specific diagnostic criteria, including a combination of hyperactivity with impulsive behavior, poor concentration and distractibility, reduced attention span and mood changes. Restless sleep and bedtime difficulties are often reported in children with ADHD. The inter-relationships between sleep disturbances, OSA, periodic limb movement disorders, and ADHD are less well-defined. Nonetheless, sleep-breathing disturbances should be considered if there is a history of snoring in a child with ADHD. There is increasing evidence that children with OSA can develop disruptive behavior and poor daytime function. Alternatively, OSA may exacerbate symptoms of coexisting ADHD.

The use of stimulant substances such as medications, in this case methylphenidate, caffeine contained in certain soft drinks or over the counter 'flu' preparations can precipitate or contribute to sleep onset difficulties (Greenhill *et al*, 1983; Tirosh *et al*, 1993). Children on dexamphetamine or methylphenidate may need to eliminate the last afternoon dose, or take it earlier.

Behavioral regimens

To implement a behavioral change in older children requires just as much persistence as with infants. Dangers for treatment failure again lie with inability to maintain consistency during a gradual change, as well as the PERB. Full explanation to the parents is paramount, along with the offer of ongoing support as they implement their new limit-setting strategies.

Night lights

No firm recommendation can be made as to the effect on children's sleep if a bedroom light is used. The need for a light may indicate bedtime fear or anxiety. If used, the intensity of the light should be low, to ensure that it does not interfere with the central role of the light–dark cycle in biological rhythms, and sleep–wake regulation. Generally, the sleep environment (with or without bedroom lighting) should be as conducive to sleep as can be feasibly achieved within the family's social and financial resources.

Summary

The pattern described for Ben shows that he is sleep-deprived during the week, and using a weekend sleep-in to catch up. To meet his sleep requirements, Ben is relying on his additional weekend sleep time. School age children generally require a sleep onset time before 9.00PM and

10 hours of sleep each night. Although stimulant medications late in the afternoon may contribute to bedtime difficulties, Ben's main reason for late bedtimes was watching television. Enlisting his cooperation in a new sleep–wake schedule is likely to require a reward system: favorite television programmes can be used as rewards for completing school work and/or maintenance of sleep–wake schedules. Ben also presents with a problem of bed-wetting (enuresis) that is persistent at the age of 9 years. This subject is discussed later in the chapter (*p. 413*).

Parasomnias

Parasomnias often occur intermittently and may be familial. A helpful classification between simple and complex movements is listed in *Table 6.1.*

Some movements are normal phenomenon of sleep, such as when body position is changed every 15–20 minutes. However, parental concern is likely to occur when a child demonstrates complex motor activity in association with sleep. The term parasomnia means 'at the time of sleep'. These events are manifestations of central nervous system activation (motor, autonomic and sensory system) that occur during transition between sleep and wake or between the sleep stages, rather than constituting abnormalities of the sleep process itself.

Case study 3

Craig, an 11-year-old boy, presents with sleep-walking. His mother describes night terrors occurring from a very early age. During these episodes, Craig would suddenly sit up in bed screaming loudly, his eyes wide open with frightened appearance, but appearing not to be awake. At times he would get out of bed or thrash about. He would normally go back to sleep after a few minutes and have no recollection of these events the following day. In the last 6 months, his behavior has become more complex and of concern to the family. At the time of presentation, Craig is regularly walking around the house in his sleep. Although he has bumped into furniture at times, he has never hurt himself. More recently, these episodes have occurred each night.

Two recent episodes have raised concern that Craig may injure himself and these have precipitated the referral. In one, he had walked in his sleep while camping and had to be brought back to the camp by an adult. In the second, about 10 days before referral, he had tried to climb out of his first floor bedroom window and his mother had found him entangled in his curtains.

His normal bedtime is 8.30PM and he wakes at 7.30AM to get ready for school. Craig is said to be 'slow in the mornings' and is easily distracted. His school performance is below average.

Craig was born after induced labour at 38 weeks' gestation because of failure to thrive, but there was no perinatal distress. He was breast fed until the age of 12 months and said to be a 'colicky' baby. He had no other significant medical problems. There was a family history of sleep-walking in the father.

Rhythmic and self-soothing behaviors are common in the first 12 months of life. Head banging (*Jactatio capitis*), head rolling, body rocking describes rhythmic movements involving the head or the entire body in a forward–backward movement or lateral rotation (*Figure 10.5*) that tend to occur in the transition to sleep.

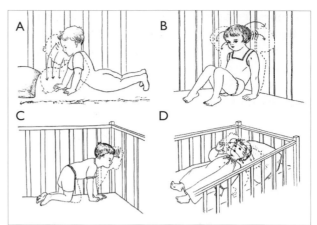

Figure 10. 5: Common forms of head banging: A. Prone position: the head is dropped or brought down with force; B. Occipital head banger: the motion may involve upper portion of body or may be primarily focused upon the head; C. Hands and knees position: rocking motion usually involving the entire body. The forehead or the cranial cap strikes the headboard on forward motion; D. Supine position: head rolling. The child strikes sides of crib.

When recorded, the EEG shows drowsiness, or stage 1 sleep. The reported incidence in childhood varies from 5% to 15%, with onset usually in the latter half of the first year of life, decreasing prevalence to 8% at the age of 4 years. The male to female ratio is approximately 4:1. Head banging generally occurs before normal sleep and varies in duration. Although typically in bouts of 10–15 minutes, the episodes may be prolonged. While head banging appears alarming, injury is rare. The management is parental reassurance (American Academy of Sleep Medicine, 2005; Rosen *et al*, 1996). Persistence into adulthood is reported in cases of mental retardation or psychopathology, but it can occur in some adults with no other abnormality (Chisholm and Morehouse, 1996). The reason for head banging is not understood, but it is hypothesized to be a form of self-soothing behavior.

Night terrors and confusional arousals (sleep drunkenness) are probably a spectrum of the same abnormality and often coexist in the same individual. They are most common between the ages of 2 and 5 years. They may be associated with a range of motor, behavioral and autonomic manifestations and share clinical and pathophysiological features. Night terrors tend to have sudden onset with intense autonomic discharge; whereas confusional arousal tends to have a more gradual onset with moaning and groaning, thrashing, and garbled talking. Sleep-walking is usually a calm automatism, although more agitated behavior is sometimes reported.

Case study 3 represents a severe but uncommon case of sleep-walking (somnambulism) with a high risk of injury. Sleep-walking, is common in young children up to 16 years of age, with a prevalence of 40% even though it is only frequent in a minority (2–3%) (Klackenberg, 1982). The occurrence of sleep-walking reduces markedly after adolescence (*Chapter 6*).

Sleep-walking, night terrors and confusional arousals are disorders of arousal that tend to occur at the transition out of deep slow-wave sleep (*Figure 10.6*). Arousal parasomnias can be seen as states of partial wakefulness and partial sleep, which means that the child is neither completely awake nor completely asleep (Bassetti *et al*, 2000). Associated motor activity can range from simple activities, such as sitting up in bed, to vocalization and complex motor actions, such as walking or running.

Night terrors are typically associated with intense autonomic nervous system activation, causing palpitation, sweating and hyperventilation. Meaningful interaction with the child is usually not possible and amnesia for the event is typical. Attempts to wake the child are often unsuccessful and may prolong the event. The episodes tend to terminate spontaneously and be quickly followed by resumption of sleep.

Vocalization and sleep-talking

The occurrence of vocalization during sleep in the form of coherent speech, barely comprehensible utterances, humming or grunting, is present in virtually all parasomnias and often during epilepsy. Sleep-talking, as a predominant parasomnia, is universal in virtually all children at some stage, and rarely of clinical significance. However in 10% it is of daily occurrence (Reimao and Lefevre, 1980). Sleep-talking appears to have no clear correlation with age, sex or socioeconomic class. It can be exacerbated by febrile illness or sleep deprivation. It often coexists with other parasomnias and occurs in all stages of sleep.

Teeth grinding

Bruxism or teeth grinding describes paroxysmal grinding of the teeth, frequently starting in young children and adolescents with no gender difference (*Chapter 6*). If a persistent or severe problem, it can be associated with facial pain, headache and sleep disruption. It is reported by 85% to 90% of the general population, even though

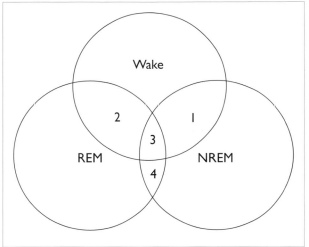

Figure 10.6: Areas of overlap among states:
1: Wake–NREM combinations
    A. Disorders of arousal (sleep-walking, sleep terror, confusional arousals)
    B. Psychogenic dissociation
2: Wake/REM combinations
    A: Cataplexy, hypnagogic hallucinations, sleep paralysis
    B: REM sleep behavior disorder
    C: Lucid dreaming (out-of-body experiences)
    D: Delirium (hallucinations – drug induced/ penduncular)
3: Wake/NREM/REM combinations
    A. Status dissociations
    B. 'Parasomnia overlap' syndromes
4: NREM/REM combinations
    Theoretically possible but not accompanied by conscious awareness
(from Mahowald and Schenck, 1992).

it is said to be a persistent problem in only about 5% of individuals (ICSD, 1990). Its prevalence in children is between 14% and 20% (Bader and Lavigne, 2000). The origin of bruxism is likely to be multifactorial, including family predisposition, dental mal-occlusion, temporomandibular problems and psychological stress.

Treatment is necessary when symptoms are persistent and/or dental and periodontal damage is occurring. Orthodontic treatment to adjust the dental bite or a dental occlusion plate may be necessary. Medications (benzodiazepines) are not used, except for a brief period as part of management of coexistent anxiety or stress. Bruxism often coexists with other parasomnias.

Nightmares

Nightmares (anxiety dreams) are associated with REM sleep and so occur more frequently in the second half of the night. Children waking after nightmares tend to be fully awake and able to describe the features of the dream that they have experienced. Autonomic manifestations with tachycardia, tachypnea and motor activity may be present, but they are not as intense as in sleep terror. The child may have difficulty going back to sleep. The prevalence of nightmares is reported to be 10–50% in 3–6-year-olds, corresponding to change in the development of dream content. Around 5 years of age, dreams contain images such as animals or familial faces and they become more active with thoughts and emotions (Foulkes, 1982; Hartmann *et al*, 1981). Studies have shown that in children with nightmares, the frequency of stressful life events and behavioral problems are not different from a control group (Hawkins and Williams, 1992).

Nightmares may need to be differentiated from REM sleep behavior disorder, which has only rarely been reported in children. This disorder is due to lack of normal muscle atonia during REM leading to 'acting out dreams'. The resulting abnormal motor activity may lead to injury (Herman *et al*, 1989; Schenck *et al*, 1986).

Vivid dreaming may involve visual (seeing things) or auditory (hearing voices or sounds) sensations, or abnormal body positions. These may occur at sleep onset rather than in the second part of night and are classified as hypnagogic hallucinations. They may occur in isolation or as part of narcoleptic syndrome.

Sleep starts (hypnic jerks)

These refer to sudden limb movements, body jerks or abnormal sensations, such as floating, which occur at sleep onset. Sleep starts are observed by the parents rather than reported by the child. At times they may be intense enough to disturb sleep onset. Although they are observed at sleep onset, sleep starts are asymmetric and jerky and easily distinguished from rhythmic movements.

Periodic limb movement disorder and restless leg syndrome

These are best known and diagnosed in adults. However symptoms have often been present since childhood. The typical sensory symptoms of cramping and creepy-crawly sensation is not a feature in children as in adults. However the consequences of sleep fragmentation during the day may negatively affect cognition and bring about behavioral difficulties. Periodic limb movement disorder is currently included among the sleep disorders that may coexist and contribute to attention deficit hyperactivity disorder, together with obstructive sleep apnea and narcolepsy. Overnight polysomnography (PSG) is usually needed to confirm the diagnosis (Picchietti and Walters, 1996; Picchietti *et al*, 1998).

Nocturnal seizures

Sleep and wake/sleep transition periods increase the risk of seizure, with 20–40% occurring only during sleep (Brown, 1996). Although generalized tonic and clonic seizures are not difficult to recognize if the event is witnessed, other forms of seizure, leading to repetitive stereotypic activity, may be confused with parasomnias. Any form of epilepsy may manifest during sleep in childhood, including *petit mal*. However the following forms of epilepsy are of special interest in the pediatric population:

❖ ***Benign rolandic epilepsy*** (benign focal epilepsy of childhood with rolandic spikes) is characterized by focal facial seizures (facial twitches and spasms) often preceded by numbness of the oral mucosa or the oropharynx. It may involve focal movement of the limbs and may spread bilaterally causing generalized seizure. Some degree of dysphasia may also be present, but the child has full awareness of the event and can describe it. It can occur both during REM and non-REM sleep. Benign rolandic epilepsy is more common in young children and tends to resolve spontaneously between the ages of 15 and 20. Diurnal EEG is usually normal.

❖ ***Juvenile myoclonic epilepsy*** (awakening epilepsy) occurs upon waking. This form of epilepsy starts in the second decade of life with manifestation of clonic movements seen soon after awakening (Janz, 1985). The patient experiences shock-like jerks in the shoulders, arms and hands, while consciousness is fully preserved. Although the focal seizure can be the only manifestation at the beginning, generalized seizure follows as a rule. Sleep deprivation is a common trigger (Grunewald and Penayiotopoulos, 1993). The occurrence in the morning upon awakening is important for suspecting the diagnosis. There are typical epileptic spikes and waves on the EEG which confirm the diagnosis if the activity is confused with REM behavior disorder, or florid periodic limb movement disorder. Typical absence seizures are also reported in one third of patients with juvenile myoclonic epilepsy, and a positive family history is common (Grunewald and Penayiotopoulos, 1993).

❖ ***Hypnogenic paroxysmal dystonia*** is characterized by stereotyped jerking movements of the limbs or trunk, with dystonic posturing of the limbs, body or face. Vocalization may be present. The episodes usually last a few minutes but may recur through the night, arising from non-REM sleep. Although hypnagogic paroxysmal dystonia was initially described in adults, it may start in childhood and can be mistaken for other forms of motor activity, including parasomnia (Montagna, 1992). Nocturnal paroxysmal dystonia is probably a form of frontal lobe epilepsy and responds to treatment with carbamazepine (Meierkord *et al*, 1992).

History

A detailed history is usually sufficient to make a diagnosis and specialised testing, such as PSG, is rarely required. The following aspects of the history are important:

❖ A careful description of the quality of motor and behavior activity will often be sufficient to make the diagnosis.

❖ Age of onset: sleep-walking, night terrors and confusional arousals typically start in toddlers and improve by school-age, but all can continue through to early teenage years.

❖ Family history: a family history is common in arousal parasomnias (Kales *et al*, 1980a).

❖ Timing during the sleep episode: arousal parasomnias are more common in the first half of the night when there is more slow-wave sleep. Nightmares are associated with REM sleep and occur more commonly in the second part of the night.

❖ As with any movement disorder, it is important to seek out any historical features suggesting seizure activity. Important features to exclude are stereotypic patterns of motor activity (repeated similar activity with each event), focal twitching suggestive of partial complex seizures, and generalized rigidity or clonic movements, suggestive of *grand mal* seizures. Video taping and polysomnography are important diagnostic tools.

❖ Precipitating events: sleep deprivation, irregular sleep schedule, fever or any other intercurrent illnesses (such as painful conditions, asthma or infection) can increase the probability of recurrent partial arousal and, therefore, increase the frequency of parasomnias. Substances such as caffeine (most commonly in soft drinks) and tricyclic antidepressants can also increase the likelihood of events. In adults, it has also been shown that external stimuli (sounding a buzzer) can elicit night terrors (Fisher *et al*, 1974).

❖ History of psychological/psychiatric problems: in children and adolescents, persistent sleep terrors and sleep-walking may be associated with anxiety disorders, depression and obsessive compulsive behavior (Dahl and Williamson, 1990; Fisher *et al*, 1974; Gau and Soong, 1999; Kales *et al*, 1980b).

Further investigations

A detailed history and examination are often sufficient to clarify the diagnosis. However, overnight PSG with a combination of videotaping, multiple sleep latency test and electroencephalogram during the day or following sleep deprivation, may be required to clarify the diagnosis when the following occur (Rosen *et al*, 1996):

● another sleep-related problem is suspected, eg. OSA
● dangerous behavior occurs
● excessive daytime sleepiness is present
● epilepsy is considered
● clinical features are unclear.

Treatment of parasomnias

Parasomnias and other paroxysmal sleep-related events often share common features. Certain aspects of management are common to all of the above syndromes:

❖ *Avoidance of precipitating factors:* A regular sleep and wake schedule is important to avoid sleep deprivation. Fever is a common aggravating factor and the underlying cause should be evaluated and treated. Substances that increase sleep fragmentation, such as caffeine or over-the-counter 'flu' preparations containing ephedrine or pseudo-ephedrine, are best avoided. Any source of stress or anxiety, either real or perceived, should be identified. Parents should be discouraged from waking infants or children with night terrors or confusional arousals.

❖ ***Prevention of injury:*** When the sleep-related behavior is potentially dangerous, such as in some cases of sleep-walking, sleep terrors or head banging, safety measures may be required, such as padding the bed, securing windows, applying gates at the top of stairs, or alarm bells at doors to alert the parents.

❖ ***Pharmacological treatment:*** When more conservative measures are ineffective or there is a danger of self-injury, benzodiazepines are usually effective. A small dose of clonazepam (0.25 mg) or temazepam (5–10 mg) at bedtime is usually effective, and can be especially useful over the short-term for events such as camping trips. Clonazepam may be associated with daytime drowsiness. In case of epilepsy or significant psychological or psychiatric conditions, specific medications and counselling are needed.

Respiratory disorders

Snoring and obstructive sleep apnea

Sleep-disordered breathing, particularly obstructive sleep apnea (OSA), is a common disorder and has significant health implications affecting about 3% of children (Kennedy and Waters, 2005). Children with OSA usually present with the symptom of snoring, but parents do not always volunteer this information. Some consider that the noisy breathing or snoring is 'normal' or harmless in a child, and others may have been reassured that there was no associated medical problem.

Case study 4

Deborah is 5 years of age and her parents have observed episodes of apnea (stopping breathing) during sleep. Deborah has a history of noisy breathing, both day and night, since her first year of life, but her mother recently noticed a recurrence of apneas lasting up to 5 seconds. The parents also describe events where Deborah coughs and then takes a big breath or moves in her sleep, after these apneas. Neither parent has ever observed cyanosis or abnormal chest movements, but they think that Deborah works harder to breath when she is asleep than when she is awake.

Deborah usually settles easily to bed between 8.00PM and 9.00PM and falls asleep within minutes. She is a restless sleeper who regularly tosses her bedclothes off during the night. She tends to wake then settle back to sleep in her parents' bed around 5.00AM. If she is not woken, she will sleep until 9.00AM or 10.00AM. However, she is usually woken at 7.30AM to get ready for school. At school, she is said to have swinging moods. Her developmental milestones are appropriate for her age but are currently being monitored by a pediatrician.

Deborah was born at term, by caesarean section because of fetal distress and had one episode of bronchiolitis in her first year of life. She suffered from tonsillitis approximately every 2 months and had one admission to hospital for tonsillitis, prior to tonsillectomy 2 years ago. Deborah had full overnight polysomnography (PSG) before her tonsillectomy and was shown to have 11.9 obstructive respiratory events per hour (apneas and hypopneas), an arousal index of 11 per hour, and minimum oxygen saturation of 88%. Sleep stage proportions and progression through the night were normal for her age. Tonsillectomy was recommended and undertaken without complications. She had immediate, post-operative symptomatic improvement. However, now, two years later, repeat polysomnography is being requested because of the recurrence of her symptoms of snoring and witnessed apneas. She has no other medical problems and is on no regular medication.

On examination, Deborah is obese, with a height of 127 cm (97 percentile) and a weight of 40 kg (well above the 97 percentile). Her pharynx is small with petechiae on the soft palate but no tonsillar tissue visible. She breathes easily through her nose when she is awake and her cardiorespiratory examination is otherwise normal.

Repeat PSG shows nineteen obstructive apneas/hypopneas per hour, with a minimum oxygen saturation of 84% and an arousal index of 19 events per hour.

Case study 5

Elizabeth is referred with snoring and daytime sleepiness at 8 years of age. Elizabeth is said to have snored since she was a toddler but recently her mother has noted increased frequency and loudness of her snoring and has started to see apneic events lasting up to 10 seconds. Elizabeth goes to bed at 8.30PM and usually reads for 30 minutes before falling asleep. She shares her bedroom with her sister. She is woken at 7.00AM on school days. Although she has never fallen asleep at school, she frequently complains of being tired and naps for about 1 hour after school 2–3 times a week.

Elizabeth's history includes premature birth at 34 weeks' gestation, followed by a 4-week admission to the neonatal intensive care (ICU). She was fed expressed breast milk in the ICU and continued breastfeeding up to 3 months of age. After having several apparent life-threatening events (ALTEs) at home, she was placed on a cardiorespiratory monitor until 12 months of age. There is no family history of SIDS.

Elizabeth is currently achieving high marks at school and plays team sports at school and at the weekends. On examination, she is 141 cm in height (97 percentile) and 34 kg (90 percentile) in weight. She has a normal pharynx, with tonsils that are visible but not large. She has no craniofacial abnormalities. She can nose breathe easily when awake, and cardiorespiratory examination is otherwise normal.

Overnight PSG reveals intermittent, soft snoring, with no clinically significant respiratory events and a minimum saturation of 94%. The arousal index was 9 events per hour with normal sleep architecture and no periodic leg movements.

Snoring is common, and occurs in 16–27% of children (Brunetti *et al*, 2001; Gislason and Benediktsdottir, 1995; Sanchez-Armengol *et al*, 2001). Habitual snoring, or snoring most nights, occurs in 4.9–12.1% of children (Ali *et al*, 1994; Brunetti *et al*, 2001; Gislason and Benediktsdottir, 1995). The estimated prevalence of OSA in children varies according to the definition being used, but lies between 0.7% and 2.9% at most ages studied to date (Ali *et al*, 1993; Brouillette *et al*, 1982; Brunetti *et al*, 2001; Gislason and Benediktsdottir, 1995; Guilleminault *et al*, 1981; Sanchez-Armengol *et al*, 2001).

Distinction is often made between 'primary snoring' and OSA. Primary snoring refers to children who do not have apneas or blood gas disturbances (oxygen desaturation or carbon dioxide retention) during sleep. However, the two cannot be distinguished without an overnight sleep study (also known as a polysomnogram, or PSG). Studies to diagnose, or exclude, OSA account for approximately 60% of referrals to pediatric sleep units (Waters *et al*, 1995).

Medical problems associated with craniofacial abnormalities or poor soft tissue or muscle tension are associated with increased risk for OSA in a child. Parents often show little concern about the symptom of snoring or noisy breathing, because it is likely to have been longstanding. Therefore, a history of snoring or noisy breathing should always be sought in children with craniofacial abnormalities, micrognathia, cleft palate or from diagnostic groups with a known, high prevalence of OSA. For groups with a very high risk for OSA, sleep studies may be recommended for routine screening eg. children with Down syndrome where at least 31% have OSA (Stebbens *et al*, 1991).

History

Snoring is the most common symptom of OSA, with chronic snoring (more than four nights per week) and witnessed apneas being the most consistent predictors for the presence of OSA. There are important differences with clinical presentation of OSA between adults and children (*Table 10.4*). However, when studied systematically, historical features of OSA have not proven to be reliable predictors of disease. Studies have shown that clinical history can distinguish normal children from those with possible OSA, but once a history of snoring is obtained, the clinical history is an unreliable predictor of OSA (Brouilette *et al*, 1984; Carroll *et al*, 1995a). Where daytime tiredness or sleepiness is a problem, it is important to exclude inadequate sleep time by checking bedtime routines and the amount of sleep being obtained, as well as nocturnal symptoms.

Factors likely to contribute to difficulty in determining the presence of OSA include cultures where children sleep independently of their parents. Some of the clinical signs that accompany OSA, such as paradoxical rib-cage movements, the use of accessory respiratory muscles, or occurrence of cyanotic episodes, require specialized knowledge in addition to careful observation.

Table 10.4: Features of adult versus childhood OSAs		
	Adult	**Child**
Snoring	Usually alternating with pauses	Often continuous
Excessive daytime sleepiness	Main presenting symptom	Minority of patients
Associated obesity	Majority of patients	Minority of patients
Underweight or failure-to-thrive	No	Minority of patients
Daytime mouth breathing	No	Minority of patients but not rare
Gender	M:F = 4:1	M:F = 1:1
Differential diagnosis	Other causes of excessive sleepiness or sleep disruption	Other causes of snoring or breathing difficulty during sleep
Enlarged tonsils and adenoids	Uncommon	Most common
Predominant obstructive pattern	Obstructive apnea	Obstructive hypoventilation
Arousal on apnea termination	Nearly always	Usually not
Sleep pattern disruption	Nearly always	Sleep stages (%) often normal
Complications	Mainly cardiopulmonary and complications of excessive daytime sleepiness (EDS)	Cardiopulmonary, growth, behavioral developmental, perioperative
Surgical correction	Only in selected cases (minority)	Successful in most cases (adenotonsillectomy)
Continuous positive airway pressure (CPAP)	Most common treatment	Only in selected cases (minority)
Mortality	Sudden death during sleep or from cardiovascular complications	Usually perioperative

Respiratory pauses (apneas) can be either obstructive or central in type. Obstructive events are generally associated with ongoing and sometimes increased respiratory effort, but many parents are only aware of the termination of the event (for example, coughing or movement) (Carroll and Loughlin, 1992). Short, central apneas are common in children of all ages, and particularly common in young infants, so a reliable history of such events may preclude the need for sleep study. It is appropriate to try and determine the frequency and length of the events if possible.

Difficulty breathing is another important clinical feature of children with upper airway obstruction. Parents often describe their child as having increased work in breathing during sleep, whether or not they see this accompanied by features such as mouth breathing, adopting unusual sleep positions with head hyperextension, or marked respiratory efforts.

Other features of OSA

Paradoxical chest movement or inward movement of the rib cage during inspiration is a normal phenomenon in infants and continues to occur during REM sleep up to the age of 6–9 months. However in older children, when accompanied by other features of OSA, it is likely to be a reflection of airway obstruction. It may also occur in children with neuromuscular abnormalities where it can reflect respiratory difficulties that should be investigated.

Restless sleep, daytime behavioral dysfunction, bed wetting, and increased night sweating are often cited as symptoms associated with OSA that tend to improve after treatment. However, these symptoms are not predictive of OSA (Ali *et al*, 1996; Carroll, 1996; Guilleminault *et al*, 1981; Swift, 1988). Insufficient sleep, sleep fragmentation due to obstructive sleep apnea, periodic limb movement disorder and narcolepsy can be associated with similar symptoms (Ali *et al*, 1993; Picchietti *et al*, 1998). Other symptoms that may indicate respiratory failure, rather than OSA, include difficulty waking and morning headaches (Brouilette *et al*, 1984). It is likely that the symptom spectrum varies among individuals and this individual variability is lost in controlled studies. The symptoms listed below may be associated with OSA, but in the clinical setting it is not currently possible to predict the individual children who will have a positive response to (resolution after) treatment.

❖ ***Night-time wakening*** is a very non-specific symptom. Wakenings can be followed by crying or moaning and are often a source of concern to the parents. Although night awakenings with or without crying and disorientation can follow apneas, they are not specific for, or predictive of, OSA. Agitated awakenings may represent parasomnias or other sleep-associated conditions.

❖ ***Behavioral problems and learning difficulties*** may be present (Gozal, 1998; Lewin *et al*, 2002, Lipton and Gozal 2003). There is increasing evidence that cognitive dysfunction occurs with OSA affecting attention, concentration and memory (Blunden *et al*, 2000). Since abnormalities have been detected even in the presence of minimal respiratory disturbance, more research is required to determine the implications for treatment. The presence of these cognitive disturbances means that OSA should be excluded in children presenting with symptoms of ADHD (together with other sleep disorders such as periodic leg movements). There is some evidence that treatment of obstructive sleep apnea by tonsillectomy and adenoidectomy, leads to improvement in behavior (Goldstein *et al*, 2000).

❖ ***Excessive daytime sleepiness (EDS)*** has not been a commonly described feature of OSA in children. The prevalence of this symptom appears to be around 30% (Carroll and Loughlin, 1995b). There is marked variability in normative sleep requirements for children, and children as old as 6 or 7 years may still have a normal requirement for daytime naps. With better study designs examining sleep time of children before and after treatment, or compared to well-matched control subjects, it seems likely that many children with OSA do have increased sleep times. Finally, the symptom profiles for children with OSA are likely to change to more adult profiles with increasing age (Sadeh *et al*, 2003).

Examination

The most common abnormality underlying sleep apnea in children is adenotonsillar hypertrophy. Nasal patency should be assessed. In selected children nasopharyngoscopy is useful to assess the retropharyngeal area (Myatt and Beckenham, 2000). The oropharyngeal area, tonsils and tongue size should be noted, as tonsillar hypertrophy is a risk factor for upper airway obstruction. Children with OSA have larger adenotonsillar size than control cases without disease, even though there is no correlation between tonsil size and symptoms of obstructive sleep apnea (Donnelly *et al*, 2003).

There is accumulating evidence that craniofacial structure is also a contributor to OSA in children. This may relate to the heritability of the disease (Palmer and Redline, 2003). As in *Case study 4* (Deborah), it appears that obesity is a risk factor for OSA in children, although it is less common in paediatric than adult sleep clinic populations (*Table 10.4*).

Growth delay appears to be as commonly documented in infants and toddlers with sleep apnea as obesity, and there is good evidence of improved growth following treatment of OSA. OSA may also be the underlying condition for young children presenting with failure to thrive, so although it is not a common cause for the condition, OSA should be part of assessment of children with such failure and growth delay (Everett *et al*, 1987; Lind and Lundell, 1982; Lipton and Gozal 2003; Stradling *et al*, 1990). Facial features, such as micrognathia and retrognathia should also be noted as they increase the risk of obstructive breathing (*Figure 10.7*). The presence of a high-arched palate and inverted bite can reflect maxillary abnormalities, which are also associated with snoring and obstructed breathing. These features are commonly called 'adenoid facies', or 'long-face syndrome'. Cleft palate increases the risk of obstructed breathing, particularly after surgical repair.

As in *Case study 4* (Deborah) the combination of obesity and tonsil hypertrophy together increase the risk of obstructive sleep apnea (Silvestri *et al*, 1993).

In childhood OSA, although severe abnormalities such as left ventricular failure, congestive heart failure and cor pulmonale have become rare presentations, there is evidence that the disease can also be associated with less marked, but nonetheless significant, cardiovascular dysfunction (Amin *et al*, 2002). It is also important to recognize that OSA may be a correctable cause for these abnormalities, especially in children with other malformations or syndromes.

Diagnostic investigations and diagnosis

Although a combination of symptoms and signs is often suggestive of obstructive sleep apnea, they are not sufficiently discriminative to be used for diagnosis. Using history, even with additional clinical assessment, one in four children presenting with a history suggestive of OSA would be misclassified, either with or without disease (Carroll *et al*, 1995; Lipton and Gozal, 2003).

The diagnosis of OSA in children requires objective documentation. A variety of methods have been proposed to document the disease, but overnight polysomnography (PSG) continues to be the gold standard for diagnosis. Other tools that have been evaluated include overnight oximetry, nap (rather than overnight) PSG and video. To date, none have negative predictive values to replace overnight PSG (Brouillette *et al*, 2000) (*Figure 10.8*). Other issues being studied and debated are the location of the investigations (sleep unit versus home), the number of parameters to be measured, and the definitions and threshold that discriminate normal from abnormal sleep studies.

The diagnostic criteria for sleep apnea in children are also being debated, as more evidence emerges that children who snore may also suffer from medical complications (Blunden *et al*, 2000). Normative data for polysomnography in children (*Table 10.5*) lacks standardization among laboratories, but guidelines have been suggested and there is work directed towards achieving this goal (American Thoracic Society, 1996; Marcus *et al*, 1992).

Points of emerging consensus include:

❖ Apneas in children are significant if they are ≥ 2 breath cycles duration, rather than a set 'time'. This means that the apnea duration increases with age and reaches a 10-second (adult) definition when adult respiratory rates of twelve breaths per minute are achieved.

❖ The threshold for considering obstructive apneas as abnormal varies, but is generally considered to be ≥ 1 per hour for research purposes. Decisions regarding the threshold for treatment tend to be made in the context of clinical presentation, with general consensus that adenotonsillectomy should be undertaken if the apnea index is ≥ 10 per hour (Lipton and Gozal, 2003). For disease that persists postoperatively, which can be as high as 20%, recommendations are more varied. This may include the use of nasal-CPAP or bi-level CPAP and supplemental oxygen, depending on the severity of OSA and associated co-morbidity, eg. growth delay, right heart failure, craniofacial malformation.

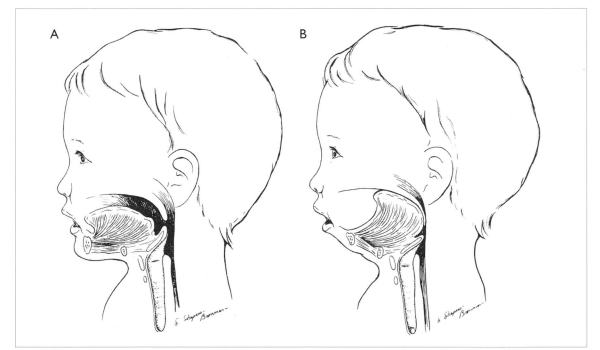

Figure 10.7: Airway anatomy in mandibular hypoplasia. A: normal child. B: child with mandibular hypoplasia. Pharyngeal obstruction results from the posterior displacement of the tongue (Potsic and Marsh, 1987).

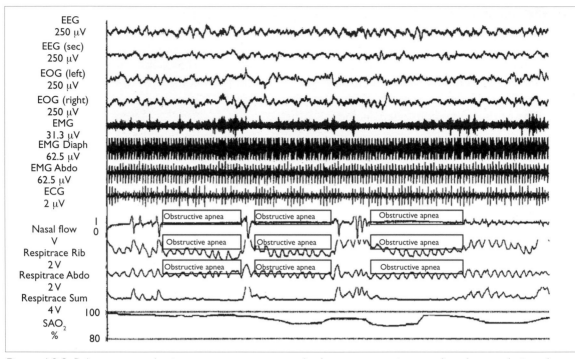

Figure 10.8: Polysomnography is necessary to accurately document respiratory disturbance during sleep. Note that oxygen desaturation is slightly delayed compared to the obstructive episode.

Definitions of central apneas are varied. Traditionally, central apneas of >20 seconds, or with bradycardia or cyanosis were considered significant, but historically this definition was used for apnea of infancy and used as the criteria for setting monitor alarms. In the context of overnight PSG, central and obstructive apneas tend to have the same baseline definition of two breath-cycles, with oxygen desaturation ≥ 3 or 4%, depending on the laboratory.

Hypopneas are events with reduced airflow generally at levels of 20–60% of baseline. This is only valid for signals that reflect the ventilatory amplitude, including respiratory flow measured by pressure or pneumotachograph, or by respiratory plethysmography, but not thermistor. Again, these events would be considered abnormal if they are terminated by oxygen desaturation >4% or arousal.

Carbon dioxide measurements (end tidal CO_2 (EtCO$_2$) or transcutaneous (TcpCO$_2$) should always be included in PSG for children. A variety of criteria are suggested, for example, an increase of >13 mmHg above the awake baseline, a peak value >53 mmHg, or >50 mmHg for more than 8% of total sleep time are considered indicative of alveolar hypoventilation.

The upper airway resistance syndrome (UARS) is a popular term. In adult sleep medicine, the events that define UARS are now called RERAs (respiratory event-related arousals), but all criteria by which these phenomena have been defined require the use of esophageal pressure catheters. Since these are quite invasive, they are not used routinely for pediatric sleep studies.

Clinically, it is useful to consider snoring, upper airway resistance syndrome and OSA as levels along a continuous spectrum of disease severity, rather than as separate syndromes with discrete boundaries between them (*Figure 10.9*).

Table 10.5: Suggested normal values for PSG in children

	Normal values	Comments
Obstructive apnea index	≤1 apnea/hour	Probably valid for children >3 months of age
	0 apneas >10 sec duration	(>3 months of age)
	0 apneas >15 sec duration	(<3 months of age)
Maximum $PaCO_2$	≤53mmHg during study	Only useful in children without underlying lung disease
%TST spent with $PETC^{O2}$ >45 mm Hg	≤10% of TST	Only useful in children without underlying lung disease
Minimum SaO_2	≥92%	Evaluate on case-by-case basis in children with lung disease
Maximum Δ SaO_2	≤8%	Does not apply to children with cyanotic heart disease

Based on data from Gaultier (1987) Respiratory adaptation during sleep from the neonatal period to adolescence. In: Guilleminault C (ed): *Sleep and its Disorders in Children*. Raven Press, New York: 67–98; Marcus CL *et al* (1992) Normal polysomnographic values for children and adolescents. *Am Rev Respir Dis* **146**: 1235; Uliel *et al* (2004) Polysomnographic respiratory values in children and adolescents. *Chest* **125**: 872–8.

The core features of pediatric overnight PSG are the study of sleep state and simultaneous measurement of ventilation. Successful recordings depend heavily on meeting the child's needs in terms of an appropriate child-friendly environment, staff experienced in dealing with children and their parents, and supervision during the recording Full PSG studies also require expert interpretation. Both the study and its interpretation should be performed by a recognized (accredited) sleep laboratory with adequate experience in interpreting pediatric studies. Sleep study results can then be interpreted in conjunction with the clinical picture, considering past treatment interventions, current symptoms and social circumstances.

The major differential diagnoses with OSA in children are associated conditions, particularly hypoventilation. However where hypoventilation is diagnosed, particularly acquired central hypoventilation, care must be taken to examine for underlying conditions. There are limited reports of acquired central hypoventilation in the literature, but it appears that underlying CNS abnormalities exist in approximately 50% of cases (Weese-Mayer *et al*, 1988). Care should also be taken when predicting the response to treatment, especially if the major concern is an atypical or non-respiratory abnormality, such as behavioral difficulties, since current information does not permit prediction of the individual's response to treatment for these symptoms.

The methods used to detect OSA in children depend in part, on the availability of local facilities and expertise.

From the current abbreviated or screening procedures, overnight oximetry has the highest specificity, so if the screen is positive for repetitive desaturations a diagnosis of OSA can be reliably made (Brouillette *et al*, 2000). However, oximetry, nap PSG, sonography and video monitoring all have poor negative predictive values, meaning that a negative screening study using any of these tools does not reliably exclude OSA. A positive diagnosis of OSA ultimately requires overnight PSG in children, and even if one of these screening studies returns a negative diagnosis, further investigations will be required in children where clinical concerns persist.

A pre-operative diagnosis of OSA is responsible for an odds ratio of 7.2 for complications after adenotonsillectomy. It is therefore prudent to determine the presence and severity of disease where possible before adenotonsillectomy is undertaken (Wilson *et al*, 2002). The relative benefits of pre- or perioperative airway management are still being investigated, but studies have shown that preoperative CPAP is beneficial in children with severe preoperative disease.

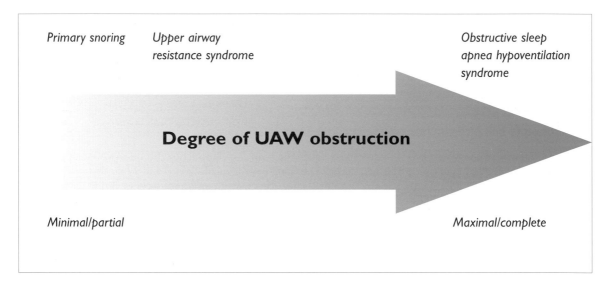

Figure 10.9: Continuum of sleep-related upper airway obstruction. UAW = upper airway (Carrol, 1996).

Management

Precise guidelines for treatment of disturbed breathing in children are not available, although with an apnea/hypopnea index of more than five events per hour, referral for adenotonsillectomy should be considered (Kennedy and Waters, 2005). The natural history of snoring is not well-defined, but the available evidence suggests that up to half the children with primary snoring stop snoring within several years (Ali *et al*, 1994; Marcus *et al*, 1998). There is no evidence to suggest that primary snoring progresses to OSA. Episodes of obstructive breathing may occur transiently, especially during periods of upper respiratory tract infections. Therefore it is often appropriate simply to observe children who only have mild or intermittent snoring.

After adenotonsillectomy, small series suggest that OSA persists in 15–20% of children who have no other underlying condition (Lipton and Gozal 2003; Pirsig and Verse, 2000; Suen *et al*, 1995). The likelihood of persisting disease increases with the severity of OSA, especially where the initial apnea index was >19 per hour. In practice, clinical follow-up is the most appropriate first step for the majority of children, with repeat investigations if symptoms persist or recur. Available evidence suggests that children with documented, severe preoperative disease should routinely have a follow-up sleep study. Treatment strategies include:

- adenotonsillectomy
- medical treatments: nasal steroids, weight loss (with mild disease)
- nasal CPAP
- other surgery, including tracheostomy, orofacial reconstruction, and distraction procedures for maxilla and mandible.

Since reports suggest that up to 15% of children fail to establish adequate CPAP therapy, other surgical options including tracheostomy, should continue to be considered under appropriate medical circumstances. Management decision requires consideration of both symptoms and polysomnography findings (*Figure 10.10*).

Decisions regarding surgery are difficult in children who have symptoms suggestive of OSA, but mild or absent abnormalities on PSG. In such children, although respiratory symptoms will almost certainly improve with surgery, the response to surgery may be better predicted on the basis of other symptoms such as recurrent tonsillitis (Darrow and Siemens, 2002) or neurobehavioral morbidity (Lipton and Gozal, 2003).

Increased perioperative risks factors include (McColley *et al*, 1992; Rosen *et al*, 1994; Walker *et al*, 1999; Wilson *et al*, 2002):

- age <2 (odds ratio (OR) 4.3, 95%CI 1.7–11) or <3 (or 9.3, 95% confidence interval [CI] 2.5–34.7)
- severity of apnea/hypopnea AHI >5 per hour
- failure to thrive (OR 5.1, CI 1.4–18.7)
- craniofacial abnormalities (OR 6.2, CI 1.5–26)
- cor pulmonale.

The question of inpatient versus outpatient surgery for OSA remains unresolved. Large studies have shown that day-stay surgery is cost-effective for adenoidectomy alone and, although preliminary data suggests that this may also be true for tonsillectomy, it is not clear whether this remains true in children who have a preoperative diagnosis of OSA (Ahmed *et al*, 1993; Shapiro *et al*, 1999). Currently, many institutions monitor all children who undergo adenotonsillectomy, but the trend is for more day-stay surgery and this will need ongoing evaluation regarding efficacy and cost-effectiveness when the indication for surgery is OSA.

Use of respiratory support (nasal CPAP and non-invasive ventilation [NIV])

Nasal CPAP is predominantly used when surgery has failed to resolve OSA in children. However, other indications include temporary airway management prior to surgery or airway management when surgery is contraindicated (Downey *et al*, 2000; Guilleminault *et al*, 1995; Marcus *et al*, 1995; McNamara and Sullivan, 2000; Waters *et al*, 1995). Regular PSG is needed in children to monitor the changing pressure requirements of CPAP with growth.

Assisted ventilation, using bi-level positive airway pressure, has also been reported in children in selected situations (Friedman *et al*, 1999). Bi-level machines allow the setting of an inspiratory and an expiratory pressure and are useful for sleep-associated respiratory failure. However they are more expensive than CPAP devices and their relevance to the treatment of OSA is still to be determined.

Critical issues in assisted ventilation with nasal CPAP or bi-level CPAP in the pediatric population include attention to proper nasal mask fitting, and education of the parents to assure compliance.

Other surgical and structural interventions

Much work is being undertaken to find surgical and other orthopedic or orthodontic interventions that could achieve permanent or long-term resolution of upper airway obstruction in children. Among the treatments currently being evaluated are maxillary expansion, maxillary or mandibular distraction procedures and facial reconstruction. Literature is accumulating regarding the effectiveness of these procedures in mild to moderate sleep apnea in adults (*Chapter 5*) but to date, most literature refers to limited series and little has been established regarding their short- or long-term efficacy in children.

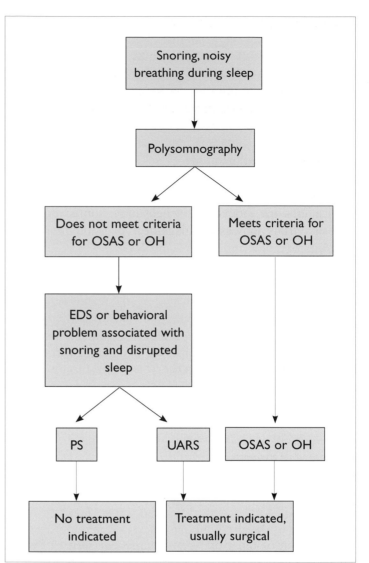

Figure 10.10: Algorithm for evaluating the snoring child. Children with obstructive sleep apnea syndrome (OSAS) may have daytime symptoms such as excessive daytime sleepiness. Children with upper airway resistance syndrome (UARS), by definition, do not meet the criteria for OSAS but have daytime symptoms believed to be due to breathing-related sleep disruption. Children with primary snoring (PS) do not meet the criteria for OSAS or obstructive hypoventilation (OH) and do not have daytime symptoms related to night-time breathing disturbance (Carroll, 1996).

Pharmacological treatment

Few studies have been undertaken regarding pharmacological treatments for OSA. Nasal steroids have been shown to improve the severity of disease in selected children (Brouillette *et al*, 2001) but the use of a brief course of oral steroid seems to be ineffective (Lipton and Gozal, 2003)

Weight reduction

As in adults, the efficacy of weight reduction is reported in individual cases. But there are no controlled trials addressing this issue.

Summary

In *Case study 4* (Deborah) the initial recommendation for tonsillectomy was appropriate based upon the constellation of symptoms and documentation of apneic events. However, even in such mild cases, this highlights the need for clinical follow-up. There is no current literature regarding the failure rate of tonsillectomy or adenoidectomy alone, so adenotonsillectomy remains the current treatment of choice.

Central sleep apnea

Central sleep apnea refers to episodes of apnea where there is absence of both airflow and respiratory efforts. Brief central apneas are commonly seen at all ages, during periodic breathing in infancy and in older children following movements or sighs in sleep or during REM sleep. To be considered pathological, central apneas must be associated with significant sequelae, including frequent or severe desaturation, bradycardia or hypoventilation.

Case study 6

Fiona is a 10-year-old girl who presents with episodes of apnea during sleep. Her mother describes episodes of change from regular nasal breathing to an episodic pattern of three to four deep mouth breathes followed by pauses of variable duration. This pattern can last for 10–30 minutes but has never been associated with cyanosis or wakening. Fiona has no symptoms to suggest respiratory compromise, such as morning headaches or daytime dysfunction. She is doing well at school.

Fiona was born at 37 weeks' gestation after an uneventful pregnancy. She currently suffers mild asthma but is otherwise well.

Medical investigations reveal no respiratory or cardiovascular pathology with normal lung function tests. EEG, head CT, and brainstem evoked potential are normal. Overnight PSG reveals seventeen central apneas per hour (*Figure 10.11*) of short duration (10 to 11 seconds) with normal sleep structure and no oxygen desaturation. MRI of the brainstem and spine showed a type 1 Chiari malformation and small syrinx.

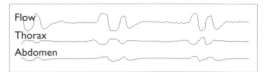

Figure 10.11: Episodes of central apnea in a child with no daytime symptoms.

No intervention was undertaken. At follow-up, at 11 years of age showed thirteen central apneas per hour, and at 13 years, eighteen apneas per hour, with Fiona remaining free of daytime symptoms.

Fiona's history (*Case study 6*) was suggestive of central apnea with PSG confirmation. Because her respiratory status was stable with no significant desaturation or retention of CO_2, and no other neurological symptoms secondary to her brainstem abnormalities, no treatment was undertaken. Periodic central apneas are abnormal at this age and investigations are appropriate. The presence of underlying pathology should be sought in such cases (Weese-Mayer *et al*, 1988).

Causes of pathological central (sleep) apnea in children include:

- congenital defects of respiratory control
- primary and secondary brainstem pathologies, including Arnold–Chiari malformation, syringomyelia, tumors, infections, and demyelinating diseases.

A diagnosis of central hypoventilation requires the presence of blood gas abnormalities (desaturation, and/or CO_2 retention), even if these only occur during sleep periods. The common definition of respiratory failure is a pO_2 <60 mmHg and pCO_2 >50 mmHg. Treatment may be required for other sequelae, such as significant sleep disruption caused by a response of high arousal frequency as a protective reflex against these respiratory abnormalities.

Abnormalities of respiratory control may be congenital or acquired, and Fiona presented with acquired central hypoventilation where underlying pathologies are common. There is much new information available about the likely genetic origin of the congenital syndrome, now known as congenital central hypoventilation syndrome, or CCHS (Amiel *et al*, 2003). This disorder tends to manifest at, or very soon after, birth, with respiratory failure occurring at each sleep onset but normal blood gases maintained during wakefulness. Many patients with CCHS also have autonomic dysfunction (Marazita *et al*, 2001), and approximately 20% have Hirschprung's disorder. The most severely affected patients also hypoventilate in the awake state (Gaultier, 2003).

Sleep, particularly slow-wave sleep, is a time of vulnerability to hypoventilation, no matter what the underlying cause, because respiratory drive is dependent upon the intact function of central chemosensory centers at this time. In contrast, where the respiratory disorder is secondary to muscle weakness or dysfunction, the most vulnerable period is during REM sleep, when drive to accessory muscles falls.

The most common treatment for hypoventilation is nocturnal, non-invasive ventilation (Fauroux *et al*, 2003), although tracheostomy may be required. The role of surgical therapy remains under debate. When cental apnea or hypoventilation occurs in the presence of the Chiari malformation, posterior fossa decompression is commonly recommended. A number of studies have demonstrated that a history of past decompression increases the risk for current respiratory abnormalities. Few studies have documented significant improvement in response to the surgery (Kirk *et al*, 2000; Pollack *et al*, 1996; Waters *et al*, 1998). Medical therapies are unlikely to be successful, but may be used if the disorder is mild and associated with less severe underlying pathologies. Respiratory stimulant medications that have been used include theophylline and medroxyprogesterone (McNicholas and Phillipson, 2002).

Apneas in the newborn and infant

When infants have apneic events the most common concern is that of sudden infant death syndrome (SIDS). However there is no clear link between these two phenomena. The presentation for apneas may differ. The definitions listed below have been refined based on the likelihood of recurrence, treatment, and prognosis for resolution. Epidemiological studies have also failed to demonstrate that home monitoring has any impact on the incidence of SIDS. Most societies and health departments now recommend that if monitors are to be used they should be able to record events that trigger alarms and should only be used in special circumstances. There is however clear evidence that SIDS risk can be reduced by the simple measure of placing infants on their back to sleep, safe sleeping environments (avoiding excessive bedclothes), and avoiding cigarette smoke exposure before and after birth.

❖ *Apnea of infancy* has been defined as 'an unexplained episode of cessation of breathing for 20 seconds or longer, or shorter respiratory pauses associated with bradycardia, cyanosis, pallor and/or marked hypotonia'. This generally refers to infants ≥37 weeks gestation at the onset of the apnea.

❖ *Apnea of prematurity* is a similar event with cessation of breathing for 20 seconds or longer, or shorter respiratory pauses associated with bradycardia, desaturation (cyanosis) in an infant younger than 37 weeks' gestation. These episodes usually cease by 37 weeks' gestational age but may persist for several weeks beyond term. Recent evidence suggests that most severe episodes in such infants cease by 43 weeks post-conceptional age (American Academy of Pediatrics, 2003; Hunt, 2001). During the period of maturation, the most common and effective treatment is the use of xanthines (theophylline, or caffeine) (Steer and Henderson-Smart, 2003).

❖ *Apparent life-threatening events (ALTEs)* is defined as 'an episode that is frightening to the observer, and is characterised by some combination of apnea (central, and occasionally obstructive), colour change (usually cyanotic or pale, but sometimes flushed), marked change in muscle tone (usually limp), and/or choking or gagging'. A large number of such infants were reviewed by Kahn who identified a cause in 61% of cases. The most common pathology was gastroesophageal reflux (Kahn *et al*, 1988).

A large collaborative study in the United States (CHIME) demonstrated that, from a group of infants who were either siblings of SIDS victims or symptomatic and asymptomatic preterm infants, only those who were born prematurely were at increased risk for apneic events. All events showed a pattern of decreasing with age and, with each event that occurred, the risk of future events decreased (Ramanathan *et al*, 2001). Another study of infants admitted to hospital with ALTEs showed that recurrence of events in hospital was also the strongest predictor of future events (Cote *et al*, 1998).

It is clear that infants may also suffer from OSA, but most reports to date are anecdotal. Obstructive apneas were documented in the CHIME study, and these may have accounted for the higher incidence of events than previously observed. Infants who have OSA may present with ALTEs, but these are not the most common cause, since all respiratory events, including OSA, accounted for less than 2% of the positive diagnoses in a unit where PSG was routinely performed. Reports of a familial link between OSA and SIDS have had methodological weaknesses, primarily because of the difficulty in obtaining a positive diagnosis of SIDS with autopsy confirmation. A positive association was, therefore, only found when all events, including ALTEs, were included (Tishler *et al*, 1996).

In summary, infants who present with apneic events should have careful documentation of their history to determine the likelihood that events will recur. There is no current evidence to support a link between apneas or ALTEs and SIDS. The recommendation is that parents should, in all cases, be diligent with SIDS prevention measures. If on history or clinical examination there are signs of snoring or craniofacial abnormalities (particularly micrognathia) then PSG is recommended to screen for OSA. Where central apneas are diagnosed, all evidence supports the likelihood that these will improve with age.

Disorders of sleep phase or sleep architecture (sleepiness and tiredness)

Diagnosis and treatment of children with sleepiness, tiredness and associated behavioral and social consequences follow the same general principles as for adults (see *Chapter 8*). Disorders of sleep and wake function represent one important cause of the 'sleepy' child, but endocrine/metabolic and psychiatric disorders should also be considered. In many cases, the symptoms that precipitate the presentation are often the personal, social, and school-related sequelae of sleepiness, rather than the sleepiness itself.

Case study 7

Grant presents at 15 years of age because of increasing sleepiness. He also has major behavioral problems, with confrontational behavior that causes problems with his teachers at school and with the local police. He admits to smoking cigarettes and using marijuana. His usual sleep time is 10.00PM and he wakes at 7.30AM on school days and 10.00AM on weekends. He is reported to snore and be a restless sleeper. He is not attentive at school, falls asleep in class and often sleeps 2 hours after school.

At the age of 10, Grant was assessed for learning difficulties and he had a history of restlessness, destructiveness and disruptive behavior in the classroom, as reported by his teachers. A diagnosis of attention deficit hyperactivity disorder was made. He was also started on up to 75 mg amitriptyline because of intercurrent sleep-related enuresis. He had a good response to dexamphetamine 7.5 mg/day, but this medication was discontinued when his mother and father separated.

Overnight sleep study shows a sleep efficiency of 95% with snoring, but only two apneas per hour. An MSLT shows mean sleep latency of 6 minutes with sleep-onset REM in four out of four naps. Urine screening for drugs is negative on the day of the MSLT, and a sleep diary kept by his father showed regular sleep patterns over the preceding 2 weeks.

A diagnosis of probable narcolepsy was made and treatment with dexamphetamine re-instated. This resulted in significant symptomatic improvement on 10 mg at breakfast and midday. A repeat MSLT on medication showed that mean sleep latency was 15 minutes with no early-onset REM periods.

Case study 8

Hilary is a 15-year-old adopted child with a diagnosis of depression following an overdose at the age 11, which was treated with cipramil. She was investigated at the age of 14 because of increased sleepiness. She falls asleep at school and her school performance is poor. She regularly naps after school. At the time of assessment, Hilary reports sleep onset at 9.30PM to 10.30PM. She wakes at 7.00AM on school days. If left undisturbed, she sleeps until midday on weekend days. She has no history of late nights on Fridays or Saturdays and denies using recreational drugs. She has none of the ancillary symptoms of narcolepsy (hypnagogic hallucinations, sleep paralysis or cataplexy).

Sleep study shows delayed sleep onset but no other abnormalities. MSLT the next day shows a mean sleep latency of 5 minutes, with two out of four sleep-onset REM periods. A diagnosis of probable narcolepsy is made and she is started on dexamphetamine up to 20 mg/day in divided doses. However, Hilary has poor symptomatic response; she remains sleepy with poor school performance and her mother describes her as an 'unhappy' child. Cipramil and dexamphetamine are withdrawn under the supervision of her psychiatrist. Actigraphy over 4 days (*Figure 10.12*) is consistent with delayed sleep phase syndrome. Her urine screen is negative for drugs.

In light of the actigraphy, the history is reviewed and reveals that although Hilary goes to bed at 9.30PM or 10.30PM, she does not settle to sleep until well past midnight on most nights. A repeat sleep study and MSLT confirmed the late sleep onset, with a mean sleep latency of 8 minutes but no sleep-onset REM periods. Hilary is treated by restriction of time spent in bed, 3 mg melatonin in the evening and bright light therapy in the mornings. These measures resulted in significant improvement in her symptoms of sleepiness, mood, school performance and improved (earlier) sleep onset (*Figure 10.13*).

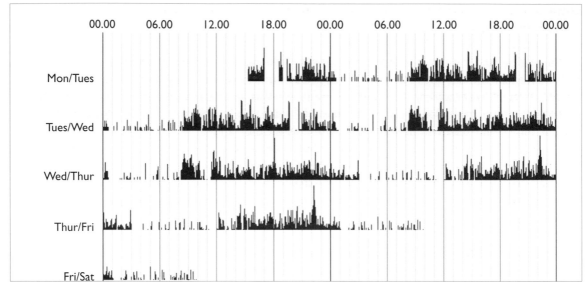

Figure 10.12: Actigraphy from a fifteen-year-old girl referred because of sleepiness and poor performance at school shows delayed sleep phase treatment.

Case study 7 (Grant) describes a child with narcolepsy who was initially diagnosed as having

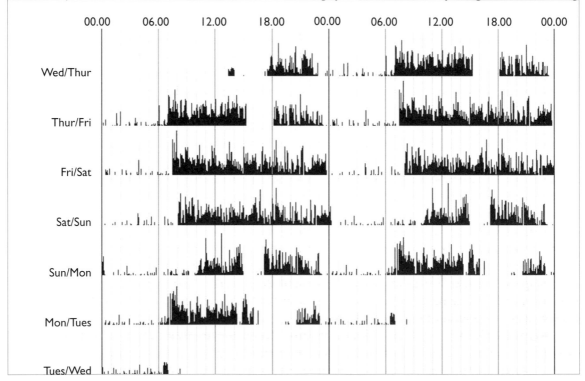

Figure 10.13: Actigraphy following treatment with melatonin, morning light therapy and restriction of time spent in bed shows normalization of sleep phase. This correlated with improvement of symptoms of sleepiness, mood and school performance.

attention deficit hyperactivity disorder (ADHD). Although his narcolepsy possibly coexisted with ADHD, the diagnosis of narcolepsy was delayed. This is a common problem with narcolepsy that commences in childhood and compounds the already psychosocial problems associated with this disorder. It is not uncommon for these children to have significant learning disabilities, personal, and social problems. The labels of 'laziness' and 'lacking motivation' may well be conferred by teachers and family alike. Despite achieving a correct diagnosis, ongoing emotional problems, lack of self-esteem, and cognitive and emotional problems are not uncommon despite symptomatic improvement on stimulant medication.

Case study 8 (Hilary) highlights the importance of keeping a high index of suspicion for abnormal sleep and wake patterns in children and teenagers who present with sleepiness. In this case, the diagnosis of delayed sleep phase syndrome (*Chapter 11*) was compounded by concurrent depression and may have contributed to her symptoms of tiredness and sleepiness.

Diagnosis and differential diagnosis

Young children rarely present with a primary problem of sleepiness. Children with increased sleepiness often present with behavioral problems, tiredness, being a 'daydreamer', or being inattentive in class and delaying tasks. The connection between sleepiness and symptoms is not straightforward and requires a high index of suspicion. The typical 'irresistible' sleep attack described in adults with narcolepsy is not common until teenage years. The differential diagnosis includes primary and secondary causes (*Table 10.6*).

Narcolepsy remains a difficult diagnosis to make in children. However, retrospective assessment of adults diagnosed with narcolepsy reveals that for approximately 50%, the symptoms started in childhood, although only 4% were diagnosed before the age of 15 (Dahl *et al*, 1994). The fact that sleepiness may often manifest in children with restlessness, motor hyperactivity and learning difficulties, and the bizarre nature of REM-related symptoms has led to many other diagnoses such as ADHD, conversion syndromes, psychotic depression and drug abuse (Dahl, 1996; Wise, 1998). Although the prevalence of narcolepsy–cataplexy in the general population is estimated at two to eighteen cases every 10,000 (American Academy of Sleep Medicine, 2005) the prevalence in the pediatric population is unknown. Hypnagogic (at the beginning of sleep) and hypnopompic (at the end of sleep) hallucinations are usually not volunteered by the young patient or are reported as frightening dreams at the time of falling asleep. Similarly, sleep paralysis may not be able to be described by a young child, although adolescents are more likely to report it when specifically asked.

Cataplexy (sudden loss of muscle power) manifests with the child falling on the ground during emotions such as laughing, as occurs in adults. It may also be described in non-typical fashion such as lack of balance or dizziness (Dahl, 1996).

Overnight sleep in children with narcolepsy tends to be disturbed with decreased sleep efficiency. Confusional arousal in the morning may be a frequent symptom (Wise, 1998). Family history of narcolepsy is useful but not common. Similarly, genetic testing for HLA DR2 and DQ1 subtypes support the diagnosis of narcolepsy but is not essential for the diagnosis.

Table 10.6: Increased sleepiness/tiredness: differential diagnosis	
Primary	**Secondary**
• Narcolepsy	• Insufficient sleep
• Idiopathic hypesomnolence	• Delayed sleep phase syndrome
• Klein–Levin syndrome	• Obstructive sleep apnea
• Primary disorder of vigilance	• Periodic limb movement disorder
	• Depression
	• Substance abuse
	• Post-infectious hypersomnolence
	• Post-traumatic hypersomnolence

Overnight sleep study and multiple sleep latency tests (MSLT) are required to make the diagnosis. The presence of early-onset REM in the overnight polysomnography or decreased mean sleep latency (less than 8 minutes) during the daytime naps, together with two or more onsets of REM, support the diagnosis of narcolepsy. However, as exemplified by *Case study 8* (Hilary) REM abnormalities may be present in chronic sleep deprivation and following withdrawal from medications such as benzodiazepines, stimulants or antidepressants.

The overnight PSG is useful for excluding other causes of sleep fragmentation such as obstructive sleep apnea and periodic limb movement disorder which may lead to increased sleepiness tendency in their own right. Supervised urine collection for drug screening is always indicated, particularly in teenagers.

The clinical evaluation of narcolepsy is made difficult by the fact that the symptoms of sleepiness, hypnagogic (at the beginning of sleep) and hypnopompic (at the end of sleep) hallucinations, sleep paralysis and cataplexy rarely occur together. The initial complaint bringing the child to medical attention varies with the age of the child (Guilleminault and Pelayo, 1998) (*Table 10.7*). Academic and learning difficulties can be a prominent feature (*Table 10.8*).

Multiple sleep latency test

Pediatric standards have been developed for the multiple sleep latency test (MSLT) as an objective measure of daytime sleepiness. A diagnosis of narcolepsy, associated with short sleep latencies, is rare. Prepubertal children are remarkably alert and they do not normally fall asleep during daytime testing. A mean sleep latency of less than 15 minutes should be considered abnormal. In normal children, mean sleep latency is 26.4 minutes, so nap opportunities should be of at least 30 minutes duration when undertaking MSLT in children. In one study evaluating MSLT in normal children, sleep propensity was similar to children with snoring alone, with values of 23.7 minutes for both groups, compared to 20.0 minutes in children with OSA where the apnea index was 14 per hour (Gozal *et al*, 2001).

Table 10.7: Initial complaint

Children up to 5 years old

Unexplained abrupt falls on the ground, with absence of abnormal movements, 'drop attacks'
Aggressive behavior, abrupt irritability, 'absent' look
Sleep terror, unresponsive with abrupt crying spells/absent during naps and nocturnal sleep
Abrupt dropping of objects

Children five to ten years old (n = 40)

Repetitive falling asleep in class, continuously asleep in class, abnormal napping
Impossible to arouse in the morning with aggressive behavior and tantrum
when awoken
Abrupt fall in school
Questions of learning disability (poor memory, low concentration, inappropriate performance
with inadequate comprehension and attention)
Abnormal behavior in school (hyperactivity with attention deficit, hyperactivity with verbal
and physical aggressiveness, hyperactivity with outbursts of strong irritability)
Abnormal behavior at home, hallucinatory behavior, repetitive nightmares
First considered diagnosis
a. neurological disorder (epilepsy, or brain tumor)
b. attention deficit disorder
c. schizophrenia
First considered diagnosis sleep disorder

Children 10–12 years old (n = 6)

Inappropriate alertness, falling asleep in class and at home, unable to wake up missing
morning classes
Abrupt unexplained falls
Significant drop in academic performance, not performing assignments, unable to
follow curriculum
First diagnosis considered: sleep disorder
Neurological disorder (epilepsy)

Children who have confirmed daytime sleepiness, especially in the absence of OSA, should be reviewed by a specialist in sleep medicine and other causes for hypersomnolence should be considered, provided that sleep insufficiency has been excluded (see later in this chapter).

Differential diagnoses

Children with insufficient sleep and delayed sleep phase syndrome can present with daytime sleepiness. A detailed history of the child's sleep habits and documentation by sleep diary and/or actigraphy is sufficient to clarify the diagnosis (as in *Case study 8,* Hilary). The differential diagnosis of narcoleptic syndrome and psychiatric illnesses is difficult as they often coexist, either as independent processes or as a complication of unrecognized narcolepsy. Hypersomnolence is a significant symptom in about 25% of children with major depressive disorder.

The diagnostic boundaries between narcolepsy and idiopathic hypersomnolence (non-REM narcolepsy) are quite blurred. Idiopathic hypersomnolence is characterized by increased sleepiness tendency documented by reduced sleep latency on MSLT, absence of cataplexy, hypnagogic hallucinations, sleep paralysis and lack of sleep-onset REM during the daytime naps. The fact that narcolepsy can present with increased sleepiness tendency as the only symptom, with REM-related manifestations occurring years later, makes the distinction between the two diagnoses difficult.

Table 10.8: School problems in children with narcolepsy
Poor attention and concentration
Irritability and emotional lability
Difficulty with longer tests and assignments
Memory problems
Embarrassment by teachers and peers because of sleepiness or cataplexy
False accusations of drug use
Tardiness and forgetfulness
Social isolation and decreased participation in after-school activities
Disciplinary problems due to sleeping in class
Difficulty with athletics due to cataplexy or sleepiness
Problems complying with stimulant-medication schedule during school hours

❖ *Post-infectious hypersomnolence:* the history of sleepiness/tiredness occurring following infective illness such as Epstein–Barr virus, cytomegalovirus, Q fever and mycoplasma is frequently associated with increased sleepiness in the absence of REM symptoms (Guilleminault and Mondini, 1986). It should not be misdiagnosed as chronic fatigue syndrome (CFS) because treatment with stimulants is effective in improving sleepiness (Ambrogetti *et al*, 1998), and spares the young patient the long series of orthodox and unorthodox investigations and treatment which usually follows a diagnosis of chronic fatigue syndrome. Post-infectious hypersomnolence tends to improve over time but is a life-long condition.

❖ *Post-traumatic hypersomnolence* varies in severity, but is a similar scenario, occurring after a head trauma (American Academy of Sleep Medicine, 2005).

❖ *Periodic hypersomnolence* is a distinct syndrome usually suspected by a typical history of sleepiness with acute or subacute onset lasting from one day to a few weeks with intervals of normal alertness. More common in males, the onset is between the ages of 10 and 20 years. It may be preceded by a viral-like infection. It tends to resolve spontaneously but symptomatic treatment with stimulants is sometimes needed if the episodes of sleepiness are prolonged. Stimulant treatment, however, is not used as prophylactic treatment. The best recognized form of periodic hypersomnolence is the Klein-Levin syndrome. During the period of sleepiness, the child may try to spend long hours in bed getting up only for a brief period during which she may be irritable and confused. In some cases overeating is an associated feature whereby the child compulsively eats whatever is within his reach. Uninhibited sexual behavior is also reported in about one third of the cases, with inappropriate sexual advances or masturbation (American Academy of Sleep Medicine, 2005).

The diagnosis of primary disorders of vigilance (Weinberg and Brumback, 1990; Weinberg and Harper, 1993) is a recently proposed finding to identify children with reported tendency to increased sleepiness, excessive napping and motor restlessness without evidence of pathological daytime sleepiness on MSLT or REM abnormalities (*Table 10.9*). Treatment is similar to narcolepsy with stimulant medications.

Treatment

The need for child and family education and support cannot be overemphasized in any disorder of excessive sleepiness. Detailed explanation of the underlying cause of the child's sleep disorder, be it insufficient sleep, circadian rhythm disorder, narcolepsy, or disorders of vigilance, is essential to treatment success. All these disorders require behavioral and lifestyle interventions, regardless of whether adjuvant medications are available. Good sleep hygiene, involving regular bed schedules, is important for all the above conditions, so consistency and discipline is important. If the same routine is not maintained on weekends and holidays, significant problems are likely to recur each time school recommences. In addition, whenever sleep times are being changed, the schedule should consider that wake-up times are often fixed according to social commitments and bedtime is more easily manipulated. Families need to understand that if their child's sleep time has been late for some time, adjustment to an earlier sleep onset may need to be implemented gradually, often by 5–20-minute intervals, which are changed every 1–2 weeks. Encouraging bright-light exposure on waking can also help maintain the circadian entrainment; breakfast on the veranda or a short walk with the family pet or family members are lifestyle changes that will assist in this (*Chapter 11*).

Enlisting the child's cooperation directly is important. However other social contacts will also need a full explanation of the child's condition and the needs that this brings to their social settings. For example, teachers can help with special arrangements for daytime naps and changes to the academic curriculum. Teenagers need to be counselled about driving, engaging in activities where sleepiness may be dangerous, and the limitations that this diagnosis will impose on their potential career paths. Jobs that require driving or high states of vigilance would not be available to them.

Table 10.9: Criteria for primary disorder of vigilance

A. Primary disorder of vigilance is a disorder of at least 1 year's duration, with symptoms from all five major symptom categories:

   1. Decreasing ability to sustain alertness, wakefulness, arousal and watchfulness during continuous mental (or other task) performance
      a. Complaints of tiredness, drowsiness, sleepiness, lethargy
      b. Yawning, stretching, sleepy-eyed ('glassy-eyed') appearance
      c. Falling asleep, excessive napping

   2. Decreasing attention to present activities
      a. Daydreaming
      b. Difficulty focusing attention; loses place in activities and conversation
      c. Poor performance
      d. Slow, delayed or incomplete tasks
      e. Disorganized

   3. Avoidance of structured or repetitive activities
      a. Loss of interest in structured activities, or complaint that they are dull, boring, monotonous, tedious, uninteresting (or no longer interesting)
      b. Preference for shifting activities that have random or irregular changes in schedule or activity (orderly randomization)

   4. Motor restlessness and behaviors to improve alertness
      a. Fidgeting
      b. Talkativeness
      c. Moving about
      d. Busyness

   5. Caring, compassionate, affectionate, kind temperament

B. This major symptom category is accepted as positive when the symptom or one or more of its behaviors is identified in a semistructured closed-end interview of patient and primary caretakers.

C. This symptom complex must precede the onset of other medical disorders (including depression, narcolepsy, various medications, alcohol and drug abuse, hypothyroidism) that can cause secondary hypovigilance.

D. Although symptoms may be identified at any age, the disorder generally becomes more symptomatic with schooling and aging, and can result in increasing maladaptation.

Medications

The use of stimulant medications, dexamphetamine, methylphenidate and modafinil (Ivanenko *et al*, 2003), are indicated for symptomatic treatment for daytime sleepiness and for primary disturbance of vigilance. The amount and time of the dose may require several trials, with all medications started at the lowest possible dose and titrated upwards to minimise side-effects (eg. 2.5 mg of dexamphetamine or 5 mg of methylphenidate). The pattern of use can be continuous on a daily basis or intermittent. However there is no evidence that drug-free days improve efficiency. It also needs to be emphasized that stimulants improve alertness but the tendency to sleepiness is not overcome completely and scheduled naps continue to play a role in maintaining daytime performance. When cataplexy is a prominent feature, the addition of a tricyclic antidepressant, clomipramine, or SSRI (fluoxetine, sertraline) may be required. In case of delayed sleep phase syndrome, the use of melatonin (0.5–5 mg) two to three hours before the desired sleep onset, can help maintain the earlier bedtime (Smits *et al*, 2003). However the safety of melatonin in prepubertal youth is not established.

Ongoing management

Regular follow-up is necessary to maintain compliance and provide support and ongoing education (*Table 10.10*).

Enuresis

Bed-wetting is widespread in children up to the age of 14 years. The organic causes listed below should be excluded before managing the significant emotional and behavioral disturbances that can be associated with bed-wetting.

Normal voiding starts with the contraction of the abdominal muscles, which cause descent of the bladder neck, followed by relaxation of the pelvic floor muscles and contraction of the bladder detrusor. Over the first few years of life, children learn to perceive bladder fullness and control micturition. The ability to inhibit micturition requires contraction of the pelvic floor muscles (Sheldon, 1996). The development of urinary continence during the day and night requires integration of both an autonomic bladder mechanism and abdominal voluntary muscle control.

Most children have acquired urinary

Table 10.10: Goals for long-term management of childhood narcolepsy

Patient and parent education and emotional support

Counseling regarding medication compliance and sleep hygiene

Monitoring medication response and side-effects

Monitoring of emergence of coexisting sleep disorders

Monitoring academic performance

Counseling regarding career planning and appropriate vocational choices

Identification of depression, family conflict, or other emotional problems

Monitoring for high-risk behaviors, such as alcohol or drug use and driving while sleepy

Assistance with documentation for academic needs, insurance or disability forms, and driver's license forms

Difficulty with athletics due to cataplexy or sleepiness

Problems complying with stimulant-medication schedule during school hours control during the day and the night by the age of 5 years. By convention, nocturnal enuresis becomes a problem because of coincident social development including starting school, having friends to sleep over and being invited to school trips or camping activities. Sleep-related enuresis can cause significant obstacles to these activities, deep embarrassment, low self-esteem and a sense of shame and stress within the family.

The prevalence of sleep-related enuresis is twice as common in boys than girls and is similar across country and ethnic groups (Caldwell *et al*, 2005; Challamel and Cochat, 1999; Sheldon, 1996). At 6 years of age, bed-wetting is reported in 8–20% of children and by the age of 12, persists in 3%, falling to approximately 1% at the age of 15 (*Figure 10.14*).

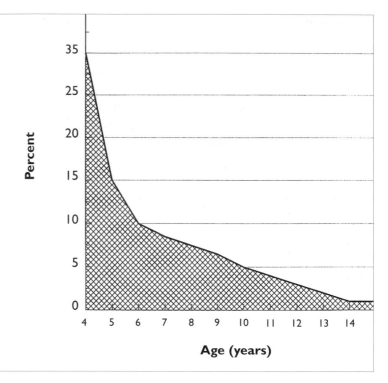

Figure 10.14: Frequency of nocturnal enuresis by age group. (Modified from Crawford JD: Introductory comments. J Pediatr 1989: 114(Part 2): 687–690; and Novello JR: Enuresis. Pediatr Clin North Am 1987; 34: 719–730 with permission). In: Sheldon et al; Pediatric Sleep Medicine 1992: 153, WB Saunders (Publishers).

It is useful to distinguish between primary enuresis and secondary enuresis. Primary enuresis refers to bed-wetting that has never ceased, ie. there have been no dry intervals. Secondary enuresis refers to bed-wetting that has recurred after a dry period of at least 3 months. Medical and psychological diagnoses are more commonly associated with cases of secondary enuresis (Robson and Leung, 2000).

In about 10% of cases of enuresis, medical or psychological causes are present (Forsythe and Redmond, 1974). History and appropriate investigation should exclude:

- urinary tract infection
- severe constipation
- urinary incontinence, that includes wakefulness
- OSA — generally accompanied by a history of snoring
- polyuria and polydipsia (indicative of diabetes mellitus or insipidus)
- evidence of family stress or poor social circumstances may suggest child neglect or abuse.

Where infections are found, urinary tract abnormalities such as vesicoureteric reflux, bladder or urethral abnormalities and intrinsic renal pathology need to be excluded. Apart from urinalysis, investigations are generally dictated by the history.

The underlying pathophysiology of primary enuresis is multifactorial and includes:

⌘ *Family history:* there is strong heritability and when both parents were affected, 77% of children have the same problem, compared to 44% of children with one affected parent and 15% of children where there is no family history (Challamel and Cochat, 1999). A twin study has confirmed these findings (Neveus *et al*, 1999).

⌘ *Functional bladder capacity:* the child needs to achieve a bladder capacity of 300–360 ml of urine to remain dry over night. Functional bladder capacity remains inadequate for longer when children have sleep-related enuresis.

⌘ *Reduced ability to wake in response to a full bladder:* the impression that enuretic children appear more difficult to wake than non-enuretic ones is not supported by objective assessments. Enuresis occurs in all stages of sleep and during daytime naps, so there is no evidence to support the assumption that it occurs during deep sleep or any particular sleep stage (Challamel and Cochat, 1999; Foxman *et al*, 1986; Kalo and Bella, 1996).

⌘ *Inadequate nocturnal secretion of antidiuretic hormone (vasopressin):* a reduction of nocturnal increase in vasopressin in enuretic children reduces the ability to concentrate urine and contributes to bed-wetting in some children.

Management

The natural history of enuresis means that spontaneous resolution occurs in 14–19% of children per year (Forsythe and Redmond, 1974). However, only 50% of children who are still bed-wetting at the age of 5 will be dry by the age of 10. Behavioral management requires prolonged follow-up, family support and multidisciplinary interventions that may involve a combination of behavioral strategies, bladder training and pharmacological intervention. Once any organic and/or psychological causes have been excluded, treatment of primary enuresis is best undertaken through specialist (dedicated) enuresis clinics whenever possible. Such programs usually enrol children aged 6 years and above.

The primary clinician can assist by explaining the nature, prevalence and anticipated outcomes to the family. The clinician is also in a position to offer ongoing support to the child and family when the condition is slow to improve (over weeks/months) or recurrences occur. Support groups like the Enuresis Resources and Information Centre (ERIC) in the UK can also be helpful.

Behavioral interventions

Behavioral intervention and conditioning are effective but time-consuming and require well-motivated families and ongoing support. Some general behavioral principles applicable to this disorder include the provision of a supportive and encouraging environment for the child and avoiding comments that lead to guilt or shame. Encouragement is provided by focusing on praise for dry nights and working with school staff to allow participation in activities such as school excursions to ensure that the child need not fear vilification. Behavioral interventions may be complemented by the short-term use of medications, for example on school excursions.

Normal fluid intake should be encouraged as there is no evidence that daytime fluid restriction is an effective intervention. The bedtime routine should include a trip to the toilet. Scheduled waking of the child late in the evening (before the parents go to bed and early hours of the morning) can also be helpful because it increases the likelihood of dry nights and, therefore, more opportunities for positive feedback.

Bladder capacity can be improved by bladder training exercises. Strategies incorporate the consumption of an adequate daytime fluid intake (1–1.5 litres per day at 6–10 years of age). To increase awareness of bladder fullness, the child should be encouraged to wait until their bladder feels full before urinating. To confirm improvement, intermittently measure voided volumes.

Enuresis alarm systems (*Figure 10.15*) are safe and effective strategies. The alarm system uses conditioning feedback and is triggered by the onset of urination. The early phase of this intervention is crucial to its ultimate success because parents often need to wake the child and ensure that micturition is finished in the toilet. The goal is that the child will wake in response to the alarm, and over a period of several days to weeks, have increased awareness of the need to void. This 'pad and bell' intervention is usually continued until 3 weeks of consecutive dry nights, and the success rate for this therapy is approximately 70% per year.

Pharmacological intervention has remained the most common form of treatment for enuresis (Tang *et al*, 2002). The most common drug in use is desmopressin. This synthetic analogue of vasopressin is delivered intranasally, one to two puffs at bed time (20–40 µ). This reduces nocturnal urine production by approximately 20%, and sleep-related enuresis improves in 50–80% of children (Brunetti *et al*, 2001; Challamel and Cochat, 1999). Side-effects are rare and include nasal congestion, nausea, abdominal cramps, nose bleeds, and headaches. A very rare side-effect is water intoxication with hyponatremia in cases of unrecognized psychogenic polydipsia. The main practical disadvantage of this therapy is that enuresis tends to recur when desmopressin is stopped.

Desmopressin can be used as an adjunct to behavioral therapies, including during times when the child wants to sleep away from home, such as at friend's houses, with school excursions, or on camping trips.

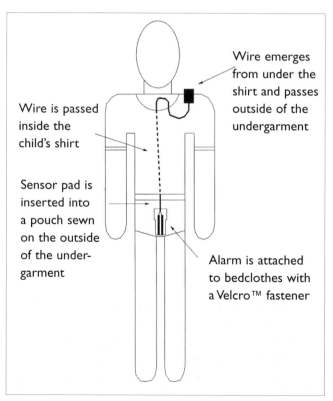

Figure 10.15: Diagram of proper placement of an enuresis alarm (From Palco Labs: Help for bed-wetting. Santa Cruz, California). With permission from Sheldon et al; Pediatric Sleep Medicine 1992, WB Saunders, Philadelphia.

Imipramine 25–50 mg at bedtime, has been widely used in the past and remains useful if desmopressin is not available, or if the side-effects of desmopressin prevent its use. However, the routine use of imipramine has essentially been superseded now that desmopressin is readily available.

References

Adair R, Bauchner H, Philipp B, Levenson S, Zuckerman B (1991) Night waking during infancy: Role of parental presence at bedtime. *Pediatrics* **87**(4): 500–4

Ahmed K, McCormick MS, Baruah AK (1993) Day-case adenoidectomy — is it safe? *Clin Otolaryngol Allied Sci* **18**(5): 406–9

Ali N J, Pitson DJ, Stradling JR (1993) Snoring, sleep disturbance, and behavior in 4–5 year olds. *Arch Dis Child* **68**(3): 360–6

Ali NJ, Pitson D, Stradling JR (1994) Natural history of snoring and related behavior problems between the ages of 4 and 7 years. *Arch Dis Child* **71**(1): 74–6

Ali NJ, Pitson D, Stradling JR (1996) Sleep-disordered breathing: Effects of adenotonsillectomy on behavior and psychological functioning. *Eur J Pediatr* **155**(1): 56–62

Ambrogetti A, Olson LG, Sutherland D, Malcolm JA, Bliss D, Gyulay S (1998) Daytime sleepiness and REM sleep abnormalities in chronic fatigue: A case series. *J Chron Fatig Syndrome* **4**(1): 23–35

American Academy of Pediatrics (2003) Apnea, sudden infant death syndrome, and home monitoring (policy statement). *Pediatrics* **111**(4): 914

American Academy of Sleep Medicine (2005) *The International Classification of Sleep Disorders. Diagnostic & Coding Manual.* 2nd edn. American Academy of Sleep Medicine, Westchester, IL

American Thoracic Society (1996) Standards and indications for cardiopulmonary sleep studies in children. *Am J Respir Crit Care Med* **153**(2): 866–78

Amiel J, Laudier B, Attie-Bitach T, Trang HT, de Pontual L, Gener B *et al* (2003) Polyalanine expansion and frameshift mutations of the paired-like homeobox gene *phox2b* in congenital central hypoventilation syndrome. *Nat Genet* **33**(4): 459–61

Amin RS, Kimball TR, Bean JA, Jeffries JL, Willging JP, Cotton RT *et al* (2002) Left ventricular hypertrophy and abnormal ventricular geometry in children and adolescents with obstructive sleep apnea. *Am J Respir Crit Care Med* **165**(10): 1395–9

Anders TF, Halpern LF, Hua J (1992) Sleeping through the night: A developmental perspective. *Pediatrics* **90**(4): 554–60

Anders TF, Keener M (1985) Developmental course of nighttime sleep-wake patterns in full-term and premature infants during the first year of life. I. *Sleep* **8**(3): 173–92

Bader G, Lavigne G (2000) Sleep bruxism; an overview of an oromandibular sleep movement disorder: Review article. *Sleep Med Rev* **4**(1): 27–43

Bassetti C, Vella S, Donati F, Wielepp P, Weder B (2000) SPECT during sleep-walking. *Lancet* **356**(9228): 484–5

Blunden S, Lushington K, Kennedy D, Martin J, Dawson D (2000) Behavior and neurocognitive performance in children aged 5–10 years who snore compared to controls. *J Clin Exp Neuropsychol* **22**(5): 554–68

Brouillette RT, Fernbach SK, Hunt CE (1982) Obstructive sleep apnea in infants and children. *J Pediatr* **100**(1): 31–40

Brouilette R, Hanson D, David R, Klemka L, Szatkowski A, Fernbach S, Hunt C (1984) A diagnostic approach to suspected obstructive sleep apnea in children. *J Pediatr* **105**(1): 10–4

Brouillette RT, Manoukian JJ, Ducharme FM, Oudjhane K, Earle LG, Ladan S, Morielli A (2001) Efficacy of fluticasone nasal spray for pediatric obstructive sleep apnea. *J Pediatr* **138**(6): 838–44

Brouillette RT, Morielli A, Leimanis A, Waters KAS, Lujciano R, Ducharme FM (2000) Nocturnal pulse oximtery as an abbreviated testing modality for pediatric obstructive sleep apnea. *Pediatr* **138**(6): 838–44

Brown LW (1996) Sleep and epilepsy. In: Dahl RE, ed. *Sleep Disorders, Child and Adolescent Psychiatric Clinics of North America*. WB Saunders, Philadelphia

Brunetti L, Rana S, Lospalluti ML, Pietrafesa A, Francavilla R, Fanelli M, Armenio L (2001) Prevalence of obstructive sleep apnea syndrome in a cohort of 1,207 children of southern Italy. *Chest* **120**(6): 1930–5

Caldwell PH, Edgar D, Hodson E, Craig J (2005) Bed-wetting and toileting problems in children. *Med J Aust* **182**(4): 190–5

Carroll JL (1996) Sleep-related upper-airway obstruction in children and adolescents. In: Dahl RE, ed. *Sleep Disorders. Child and Adolescent Psychiatric Clinics of North America*. Saunders, Philadelphia

Carroll JL, Loughlin GM (1992) Diagnostic criteria for obstructive sleep apnea syndrome in children. *Pediatr Pulmonol* **14**(2): 71–4

Carroll JL, Loughlin GM (1995a) Obstructive sleep apnea syndrome in infants and children: Diagnosis and Management. In: Ferber C, Kryger MH, eds. *Principles and Practice of Sleep Medicine in the Child*. Saunders, Philadelphia

Carroll JL, Loughlin GM (1995b) Obstructive sleep apnea syndrome in infants and children: Clinical features and pathophysiology. In: Ferber C, Kryger MH, eds. *Principles and Practice of Sleep Medicine in the Child*. Saunders, Philadelphia

Carroll JL, McColley SA, Marcus CL, Curtis S, Loughlin GM (1995) Inability of clinical history to distinguish primary snoring from obstructive sleep apnea syndrome in children. *Chest* **108**(3): 610–8

Challamel MJ, Cochat P (1999) Review article: Enuresis: Pathophysiology and treatment. *Sleep Med Rev* **3**(4): 313–24

Chisholm T, Morehouse RL (1996) Adult headbanging: Sleep studies and treatment. *Sleep* **19**(4): 343–6

Cote A, Hum C, Brouillette RT, Themens M (1998) Frequency and timing of recurrent events in infants using home cardiorespiratory monitors.[comment]. *J Pediatr* **132**(5): 783–9

Dahl RE (1996) Narcolepsy in children and adolescents. In: Dahl RE, editor. *Sleep Disorders, Child and Adolescent Psychiatric Clinics of North America*. Saunders, Philadelphia: 649-660

Dahl RE, Holttum J, Trubnick L (1994) A clinical picture of child and adolescent narcolepsy. *J Am Acad Child Adolescent Psychiatry* **33**(6): 834–41

Dahl RE, Williamson DJ (1990) Aggressive partial arousals proceeding competitive football games. *Sleep Res* **19**: 116

Darrow DH, Siemens C (2002) Indications for tonsillectomy and adenoidectomy. *Laryngoscope* **112**(8 Pt 2): 6–10

de Veerd AW, van den Bossche RA (2003) The development of sleep during the first months of life. *Sleep Med Rev* **7**(2): 179–91

Donnelly LF, Surdulescu V, Chini BA, Casper KA, Poe SA, Amin RS (2003) Upper airway motion depicted at cine MR imaging performed during sleep: Comparison between young patients with and those without obstructive sleep apnea. *Radiology* **227**(1): 239–45

Downey R, III, Perkin RM, MacQuarrie J (2000) Nasal continuous positive airway pressure use in children with obstructive sleep apnea younger than 2 years of age. *Chest* **117**(6): 1608–12

Everett AD, Koch WC, Saulsbury FT (1987) Failure to thrive due to obstructive sleep apnea. *Clin Pediatr* **26**(2): 90–2

Fauroux B, Boffa C, Desguerre I, Estournet B, Trang H (2003) Long-term noninvasive mechanical ventilation for children at home: A national survey. *Pediatr Pulmonol* **35**(2): 119–25

Fisher C, Kahn E, Edwards A, Davis DM, Fine J (1974) A psychophysiological study of nightmares and night terrors. 3. Mental content and recall of stage 4 night terrors. *J Nerv Ment Dis* **158**(3): 174–88

Forsythe WI, Redmond A (1974) Enuresis and spontaneous cure rate. Study of 1129 enuretics. *Arch Dis Child* **49**(4): 259–63

Foulkes D (1982) *Children's Dreams: Longitudinal Studies*. Wiley, New York

Foxman B, Valdez RB, Brook RH (1986) Childhood enuresis: Prevalence, perceived impact, and prescribed treatments. *Pediatrics* **77**(4): 482–7

France KG, Henderson JMT, Hudson SM (1996) Fact, act and tact: A three-stage approach to treating the sleep problems of infants and young children. In: Dahl RE, ed. *Sleep Disorders, Child and Adolescent Psychiatric Clinics of North America*. Saunders, Philadelphia

Friedman O, Chidekel A, Lawless ST, Cook SP (1999) Postoperative bilevel positive airway pressure ventilation after tonsillectomy and adenoidectomy in children — a preliminary report. *Int J Ped Otolaryngol* **51**(3): 177–80

Gau SF, Soong WT (1999) Psychiatric comorbidity of adolescents with sleep terrors or sleep-walking: A case control study. *Aust N Z J Psychiat* **33**(5): 734–9

Gaultier C, Dauger S, Simonneau M, Gallego J (2003) Genes modulation chemical breathing control: lessons from mutant animals. *Resp Physiol Neurobiol* **136**: 105–14

Gislason T, Benediktsdottir B (1995) Snoring, apneic episodes, and nocturnal hypoxemia among children 6 months to 6 years old. An epidemiologic study of lower limit of prevalence. *Chest* **107**(4): 963–6

Goldstein NA, Post JC, Rosenfeld RM, Campbell TF (2000) Impact of tonsillectomy and adenoidectomy on child behavior. *Arch Otolaryngol Head Neck Surg* **126**(4): 494–8

Gozal D (1998) Sleep-disordered breathing and school performance in children. *Pediatrics* **102**(3 part I): 616–20.

Gozal D, Wang M, Pope DW, Jr (2001) Objective sleepiness measures in pediatric obstructive sleep apnea. *Pediatrics* **108**(3): 693–7

Greenhill L, Puig-Antich J, Goetz R, Hanlon C, Davies M (1983) Sleep architecture and REM sleep measures in prepubertal children with attention deficit disorder with hyperactivity. *Sleep* **6**(2): 91–101

Grunewald RA, Penayiotopoulos CP (1993) Juvenile myoclonic epilepsy — a review. *Arch Neurol* **50**: 594–8

Guilleminault C, Korobkin R, Winkle R (1981) A review of 50 children with obstructive sleep apnea syndrome. *Lung* **159**(5): 275–87

Guilleminault C, Mondini S (1986) Mononucleosis and chronic daytime sleepiness. A long-term follow-up study. *Arch Intern Med* **146**(7): 1333–5

Guilleminault C, Pelayo R, Clerk A, Leger D, Cobian RC (1995) Home nasal continuous positive airway pressure in infants with sleep-disordered breathing. *J Pediatr* **127**(6): 905–12

Guilleminault C, Pelayo R (1998) Narcolepsy in prepubertal children. *Ann Neurol* **43**(1): 135–42

Hartmann E, Russ D, van der Kolk B, Falke R, Oldfield M (1981) The preliminary study of the personality of the nightmare sufferer: Relationship to schizophrenia and creativity? *Am J Psychiat* **138**(6): 794–7

Hawkins C, Williams TI (1992) Nightmares, life events and behavior problems in preschool children. *Child: Care, Health Dev* **18**(2): 117–28

Herman JH, Blawme, Steinberg JB (1989) REM behavior disorder in a 2-year-old male with evidence of brain stem pathology. *Sleep Res* **18**: 242

Hunt CE (2001) Sudden infant death syndrome and other causes of infant mortality . Diagnosis, mechanisms, and risk for recurrence in siblings. *Am J Respir Crit Care Med* **164**(3): 346–57

Ivanenko A, Tauman R, Gozal D (2003) Modafinil in the treatment of excessive daytime sleepiness in children. *Sleep Med* **4**: 579–82

Janz D (1985) Epilepsy with impulsive petit mal (juvenile myoclonic epilepsy). *Acta Neurol Scand* **72**(5): 449–59

Kahn A, Rebuffat E, Sottiaux M, Blum D (1988) Management of an infant with an apparent life-threatening event. *Pediatrician* **15**(4): 204–11

Kales A, Soldatos CR, Bixler EO, Ladda RL, Charney DS, Weber G, Schweitzer PK (1980) Hereditary factors in sleep-walking and night terrors. *Br J Psychiat* **137**: 111–8

Kales A, Soldatos CR, Caldwell AB, Kales JD, Humphrey FJ, II, Charney DS, Schweitzer PK (1980b) Somnambulism. Clinical characteristics and personality patterns. *Arch Gen Psychiat* **37**(12): 1406–10

Kalo BB, Bella H (1996) Enuresis: Prevalence and associated factors among primary school children in Saudi Arabia. *Acta Paediatr* **85**(10): 1217–22

Kennedy DJ, Waters KA (2005) Investigation and treatment of upper-airway obstruction: childhood sleep disorders 1. *Med J Aust* **182**(8): 419–23

Kirk VG, Morielli A, Gozal D, Marcus CL, Waters KA, D'Andrea LA *et al* (2000) Treatment of sleep-disordered breathing in children with myelomeningocele. *Pediatr Pulmonol* **30**(6): 445–52

Klackenberg G (1982) Somnambulism in childhood — prevalence, course and behavioral correlations. A prospective longitudinal study (6–16 years). *Acta Paediatr Scand* **71**(3): 495–9

Kleitman N (1987) *Sleep and Wakefulness.* The University of Chicago Press, Chicago

Lewin DS, Rosen RC, England SJ, Dahl RE (2002) Preliminary evidence of behavioral and cognitive sequelae of obstructive sleep apnea in children. *Sleep Med* **3**: 5–13

Lind MG, Lundell BP (1982) Tonsillar hyperplasia in children. A cause of obstructive sleep apneas, CO_2 retention, and retarded growth. *Arch Otolaryngol* **108**(10): 650–4

Lipton AJ, Gozal D (2003) Treatment of obstructive sleep apnea in children: do we really know how? *Sleep Med Rev* **7**(1): 61–80

Lozoff B (1995) Culture and family: Influences on childhood sleep practices and problems. In: Ferber C, Kryger MH, eds. *Principles and Practice of Sleep Medicine in the Child.* Saunders, Philadelphia

Madansky D, Edelbrock C (1990) Cosleeping in a community sample of 2- and 3-year-old children. *Pediatrics* **86**(2): 197–203 [erratum in *Pediatrics* 1990 **86**(5): 702]

Mahowald MW, Schenck CH (1992) Dissociated states of wakefulness and sleep. *Neurology* **42**(suppl 6): 44–52

Marazita ML, Maher BS, Cooper ME, Silvestri JM, Huffman AD, Smok-Pearsall SM *et al* (2001) Genetic segregation analysis of autonomic nervous system dysfunction in families of probands with idiopathic congenital central hypoventilation syndrome. *Am J Med Genet* **100**(3): 229–36

Marcus CL, Hamer A, Loughlin GM (1998) Natural history of primary snoring in children. *Pediatr Pulmonol* **26**(1): 6–11

Marcus CL, Omlin KJ, Basinki DJ, Bailey SL, Rachal AB, Von Pechmann WS *et al* (1992) Normal polysomnographic values for children and adolescents. *Am Rev Respir Dis* **146**(5 pt 1): 1235–9

Marcus CL, Ward SL, Mallory GB, Rosen CL, Beckerman RC, Weese-Mayer DE *et al* (1995) Use of nasal continuous positive airway pressure as treatment of childhood obstructive sleep apnea. *J Pediatr* **127**(1): 88–94

McColley SA, April MM, Carroll JL, Naclerio RM, Loughlin GM (1992) Respiratory compromise after adenotonsillectomy in children with obstructive sleep apnea. *Arch Otolaryngol Head Neck Surg* **118**(9): 940–3

McGraw K, Hoffmann R, Harker C, Herman JH (1999) The development of circadian rhythms in a human infant. *Sleep* **22**(3): 303–10

McNamara F, Sullivan CE (2000) Treatment of obstructive sleep apnea syndrome in children. *Sleep* **23** (suppl 4): S142–S146

McNicholas WT, Phillipson EA (2002) *Breathing Disorders in Sleep*. Harcourt Publishers Limited, London

Meier-Koll A, Hall U, Hellwig U, Kott G, Meier-Koll V (1978) A biological oscillator system and the development of sleep–waking behavior during early infancy. *Chronobiologia* **5**(4): 425–40

Meierkord H, Fish DR, Smith SJ, Scott CA, Shorvon SD, Marsden CD (1992) Is nocturnal paroxysmal dystonia a form of frontal lobe epilepsy? *Move Disord* **7**(1): 38–42

Meirs PJ (1994) Chronobiology of pergnancy and the perinatal TIME span. In: Hans TY, ed. *Biologic Rhythms in Clinical and Laboratory Medicine*. Springer Verlag, Berlin

Mindell JA, Owens JA, Carskadon MA (1999) Developmental features of sleep. *Child Adolesc Psychiatric Clin N Am* **8**(4):695–725

Montagna P (1992) Nocturnal paroxysmal dystonia and nocturnal wandering. *Neurology* **42**(7) (suppl 6): 61–7

Myatt HM, Beckenham EJ (2000) The use of diagnostic sleep nasendoscopy in the management of children with complex upper airway obstruction. *Clin Otolaryngol Allied Sci* **25**(3): 200–8

Neveus T, Hetta J, Cnattingius S, Tuvemo T, Lackgren G, Olsson U, Stenberg A (1999) Depth of sleep and sleep habits among enuretic and incontinent children. *Acta Paediatr* **88**(7): 748–52

Owens JA (2001) The practice of pediatric sleep medicine: Results of a community survey. *Pediatrics* **108**(3): E51

Owens JA, Spirito A, McGuinn M, Nobile C (2000) Sleep habits and sleep disturbance in elementary school-aged children. *J Dev Behav Pediatr* **21**(1): 27–36

Palmer LJ, Redline S (2003) Genomic approaches to understanding obstructive sleep apnea. *Respir Physiol Neurobiol* **135**(2–3): 187–205

Picchietti DL, Walters AS (1996) Restless legs sydrome and periodic limb movement disorder in children and adolescents: Comorbidity with attention-deficit hyperactivity in sleep disorders. In: Dahl RE, ed. Sleep Disorders. *Child and Adolescent Psychiatric Clinics in North America*. WB Saunders, Philadelphia

Picchietti DL, England SJ, Walters AS, Willis K, Verrico T (1998) Periodic limb movement disorder and restless leg syndrome in children with attention-deficit hyperactivity disorder. *J Child Neurol* **13**(12): 588–94

Pirsig W, Verse T (2000) Long-term results in the treatment of obstructive sleep apnea. *Eur Arch Oto-Rhino-Laryngol* **257**(10): 570–7

Pollack IF, Kinnunen D, Albright AL (1996) The effect of early craniocerviocervical decompression on functional outcome in neonates and young infants with myelodysplasia and symptomatic Chiari II malformations: Results from a prospective series. *Neurosurgery* **38**(4): 703–10

Ramanathan R, Corwin MJ, Hunt CE, Lister G, Tinsley LR, Baird T, The Collaborative Home Infant Monitoring Evaluation Study G (2001) Cardiorespiratory events recorded on home monitors: Comparison of healthy infants with those at increased risk for sids. *JAMA* **285**(17): 2199–207

Ramchandani P, Wiggs L, Webb V, Stores G (2000) A systematic review of treatments for settling problems and night waking in young children. *Br Med J* **320**(7229): 209–13

Reimao RN, Lefevre AB (1980) Prevalence of sleep-talking in childhood. *Brain Development* **2**(4): 353–7

Robson WL, Leung AK (2000) Secondary nocturnal enuresis. *Clin Pediatr* **39**(7): 379–85

Rosen GM, Ferber R, Mahowald MW (1996) Evaluation of parasomnias in children. In: Dahl RE, ed. *Sleep Disorders. Child and Adolescent Psychiatric Clinics of North America.* WB Saunders, Philadelphia

Rosen GM, Robert P, Mahowald MW, Goding GS, Ullevig C (1994) Postoperative respiratory compromise in children with obstructive sleep apnea syndrome: Can it be anticipated? *Pediatrics* **93**(5): 784–8

Sadeh A, Gruber R, Raviv A (2003) The effects of sleep restriction and extension on school-age children: What a difference an hour makes. *Child Development* **74**(2): 444–55

Sanchez-Armengol A, Fuentes-Pradera MA, Capote-Gil F, Garcia-Diaz E, Cano-Gomez S, Carmona-Bernal C, Castillo-Gomez J (2001) Sleep-related breathing disorders in adolescents aged 12 to 16 years: Clinical and polygraphic findings. *Chest* **119**(5): 1393–400

Schenck CH, Bundlie SR, Smith SA *et al* (1986) REM behavior disorder in a 10-year-old girl and aperiodic REM and non-REM sleep movement in her 8-year old brother. *Sleep Res* **15**(162)

Shapiro NL, Seid AB, Pransky SM, Kearns DB, Magit AE, Silva P (1999) Adenotonsillectomy in the very young patient: Cost analysis of two methods of postoperative care. *Int J Pediatr Otorhinolaryngol* **48**(2): 109–15

Sheldon SH (1996) Sleep-related enuresis. In: Dahl RE, ed. *Sleep Disorders. Child and Adolescent Psychiatric Clinics of North America.* WB Saunders, Philadelphia

Sheldon SH, Spire J-P, Levy HB (1992) *Pediatric Sleep Medicine.* WB Saunders, Philadelphia

Silvestri JM, Weese-Mayer DE, Bass MT, Kenny AS, Hauptman SA, Pearsall SM (1993) Polysomnography in obese children with a history of sleep-associated breathing disorders. *Pediatr Pulmonology* **16**(2): 124–9

Smedje H, Broman JE, Hetta J (2001) Short-term prospective study of sleep disturbances in 5–8-year-old children. *Acta Paediatr* **90**(12): 1456–63

Smits MG, van Stel H, van der Heijden K, Meijer AM, Coenene AM, Kerkhof GA (2003) Melatonin improves health status and sleep in children with idiopathic chronic sleep-onset insomnia: a randomised placebo-controlled trial. *J Am Child Adolesc Psychiat* **42**(11): 1286–93

Stebbens VA, Dennis J, Samuels MP, Croft CB, Southall DP (1991) Sleep-related upper airway obstruction in a cohort with Down's syndrome. *Arch Dis Childhood* **66**(11): 1333–8

Steer PA, Henderson-Smart DJ (2003) Caffeine versus theophylline for apnea in preterm infants. Cochrane Review. Update Software, Oxford

Stein MA, Mendelsohn J, Obermeyer WH, Amromin J, Benca R (2001) Sleep and behavior problems in school-aged children. *Pediatrics* **107**(4): E60

Stradling JR, Thomas G, Warley AR, Williams P, Freeland A (1990) Effect of adenotonsillectomy on nocturnal hypoxaemia, sleep disturbance, and symptoms in snoring children. *Lancet* **335**(8684): 249–53

Suen JS, Arnold JE, Brooks LJ (1995) Adenotonsillectomy for treatment of obstructive sleep apnea in children. *Arch Otolaryngol Head Neck Surg* **121**(5): 525–30

Swift AD (1988) Upper-airway obstruction, sleep distrubance and adenotonsillectomy in children. *J Laryngol Otol* **102**: 419–22

Tang JP, Rosen CL, Larkin EK, DiFiore JM, Arnold JL, Surovec SA *et al* (2002) Identification of sleep-disordered breathing in children: Variation with event definition. *Sleep* **25**(1): 72–9

Tirosh E, Sadeh A, Munvez R, Lavie P (1993) Effects of methylphenidate on sleep in children with attention-deficit hyperactivity disorder. An activity monitor study. *Am J Dis Children* **147**(12): 1313–5

Tishler PV, Redline S, Ferrette V, Hans MG, Altose MD (1996) The association of sudden unexpected infant death with obstructive sleep apnea. *Am J Respir Crit Care Med* **153**(6 Pt 1): 1857–63

Tomioko K, Tomioko F (1991) Development of circadian sleep-wakefulness rhythmicity of three infants. *J Interdisciplin Cycle Res* **22**(1): 71–80

Uliel S, Tauman R, Greenfeld M, Sivan Y (2004) Normal polysomnographic respiratory values in children and adolescents. *Chest* **125**: 872–8

Walker P, Temperley A, Bradshaw R (1999) A 5-year prospective audit of the complications of paediatric diathermy tonsillectomy, adenoidectomy and adeno-tonsillectomy. *Aus J Otolaryngol* **3**(4): 317–23

Waters KA, Everett FM, Bruderer JW, Sullivan CE (1995) Obstructive sleep apnea: The use of nasal CPAP in 80 children. *Am J Respir Crit Care Med* **152**(2): 780–5

Waters KA, Forbes P, Morielli A, Hum C, O'Gorman AM, Vernet O *et al* (1998) Sleep-disordered breathing in children with myelomeningocele. *J Pediatr* **132**(4): 672–81

Weese-Mayer DE, Brouillette RT, Naidich TP, McLone DG, Hunt CE (1988) Magnetic resonance imaging and computerized tomography in central hypoventilation. *Am Rev Respir Dis* **137**(2): 393–8

Weinberg WA, Brumback RA (1990) Primary disorder of vigilance: A novel explanation of inattentiveness, daydreaming, boredom, restlessness, and sleepiness. *J Pediatr* **116**(5): 720–5

Weinberg WA, Harper CR (1993) Vigilance and its disorders. *Neurologic Clin* **11**(1): 59–78

Weissbluth M (1995) Naps in children: 6 months–7 years. *Sleep* **18**(2): 82–7

Wilson K, Lakheeram I, Morielli A, Brouillette R, Brown K (2002) Can assessment for obstructive sleep apnea help predict postadenotonsillectomy respiratory complications? *Anesthesiology* **96**(2): 313–22

Wise MS (1998) Childhood narcolepsy. *Neurology* **50** (2 suppl 1): S37–S42

Wolfson AR (1996) Sleeping patterns of children and adolescents: Developmental trends, disruptions and adaptation. In: Dahl RE, ed. Sleep Disorders. *Child and Adolescent Psychiatric Clinics in North America.*WB Saunders, Philadelphia

CHAPTER 11

Circadian rhythm sleep disorder

Liat Ayalon and Yaron Dagan

Normal sleep–wake rhythm

Underlying rhythmicity is a fundamental property inherent to all living organisms. Since rotation of the earth causes predictable variations in light and temperature, natural selection has favored the evolution of circadian (from the latin circa, meaning 'about', and dies, meaning 'day') rhythms. Many behavioral and physiological processes are characterized by this temporal structure that matches the 24-hour day–night cycle, sleep and wakefulness having the most conspicuous rhythm. The cues from the environment serve as 'zeitgebers' (time givers) and include exogenous heuristics such as light and temperature of the environment, as well as concurrent fluctuations of social contacts.

The mechanism by which the environmental variables influence the phase of the endogenous pacemaker is referred to as entrainment. Entrainment synchronizes the intrinsic circadian cycle, which is generally not equivalent to 24 hours, to the environmental 24-hour period. Absence of zeitgebers releases the endogenous rhythms from exogenous constraints, resulting in a free-running rhythm. Rhythms allowed to free-run demonstrate a persistent periodicity ranging from 23.8 to 27.1 hours (Wever, 1979), implicating a biological clock in control of these events.

Most circadian rhythms are controlled by the suprachiasmatic nucleus (SCN) of the hypothalamus (Turek, 1999). The synchronizing effects of light are mediated via a direct pathway from the retina to the SCN, and by an indirect pathway through the thalamus (Card, 1982; Friedman, 1991; Hendrickson, 1972). In response to input from the SCN, the pineal gland secretes melatonin during the night. Melatonin is synthesized from tryptophan within the pineal gland via hydroxylation and decarboxylation to serotonin (5-HT) (Axelrod, 1974). Subsequent N-acetylation of serotonin by serotonin N-acetyltransferase is thought to be the rate-limiting step in melatonin synthesis (Klein, 1979; 1985). The activity of this enzyme is increased during the dark phase of the day, leading to melatonin production almost exclusively at night. In individuals with a normal sleep–wake cycle, melatonin secretion follows a circadian rhythm: higher levels occur at night and reach a maximum level between 3.00AM and 5.00AM. This light–dark variation in melatonin synthesis may play a role in the translation of changes in environmental lighting to circadian rhythms, sleep–wake rhythm being one of the most significant phenomena.

Other biological rhythms that work in harmony with the circadian rhythm of sleep and wakefulness are body temperature and the secretion of growth hormone and cortisol. Daily rhythms of body temperature and endocrine secretion have been the focus of much research.

Body temperature decreases during sleep and increases during activity and wakefulness. Sleep tends to terminate when our bodies are warming (Zulley, 1981), and the length of our sleep is partially dependent on the circadian rhythm of our body temperature (Carskadon, 1994). In subjects with synchronized sleep–wake and body temperature rhythms, sleep onset is far more likely to be initiated when body temperature is getting close to, or is at, its nadir. The circadian rhythm of core body temperature has a nadir at 3.00AM to 6.00AM and amplitude of about 0.4°C. It is considered to be one of the more rigid endogenous oscillating systems in the human body, often showing difficulty in re-adjusting and entraining itself to other circadian rhythms that may have undergone a phase-shift (Cagnacci, 1992).

Internal desynchronization occurs during free-running experiments and body temperature rhythm dissociates from sleep rhythm as a result of that desynchronization. The nocturnal decline of core body temperature is completely opposite to the nocturnal rise of melatonin. Peak melatonin values are associated with the core body temperature nadir, while the subsequent decline of melatonin is immediately followed by the increase of body temperature (Cagnacci, 1992).

Pathologies of sleep–wake rhythm

Since both endogenous cues and environmental factors influence biological rhythms, the sleep–wake cycle is highly sensitive to environmental disturbance and intrinsic pathology (Hayes, 1992). The normal sleep–wake rhythm that is taken for granted by most people can, in some people, become chronically impaired, leading to a group of disorders called circadian rhythm sleep disorders (CRSD). CRSD are characterized by a misalignment between the patient's sleep pattern and the sleep pattern that is desired or regarded as the societal norm (American Academy of Sleep Medicine, 2005).

The underlying problem is that the patient cannot sleep when sleep is expected. As a result of sleep episodes occurring at inappropriate times, the corresponding wake periods may occur at undesired times. Consequently, the patient complains of insomnia or excessive daytime sleepiness and impairment in alertness, concentration, and performance. An important factor in CRSD is the inflexibility of the sleep–wake cycle and the subjective distress of the patient (Dagan, 1994).

The International Classification of Sleep Disorders (American Academy of Sleep Medicine, 2005) categorizes circadian rhythm sleep disorders separately, in part to acknowledge that in most cases the etiology of circadian disorders is a mixture of internal and environmental factors or a temporal mismatch between the two (*Table 11.1*).

Delayed sleep-phase syndrome (DSPS)

DSPS is a disorder in which the major sleep episode is delayed in relation to the desired clock time, resulting in symptoms of sleep-onset insomnia or difficulty in awakening at the desired time. DSPS is marked by:

- sleep-onset and wake times that are intractably later than desired
- actual sleep-onset times at nearly the same daily clock hour

- little or no reported difficulty in maintaining sleep once sleep has begun
- extreme difficulty awakening at the desired time in the morning
- relatively severe to absolute inability to advance the sleep phase to earlier hours by enforcing conventional sleep and wake times.

Table 11.1: Circadian rhythm sleep disorders
• Delayed sleep phase syndrome (DSPS)
• Advanced sleep phase syndrome (ASPS)
• Non-24-hour sleep–wake syndrome
• Irregular (disorganized) sleep–wake pattern (ISWP)
• Jet lag disorder
• Shift work sleep disorder
• Circadian rhythm sleep disorder due to medical condition: dementia Parkinson's disease blindness hepatic encephalopathy head trauma
• Circadian rhythm sleep disorder due to drug or substance abuse

Typically, patients complain primarily of chronic difficulty in falling asleep until between 2.00AM and 6.00AM, or difficulty awakening at the desired or necessary time in the morning to fulfil social or occupational obligations. The patients' efforts to advance the timing of sleep onset (early bedtime, help from family or friends in getting up in the morning, relaxation techniques, or the ingestion of hypnotic medications) yield little permanent success. In addition, unsuccessful efforts to fall asleep at earlier times may produce prolonged periods of time awake in bed, resulting in development of secondary conditioned insomnia that further compounds the phase delay.

Hypnotics in normal doses are often described as having little or no effect in advancing sleep onset, and may only aggravate the daytime symptoms of difficulty awakening and sleepiness. Individuals with DSPS who use alcohol or sedative-hypnotics in an attempt to induce sleep sometimes develop alcohol or drug dependence.

Patients with DSPS typically score high as 'evening people' on the morningness–eveningness questionnaire (Jan, 1994), and state that they feel and function best, and are most alert, during the late evening and night hours. Most of these patients experience profound sleepiness and functional disability during the morning hours. A sleep–wake log documents a consistent pattern of sleep-onsets (usually later than 2.00AM), few to no awakenings once sleep is achieved, with late morning to mid-afternoon rising times on weekends. Sleep–wake logs obtained during periods when morning social obligations are lessened or absent show consistently late sleep and rising times.

The exact prevalence of DSPS is unknown. Five to ten per cent of patients present at sleep disorders centers with the complaint of insomnia. DSPS is more common in adolescents and young adults, with a reported prevalence of 7% (Pelayo, 1988). The prevalence in middle-aged adults is estimated at 0.7% (Ando *et al*, 1995). Onset after the age of 30 is reported to be rare. No sex differences were found (Dagan and Eisenstein, 1999; Kamei *et al*, 1998).

Differential diagnosis includes: irregular sleep–wake syndrome, non-24-hour sleep–wake pattern (see below), psychiatric disorders associated with disturbed sleep and a volitional sleep–wake schedule adopted by an individual as a result of work or other social factors.

The current understanding of the pathophysiology of DSPS rests on the application of the principles of phase-response curves, largely derived from experiments in lower animals, to the human sleep–wake cycle. Patients with DSPS are thought to have a relatively weak ability to phase advance their circadian systems in response to normal environmental time cues.

Several studies suggest altered phase relationships in patients with DSPS. A delayed sleep onset, sleep offset, temperature nadir, and melatonin rhythm were found, as well as prolonged sleep periods from temperature nadir and melatonin onset and offset to sleep offset (Ozaki *et al*, 1996; Uchiyama *et al*, 2000).

Although no genetic inheritance pattern has been described, familial DSPS has been reported (Ancoli-Israel *et al*, 2001; Takahashi *et al*, 2000). Mammalian genes that confer altered circadian periodicity have been cloned and characterized in mice (King *et al*, 1997). Research suggests that structural polymorphisms in the human period 3 gene (*hPer3*) may be implicated in the pathogenesis of DSPS. Six sequence variations with amino acid changes have been identified; five of which were common and predicted four haplotypes of the *hPer3* gene. One of the haplotypes was significantly associated with DSPS (Ebisawa *et al*, 2001). In addition, a possible association of human leukocyte antigen DR1 with delayed sleep phase syndrome was also reported (Hohjoh, 1999).

Case study 1

Danny Meyers, a 24-year-old medical student, is seeking treatment for his inability to fall asleep before 4.00AM and wake up before noon. Because of his delayed sleep–wake cycle he misses anatomy labs that take place in the morning, and complains of chronic fatigue that impairs his alertness and concentration. When on holidays, he stays awake until 5.00AM and sleeps until the afternoon, resulting in the disappearance of his fatigue and improvement in his functioning.

Careful medical history reveals that this pattern of delayed sleep onset and sleep offset times has been evident during the last several years, since the onset of puberty. In high school, Danny experienced extensive disciplinary problems with his teachers and parents on the issue of his tardiness. He also had conflicts with his parents over staying awake until very late hours on the Internet. Danny was always described as being an intelligent and good student, although not achieving his full potential.

Further inquiry reveals that Danny is more alert during the evening and, even when awake, he never eats before noon, usually eating big meals at around midnight. Apparently, both his mother and younger brother (a high school student) had similar patterns.

Monitoring of his sleep–wake schedule by an actigraph (for detailed description see Diagnosis of CRSD, *p. 436*) supported the late bedtime and late wake-up times (*Figure 11.1*). Melatonin and temperature rhythms were also delayed, with salivary melatonin peak and temperature nadir at around 7.00AM to 8.00AM (*Figure 11.2*).

Advanced sleep-phase syndrome (ASPS)

ASPS is a disorder in which the major sleep episode is advanced in relation to the desired clock time, resulting in symptoms of compelling evening sleepiness, an early sleep onset, and an awakening that is earlier than desired. Typical sleep-onset times are between 6.00PM and 8.00PM and no later than 9.00PM, and wake times are between 1.00AM and 3.00AM and no later than 5.00AM. These sleep-onset and wake times occur despite the patient's best efforts to delay sleep to later hours (American Academy of Sleep Medicine, 2005).

ASPS is thought to be less common than DSPS and rare in adolescents and young adults. A prevalence of 1% was reported in middle-aged adults (Ando *et*

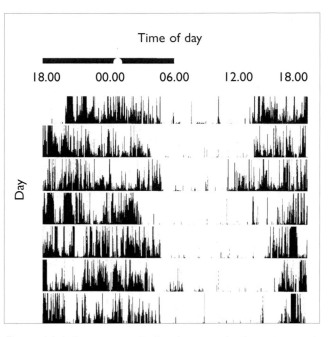

Figure 11.1: Rest–activity rhythm (actogram) of a patient with delayed sleep phase syndrome (DSPS).

al, 1995). However, because societal constraints on sleep time are less rigid than on wake time, the prevalence of this disorder might be underestimated. The elderly are at a greater risk of developing the syndrome but, because advanced sleep–wake cycles are a common characteristic in this group, ASPS may be considered as being part of the normal aging process, rather than as a disorder.

Familial ASPS was reported with an advanced melatonin onset in affected family members (Reid *et al*, 2001). Although the gene of familial ASPS, an autosomal dominant variant near the telomere of chromosome 2q, has been localized (Toh *et al*, 2001), the exact mechanisms by which it causes ASPS remain to be elucidated.

The differential diagnosis includes psychiatric disorders. Early morning awakenings are often mistakenly interpreted as a manifestation of major depression. In addition, the early evening sleepiness may be misinterpreted as hypersomnia resulting from sleep apnea or narcolepsy.

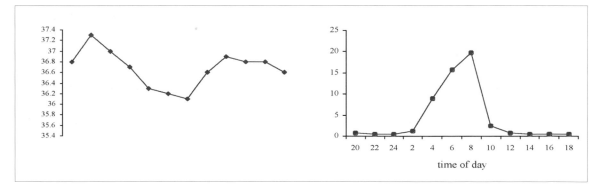

Figure 11.2: Salivary melatonin (pg/ml) and oral temperature (C°) rhythms of a patient with delayed sleep phase syndrome (DSPS).

Case study 2

Dana Wehr, a 39-year-old woman, is referred by her physician. She works in a bank where she arrives at work very early in the morning and she is regarded as a diligent and highly motivated worker. She reports a short period of sleepiness at around 9.00AM to 10.00AM but overall feels quite refreshed until late afternoon. Dana had always been a morning person and says she likes to get up early (at about 4.00AM). In the last several years, however, she has found it almost impossible to stay awake after 9.00PM (*Figure 11.3*). When she attempts to go to bed later than usual (eg. at weekends, when her children come home) she finds it difficult, and because she wakes up at her habitual time, this results in her being sleep deprived. On weekdays she usually goes to bed between 7.00PM and 8.00PM often only one hour after her husband returns home from work. She complains of a limited social life.

Careful examination rules out sleep disorders, such as sleep apnea, restless leg syndrome, and early wakening insomnia. No complaints or symptoms of depression are evident.

Non-24-hour sleep–wake syndrome (free-running type)

Non-24-hour sleep–wake syndrome (hypernychthemeral syndrome) consists of a chronic steady pattern, comprising 1- to 2-hour daily delays in sleep onset and wake times. Patients with non-24-hour sleep–wake syndrome exhibit a sleep–wake pattern reminiscent of that found in individuals living without environmental time cues. However, freed of exogenous influences, the free-running internal rhythms behave with a periodicity of more than 24 hours. Because an incremental phase delay in sleep occurs, and the relationship between the internal clock and the external clock tends to vary from complete synchrony to total asynchrony, the complaints will consist of difficulty initiating sleep at night, coupled with daytime sleepiness. Patients may alternate between being symptomatic and asymptomatic, depending on the degree of synchrony between their internal biological rhythm and the 24-hour world. This total disregard for environmental time cues makes entrainment to a scheduled lifestyle almost impossible and leads to educational and occupational problems. Despite variations in sleep onset and offset, sleep efficiency is usually normal (American Academy of Sleep Medicine, 2005).

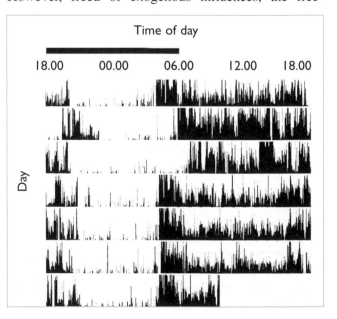

Figure 11.3: Rest–activity rhythm (actogram) of a patient with advanced sleep phase syndrome (ASPS).

Non-24-hour sleep–wake syndrome occurs most often in totally blind individuals (Klein *et al*, 1993; Lapierre and Dumont, 1994; Palm *et al*, 1997; Sack *et al*, 1992). Sleep–wake schedule disorders have been reported in 70% of totally blind people (Wagner, 1996) as well as free-running plasma melatonin rhythms (Sack *et al*, 1992). This syndrome is rarely encountered in sighted individuals.

Several mechanisms have been hypothesized to account for the syndrome, including: weakness of environmental time cues; reduced sensitivity to the entraining influences of light; and a circadian system period that is longer than 24 hours. Melatonin rhythm may be deficient (Kamgar-Parsi *et al*, 1983), delayed (McArthur *et al*, 1996; Palm *et al*, 1997) or free running (Lappierre and Dumont, 1995). Altered interval between sleep onset and body temperature trough was also reported (Kokkoris *et al*, 1978). Non-24-hour sleep–wake syndrome associated with lesions of the central nervous system, specifically hypothalamic tumors, as well as impairment of the hypothalamic pathway is classified as circadian rhythm sleep disorder due to medical conditions (American Academy of Sleep Medicine, 2005).

The differential diagnosis includes irregular sleep–wake pattern. In addition, a mutation in the human melatonin 1a (*hMel1a*) receptor gene was identified in patients with non-24-hour sleep–wake syndrome, suggesting a genetic predisposition toward this CRSD (Ebisawa *et al*, 1999).

Case study 3

Christian Rudd is a 14-year-old boy referred by his psychiatrist. During the 4 years prior to this consultation, Christian suffered from major functioning difficulties and conflicts with teachers, parents, and peers. He is described by his psychologist as being extremely introverted with very severe narcissistic damage, poverty of thought and disturbed thinking, anhedonia, social isolation and withdrawal, and thoughts with persecutory content and self-destruction that have led to a paralysing anxiety. In addition, various learning disabilities with high intelligence were diagnosed. Two years ago, Christian quit school and was sent to a child-psychiatry center.

Three months of psychiatric evaluation yielded a diagnosis of depression, schizotypal personality disorder, developmental disorder, and possible psychosis. He was described as sleepy, passive, and lacking motivation. The boy was sent to a special boarding school, subsequent to his running away from the school after one day, his psychiatrist suggested further examination to include assessment of sleep disorders.

Careful medical history taken by a sleep physician raises the possibility of sleep–wake schedule disorder. Three weeks of wrist actigraphy (*Figure 11.4*) reveals a non 24-hour sleep–wake pattern with a period of approximately 26 hours. In addition, 24-hour evaluation of oral temperature and salivary melatonin reveals a delay in temperature rhythm and dissociation between oral temperature and melatonin rhythms. Treatment with oral melatonin (5 mg at 20:00) restores normal sleep–wake schedule within a month, and follow up actigraphy at 6 months reveals a full entrainment to a 24-hour day (*Figure 11.5*).

The patient returned to school a year later and succeeded in filling the gap of missing studies, returning to the class that he had left a year previously. At the end of the first semester his school report showed excellent results. His parents also reported a good relationship with his family and peers. Neither of the previously described severe diagnoses was apparent, and the boy showed no evidence of the previously diagnosed severe psychopathology.

This case study presents a grave psychiatric misdiagnosis of a sleep–wake schedule disorder. This wrong diagnosis caused harmful psychological distress to a young boy whose sleep disorder was easily diagnosed and treated by melatonin.

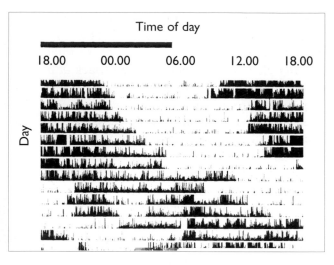

Figure 11.4: Rest–activity rhythm (actogram) of a patient with non-24-hour sleep–wake pattern before treatment with melatonin.

Irregular (disorganized) sleep–wake pattern (ISWP)

ISWP consists of temporally disorganized and variable episodes of sleeping and waking behavior. Patients may have a total 24-hour average sleep time that is within normal limits for age: however, no single sleep period is of normal length, and the likelihood of being asleep at any particular time of day is unpredictable. The clinical manifestation may be inability to initiate and maintain sleep at night, frequent daytime napping, or both.

Unlike patients with advanced sleep-phase, delayed sleep-phase, or non-24-hour syndromes, a well-kept sleep–wake log by patients with this disorder shows no recognizable ultradian or circadian patterns of sleep onset or wake time. Instead, sleep is broken up into three or more short blocks in each 24 hours, with marked day-to-day variability in the timing of sleep and wakefulness. Sleep onsets and wake times throughout the day are

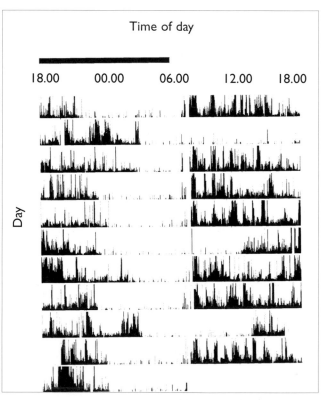

Figure 11.5: Rest–activity rhythm (actogram) of a patient with non-24-hour sleep–wake pattern after treatment with melatonin.

unpredictable (*Figure 11.6*). Rhythms of endocrine, temperature and other functions that normally display regular circadian periodicity may lose their expected fluctuations and show flattened amplitudes.

ISWP is rare and is sometimes associated with brain dysfunction. It appears to affect both genders equally and has no identified familial pattern (American Academy of Sleep Medicine, 2005).

We human beings, being able to lighten the night and darken the day, are not slaves to our biological clock. We are often awake when our internal clocks are telling us it is time to sleep and sometimes try to sleep when our biological clocks signal that it is time to be awake. This freedom to fool Mother Nature leads to two other disorders of chronobiology: shift work and jet lag. In these two disorders, human beings usually voluntarily choose to create temporal de-synchronization between their biological clocks and their environment.

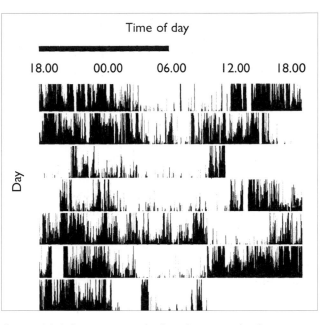

Figure 11.6: Rest–activity rhythm (actogram) of a patient with irregular sleep–wake pattern (ISWP).

Time zone change (jet lag) syndrome

In jet lag, endogenous rhythms are out of phase with local time; however, since environmental cues promote adjustment of the circadian system, the sleep–wake disturbances generally abate after two to three days in the arrival location. On average, it takes about a day per time zone for the circadian rhythm to catch up the local time. Following rapid travel across multiple time zones, people exhibit varying degrees of difficulty in initiating or maintaining sleep, excessive sleepiness, decrements in subjective daytime alertness and performance, and somatic symptoms. Gastrointestinal symptoms are also common. Symptoms are often associated with, but not entirely dependent upon, sleep deprivation and are aggravated by excitement or stress and by heavy alcohol or caffeine use.

Shift work sleep disorder

Shift work sleep disorder consists of symptoms of insomnia or excessive sleepiness that occur as transient phenomena in relation to work schedules. The sleep complaint typically consists of an inability to maintain a normal sleep duration when the major sleep episode is begun in the morning (6.00AM to 8.00AM) after a night shift. The reduction in sleep length usually amounts to one to four hours. Subjectively, the sleep period is perceived as unsatisfactory and non-restorative. Early morning work shifts may also be associated with complaints of difficulty in sleep initiation as well as difficulty in awakening. The condition is directly related to the circadian interference with sleep during the morning and evening that conflicts with the shift workers' need to sleep at these times.

Primary and secondary circadian rhythm sleep disorders

A distinction can be made between primary and secondary CRSD. DSPS, ASPS, non-24-hour sleep–wake syndrome, and ISWP are considered to be malfunctions of the biological clock *per se* and are, therefore, primary; while jet lag and shift work are considered to result from environmental effects and are, therefore, secondary. In primary CRSD, the endogenous circadian clock may change relative to the terrestrial light–dark cycle, while in secondary CRSD, the terrestrial light–dark cycle may change relative to the endogenous circadian clock. Another distinction, mentioned earlier, views the first four subgroups as involuntary while the latter two are considered to be situations where the person voluntarily chooses to create a temporal mismatch between internal and environmental factors.

Since sleep–wakefulness problems resulting from shift work and jet lag are not pathological, but rather normal responses to abnormal situations, the rest of the chapter will focus on the characteristics, diagnosis, treatment, and possible etiology of primary CRSD.

Diagnosis of CRSD

Diagnosis of CRSD is largely based on recognizing the characteristics and patterns described above. A careful history together with 7–14 days of sleep logs and/or actigraphic monitoring is recommended. The actigraph is a watch-sized device worn on the wrist sampling hand motion. A computerized algorithm can provide highly reliable data on sleep and wake periods of the patient (Sadeh *et al*, 1989; 1995).

Actigraphic monitoring should be an indispensable diagnostic tool for CRSD. Generally, polysomnography (PSG) is an inadequate tool for the assessment of CRSD, since the nature of these disorders requires that monitoring be conducted for at least several days for the patient's sleep–wake pattern to be manifested. This cannot be achieved with PSG, but can be perfectly demonstrated by actigraphy. Importantly, actigraphic monitoring must be done under free-running conditions: the sleep–wake schedule that is usually achieved under forced conditions can mask the pattern of the schedule, thereby misleading the diagnosis. Melatonin secretion and/or temperature measurements for a 24–36-hour period, whether continuous or sampled every two to three hours, can also be used as diagnostic tools. Inclusion of these measures is usually at the discretion of the medical professional and not always necessary.

Other characteristics may also aid in the formulation of CRSD diagnosis. Questioning the patient about hunger times, hours of alertness, heredity, sensitivity to light, and rigidity of the endogenous biological rhythm, may help focus a diagnosis (*Table 11.1*).

Table 11.1: History-taking in CRSD

Hunger times	The patient should be questioned about his/her preferable eating hours — whether he/she eats or is hungry during the night, and whether he/she ever eats early in the morning.
Hours of alertness	DSPS patients, even when they wake up early and should thus become more and more tired as the day passes, may paradoxically become more alert as evening approaches.
Hereditary	Patients should be asked about family members with the same characteristics.
Sensitivity to light	Many CRSD patients will spontaneously report high sensitivity to light and extensive use of sunglasses.
Functional difficulties	CRSD patients often have trouble functioning in everyday life — keeping a steady job usually requires in a pre-determined timeframe with rigid working hours, which for most of them is impossible. The hallmark of their problem is severe difficulty in waking up in the morning. A patient suffering from ASPS, non-24-hour sleep–wake syndrome, and ISWP may also find it difficult to have a normal social life, etc.
Rigidity of biological rhythm	Rigidity of biological rhythm: CRSD patients have, unlike most people, very rigid biological clocks. Therefore, it is extremely difficult for them to adjust to environmental demands, even for a very limited period of time. Questioning about sleep–wake habits during vacation time may be informative.
Head injury	Patients displaying symptoms of an ISWP or DSPS should be questioned about prior head injuries.

An important distinction should be made between DSPS and other sleep-onset insomnias. Difficulties in initiating sleep can be due to primary (psychophysiologic insomnia) or secondary insomnia (eg. due to psychiatric conditions). The main distinguishing feature is that DSPS patients, once asleep, will typically have sleep of normal duration and architecture if allowed to sleep on their habitual schedule. Having slept at their habitual times, most CRSD patients would show an adequate daytime alertness and function. DSPS should also be distinguished from irregular sleep–wake syndrome, psychiatric disorders associated with disturbed sleep, and a volitional sleep–wake schedule adopted by an individual as a result of work or other social factors.

Early morning awakenings in ASPS patients are often mistakenly interpreted as being manifestations of major depression. In addition, the early evening sleepiness may be misinterpreted as hypersomnia resulting from sleep apnea or narcolepsy. Hence, differential diagnosis for ASPS includes psychiatric disorders. An important distinction should be also made between non-24-hour sleep–wake syndrome and irregular sleep–wake pattern. This can be easily achieved by actigraphic monitoring.

Treatment

The goal of the therapy in CRSD is to resynchronize the circadian clock with the terrestrial light–dark cycle. This can be done by chronotherapy (Czeisler *et al*, 1981), light therapy (Czeisler *et al*, 1989; Lewy *et al*, 1987), or melatonin administration (Dagan *et al*, 1998b; Dahlitz *et al*, 1991). Other treatments, such as vitamin B_{12}, have also been suggested (Okawa *et al*, 1990).

Chronotherapy

In sleep medicine, chronotherapy refers to a behavioral technique in which sleep onset is systematically delayed or advanced by a few hours every day, until the sleep onset occurs at the desired time (Czeisler *et al*, 1981). Once the desired sleep time is achieved, a rigid adherence to a set sleep–wake schedule is required. The main disadvantage of this technique is that the phase-shifting procedure requires several days of free time. In addition, patients often find chronotherapy demanding and difficult to maintain. An important advantage of this treatment modality is its basis in the natural tendency of patients with ASPS or DSPS to phase advance or phase delay their sleep–wake cycle, respectively.

Phototherapy

Phototherapy, also known as light therapy, became increasingly popular as the importance of light in resetting the circadian system was recognized (see *Chapter 2* and *Chapter 8, Table 8.6, p. 306*) Light is the most potent external factor that can alter the period of the SCN. Light pulses reach the SCN and induce changes in the firing rates of neurons that affect circadian rhythms (Dijk *et al*, 1995). Exposure to bright light at specific times of the sleep–wake cycle can result in a phase-shift (Lewy *et al*, 1985a; 1985b). Morning bright-light exposure may induce a phase advance, while evening bright light exposure may induce phase delay. Light pulse given slightly before the time of body temperature nadir has been shown to result in phase delay, while a pulse slightly after the nadir advances it (Minors *et al*, 1991). Apart from phase-shifting effects, light exposure at night also suppresses melatonin secretion (Lewy *et al*, 1980).

Bright light has been successfully used to realign the circadian phase of DSPS patients (Rosenthal *et al*, 1990; Watanabe *et al*, 1999; Weyerbrock *et al*, 1996) and shift workers (Baehr *et al*, 1999; Yoon *et al*, 2002). In addition, it has been shown to be effective in delaying the peak of the activity rhythm and increasing the mean activity level in demented patients (Ancoli-Israel *et al*, 2002). However, this treatment demands a total control of light and dark exposure over the whole day, making it complicated to manage.

Bright light treatment has also been found to be effective in reducing symptoms of seasonal affective disorder (SAD) (Rosenthal *et al*, 1984; Terman *et al*, 1989). The pathogenesis of SAD and mechanism of action of light remain uncertain despite numerous investigations. A potential role for abnormal circadian timing has been suggested. Lewy *et al* (Lewy *et al*, 1987; 1988; Sack *et al*, 1990) proposed that morning light would be effective because it provides corrective phase advances of delayed circadian rhythms in patients with winter depression.

Recently, commercial devices have become available to provide artificial external light for varying intensities to treat a variety of sleep disorders. Recommended intensities and time limits for phototherapy in the treatment of DSPS, ASPS, non-24-hour sleep–wake syndrome, jet lag, shift work, dementia, and sleep complaints in the healthy elderly are provided by the American Academy of Sleep Medicine (Chesson, 1999).

Interestingly, recent studies suggested that extraocular light (such as behind the knee) may also affect circadian rhythms (Campbell and Murphy, 1998), although other workers could not replicate this finding (Koorengevel *et al*, 2001; Lindblom *et al*, 2000a; 2000b) or found no phase-shifting effect on melatonin rhythm (Eastman *et al*, 2000).

Although promising, ocular light treatment demands a total control of light and dark exposure over the whole day, making it complicated to manage.

Pharmacotherapy

While chronotherapy and phototherapy are demanding treatments that are typically accompanied by compliance problems, pharmacological manipulation is a relatively simple treatment modality. Of the various neurotransmitters and peptides that affect the circadian rhythm (Dawson and Armstrong, 1996), one of the most promising treatments is melatonin.

Studies have shown that exogenous melatonin administration has a sleep-promoting and entraining action when taken in the evening. While phase advance is produced by melatonin administered in the evening, phase delay appears when it is administered in the early morning (Lewy *et al*, 1995; 1996). It has also been shown that melatonin induces temperature suppression (Cagnacci *et al*, 1992) and that there is a direct relationship between the ability of melatonin to phase shift the endogenous circadian clock and its temperature-suppressing quality (Deacon and Arendt, 1995). Melatonin has been shown to be effective in the treatment of jet lag (Petrie *et al*, 1989), shift work induced sleep disorders (Folkard *et al*, 1993), and sleep disturbances caused by a desynchronization of the endogenous sleep–wake cycle from lighting cues in blind, geriatric and brain-damaged subjects (Jan *et al*, 1994) and CRSD (Dagan *et al*, 1998b; Dahlitz *et al*, 1991).

It has been shown that melatonin has an extremely wide margin of safety, at least in terms of short-term side-effects. In a study that examined the effects of oral melatonin on skin colour and the release of pituitary hormones, five patients with hyperpigmented skin were given 1 g per day of melatonin orally for a period of 30 days, with minimal adverse effects. These patients did complain of increased drowsiness but a thorough examination did not reveal any evidence of toxicity (Nordlund and Lerner, 1977). Although the dosage used in this study was 200–2000 times greater than that generally used for the treatment of circadian disorders, it should be noted that even a 0.5–5.0 mg dose of melatonin is higher than normal nocturnal levels of melatonin in the blood.

Dahlitz *et al* (1991) illustrated that an oral dose of 5 mg of melatonin taken in the evening caused a significant phase advance toward conventional times of both sleep onset and awakening, with no significant changes in sleep duration or architecture. Oldani *et al* (1994) treated six DSPS patients with 5 mg of melatonin for a period of 1 month with similarly positive results, and without effects on sleep architecture or duration. However, patients reverted to their previous sleep–wake cycle upon cessation of melatonin treatment (Alvarez *et al*, 1992).

Most studies that support the efficiency of melatonin treatment for CRSD were carried out on a relatively small number of patients. A subjective follow-up study (Dagan *et al*, 1998) examined the efficiency of melatonin treatment in a relatively large population of DSPS subjects; 61 subjects, 37 males and 24 females, were diagnosed with DSPS by means of clinical assessment and actigraphy. Their mean pre-treatment falling asleep and waking times were 3.09AM and 11.31AM respectively. All patients underwent a 6-week course of treatment comprised of 5 mg of oral melatonin, taken daily at 10.00PM based on the principles suggested by Dahlitz *et al* (1991).

A survey questionnaire administered 12–18 months after the completion of the treatment revealed that 96.7% of the patients found melatonin treatment to be effective, with almost no side-effects. Of these respondents, 91.5% reported a relapse to their pre-treatment sleeping patterns within one year of cessation of treatment. Only 28.8% reported that the relapse occurred within one week. The pre-treatment falling asleep and waking times of patients in whom the changes were retained for a relatively long period of time were significantly earlier than those of patients whose relapse was immediate, with no difference in sleep duration (Dagan *et al*, 1998b).

In a randomized, double-blind, placebo-controlled crossover trial, subjects received either placebo or melatonin (5 mg) daily for 4 weeks, underwent a 1-week washout period, and then were given the other treatment for an additional four weeks. It was found that melatonin ameliorated some symptoms of delayed sleep phase syndrome, as confirmed by both objective and subjective measures, and no adverse effects of melatonin were noted during the 4-week treatment period (Kayumov *et al*, 2001).

Since few studies systematically assessed the side-effects of melatonin treatment (Seabra *et al*, 2000) and no data is available regarding its long-term effects in humans, issues of safety have yet to be fully researched and resolved.

Administration of B_{12} has been anecdotally reported to normalize human sleep–wake rhythm disorders, such as non-24-hour sleep–wake syndrome and DSPS (Ohta *et al*, 1990; 1991). However, the mechanisms of action of B_{12} on these rhythm disorders are unknown (Ebihara *et al*, 1996). It may act by changing the ocular receptors' affinity to light or by exerting a direct influence on melatonin (Mayer *et al*, 1996). At present, there is little experience with this treatment and very few accounts appear in the literature.

Exercise

Physical exercise was shown to be effective in promoting circadian adaptation to night shift work (Eastman *et al*, 1995), jet lag (Shiota *et al*, 1996) and in phase-delaying plasma thyrotropin and melatonin rhythms (Buxton *et al*, 1997). Combined therapies of exercise and bright light were also proposed (Miyazaki *et al*, 2001; Youngstedt *et al*, 2002).

CRSD as a possible side-effect of CNS drugs

Although CRSD are usually perceived as endogenous conditions, accumulating evidence supports the suggestion that CRSD may appear as iatrogenic, resulting from the use of certain drugs. A few reports of CRSD as a possible side-effect of psychotropic drugs have been published and the differential effects of typical *vs* atypical neuroleptics on sleep–wake schedule have been explored. Actigraphic data in hospitalized schizophrenia patients indicated that changing the antipsychotic medication of a patient with a near-arrhythmic circadian sleep–wake (disorganized) cycle from haloperidol (a typical neuroleptic) to clozapine (an atypical neuroleptic) improved the organization of his sleep–wake cycle (Wirz-Justice *et al*, 1997). They also found that schizophrenic patients treated with the atypical neuroleptic, clozapine, had more stable sleep–wake cycle than patients treated with the typical neuroleptics, haloperidol or flupentixol (Wirz-Justice *et al*, 2001).

Similarly, in 2000 Wirz-Justice *et al* described a patient with early-onset alzheimer's disease. After initiation of haloperidol treatment, the patient's sleep–wake cycle became completely arrhythmic for a period of two months, together with a marked worsening of cognitive state. When the patient's medication was changed to clozapine, the circadian sleep–wake cycle normalized and his clinical state improved. In addition, Dursun *et al* (Dursun *et al*, 1999) reported that compared with patients treated with typical antipsychotic drugs, patients treated with risperidone reported significantly better sleep quantity and quality as well as general functioning.

Circadian rhythm sleep disorders were also documented in humans as a side-effect of the selective serotonin reuptake inhibitor (SSRI) fluvoxamine on ten patients, while fluoxetine (another SSRI) and clomipramine (a tricyclic antidepressant) had no adverse effect on sleep–wake cycles (Hermesh *et al*, 2001). The differential effects of these drugs on sleep–wake schedule may be attributed to their different effects on serum melatonin levels (Demisch *et al*, 1987; Skene *et al*, 1994).

Ayalon *et al* (2001) described a patient with Gilles de la Tourette syndrome treated with haloperidol who exhibited an ISWP with a free-running component. Transfer to risperidone improved his sleep–wake schedule and treatment with melatonin, in addition to risperidone, resulted in complete resynchronization (*Case study 4*).

Case study 4

Julian Hoffman has Gilles de la Tourette syndrome treated with haloperidol, ingested once daily after awakening from sleep, and exhibits an irregular sleep–wake pattern with a free-running component of approximately 48 hours (*Figure 11.7a*). Transfer to risperidone, ingested once daily after awakening from sleep proves beneficial and results in a sleep–wake cycle more synchronized in the appropriate phase to external zeitgebers, and fewer nocturnal disturbances (*Figure 11.7b*). The circadian sleep–wake schedule is fully synchronized when the patient is subsequently treated with melatonin at 21.00 hours, before intended nocturnal sleep, in addition to risperidone in the morning (*Figure 11.7c*). Restoration of the sleep–wake circadian pattern is accompanied by the patient's subjective report of significant improvement in his quality of life, social interactions, and occupational status. This observation suggests that circadian rhythm sleep disorders can be related to the typical neuroleptic haloperidol and restored by the atypical neuroleptic risperidone.

CRSD and minor head trauma (MHT)

Following MHT some patients complain of sleep disorders and changes in normal sleep-schedule habits. These complaints are often diagnosed as psychophysiological insomnia attributed to trauma. Several single-case studies have indicated that CRSD may occur following head trauma (Nagtegaal *et al*, 1997; Patten and Lauderdale, 1992, Quinto *et al*, 2000) but, to date, no integrative assessment of a group of subjects with CRSD has been published.

In an exploratory study, fifteen of forty-two patients (35.7%) complaining of insomnia following MHT, with no pathological findings in CT and MRI, were clinically diagnosed as suffering from CRSD. Four patients with no clinical evidence of CRSD, but complaining of insomnia following MHT, served as controls. All subjects underwent 14-day 24-hour free-running actigraphic recording, 24-hour monitoring of body temperature and melatonin secretion, and polysomnography. Actigraph analysis of the fifteen subjects indicated that eight were suffering from DSPS, and seven were suffering from ISWP. CRSD within the control group was ruled out. Analysis of 24-hour data revealed a change in the biological rhythm following MHT. DSPS and ISWP patients both exhibited 24-hour periodicity, with a significant phase delay in the chronobiological parameters of temperature and melatonin secretion, with no difference between the two groups on the amplitude of the rhythms.

The only difference between the groups was portrayed on a behavioral level of the sleep–wake schedule, according to actigraph recording. DSPS patients fell asleep and woke up at relatively late clock hours. Patients with ISWP exhibited a fragmented pattern of polyphasic sleep with a tendency to phase delay. Five of seven subjects in the ISWP group were diagnosed as suffering from post-traumatic stress disorder (PTSD), as opposed to only two PTSD patients out of eight in the DSPS group. Higher occurrence of CRSD among post-MHT patients than patients referred to sleep centres (35.7% versus 5–10%) suggests that MHT may be an etiological factor in CRSD.

Although the mechanisms underlying this co-occurrence of MHT and CRSD are not clear, the finding of this study reiterates previous postulations put forth in single-case studies, revealing impairment in the biological rhythm following MHT. Since complaints about insomnia are

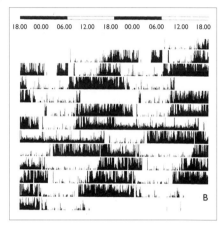

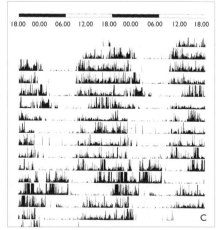

Figure 11.7: Rest–activity rhythm (actogram) of a patient during treatment with haloperidol (A); risperidone (B); and risperidone with melatonin (C).

common following MHT, it is possible that in some cases, CRSD are misdiagnosed, and hence, wrongly treated (Ayalon *et al*, 2001).

CRSD and psychopathology

Several investigators have noted a relationship between circadian rhythms and psychiatric disorders, particularly affective disorders (Dagan, 2002), and personality disorders. A high rate of depression and affective lability were noted in patients with DSPS (Dagan *et al*, 1998a; Kamei *et al*,1998). Regestein and Monk (1995) reported that twenty-five of thirty-three DSPS patients had past history and/or current episodes of depression. However, it should be considered that sleep architecture and sleep–wake rhythms are affected by many of the treatment modalities for affective disorder and obviously no conclusions regarding a causal relationship can be inferred.

Personality disorders have also been associated with CRSD. High prevalence of personality disorders (22.4%) has been found in CRSD patients (Dagan and Eisenstein, 1999). This high prevalence has been confirmed in a controlled study, which found that individuals suffering from CRSD are characterized to a greater extent by personality disorders than a control group (Dagan *et al*, 1996). In a complementary study the sleep–wake rhythm of hospitalized psychiatric patients was evaluated. Ten of sixty-three hospitalized adolescents (16%) were diagnosed as suffering from DSPS following a sleep–wake schedule structured interview, and subjects diagnosed as suffering from personality disorders had a significantly higher probability of also suffering from DSPS. In addition, patients with DSPS were more likely to have received an Axis II diagnosis only, and were more likely to be diagnosed as suffering from a distinct group of disorders characterized by affective lability (Dagan *et al*, 1998a).

The association between DSPS and personality disorders may lend some support to the hypothesis that inborn peculiarities in the sleep–wake rhythm lead to the social and functional difficulties characteristic of personality disorders.

High prevalence of learning disorders (19.3%) has been reported in CRSD patients (Dagan and Eisenstein, 1999). In addition, Tomoda *et al* (1997) describe disturbed circadian core body-temperature rhythm and sleep disturbance in school-refusal children and adolescents without physical or psychiatric disorders or clinical psychosomatic symptoms. Importantly, instability of the sleep–wake system was found in children with attention-deficit/hyperactivity disorder (Gruber *et al*, 2000).

Learning and attention deficits as well as personality disorders are related to, or may even be an outcome of, CRSD. A child without adequate sleep at night will not be alert the following day in school and is prone to difficulty in keeping up with the other children. Frequently, the child's parents, teachers, doctors, or psychologists believe that his/her biological sleep–wake problem and the accompanying dysfunction at school are motivational or psychological in nature and presume that, over a period of time, the children tend to adapt themselves. This environmental attitude towards CRSD patients since early childhood or adolescence adds psychological distress to the existing difficulties of coping with life.

Conclusions

In 1981, Weitzman *et al* first noticed that thirty of their insomnia patients (7%) were suffering from DSPS. These patients had a tendency to fall asleep late at night and experienced difficulty rising at a desired time in the morning (Weitzman *et al*, 1981). When these patients were allowed to sleep without external restrictions, they slept for a normal length of time and exhibited no pathology in their sleep architecture. These patients were younger than other insomniacs, without differences of sex prevalence, displayed no specific psychiatric disorders, and evidenced various ages at onset of insomnia. This pioneer report published in 1981 was followed by a few studies based on small numbers of patients with no more than thirty participants (Regestein and Monk, 1995).

A single large study on CRSD patients that included a survey of the characteristics of 322 patients suffering from CRSD revealed that a great majority (84.6%) of the patients were diagnosed as suffering from DSPS. Of these patients, 12.3% had a non-24-hour sleep–wake syndrome, and only a handful of patients were diagnosed with either ISWP (1.9%) or ASPS (1.3%). The majority of patients (89.6%) reported onset of CRSD in early childhood or adolescence; no sex differences were evident; a familial trait existed in 44% of patients (Dagan and Eisenstein, 1999). Similar data was reported in a sleep clinic in Japan (Kamei *et al*, 1998). The reported prevalence of CRSD in these studies reflects the population of patients who approach sleep specialists for help. There is, at the present time, limited data available regarding the prevalence of CRSD in the general population. The prevalence of the disorder was estimated to be 0.13% in Japan (Yazaki *et al*, 1999), 0.17% in Norway (Schrader *et al*, 1993) and 7.3% of adolescents in the western population (Pelayo *et al*, 1988).

It is now well known that CRSD patients differ from night- or morning-type people ('owls' and 'larks') in the rigidity of their maladjusted biological clock. While 'owls' and 'larks' prefer morning or evening, they are flexible and can adjust to the demands of the environmental clock. CRSD patients, on the other hand, appear to be unable to change their clock by means of motivation or education. In the future, this clinical impression should be empirically examined and the relevant physiological component identified, in the same way that daily body temperature was identified as a physiological component in adjustment to shift work and jetlag (Kryger *et al*, 1994).

Circadian rhythm sleep disorders are sleep pathologies largely unfamiliar to doctors. Many of the patients with CRSD have, for years, been inaccurately diagnosed by neurologists, paediatricians, and psychiatrists as psychophysiological insomniacs, and, therefore have been unsuccessfully treated, usually with sedative-hypnotic drugs. The combination of the early onset of CRSD, the ease of diagnosis, and the high frequency of misdiagnosis and erroneous treatment resulting in the potentially harmful psychological and adjustment consequences, together with the availability of promising treatments, all indicate the importance of greater awareness of these disorders on the part of paediatricians, family doctors, psychiatrists and neurologists, as well as psychologists and teachers.

References

Alvarez B, Dahlitz MJ, Vignau J, Parkes JD (1992) The delayed sleep phase syndrome: clinical and investigative findings in 14 subjects. *J Neurol Neurosurg Psychiat* **55**: 665–70

American Academy of Sleep Medicine (2005) *The International Classification of Sleep Disorders*. 2nd edn. American Academy of Sleep Medicine, Westchester, IL

Ancoli-Israel S, Martin JL, Kripke DF, Marler M, Klauber MR (2002) Effect of light treatment on sleep and circadian rhythms in demented nursing home patients. *J Am Geriatr Soc* **50**: 282–9

Ancoli-Israel S, Schnierow B, Kelsoe J, Fink R (2001) A pedigree of one family with delayed sleep phase syndrome. *Chronobiol Int* **18**: 831–40

Ando K, Kripke DF, Ancoli-Israel S (1995) Estimated prevalence of delayed and advanced sleep phase syndrome among adolescents. *Sleep Res* **24**: 509

Axelrod J (1974) The pineal gland: a neurochemical transducer. *Science* **184**: 1341–8

Ayalon L, Dishon L, Dagan Y (2001) Circadian rhythm sleep disorders following minor head trauma. *Chronobiol Int* **18**: A1065–A1066

Ayalon L, Hermesh H, Dagan Y (2002) Case study of circadian rhythm sleep disorder following haloperidol treatment: reversal by risperidone and melatonin. *Chronobiol Int* **19**: 947–59

Baehr EK, Fogg LF, Eastman CI (1999) Intermittent bright light and exercise to entrain human circadian rhythms to night work. *Am J Physiol* **277**: R1598–R1604

Buxton OM, Frank SA, L'Hermite-Baleriaux M, Leproult R, Turek FW, Van Cauter E (1997) Roles of intensity and duration of nocturnal exercise in causing phase delays of human circadian rhythms. *Am J Physiol* **273**: E536-E542

Cagnacci A, Elliott JA, Yen SS (1992) Melatonin: a major regulator of the circadian rhythm of core temperature in humans. *J Clin Endocrinol Metab* **75**: 447–52

Campbell SS, Murphy PJ (1998) Extraocular circadian phototransduction in humans. *Science* **279**: 396–9

Card JP, Moore RY (1982) Ventral lateral geniculate nucleus efferents to the rat suprachiasmatic nucleus exhibit avian pancreatic polypeptide-like immunoreactivity. *J Comp Neurol* **206**: 390–6

Carskadon MA, Dement WC (1994) Normal human sleep: an overview. In: Kryger MH, Roth T, Dement WC, eds. *Principles and Practice of Sleep Medicine*. WH Saunders, Philadelphia: 16–25

Chesson AL Jr, Littner M, Davila D, Anderson WM, Grigg-Damberger M, Hartse K *et al* (1999) Practice parameters for the use of light therapy in the treatment of sleep disorders. Standards of Practice Committee, American Academy of Sleep Medicine. *Sleep* **22**: 641–60

Czeisler CA, Kronauer RE, Allan JS, Duffy JF, Jewett ME, Brown EN, Ronda JM (1989) Bright light induction of strong (type 0) resetting of the human circadian pacemaker. *Science* **244**: 1328–33

Czeisler CA, Richardson GS, Coleman RZ, Zimmerman JC, Moore-Ede MC *et al* (1981) Chronotherapy: resetting the circadian clocks of patients with delayed sleep phase insomnia. *Sleep* **4**: 1–21

Dagan Y (2002) Circadian rhythm sleep disorders (CRSD) in psychiatry — a review. *Israel J Psychiat Rel Sci* **39**(1): 19–27

Dagan Y, Eisenstein M (1999) Circadian rhythm sleep disorders: toward a more precise definition and diagnosis. *Chronobiol Int* **16**: 213–22

Dagan Y, Lavie P (1994) Characteristics of sleep–wake schedule disorders (SWSD) patients. *Sleep Res* **3**: 53

Dagan Y, Sela H, Omer H, Hallis D, Dar R (1996) High prevalence of personality disorders among circadian rhythm sleep disorders (CRSD) patients. *J Psychosom Res* **41**: 357–63

Dagan Y, Stein D, Steinbock M, Yovel I, Hallis D (1998a) Frequency of delayed sleep phase syndrome among hospitalized adolescent psychiatric patients. *J Psychosom Res* **45**: 15–20

Dagan Y, Yovel I, Hallis D, Eisenstein M, Raichik I (1998b) Evaluating the role of melatonin in the long-term treatment of delayed sleep phase syndrome (DSPS). *Chronobiol Int* **15**: 181–90

Dahlitz M, Alvarez B, Vignau J, English J, Arendt J, Parkes JD (1991) Delayed sleep phase syndrome response to melatonin. *Lancet* **337**: 1121–4

Dawson D, Armstrong SM (1996) Chronobiotics — drugs that shift rhythms. *Pharmacol Ther* **69**: 15–36

Deacon S, Arendt J (1995) Melatonin-induced temperature suppression and its acute phase-shifting effects correlate in a dose-dependent manner in humans. *Brain Res* **688**: 77–85

Demisch K, Demisch L, Nickelsen T, Rieth R (1987) The influence of acute and subchronic administration of various antidepressants on early morning melatonin plasma levels in healthy subjects: increases following fluvoxamine. *J Neural Transm* **68**: 257–70

Dijk DJ, Boulos Z, Eastman CI, Lewy AJ, Campbell SS, Terman M (1995) Light treatment for sleep disorders: consensus report. II. Basic properties of circadian physiology and sleep regulation. *J Biol Rhythms* **10**: 113–25

Dursun SM, Patel JK, Burke JG, Reveley MA (1999) Effects of typical antipsychotic drugs and risperidone on the quality of sleep in patients with schizophrenia: a pilot study. *J Psychiat Neurosci* **24**: 333–7

Eastman CI, Hoese EK, Youngstedt SD, Liu L (1995) Phase-shifting human circadian rhythms with exercise during the night shift. *Physiol Behav* **58**: 1287–91

Eastman CI, Martin SK, Hebert M (2000) Failure of extraocular light to facilitate circadian rhythm reentrainment in humans. *Chronobiol Int* **17**: 807–26

Ebihara S, Mano N, Kurono N, Komuro G, Yoshimura T (1996) Vitamin B_{12} affects non-photic entrainment of circadian locomotor activity rhythms in mice. *Brain Res* **727**: 31–9

Ebisawa T, Kajimura N, Uchiyama M, Katoh M, Sekimoto M, Watanabe T *et al* (1999) Alleic variants of human melatonin 1a receptor: function and prevalence in subjects with circadian rhythm sleep disorders. *Biochem Biophys Res Commun* **262**: 832–7

Ebisawa T, Uchiyama M, Kajimura N, Mishima K, Kamei Y, Katoh M *et al* (2001) Association of structural polymorphisms in the human period 3 gene with delayed sleep phase syndrome. *EMBO Rep* **2**: 342–6

Folkard S, Arendt J, Clark M (1993) Can melatonin improve shift workers' tolerance of the night shift? Some preliminary findings. *Chronobiol Int* **10**: 315–20

Friedman DI, Johnson JK, Chorsky RL, Stopa EG (1991) Labeling of human retinohypothalamic tract with the carbocyanine dye, DiI. *Brain Res* **560**: 297–302

Gruber R, Sadeh A, Raviv A (2000) Instability of sleep patterns in children with attention-deficit/hyperactivity disorder. *J Am Acad Child Adolesc Psychiat* **39**: 495–501

Hayes B, Czeisler CA (1992) Chronobiology of human sleep and sleep disorders. In: Touitou Y, Haus E, eds. *Biologic Rhythms in Clinical and Laboratory Medicine*. Springer-Verlag, Berlin: 263–4

Hendrickson AE, Wagoner N, Cowan WM (1972) An autoradiographic and electron microscopic study of retino-hypothalamic connections. *Z Zellforsch Mikrosk Anat* **135**: 1–26

Hermesh H, Lemberg H, Abadi J, Dagan Y (2001) Circadian rhythm sleep disorders as a possible side-effect of fluvoxamine. *CNS Spectrum* **6**: 511–13

Hohjoh H, Takahashi Y, Hatta Y, Tanaka H, Akaza T, Tokunaga K *et al* (1999) Possible association of human leucocyte antigen DR1 with delayed sleep phase syndrome. *Psychiat Clin Neurosci* **53**: 527–9

Jan JE, Espezel H, Appleton RE (1994) The treatment of sleep disorders with melatonin. *Dev Med Child Neurol* **36**: 97–107

Kamei Y, Urata J, Uchiyaya M, Hayakawa T, Ozaki S, Shibui K, Okawa M (1998) Clinical characteristics of circadian rhythm sleep disorders. *Psychiat Clin Neurosci* **52**: 234–5

Kamgar-Parsi B, Wehr TA, Gillin JC (1983) Successful treatment of human non-24-hour sleep–wake syndrome. *Sleep* **6**: 257–64

Kayumov L, Brown G, Jindal R, Buttoo K, Shapiro CM (2001) A randomized, double-blind, placebo-controlled crossover study of the effect of exogenous melatonin on delayed sleep phase syndrome. *Psychosom Med* **63**: 40–8

King DP, Zhao Y, Sangoram AM, Wilsbacher LD, Tanaka M, Antoch MP *et al* (1997) Positional cloning of the mouse circadian clock gene. *Cell* **89**: 641–53

Klein DC (1979) Circadian rhythms in the pineal gland. In: Krieger DT, ed. *Endocrine Rhythms* Ravan Press, New York: 203–23

Klein DC (1985) Photoneural regulation of the mammalian pineal gland. In:Everd D, Clark S, eds, *Photoperiodism, Melatonin and the Pineal*. Ciba Foundation Symposium 17. Pitman, London: 38–56

Klein T, Martens H, Dijk DJ, Kronauer RE, Seely EW, Czeisler CA (1993) Circadian sleep regulation in the absence of light perception: chronic non-24-hour circadian rhythm sleep disorder in a blind man with a regular 24-hour sleep–wake schedule. *Sleep* **16**: 333–43

Kokkoris CP, Weitzman ED, Pollak CP, Spielman AJ, Czeisler CA, Bradlow H (1978) Long-term ambulatory temperature monitoring in a subject with a hypernychthemeral sleep–wake cycle disturbance. *Sleep* **1**: 177–90

Koorengevel KM, Gordijn MC, Beersma DG, Meesters Y, den Boer JA, van den Hoofdakker RH, and Daan S. (2001) Extraocular light therapy in winter depression: a double-blind placebo- controlled study. *Biol Psychiat* **50**: 691–8

Kryger MH, Roth T, Dement WC (1994) *Principles and Practice of Sleep Medicine*. 2nd ed. edn. Saunders Company, Pennsylvania

Lapierre O, Dumont M (1995) Melatonin treatment of a non-24-hour sleep–wake cycle in a blind retarded child. *Biol Psychiat* **38**: 119–22

Lewy AJ, Ahmed S, Sack RL (1996) Phase shifting the human circadian clock using melatonin. *Behav Brain Res* **73**: 131–4

Lewy AJ, Sack RL, Blood ML, Bauer VK, Cutler NL, Thomas KH (1995) Melatonin marks circadian phase position and resets the endogenous circadian pacemaker in humans. *Ciba Found Symp* **183**: 303–17

Lewy AJ, Sack RL, Miller LS, Hoban TM (1987) Antidepressant and circadian phase-shifting effects of light. *Science* **235**: 352–4

Lewy AJ, Sack RL, Singer CM (1985a) Melatonin, light and chronobiological disorders. *Ciba Found Symp* **117**: 231–52

Lewy AJ, Sack RL, Singer CM (1985b) Treating phase typed chronobiologic sleep and mood disorders using appropriately timed bright artificial light. *Psychopharmacol Bull* **21**: 368–72

Lewy AJ, Sack RL, Singer CM, White DM, Hoban TM (1988) Winter depression and the phase-shift hypothesis for bright light's therapeutic effects: history, theory, and experimental evidence. *J Biol Rhythms* **3**: 121–34

Lewy AJ, Wehr TA, Goodwin FK, Newsome DA, Markey SP (1980) Light suppresses melatonin secretion in humans. *Science* **210**: 1267–9

Lindblom N, Hatonen T, Laakso M, Alila-Johansson A, Laipio M, Turpeinen U (2000A) Bright light exposure of a large skin area does not affect melatonin or bilirubin levels in humans. *Biol Psychiat* **48**: 1098–104

Lindblom N, Heiskala H, Hatonen T, Mustanoja S, Alfthan H, Alila-Johansson A, Laakso ML. (2000B) No evidence for extraocular light induced phase shifting of human melatonin, cortisol and thyrotropin rhythms. *Neuroreport* **11**: 713–7

Mayer G, Kroger M, Meier-Ewert K (1996) Effects of vitamin B_{12} on performance and circadian rhythm in normal subjects. *Neuropsychopharmacology* **15**: 456–64

McArthur AJ, Lewy AJ, Sack RL (1996) Non-24-hour sleep–wake syndrome in a sighted man: circadian rhythm studies and efficacy of melatonin treatment. *Sleep* **19**: 544–53

Minors DS, Waterhouse JM, Wirz-Justice A (1991) A human phase-response curve to light. *Neurosci Lett* **133**: 36–40

Miyazaki T, Hashimoto S, Masubuchi S, Honma S, Honma KI (2001) Phase-advance shifts of human circadian pacemaker are accelerated by daytime physical exercise. *Am J Physiol Regul Integr Comp Physiol* **281**: R197–R205

Nagtegaal JE, Kerkhof GA, Smits MG, Swart AC, van der Meer YG (1997) Traumatic brain injury-associated delayed sleep phase syndrome. *Funct Neurol* **12**: 345–8

Nordlund JJ, Lerner AB (1977) The effects of oral melatonin on skin color and on the release of pituitary hormones. *J Clin Endocrinol Metab* **45**: 768–74

Ohta T, Ando K, Iwata T, Ozaki N, Kayukawa Y, Terashima M, Okada T, Kasahara Y (1991) Treatment of persistent sleep–wake schedule disorders in adolescents with methylcobalamin (vitamin B$_{12}$). *Sleep* **14**: 414–8

Okawa M, Mishima K, Nanami T, Shimizu T, Iijima S, Hishikawa Y, Takahashi K (1990) Vitamin B$_{12}$ treatment for sleep–wake rhythm disorders. *Sleep* **13**: 15–23

Oldani A, Ferini-Strambi L, Zucconi M, Stankov B, Fraschini F, Smirne S (1994) Melatonin and delayed sleep phase syndrome: ambulatory polygraphic evaluation. *Neuroreport* **6**: 132–4

Ozaki S, Uchiyama M, Shirakawa S, and Okawa M (1996) Prolonged interval from body temperature nadir to sleep offset in patients with delayed sleep phase syndrome. *Sleep* **19**: 36–40

Palm L, Blennow G, Wetterberg L (1997) Long-term melatonin treatment in blind children and young adults with circadian sleep–wake disturbances. *Dev Med Child Neurol* **39**: 319–25

Patten SB, Lauderdale WM (1992) Delayed sleep phase disorder after traumatic brain injury. *J Am Acad Child Adolesc Psychiat* **31**: 100–2

Pelayo RP, Thorpy MG, Glovinsky P (1988) Prevalence of delayed sleep phase syndrome among adolescents. *Sleep Res* **17**: 392

Petrie K, Conaglen JV, Thompson L, Chamberlain K (1989) Effect of melatonin on jet lag after long haul flights. *Br Med J* **298**: 705–7

Quinto C, Gellido C, Chokroverty S, Masdeu J (2000) Posttraumatic delayed sleep phase syndrome. *Neurology* **54**: 250–2

Regestein QR, Monk TH (1995) Delayed sleep phase syndrome: a review of its clinical aspects. *Am J Psychiatry* **152**: 602–8

Reid KJ, Chang AM, Dubocovich ML, Turek FW, Takahashi JS, Zee PC (2001) Familial advanced sleep phase syndrome. *Arch Neurol* **58**: 1089–94

Rosenthal NE, Joseph-Vanderpool JR, Levendosky AA, Johnston SH, Allen R, Kelly KA *et al* (1990) Phase-shifting effects of bright morning light as treatment for delayed sleep phase syndrome. *Sleep* **13**: 354–61

Rosenthal NE, Sack DA, Gillin JC, Lewy AJ, Goodwin FK, Davenport Y *et al* (1984) Seasonal affective disorder. A description of the syndrome and preliminary findings with light therapy. *Arch Gen Psychiat* **41**: 72–80

Sack RL, Lewy AJ, Blood ML, Keith LD, Nakagawa H (1992) Circadian rhythm abnormalities in totally blind people: incidence and clinical significance. *J Clin Endocrinol Metab* **75**: 127–34

Sack RL, Lewy AJ, White DM, Singer CM, Fireman MJ, Vandiver R (1990) Morning vs evening light treatment for winter depression. Evidence that the therapeutic effects of light are mediated by circadian phase shifts. *Arch Gen Psychiat* **47**: 343–51

Sadeh A, Aesler DU, Lawre P (1989) Actigraphically based automatic bedtime sleep–wake recording: Validity and clinical applications. *J Ambulat Monitor* **2**: 209–16

Sadeh A, Hauri PJ, Kripke DF, Lavie P (1995) The role of actigraphy in the evaluation of sleep disorders. *Sleep* **18**: 288–302

Schrader H, Bovim G, Sand T (1993) The prevalence of delayed and advanced sleep phase syndromes. *J Sleep Res* **2**: 51–5

Seabra ML, Bignotto M, Pinto LR Jr, Tufik S (2000) Randomized, double-blind clinical trial, controlled with placebo, of the toxicology of chronic melatonin treatment. *J Pineal Res* **29**: 193–200

Shiota M, Sudou M, Ohshima M (1996) Using outdoor exercise to decrease jet lag in airline crewmembers. *Aviat Space Environ Med* **67**: 1155–60

Skene DJ, Bojkowski CJ, Arendt J (1994) Comparison of the effects of acute fluvoxamine and desipramine administration on melatonin and cortisol production in humans. *Br J Clin Pharmacol* **37**: 181–6

Takahashi Y, Hohjoh H, Matsuura K (2000) Predisposing factors in delayed sleep phase syndrome. *Psychiat Clin Neurosci* **54**: 356–8

Terman M, Terman JS, Quitkin FM, McGrath PJ, Stewart JW, Rafferty B (1989) Light therapy for seasonal affective disorder. A review of efficacy. *Neuropsychopharmacology* **2**: 1–22

Toh KL, Jones CR, He Y, Eide EJ, Hinz WA, Virshup DM *et al* (2001) An *hPer2* phosphorylation site mutation in familial advanced sleep phase syndrome. *Science* **291**: 1040–3

Tomoda A, Miike T, Yonamine K, Adachi K, Shiraishi S (1997) Disturbed circadian core body temperature rhythm and sleep disturbance in school refusal children and adolescents. *Biol Psychiatry* **41**: 810–3

Turek FW, Zee PC (1999) Regulation of sleep and circadian rhythms. In: Lenfant C, ed. *Lung Biology in Health and Disease*, vol. 133. Marcel Dekker, New York

Uchiyama M, Okawa M, Shibui K, Kim K, Tagaya H, Kudo Y *et al* (2000) Altered phase relation between sleep timing and core body temperature rhythm in delayed sleep phase syndrome and non-24-hour sleep–wake syndrome in humans. *Neurosci Lett* **294**: 101–4

Wagner DR (1996) Disorders of the circadian sleep–wake cycle. *Neurol Clin* **14**: 651–70

Watanabe T, Kajimura N, Kato M, Sekimoto M, Takahashi K (1999) Effects of phototherapy in patients with delayed sleep phase syndrome. *Psychiat Clin Neurosci* **53**: 231–3

Weitzman ED, Czeisler CA, Coleman RM, Spielman AJ, Zimmerman JC, Dement W *et al* (1981) Delayed sleep phase syndrome. A chronobiological disorder with sleep- onset insomnia. *Arch Gen Psychiat* **38**: 737–46

Wever R, ed (1979) *The Circadian System of Man*. Springer-Verlag, New York

Weyerbrock A, Timmer J, Hohagen F, Berger M, Bauer J (1996) Effects of light and chronotherapy on human circadian rhythms in delayed sleep phase syndrome: cytokines, cortisol, growth hormone, and the sleep–wake cycle. *Biol Psychiat* **40**: 794–7

Wirz-Justice A, Cajochen C, Nussbaum P (1997) A schizophrenic patient with an arrhythmic circadian rest–activity cycle. *Psychiat Res* **73**: 83–90

Wirz-Justice A, Haug HJ, Cajochen C (2001) Disturbed circadian rest-activity cycles in schizophrenia patients: an effect of drugs? *Schizophr Bull* **27**: 497–502

Wirz-Justice A, Werth E, Savaskan E, Knoblauch V, Gasio PF, Muller-Spahn F (2000) Haloperidol disrupts, clozapine reinstates the circadian rest–activity cycle in a patient with early-onset alzheimer disease. *Alzheimer Dis Assoc Disord* **14**: 212–5

Yazaki M, Shirakawa S, Okawa M, Takahashi K (1999) Demography of sleep disturbances associated with circadian rhythm disorders in Japan. *Psychiat Clin Neurosci* **53**: 267–8

Yoon IY, Jeong DU, Kwon KB, Kang SB, Song BG (2002) Bright light exposure at night and light attenuation in the morning improve adaptation of night shift workers. *Sleep* **25**: 351–6

Youngstedt SD, Kripke DF, Elliott JA (2002) Circadian phase-delaying effects of bright light alone and combined with exercise in humans. *Am J Physiol Regul Integr Comp Physiol* **282**: R259–R66

Zulley J, Wever R, Aschoff J (1981) The dependence of onset and duration of sleep on the circadian rhythm on rectal temperature. *Pflugers Arch* **391**: 314–18

CHAPTER 12

Medications and sleep

Lata Jayaram

The quantity of pharmacological substances, prescriptions, over-the-counter and complementary medicines is quite large and is increasing. Although most medications are targeted at specific conditions and functions, they often have actions beyond their intended ones. Their effects on sleep and wake function are both poorly understood and studied. The effects on sleep of normal subjects may be different to the changes seen in unwell people. For example, benzodiazepine hypnotics may have a detrimental effect on the sleep structure on a normal volunteer but may improve it in patients with insomnia. For information to be clinically useful, it is important that drug evaluation on the sleep and wake function is described in both normal volunteers and subjects with specific medical and psychiatric conditions.

A new understanding of the importance of chronopharmacology (*Chapter 2*) on the effects of medications needs to be considered. Some of the issues concerning sleep and wake function and medications, including complementary substances, are discussed below. All medications considered in this chapter should be used with caution in pregnancy and lactation.

Substance dependence (addiction), tolerance and withdrawal

In the management of sleep and wake disorders, health practitioners often use medication with abuse liability (eg. benzodiazepines, amphetamines, opioids) and many patients are concerned about the addictive or habit-forming nature of these medications.

⌘ **The term drug dependence**, both psychological and physical dependence, is used in preference to *drug addiction* (Camí and Farré, 2003).

⌘ **Physical drug dependency** is characterized by the development of intense physical symptoms when the administration of the drug is stopped, or, following the administration of a specific antagonist (Brust, 1993; Eddy *et al*, 1965). Psychological dependence is characterized by the psyche drive to continue to use the drugs to produce pleasure or avoid discomfort. Criteria for substance dependence have been published in the *Statistical Manuals of Mental Disorders* (DSM-IV) (*Table 12.1*). It should be emphasized that addiction (drug dependence) is a state where the use of a drug is compulsive and repetitive despite negative consequences to the user.

⌘ ***Tolerance*** is a state in which the action of the medication decreases over time after repeated administration and may lead the patient to seek an increase in dosage to maintain an equivalent effect. It also forms the basis for withdrawal when the medication is stopped suddenly. The underlying mechanism of tolerance is complex and involves increased metabolism with reduction of the active substance at the site of action, as well as down-regulation of the drug receptors at cellular level.

⌘ ***Withdrawal symptoms and signs*** vary in intensity depending on the specific drug and its pharmacological characteristics (duration of action). Symptoms and signs include mood changes, with anxiety, irritability and depression; sleep disturbance with insomnia or hypersomnia; and altered motor activity with restlessness and irritability. Withdrawal symptoms are thought to be important contributors to medication-seeking behavior and physical drug dependency.

Given the above considerations, a therapeutic situation where medications like benzodiazepines, amphetamines or opioids are prescribed for a specific medical disorder, under medical supervision to improve the patient's symptoms, should not be construed as drug dependency. In a controlled and supervised clinical situation, drug dependency is a rare event. However, before medications with potential abuse liability are prescribed, particularly on a chronic basis, prior drug abuse should be ascertained as accurately as possible. A supervised drug screen should also be undertaken during the diagnostic process in the appropriate circumstances.

Stimulant medications

The stimulants available in clinical practice include amphetamines, amphetamine-like medications and a new group of compounds, stimulant non-amphetamines (modafinil).

Amphetamines and related stimulants

The stimulants commonly used in clinical practice include dexamphetamine and methylphenidate; mazindol and pemoline are also available in certain countries. Amphetamines act by increasing noradrenergic and dopaminergic activity within the central nervous system. The effect on the metabolism of serotonin does not appear to be important to the alerting effect. Stimulation of peripheral noradrenergic terminals and of CNS dopaminergic pathways is responsible for some of the undesirable side-effects of amphetamines (tremor, palpitations, hypertension and sweating).

Methylphenidate and mazindol increase adrenergic neurotransmitters blocking the reuptake of noradrenaline (norepinephrine) and dopamine. Dexamphetamine and pemoline also increase the release of these neurotransmitters in the synaptic cleft.

Table 12.1: Substance dependence
Substance dependence is present when three (or more) of the following, occur at any time over a period of 12 months:
1 Tolerance, defined by the need to increase the dose to maintain the desired effect and/or increase effect after continuous use of the same amount
2 Withdrawal symptoms (specific for different drugs)
3 The substance is often taken in larger amounts or over a longer period than was intended
4 There is a persistent desire or unsuccessful efforts to cut down or control substance abuse
5 The person spends a large part of his time on activities necessary to obtain the substance, use the substance, or recover from its effects, which results in neglecting important social, occupational or recreational activities
7 The substance use is continued and repetitive despite knowledge of having a persistent or recurrent physical or psychological problem from its use

(modified from American Psychiatry Association, *Diagnostic and Statistical Manual of Mental Disorders*, 1995)

Dexamphetamine and methylphenidate are well absorbed orally and food has little impact on the irpharmacokinetic profile. Peak levels occur within 2 hours for both medications with the duration of action of 6–10 hours for dexamphetamine and 3–6 hours for methylphenidate (Patrick *et al*, 1987). The difference in duration between the 2 agents relates clinically to the apparently more abrupt cessation of the alerting effect in patients on methylphenidate. This problem, in part, can be controlled by the use of a slow-release formulation of methylphenidate.

Clinical effects

The response to stimulants is highly variable from one patient to another, with little correlation between plasma levels and response. Occasionally, patients respond with increased sleepiness (paradoxical effect) an hour or two after ingestion (Tecce and Cole, 1974).

Effects on sleep and wakefulness

Dexamphetamine and methylphenidate promote wakefulness and activity in volunteer subjects, particularly if they are sleep deprived. The benefits should be more obvious in patients with hypersomnolence syndromes. Mood is also affected with an increased sense of well being. Stimulants are useful in depression and even normal volunteers report a sense of euphoria, contentment and increased proficiency (Martin *et al*, 1971).

Effects on sleep

In normal volunteers, stimulants reduce total sleep time and structures, and stages of sleep. There is reduction in the percentage of REM sleep and latency to REM stage during acute use, with partial adaptation during prolonged use. During abrupt withdrawal of the medication there is rebound of REM sleep. This is relevant when performing studies in patients who are or have been on prescribed stimulants or have taken them for recreational use (Rechtschaffen *et al*, 1964). We require patients to be off the medication for at least 1 week before performing a sleep study and longer periods are recommended by other authors. Slow-wave sleep is usually not affected at therapeutic dose.

Other effects and side-effects

Other effects of dexamphetamine and methylphenidate are related to stimulation of the autonomic nervous system and include a dose-related increase in systolic and diastolic blood pressure, increased respiratory rate and increase in body temperature. In clinical practice, hypertension, however, is not a common problem and the changes in blood pressure value are subject to adaptation.

⌘ *Anorexia* occurs in some patients but significant weight reduction is rare and usually controlled by appropriate attention to diet.

⌘ *Psychosis* is uncommon at the doses used in clinical practice for treatment of narcoleptic syndromes. However, the risk is increased in patients with pre-existing psychiatric illness. Psychotic symptoms caused by amphetamines (hallucination, aggression, paranoid ideation) resolve after stopping the medication (Parkes, 1985).

⌘ *Increased motor activity*, such as tremors, tics and dyskinesias are seen in some patients, even with a small dose.

⌘ *Myopathy and cardiomyopathy* are potentially life-threatening complications documented in drug addicts (Karch, 1996) but there is no documented evidence in the clinical population.

⌘ *Violent aggressive behavior* is seen at therapeutic doses and requires stopping the medication. Modafinil would be an alternative, although re-introduction of an amphetamine at a low dose can be tried.

⌘ *Liver abnormalities* have been reported in people abusing methylphenidate intravenously.

⌘ *Insomnia* in sensitive patients or following late-evening administration of stimulants can be a problem. Side-effects reported by at least 5% of the patients in a survey of 150 is reported in *Table 12.2*.

Table 12.2: Reported side-effects of stimulant medication	
Appetite loss	12.2%
Migraine/headaches	9.6%
Mood problems	8.7%
Shakiness/tremor	7.8%
Weight loss	7.0%
Palpitations	6.1%
Still sleepy	5.2%
Lack of concentration	5.2%

Clinical use of stimulants

It is safe to start treatment with half a tablet twice a day (2.5 mg of dexamphetamine or 5 mg of methylphenidate) at breakfast and lunch with or without food. The dose can be increased to a full tablet within 2–3 days and then adjusted upwards slowly over the following 2-week period. It is not advisable to take the medication after 4.00PM–5.00PM because of the increased risk of insomnia. Exceptions include patients who have to drive or are engaged in important activities in the evening hours. In shift workers, the medication needs to be scheduled according to the work practice.

It is important to give written information to the patient (see the example at the end of this chapter). The medicolegal implications of being on stimulants should be explained as well as special arrangements needed in case of traveling, particularly overseas. The Road and Traffic Authority often requires notification when a patient is on stimulants.

Pattern of use

The pattern of use depends on the clinical response. Some patients have the medication spread through the day in various amounts; others take a full dose once in the morning only. Some patients use the medication every day; others only when they work or when driving.

There is no evidence that drug-free days are necessary or useful to reduce tolerance. As a narcoleptic patient said: 'What justification can be given for a patient to virtually withdraw from existence for two days out of seven?' (Piscopo *et al*, 1992).

Contraindications

Contraindications to the use of amphetamines or methylphenidate are predominantly minor, but the following conditions require particular attention:

- *Previous drug abuse:* Prior drug abuse increases the risk of drug dependency and a different stimulant (modafinil) may need to be considered if clinically indicated. Occasionally patients with undiagnosed narcolepsy have used illegally obtained stimulants to improve their alertness and these patients should not be denied treatment. Psychiatric consultation and liaison with the drug and alcohol services is always necessary in this situation.

- *Psychiatric syndromes:* Anxiety state, emotional instability and schizophrenia can be made worse by stimulants and the concomitant use of psychotropic drugs can cause diagnostic as well as treatment difficulties. However, stimulants do have a potential role in depressed patients and close liaison with a psychiatrist is always necessary if treatment is to be undertaken.

- *Hypertension and cardiac disease:* Difficult-to-control blood pressure and arrhythmia are relative contraindications to the use of stimulants, particularly if high doses are needed.

❖ ***Glaucoma:*** Because of the mydriatic effect of the sympathomimetic action of stimulants, narrow angle glaucoma needs particular attention.

❖ ***Epilepsy:*** Amphetamines are said to decrease seizure threshold and their use in patients with epilepsy has to be evaluated on an individual basis. Interaction between stimulant medications and antiepileptics such as phenytoin (Dilantin™) also needs to be considered.

❖ ***Pregnancy:*** The use of stimulants should be avoided in pregnancy and when the patient is attempting to conceive. Although prematurity and low birth weight has been reported in amphetamine users, other studies have reported no ill effects in children of mothers who have used or abused amphetamines during pregnancy (Briggs GG *et al* 1975; Eriksson *et al*, 1978; Little *et al*, 1988).

❖ ***Breastfeeding:*** Breastfeeding mothers need to be informed that stimulants concentrate in breast milk even though there is no evidence of harm to the infant.

❖ ***Tolerance and dependence:*** Tolerance to the sense of euphoria, anorexia, hyperthermia and hypertension develops quickly; within 3–4 weeks. However, in clinical practice there appears to be little tolerance to the anti-sleepiness action.

In a follow-up survey in our centre of 115 patients on either dexamphetamine or methylphenidate (unpublished data) twenty-nine (26%) had stopped the medication because of no beneficial effect (US Modafinil in Narcolepsy Multicentre Study Group, 1998) or side-effects. None had difficulty stopping the medications. Twenty-eight patients (24%) reported decreased efficacy over time (average duration of treatment 63 weeks, range 4–260 weeks). However, nineteen patients reported increased efficacy over time. The patients who reported decreased efficacy still found the medication beneficial to their everyday functioning compared to having no treatment. Dose escalation was not seen in any of the patients. The mean consumption of dexamphetamine was 15 mg/day (range 2.5–45 mg/day).

Follow-up

After the initial dose titration period, a follow-up every 6–12 months is usually sufficient. Because of the potential risk of myopathy, including cardiomyopathy and liver abnormalities, it is recommended that a creatine kinase and liver function test is performed at each follow-up visit.

Drug interactions

Stimulants and tricyclic antidepressants are often used in combination for the management of cataplexy in narcoleptic patients. Imipramine and desipramine levels are increased by concomitant use of methylphenidate and amphetamine. The concomitant use of amphetamine and monoamine oxidase inhibitors (MAOIs) may lead to hypertensive crisis and should be avoided.

The use of lithium and beta-blockers tends to reduce the stimulant action of amphetamine. Chlorpromazine tends to increase the half-life of amphetamine and the use of both medications at the same time should be avoided, although they are hardly likely to be used together.

Modafinil

Modafinil (Modadiol™, Provigil™, Modavigil™, 100 mg tablets) is a non-amphetamine stimulant medication with a safer profile than amphetamine and methylphenidate. Developed by the French company LaFon, it was initially used in narcoleptic patients in the 1980s (Laffont *et al*, 1987). Subsequent clinical trials have confirmed that modafinil reduces sleepiness and maintains wakefulness in patients with pathological sleepiness (Broughton *et al*, 1997; US Modafinil in Narcolepsy Multicentre Study Group, 1998). Modafinil increases the sense of energy and mental efficiency but does not induce elation and euphoria like amphetamines, and this may explain the reduced risk for abuse and dependency (Warot *et al*, 1993).

Mode of action

Animal studies suggest that, at least in part, the wakefulness activity of modafinil is mediated by the inhibition of gamma-aminobutyric acid (GABA) activity (GABA being the most important inhibitory neurotransmitter in the central nervous system) (Ferraro *et al*, 1997). Modafinil is also shown to increase the activity of neurons containing orexin, a neurotransmitter associated with regulation of sleep and wakefulness in the lateral hypothalamus (Chemelli *et al*, 1999; Scammell *et al*, 2000).

Compared to amphetamines, modafinil has a more restricted pattern of activity. In autoradiographic studies in rats, modafinil increases activity in the hyppocampus, thalamic areas and amygdala. Unlike amphetamines, modafinil does not activate the extrapyramidal system, in keeping with the observation that the dopaminergic system is not activated by this stimulant (Engber *et al*, 1998).

Clinical use

Modafinil is well absorbed, with a half-life of about 11–14 hours, and excreted predominantly as modafinil acid in the urine. The presence of food does not interfere significantly with its absorption. In the presence of significant renal impairment (creatinine clearance less than 16 ml/min) a dose reduction is needed, starting with 100 mg/day rather than 200 mg. Similarly, with significant hepatic impairment a dose reduction is warranted. It can be given as a single or twice daily dose (morning and midday). The dose is between 200 and 400 mg/day. On occasion, doses of up to 600 mg have been used but this is not recommended.

Side-effects

Headache has been reported by up to 51% of patients and is the only difference from side-effects reported by patients on placebo (US Modafinil in Narcolepsy Multicentre Study Group, 1998).

The use of modafinil in the evening should be avoided as it can lead to insomnia.

Modafinil is likely to become the first-line medication in the treatment of narcoleptic syndromes, given the equivalent efficacy of amphetamines in increasing alertness and its safer profile, lack of peripheral side-effects, and low potential for dependency. Modafinil does not reduce total sleep time or change sleep structure. In particular, it does not reduce REM sleep. This helps to explain modafinil's lack of efficacy in controlling cataplexy, as opposed to dexamphetamines which are effective, at least in part. Other uses of modafinil include improvement in:

- the residual sleepiness in patients with obstructive sleep apnea while on nasal CPAP (Kingshott *et al*, 2001
- sleepiness in myotonic dystrophy (Damian *et al*, 2001) in children with attention deficit disorder (Rugino and Copley, 2001; Rugino and Samsock, 2003)
- fatigue in patients with multiple sclerosis.

Combined use of modafinil and amphetamine is possible and well tolerated in normal volunteers, even though there is an increased incidence of side-effects (Wong *et al*, 1998). However, it should be noted that in a clinical population of patients with narcoleptic syndrome, the decision to use both amphetamine and modafinil is usually taken because neither has been effective on their own in improving hypersomnolence. Anecdotal experience of combintion therapy is usually disappointing.

Drug interactions

Female patients should be warned of the risk of oral contraceptives being less effective and formulation with a higher dose of estrogen may be needed. As modafinil becomes more widely used, other clinically significant interactions may become apparent.

Pemolin and mazindol

Pemoline and mazindol are synthetic analogues with a mode of action similar to methylphenidate and amphetamine respectively. Although not commonly seen in the treatment of narcolepsy, Pemolin can cause a rare but important liver necrosis, which is due to an idiosyncratic metabolic reaction. Mazindol is an anorectic medication found to be effective in narcoleptic patients at doses of 3–8 mg daily (Parkes and Schachter, 1979).

Mazindol has a stimulant effect similar to amphetamine with no effect on cataplexy. Side-effects are similar to amphetamine even though it is said to have low abuse potential. It is predominantly used in the UK and not available in Australia. The potential risk of pulmonary hypertension (Hagiwara *et al*, 2000) and the availability of medications with a safer profile will reduce the use of mazindol in the future.

Gamma-hydroxybutyrate (GHB)

Gamma-hydroxybutyrate (GHB) is a fatty acid derivative of gamma-aminobutyric acid (GABA) with nervous system inhibitory activity. It is of interest in sleep medicine for its potential role in the management of narcolepsy. However, because of its use as recreational drugs and potential abuse, it is not available for routine use in many countries.

Because of its amnestic and euphoric effects, GHB has been used illegally and for recreational purposes. Observations that GHB increases growth hormone release have led to inappropriate use by body builders as a dietary supplement. GHB also has a short half-life (1.5–2 hours), which means multiple administrations every 3–4 hours, making it somewhat impractical.

GHB is an endogenous compound and constituent of the brain, with the hypothalamus, thalamus and substantia nigra having the highest concentrations (Tunnicliff, 1997). Its action may be mediated through specific receptors, as well as GABA receptors, with an indirect decrease in dopamine level.

GHB was initially used as an agent to induce general anesthesia but it has been investigated in the management of narcolepsy over the last 26 years (Broughton and Mamelak, 1979; Lammers *et al*, 1993; Mamelak and Webster, 1981; Scrima *et al*, 1990; Sharf *et al*, 1998). In narcoleptic patients, GHB improves night sleep quality, decreases frequency of cataplexy and may marginally reduce daytime sleepiness, probably by improving nighttime sleep.

The effects of GHB on sleep variables in narcolepsy patients (Lammers *et al*, 1993) include reduction in awakenings during REM sleep without affecting the total amount of REM sleep itself. Slow-wave sleep amount is increased with some reduction in stage 1 (Scrima *et al*, 1990).

Natural stimulants

Caffeine

Caffeine is a mild stimulant found in plants such as coffee, tea, cola, and guarana.

Mode of action

Caffeine, a methylxanthine, is an adenosine receptor antagonist which inhibits the hypnogenic actions of adenosine on the brain. Caffeine also increases catecholamine availability by reducing the reuptake of noradrenaline (norepinephrine) and adrenaline (epinephrine). It is rapidly absorbed, reaching peak blood levels within 15–45 minutes. Caffeine is metabolized by the liver and primarily excreted by the kidneys with a half-life of 5–7 hours. This is increased in liver diseases, pregnancy, and with certain medications, and is reduced in smokers.

Dose

The various doses of caffeine in selected beverages, food and medications are illustrated in *Table 12.3*.

Table 12.3: Estimated caffeine dose found in selected beverages, foods and medications		
Substance	**Serving size**	**Caffeine dose per serving**
Coffee		
Filter	1 cup (5 oz)	110–150 mg
Percolated	1 cup (5 oz)	60–125 mg
Espresso	1 oz	30–50 mg
Instant	1 cup (5 oz)	40–105 mg
Decaffeinated (brewed or instant)	1 cup (5 oz)	1–4 mg
Tea (bag or loose)	1 cup (5 oz)	20–100 mg
Hot cocoa	1 cup (5 oz)	10 mg
Carbonated drinks (national brands)	12 oz	30–49 mg
Cola (regular or diet)	12 oz	18–43 mg
Pepper (regular or diet)	12 oz	43–56 mg
Citrus (regular or diet)		
Milk chocolate bar	1 oz	6 mg
Bittersweet chocolate	1 oz	5–35 mg
Guarana	Variable	25–50 mg
Mate	Variable	25–50 mg
Excedrin™	2 tablets	130 mg
NoDoz™	2 capsules	200 mg
Dexatrim™	1 capsule	200 mg

(reprinted from Gyllenhaal *et al*, 2000, *Sleep Medicine Reviews* **4**(3), with permission from Elsevier Ltd)

Effect on sleep and polysomnography

In normal volunteers, caffeine reduces total sleep time and REM sleep, and increases sleep latency. The effects appear to be dose related, although responses between individuals vary depending on the amount and frequency of caffeine use. Caffeine ingested 3–4 hours prior to sleep rather than throughout the day can similarly impair sleep (Gyllenhall *et al*, 2000). Caffeine in doses of 250–

400 mg, one to three times a day has been shown to increase wakefulness based on mean sleep latency time (MSLT) recordings, when compared with placebo. As expected, narcoleptics with a moderate (two to four cups a day) caffeine intake have demonstrated a shorter sleep latency than those with light use (one to two cups a day) as measured by the mean wakefulness test (MWT) (Duffy and Milin, 1996; Milter *et al*, 1998). In chronic marijuana use there is an increase in sleep latency and REM percentage (Karacan *et al*, 1976).

Side-effects

Excessive caffeine intake leads to symptoms of sympathetic stimulation such as tachycardia, arrhythmias, tremor, insomnia, anxiety, and agitation. Tolerance, dependence and withdrawal symptoms, primarily of irritability headache and lethargy, to caffeine, have been documented. Caffeine in doses greater than 100 mg per day has been associated with spontaneous abortion (Cnattingus *et al*, 2000).

Ephedrine

Ephedrine is a sympathomimetic amine derived from the plant ephedra or Ma Huang. Ephedrine can be bought over the counter for the purposes of weight loss, increasing energy, as a decongestant, and for use in asthma (Gyllenhall *et al*, 2000).

Mode of action

Ephedrine acts mainly through the release of catecholamines with some direct effect on the adrenoreceptors.

Effect on sleep and polysomnography

There are no polysomnographic studies to date examining the effect of ephedrine on the sleep–wake cycle.

Side-effects and drug interactions

There are numerous serious side-effects related to ephedrine. Due to sympathetic stimulation, it can cause symptoms similar to caffeine including heart attack, stroke, psychosis, seizure and death. Ephedrine should not be used with other sympathomimetic agents or in cardiac, renal, thyroid and seizure disorders, or psychiatric conditions (MIMS, 2002).

Ginseng and Siberian ginseng

Ginseng or panax ginseng is used as a 'pick me up' to increase energy or deal with stressors. It contains ginsenosides, triterpenoid saponin glycosides and other compounds. Siberian ginseng, also called eleuthero, is related to Panax ginseng. It, too, is a performance enhancer (Gyllenhall *et al*, 2000).

Mode of action (underlying substances)

Ginsenosides, the active compounds, increase acetylcholine synthesis and decrease serotonin synthesis in the brain.

Effect on sleep and polysomnography

There is evidence supporting an antifatigue role for ginseng. Standardized extracts of ginseng have been shown to improve aerobic capacity and decrease blood lactate and heart rate during exercise compared with placebo (Pieralisi *et al*, 1991.) Conflicting results are noted in studies examining the effects of ginseng on mood, quality of life and alertness.

Placebo controlled studies have shown that Siberian ginseng increases physical endurance and work capacity. To date, there is no polysomnographic evidence on the effects of ginseng and Siberian ginseng on the sleep–wake cycle

Side-effects and drug interactions

Ginseng can have an estrogenic effect and inhibit clotting. A syndrome of hypertension, nervousness, insomnia and morning diarrhea has been attributed to ginseng use (Gyllenhall *et al*, 2000). However, several of the subjects in the case series from which this information was derived were drug addicts using other substances. The symptoms also occurred after the use of high doses of products that contained ginseng, the dose of which was not specified (Siegel, 1979). Ginseng can interact with the monoamine oxidase inhibitor phenelzine. Documented side-effects of Siberian ginseng include insomnia and arrhythmias in the elderly.

Yohimbine

Yohimbine bark is used as a stimulant and aphrodisiac.

Mode of action

Yohimbine, the active compound, is an alpha-2 antagonist which increases synaptic noradrenaline (norepinephrine) levels.

Effect on sleep and polysomnography

Yohimbine has been successfully used to treat narcolepsy in a small, uncontrolled study (Wooten, 1994). There are few polysomnographic studies examining the effects of yohimbine on sleep, however it has a similar effect to placebo on sleep study outcomes in healthy men (Gentili *et al*, 1996).

Side-effects and drug interactions

Side-effects include nausea, vomiting, and symptoms of sympathetic stimulation. Contraindications are similar to ephidrine. A lupus-like syndrome has been reported with yohimbine.

Sedative hypnotics

Benzodiazepines

Mode of action

These drugs are gamma-aminobutyric acid (GABA) receptor agonists. GABA receptors are located in the limbic, thalamic, and hypothalamic areas of the brain — all of which are involved in coordinating sleep (*Figure 12.1*). Benzodiazepines bind to these receptors and, by opening the associated chloride channels and enhancing post-synaptic inhibition, produce the well-known anxiolytic, sedating, muscle relaxant and anti-convulsant effects.

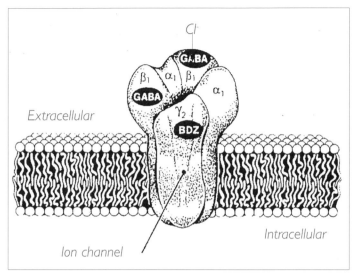

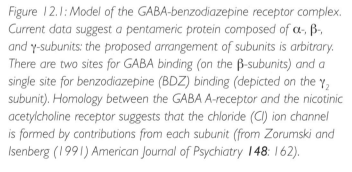

*Figure 12.1: Model of the GABA-benzodiazepine receptor complex. Current data suggest a pentameric protein composed of α-, β-, and γ-subunits: the proposed arrangement of subunits is arbitrary. There are two sites for GABA binding (on the β-subunits) and a single site for benzodiazepine (BDZ) binding (depicted on the γ$_2$ subunit). Homology between the GABA A-receptor and the nicotinic acetylcholine receptor suggests that the chloride (Cl) ion channel is formed by contributions from each subunit (from Zorumski and Isenberg (1991) American Journal of Psychiatry **148**: 162).*

Pharmacokinetics

The clinical and side-effect profile of a particular benzodiazepine depends on its pharmacological properties. Factors that need to be considered include the dose, rate of absorption, lipophilicity of the drug (which determines the rate of entry into the brain and produces the central nervous system effects) rate of tissue distribution, elimination half-life and the presence or absence of active metabolites. Most benzodiazepines are rapidly absorbed achieving peak plasma levels in 1–1.5 hours (American Formulary Hospital Services, 2002). It is important to note that peak plasma levels and the half-life of benzodiazepines are increased in the elderly. Benzodiazepines are highly protein bound and metabolized by the liver.

Effect on sleep and polysomnography

In healthy volunteers, benzodiazepines generally increase total sleep time and efficiency, reduce sleep latency, waking after sleep onset, and slow-wave sleep (stages 3 and 4), with a variable (mainly suppressant) effect on REM sleep (*Figure 12.2*). Performance impairment has also been noted (Wesensten *et al*, 1995; Roehrs *et al*, 1994).

Insomnia

While there is accumulating evidence that non-pharmacological therapies are the treatment of choice in insomnia, benzodiazepines are the preferred pharmacological agents. Anti depressants are preferred in patients with secondary insomnia due to depression and melatonin may have a role in insomnia due to circadian rhythm disturbances. Antihistamines have been used in the past but do not have a sufficient sedating effect.

		SL	TST	SE	WASO	TWT	S1	S2	S3	S4	SWS	SREM	REM-L
Temazapam 7, 15, 20, 30mg	H	↓	↑	↑	↓		↓	↑	=	↓		↓↑	
	I	↓	↑	↑	↓PLMD	↓30mg	↓	↑	=	=	↓	↓30mg	
Flunitrazepam 0.25, 0.5, 2.0mg	H	↓	↑	↑	↓			↑		↓		↓	↑
	I	↓	↑		↓			↑			↓	↓	
Flurazepam 15, 20, 30, 45mg	H	↓	↑		↓	↓		↑		↓	↓	↓	↑
	I	↓	↑ (R)	↑	↓ (R)		↓	↑		↓	↓	↓ (C)	↑ (R)
Triazolam 0.125, 0.25, 0.5mg	H	↓	↑ (R)		↓ (R)		↓	↑			↓ (C)	↓	↓↑
	I	↓ (R)	↑ (R)	↑	↓ (R)	↓	↓	↑			↓	↓ (C)	↑
Zopiclone 3.75–5, 7.5–10mg	H	↓	↑	↑	↓	↓	↓	↑			↓	↓	↑
	I	↓	↑	↑	↓	↓	↓	↑			=	↓	↑
Zolpidem 5–10, 15–20, 30–40mg	H	↓	=	↑	↓	↓	↓	=	=	=	↓	↓20mg	=
	I	↓	↑ (C)	↑	↓	↓		↑ (C)		↑	↑ (C)	↓↑	↓20mg

Figure 12.2: Effects of hypnotic drugs on sleep structure. (SL = sleep latency; TST = total sleep time; SE = sleep efficiency; WASO = wake after sleep onset; TWT = total wake time; S1 = stage 1; S2 = stage 2; S3 = stage 3; S4 = stage 4; SWS = slow-wave sleep; SREM = REM sleep; REM-L = latency to REM sleep; PLM = periodic limb movement disorder; RL = rebound; C = carry over; H = healthy volunteers; I = insomniac patients; ↑ = increase; ↓ = decrease; = = no change; ↑↓ = decrease or increase. (Parrino and Terzano, 1996).

Benzodiazepines increase polysomnographic total sleep time and decrease sleep latency minimally (means of 61 minutes and 4.2 minutes) in insomnia compared with placebo, with patient-reported outcomes yielding similar but less conservative results (Holbrook *et al*, 2000), including a lower number of awakenings and improved quality of sleep (Nowell *et al*, 1997). Most studies examining the effects of hypnotics in insomnia are of short duration (less than 6 weeks), with a mean duration of 12 days. Longer term studies are required to assess the efficacy of these drugs in chronic insomnia. Current recommendations suggest a possible role for benzodiazepines in transient (few days) or short-term (few weeks) insomnia associated with a stressor.

Which benzodiazepine?

The choice of a benzodiazepine depends on its pharmacological properties (see above). A benzodiazepine with a short half-life and no active metabolite, such as lorazepam, triazolam or oxazepam, is preferred, in conjunction with behavioral modification. Benzodiazepines are also used as muscle relaxants in skeletal muscle spasticity, as anti-convulsants, anaesthetic agents, and as an adjunct to antipsychotic or antiemetic therapy.

Side-effects

Benzodiazepines are associated with minor side-effects such as drowsiness, dizziness or light-headedness, headaches, impaired coordination, nervousness, anxiety, difficulty in concentrating, and lethargy. Major side-effects include the development of rebound insomnia, withdrawal, tolerance and dependence (MIMS, 2002). The development of side-effects is determined by the dose of the drug and the presence of active metabolites. Benzodiazepines have a significantly greater side-effect profile compared with placebo, in particular, daytime drowsiness and dizziness or light-headedness (Holbrook *et al*, 2000).

Tolerance, defined as the need to increase the dose of a drug to achieve the same therapeutic effect, dependence, which has a pharmacological and psychological basis, and rebound insomnia can all develop within 1–2 weeks of therapy. However, rebound insomnia is also seen after placebo administration (Roehrs *et al*, 1992). It is for these reasons that benzodiazepines are best recommended for short-term (less than 2–4 weeks) use only. Polysomnographic and subjective rebound insomnia is greater if the benzodiazepine is stopped suddenly, rather than tapered to cessation (Roehrs *et al*, 1992). Rebound insomnia, in general, is more likely to occur with higher doses, and more potent and shorter-acting benzodiazepines due to their reduced half-life. It can occur with regular or intermittent use.

Common withdrawal symptoms with benzodiazepines include anxiety, headache, insomnia, tension, sweating, difficulty in concentrating, tremor, sensory disturbance, fear and fatigue. The timing and duration of the withdrawal syndrome associated with benzodiazepines is related to their kinetics. The onset of withdrawal symptoms occurs a day after stopping a short- or intermediate-acting benzodiazepine, but 3–8 days following cessation of a long-acting benzodiazepine. Symptoms are reported to be at their worst 1 ± 0.5 day after stopping a short-acting benzodiazepine, but 9.6 ± 5.6 days after stopping a long-acting benzodiazepine. Withdrawal symptoms usually settle within 4 weeks of drug cessation. Persistent tinnitus for 6–8 months after stopping benzodiazepines has been documented (Busto *et al*, 1986).

Drug interactions

Benzodiazepines have an additive central nervous system effect with alcohol and other sedating agents, such as antidepressants, antihistamines, analgesics and anticonvulsants. Increased concentrations may be observed if taken with other drugs that are also metabolized by the liver. The anticholinergic effect of certain drugs such as atropine and antidepressants may be enhanced if taken with benzodiazepines.

Non-benzodiazepine hypnotics

These include the 'Z' drugs: zoplicone (a cyclopyrrolone), zolpidem (an imidazopyridine) and zaleplon (a pyrazolopyrimidine). They, like the conventional benzodiazepines, act on the GABA receptors in the brain but are thought to be subreceptor specific. While the former bind to the entire GABA receptor, the 'Z' drugs attach specifically to the $GABA_A$ receptor – chloride ionophore complex (*Figure 12.1*). This specificity is thought to be responsible for their non-sedating effects.

Pharmacokinetics

The 'Z' drugs are rapidly absorbed, achieving peak plasma levels within 0.5–2 hours. They are lipophilic and highly protein bound. Zoplicone has a half-life of 3.5–6 hours and is primarily excreted by the liver cytochrome P450 system and kidneys. It has two main metabolites, both with little or no pharmacological activity (AFHS, 2002; Kryger *et al*, 2000). Zolpidem has a half-life of 1.5 to 2.4 hours. Both zolpidem and zaleplon are eliminated similarly to zoplicone, but without residual active metabolites.

Effect on sleep and polysomnography

In healthy volunteers, the 'Z' drugs have little or no effect on REM sleep and do not alter slow-wave sleep. They reduce sleep latency.

In insomnia, zoplicone increases total sleep time and REM latency, and reduces nocturnal awakenings and sleep latency. The changes in sleep stages are dose dependent. Zolpidem acts similarly to zoplicone but also increases stage 2 and slow-wave sleep. Interestingly, in a meta-analysis with limited numbers comparing the efficacy of zoplicone with benzodiazepines, zoplicone was not found to be superior to benzodiazepines in polysomnographically measured sleep latency or total sleep time (Holbrook *et al*, 2000). Zaleplon has been shown to reduce sleep latency without significant effects on sleep time or number of awakenings (AFHS, 2002).

Side-effects and drug interactions

The side-effect profile of the 'Z' drugs is not well established due to their recent availability. Lower doses are recommended in the elderly and those with hepatic or renal impairment. Common side-effects include a bitter taste, dry mouth, drowsiness, headaches, and fatigue. While the specificity of the 'Z' drugs to the GABAA receptor suggest that they may have less central nervous system side-effects compared with the benzodiazepines, this needs to be conclusively demonstrated in further trials. All the 'Z' drugs have demonstrated some sedative effects, potential for dependence, and mild withdrawal symptoms (AFHS, 2002; Lader, 1998; MIMS, 2002), but the risk of abuse and dose escalation is minimal (Wohlgemuth and Krystal, 2005). It is unclear, due to the short duration of most studies, if tolerance develops with these drugs.

Clinical use

The 'Z' drugs are mainly used in the short-term (less than 1 month) management of insomnia. However, in the appropriate clinical setting long-term use appears to be safe (Ancoli-Israel *et al*, 2005). There is evidence that they are useful in reducing nightmares associated with the post-traumatic stress disorder (Alderman *et al*, 2000).

Interactions

Caution is advised with using the 'Z' drugs in combination with other CNS agents, such as alcohol and barbiturates, and with drugs that induce or inhibit the liver cytochrome P450 system, such as phenytoin, rifampicin, erythromycin, and cimetidine.

Natural hypnotics

Valerian

Known from ancient Greece, the roots of valerian are used in different preparations including infusion, tincture or in tablets in standardized formulation as mild sedatives.

Mode of action

Valepotriates are the chemicals from valerian extracts which are said to act by increasing GABA activity in a benzodiazepine-like fashion. A possible effect on melatonin secretion is also reported (Donath *et al*, 2000; Gyllenhaal *et al*, 2000).

Effect on sleep and polysomnography

Although studies in normal volunteers show no significant differences from placebo, the use in patients with psychophysiological insomnia seems to improve both self-reported quality of sleep as well as polysomnographic variables.

Long-term use (15 days) of 300 mg of dry extract of valerian increases the percentage of slow-wave sleep and there is a trend in reducing slow-wave sleep latency. Other polysomnographic variables, including arousals index, are not different from placebo. Subjective sleep latency, however, is reduced after two weeks on valerian suggesting that the element of sleep misperception, often present in psychophysiological insomnia, might be improved (Balderer *et al*, 1985; Donath *et al*, 2000; Schulz *et al*, 1994). Patients using valerian should be told that it may take several weeks before an effect is seen.

Side-effects and drug interactions

Valerian extracts seem to be free of side-effects with no residual sedation in the morning (Kuhlmann *et al*, 1999) and no withdrawal symptoms. There appears to be no interaction with other sedatives or alcohol. Metabolites of valepotriates have mutagenic activity *in vitro* and it seems prudent to avoid the use of valerian at conception and during lactation.

Use

Available evidence suggests that the use of valerian in acute situations (for a few nights) is not likely to be beneficial. However, the use for a few weeks, together with other non-pharmacological measures (eg. sleep hygiene) has beneficial effects in patients with psychophysiological insomnia.

Kava

Kava is a common beverage in the South Pacific. It is used as an herbal anxiolytic and sedative in Western countries. The dosage of kava in the beverage is 10 to 100 times that used clinically.

Mode of action

Kava contains kavapyrones or kavalactones which are responsible for the anti-anxiety and sedative effects, possibly via GABA receptors.

Clinical use

Kava has been shown to reduce anxiety in placebo-controlled studies (Volz and Kieser, 1997).

Effect on sleep and polysomnography

Some studies have demonstrated that kava does reduce sleep latency and stage 1 sleep without altering REM sleep, in addition to improving subjective variables and, therefore, possibly having an effect on sleep misperception associated with insomnia (Cauffield and Forbes, 1999).

Side-effects and drug interactions

There have been reports of kava-containing medications causing liver failure. Its use is currently not recommended (Centers for Disease Control and Prevention, 2003) pending an FDA investigation. Kava in doses up to 600 mg does not impair cognitive function in study patients. Cutaneous allergic reactions have been reported from the use of kava, including a severe but reversible dermopathy and yellowish skin discoloration in Pacific Islanders who drink kava due to the deposition of a pigment. The discoloration resolves when kava is stopped (Gyllenhaal *et al*, 2000).

Lavender

Lavender is an essential oil that is thought to have relaxant properties.

Mode of action

The active compounds in lavender, linaloyl acetate and linalool, are thought to act as central nervous system depressants. Lavender is prepared as an oil and is effective when inhaled (Gyllenhaal *et al*, 2000).

Effect on sleep and polysomnography

There is little polysomnographic information on the effect of lavender on the sleep–wake cycle.

In a crossover trial of twenty-three subjects using lavender, central nervous system depressant activity was documented on EEG recordings and the subjects were less restless during sleep. In another study, forty subjects given three minutes of lavender aromatherapy were found to be more relaxed, based on a Profile of Moods Scale (POMS), less depressed and faster and more accurate at solving math problems than prior to the inhalation.

Side-effects and drug interactions

Toxicity has not been reported with lavender aromatherapy.

Chamomile

Chamomile is ingested as a tea and is considered to be a relaxant. It is a flavonoid apigenin which is a natural benzodiazepine receptor agonist. It has been found to have a central nervous system depressant effect in animal studies.

Side-effects and drug interactions

Allergic reactions on ingestion are not common but contact allergy to the plant has been reported (Gyllenhaal *et al*, 2000).

Melatonin

Melatonin is a hormone produced by the pineal gland. It has a role in regulating the sleep–wake cycle. Melatonin has been found to be useful in jet lag, sleep disorders of the blind, and in insomnia where circadian rhythm disturbances are a factor.

Mode of action

Melatonin is purported to have a direct inhibitory effect on the suprachiasmatic nucleus (SCN) which is responsible for maintaining wakefulness. The low levels of melatonin produced during daytime are thought to enhance wakefulness, while the large amounts produced at night are thought to diminish alertness by binding to melatonin receptors in the SCN.

Effect on sleep and polysomnography

In healthy volunteers there is increasing polysomnographic information on the effect of melatonin on the sleep–wake cycle. Doses ranging from 0.3–0.8 mg administered during the day have been shown to reduce sleep latency (Zhdanova *et al*, 1996). Melatonin in doses of 1–80 mg administered before sleep at night have produced varying results, with some studies showing a reduction in sleep onset and others having no effect (Kryger *et al*, 2000; Olde Rikkert *et al*, 2001; Pires *et al*, 2001).

There is evidence to support the selected use of melatonin in the elderly population with insomnia; specifically in those who used benzodiazepines chronically and those with low melatonin levels during sleep (Olde Rikkert *et al*, 2001). Melatonin doses ranging from 0.5 mg to 6 mg, 30–120 minutes before bed improve sleep latency, sleep efficiency, total sleep time and wake during sleep, as measured by polysomnography or actigraphy (Olde Rikkert *et al*, 2001; Zhdanova *et al*, 2001). Further studies with polysomnographic endpoints need to be performed to compare the efficacy of melatonin with conventional hypnotics, and behavioral therapy in insomnia.

Circadian rhythm disturbances

⌘ *Jet lag:* Melatonin has been shown to reduce jet lag based on subjective assessments (Arendt *et al*, 1997). There are no studies using objective outcomes.

⌘ *Delayed sleep phase syndrome:* Melatonin has been shown to advance sleep onset and wake time compared with placebo (Dagan *et al*, 1998; Dagan, 2002; Dahlitz *et al*, 1991).

Side-effects and drug interactions

The short- and long-term toxicity associated with melatonin is unknown. Melatonin has been shown to adversely affect the reproductive system of other mammals (Kryger *et al*, 2000).

Alcohol

Alcohol contains ethanol, a direct central nervous system depressant, in varying amounts.

Mode of action

Alcohol has a direct depressant effect on brain tissue, especially cell membrane function and enzymes and on myocardial contractility. It is a smooth muscle vasodilator.

Effect on sleep and polysomnography

❖ *In healthy volunteers:* Following ingestion, alcohol tends to increase sleep at the beginning of the night by reducing sleep latency, and increase non-REM sleep while reducing REM sleep (Kryger *et al*, 2000). It is, however, metabolized quickly (a glass of wine per hour on average) and so, as the night progresses, the individual experiences 'withdrawal effects' comprising of shallow sleep, increased REM sleep, dream recall or nightmares and symptoms of sympathetic arousal. Alcohol increases the likelihood of snoring, inspiratory resistance and apneic events by reducing airway tone (Mitler *et al*, 1988) in normal subjects without a preceding history of a sleep disorder. Alcohol can sometimes increase the periodic limb movements noted with sleep.

❖ ***In insomnia:*** The use of alcohol as a hypnotic to induce sleep in insomnia is not well studied. In a small trial of nineteen adults (eleven with insomnia and nine normal subjects), alcohol reduced REM sleep for the entire sleep period and increased stages 3 and 4 sleep, while reducing stage 1 sleep during the first half of the night to levels comparable with normal subjects (Roehrs *et al*, 1999).

❖ ***In alcoholics:*** Subjects commonly report insomnia or hypersomnia, circadian rhythm disturbances or parasomnias. As alcohol dependence develops, sleep latency increases, sleep efficiency worsens and total sleep time and slow-wave sleep is reduced. In addition, the expected age-related increase in sleep-disordered breathing in alcoholics is greater than in healthy subjects (Aldrich *et al*, 1993).

❖ ***In recovering alcoholics:*** Sleep is short and fragmented early with reduced non-REM sleep and increased REM density (a measure of ocular activity during sleep). These findings usually improve over the first year of abstinence, but some features of sleep may remain abnormal for as long as 27 months (Drummond *et al*, 1998). Persisting abnormalities in REM sleep (short REM latency, increased REM density and percentage) after 2 weeks of abstinence appear to predict relapse at 3 months after discharge (Clark *et al*, 1999). Ongoing insomnia and sleep fragmentation persisting after 5 months can also be associated with relapse by 14 months (Drummond *et al*, 1998).

Side-effects and drug interactions

The side-effects associated with alcohol are well documented and a detailed description is beyond the scope of this chapter. Minor adverse effects include loss of judgment, emotional lability, slurred speech, headache, amnesia, ataxia, nausea and vomiting. Alcohol targets most organs and some major side-effects especially with chronic consumption include coma, tolerance, physical and psychological dependence, peripheral neuropathy, Wernicke–Korsakoff syndrome, cardiomyopathy, liver impairment or cirrhosis, peptic ulcer disease, and pancreatitis.

Drug interactions

Alcohol has an additional sedating effect when used with other CNS depressants such as hypnotics, anticonvulsants, antidepressants and phenothiazines. It potentiates the action of oral hypoglycemics, anticoagulants, and vasodilators.

Marijuana

Marijuana or cannabis is a recreational drug that is considered to have relaxant properties. It is used as an antiemetic following chemotherapy and other medical uses, such as reducing tremor in a variety of neurological disorders, is currently being explored.

Mode of action

Marijuana contains three main cannabinoids: cannabidiol (CBD), tetrahydrocannabinol (THC) and cannabinol (CBN). Cannabidiol is synthesized to THC which is then degraded to cannabinol. THC is responsible for the psychoactive properties of marijuana. It binds to receptors in the substantia nigra, globus pallidus, hippocampus, cerebellum and forebrain.

Effect on sleep and polysomnography

A single marijuana cigarette is estimated to have 20 mg of THC. Early studies examining the effects of marijuana on sleep used low doses of THC (10–30 mg) that produced equivocal results. Later studies found no difference in total sleep time and sleep latency following 70 mg and 210 mg doses of THC compared with baseline. A significant increase in slow-wave sleep and reduction in REM sleep was noted with THC. Cessation of THC leads to withdrawal symptoms manifested by increased sleep latency and reduced total sleep time, REM rebound and decreased slow-wave sleep. It must be noted that these doses exceed those used socially (Barratt *et al*, 1974; Duffy and Milin, 1996; Feinberg *et al*, 1975; 1976; Freemon, 1972).

Side-effects and drug interactions

Side-effects of heavy marijuana use may include chronic bronchitis, worsening of angina pectoris due to tachycardia, and lack of motivation. High doses can result in tolerance and withdrawal symptoms. Frank psychosis or delerium is rare.

Smoking and nicotine

Tobacco leaves contain nicotine, a naturally occurring stimulant and relaxant. Tobacco leaves can be chewed or prepared for inhalation as cigarettes or via a pipe.

Mode of action

Nicotine is an acetylcholine receptor agonist that exerts its effect via nicotinic receptors. Nicotine has an initial relaxant effect at low blood concentrations and a subsequent stimulant effect at higher blood concentrations (Stradling, 1993). It has a half-life of 1–2 hours.

Effect on sleep wake cycle

Nicotine's effects on the sleep–wake cycle are similar to caffeine. Abstinence following chronic consumption of nicotine can lead to psychological and polysomnographic withdrawal (Kryger *et al*, 2000).

Side-effects and drug interactions

Side-effects include nausea and vomiting, anticholinergic effects, withdrawal and psychological and physical dependence.

Antidepressants

Antidepressants are used to treat depression, obsessive-compulsive and anxiety or panic disorders. They include tricyclic antidepressants, monoamine oxidase inhibitors, selective serotonin reuptake inhibitors, 5-hydroxytryptamine antagonists, and noradrenaline uptake inhibitors. Both the underlying disorder and its treatment may affect sleep quality and duration and it is often difficult to determine the contribution of each to poor sleep.

Tricyclic antidepressants

The tricyclics are first-generation antidepressants and include amitryptyline, doxepin, imipramine, triimpramine, clomipramine (tertiary amines), desipramine, nortriptyline, and protriptyline (secondary amines).

Mode of action

Tricyclic antidepressants work by inhibiting the post-synaptic uptake of noradrenaline, and 5-hydroxytryptamine, blocking acetylcholine receptors and inhibiting fast sodium channels. The cumulative effect of these actions is to raise the circulating concentration of catecholamines.

Effect on sleep and polysomnography

Tricyclic antidepressants improve sleep and tend to increase total sleep time, reduce the number of awakenings, with variable (both enhancing and suppressant) effects on REM sleep in healthy individuals and in depressed patients. Interestingly, as the depression improves on treatment, REM rebound has been documented (*Table 12.4*) (Gursky *et al*, 2000; Kryger *et al*, 2000; Roth *et al*, 1982; Sharpley and Cowen, 1995; Thase, 1998). Antidepressants may worsen the periodic leg movements associated with sleep.

Antidepressants are not first-line therapy for insomnia unless depression is thought to be an underlying factor. Doxepin has been shown to improve sleep efficiency in depressed subjects (Roth *et al*, 1982).

Side-effects and drug interactions

Owing to their non-specific mechanism of action, tricyclic antidepressants have more side-effects than the later developed, more selective, antidepressants. Their main side-effect is sedation and this is more common with the tertiary rather than secondary amines. They may impair cognitive function and psychomotor performance (Kryger *et al*, 2000). Altered mentation from anxiety to psychosis, extrapyramidal symptoms, parasthesiae, ataxia, incoordination and seizures have been reported. Cardiovascular side-effects, including tachycardia, arrhythmias, hyper- and hypotension, anticholinergic, dermatological and hematological side-effects are documented (MIMS, 2002). Abrupt withdrawal of treatment may result in nausea, headache and malaise.

Table 12.4: Overview of the effects of antidepressants on sleep

| Drug | Effects on sleep | | | |
	Continuity	Slow-wave sleep	REM sleep %	REM latency
TCAs	Increased?	Unchanged	Decreased	Increased
MAOIs	?	?	Decreased	?
SSRIs*	Decreased	Unchanged	Decreased	Increased
Bupropion	Unchanged	Unchanged	Increased	Decreased
Venlafaxine	Decreased	Unchanged	Decreased	Increased
Nofazodone	Increased	Unchanged	Increased?	Decreased
Mirtazapine	Increased	Increased?	Unchanged	Unchanged
Trazodone	Increased	Increased	Decreased	Increased

REM, rapid eye movement; TCA, tricyclic antidepressants; MAOI, monoamineoxidase inhibitor; SSRI, selective serotonin reuptake inhibitor.
*When taken at bedtime, paroxetine potentially decreases sleep continuity less than other selective serotonin reuptake inhibitors.

(modified from Gursky and Krohn, 2000)

Drug interactions

Tricyclic antidepressants may interact with other antidepressants and drugs that induce or inhibit the cytochrome P450 system such as cimetidine, phenothiazines, carbamazepine, or quinidine. Dosage needs to be adjusted in these situations.

Monoamine oxidase inhibitors (MAOIs)

These include the older irreversibly binding agents such as phenelzine and tranylcypromine and the newer reversibly binding drugs such as moclobemide and brofaromine.

Mode of action

The drugs inhibit (either reversibly or irreversibly) the monoamine oxidase A and/or B enzymes that metabolize noradrenaline, 5-hydroxytryptamine and dopamine, thus increasing their circulating concentrations. The drugs are absorbed rapidly and acetylated by the liver.

Effect on sleep and polysomnography

Monoamine oxidase inhibitors usually reduce total sleep time and increase the number of wakenings in depressed patients. REM sleep is markedly reduced (Gursky *et al*, 2000; Sharpley *et al*, 1995; Thase, 1998). However, moclobemide in depressed patients has been reported to improve sleep continuity with only mild reduction in REM sleep (Monti, 1989).

Side-effects

The MAOIs do not appear to impair cognitive function, but there is only a limited number of studies. Adverse effects are less frequent with the newer MAOIs. The most serious side-effect is the occurrence of a hypertensive crisis, precipitated by the interaction of the monoamine oxidase inhibitor with certain foods that contain high concentrations of tyramine or dopamine, ie. cheese, yoghurt, caffeine, alcohol, meat and fish, and sympathomimetic medications, eg. decongestants. Other adverse effects include hypotension, dizziness, headache, fatigue, agitation, hypomania, gastrointestinal disturbances, elevated serum transaminases, weight gain, urinary retention, rash, blurred vision or glaucoma. Carcinogenicity and infertility in mice have been documented (MIMS, 2002).

Drug interactions

Monoamine oxidase inhibitors should be used cautiously, if at all, with other antidepressants and sedatives. Serious reactions such as hyperthermia, rigidity, and death have been reported when serotonin reuptake inhibitors or venlafaxine hydrochloride have been used in conjunction with a MAOI. The combination of a MAOI with tryptophan has resulted in behavioral and neurological symptoms and signs. Elevation of blood pressure has been documented in patients on a MAOI who were then commenced on buspirone (MIMS, 2002).

Selective serotonin reuptake inhibitors (SSRIs)

This is a new group of agents (eg. fluoxetine, paroxetine, sertraline, fluvoxamine and citalopram) with few side-effects.

Mode of action

SSRIs inhibit the reuptake of 5-hydroxytryptamine (*Figure 12.3*).

Pharmacokinetics

Peak plasma concentrations are achieved 6–8 hours after ingestion. SSRIs are highly protein bound and are extensively metabolized by the liver (cytochrome P450 system) to active and inactive compounds. SSRIs are eliminated slowly, and this, along with the presence of active metabolites, leads to persisting drug effects.

Effect on sleep and polysomnography

SSRIs tend to improve subjective sleep quality. Polysomnographic evidence, however, shows a reduction in total sleep time and efficiency, increase in sleep latency, the number of wakenings, and stage 1 sleep in normal and depressed patients with these agents with the exception of citralopram (Hendrickse *et al*, 1994; Kryger *et al*, 2000; Vasar *et al*, 1994). Alteration with REM sleep has been noted with the SSRIs. In depressed outpatients, fluoxetine reduces REM sleep and increases REM latency during the acute phase of treatment, with REM rebound occurring following discontinuation of the drug (Trivedi *et al*, 1999). In normal subjects, paroxetine decreases REM sleep and increases REM latency (Sharpley *et al*, 1996).

Side-effects

Insomnia in the order of 5–10% and daytime sedation in up to 26% of cases has been reported in clinical trials with SSRIs. These effects appear to be dose dependent with fluoxetine. SSRIs do not impair (and, indeed, may actually improve) cognitive function or performance. Anxiety, nervousness, dizziness, mania/emotional lability, gastrointestinal symptoms, myalgias, myopathy, abnormal urination, impotence, rash, hyponatremia and elevation of hepatic enzymes have been documented. Withdrawal effects are rare because of the long elimination half-life of these drugs (MIMS, 2002). Circadian rhythm sleep disorder (*Chapter 11*) can be associated with some SSRIs use, eg. fluvoxamine (Dagan and Lemberg, 1999; Dagan, 2002).

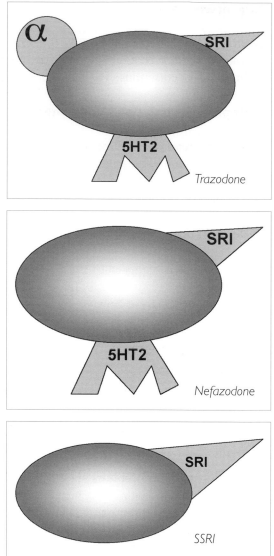

Figure 12.3: Mechanism of action of trozodone, nefazodone and SSRIs. Trazodone and nefazodone are serotonin receptor modulators (SRMs) in that they have a dual mechanism of modulating serotonin receptors (5-HT$_{2A}$) combined with lesser but necessary serotonin uptake inhibition (SRI). Trazodone also has alpha-adrenergic blocking properties which may account for undesired side effects which nefazodone lacks. The SSRIs have potent serotonin reuptake inhibition (SRI) but no other actions (Stahl and Frakes, 1995, International Review of Psychiatry 7: 30 with permission from Taylor & Francis Ltd).

Drug interactions

SSRIs must be used cautiously, if at all, in patients already on antidepressants, especially monoamine oxidase inhibitors (see monoamine oxidase inhibitors section, *pp. 474–475*). An interval of 5 weeks minimum should be allocated between stopping a SSRI and commencing a monoamine oxidase inhibitor. SSRIs interact with drugs that inhibit or induce the cytochrome P450 system. As SSRIs are highly protein bound, they may alter plasma concentrations of other highly protein bound drugs.

Trazodone and nefazodone

These drugs are synthetically derived phenylpiperazine antidepressants.

Mode of action

They block 5-hydroxytryptamine 1 and 2 receptors and block serotonin reuptake pre-synaptically to increase serotonin levels centrally. Trazodone has also an alpha-adrenergic blocking property (*Figure 12.3*) (Stahl and Frakes, 1995).

Pharmacokinetics

Nefazodone and trazodone are rapidly absorbed and reach peak plasma concentrations between 1–3 hours. They are highly protein bound and eliminated primarily by hepatic metabolism (CYPA3A4 system).

Effect on sleep and polysomnography

Trazadone and nefazodone increase total sleep time. Nefazodone has been shown to decrease or not affect the number of awakenings and reduce stage 2 sleep, while trazodone reduces stage 1 and 2 sleep and increases slow-wave sleep in normal and depressed subjects. Both drugs do not alter REM sleep or latency (MIMS, 2002; Sharpley *et al*, 1996). A direct comparison of nefazodone with fluoxetine demonstrated an equivalent antidepressant effect, but improved sleep quality measured both subjectively and objectively with nefazodone (Gillin *et al*, 1997).

Side-effects

Data is limited, but variable effects on performance have been reported with these drugs. Common side-effects include headache, dizziness, emotional lability/mania, confusion, daytime somnolence, postural hypotension, dyspnea, gastrointestinal symptoms, and impotence. Rare cases of liver necrosis and liver failure and seizures have been reported with nefazodone.

Drug interactions

These include an interaction with monoamine oxidase inhibitors and buspirone, as noted with other SSRIs and with drugs that are metabolized by the CYPA3A4 system of the liver such as terfenadine, astemzole, pimozide and cisapride. Rhabdomyolysis has been reported with nefazodone and HMG-CoA reductase inhibitors. The concurrent use of alcohol and other CNS sedatives should be avoided. Trazodone and nefazodone may alter plasma concentrations of other highly protein bound drugs.

Venlafaxine

Venlafaxine, phenethylamine, is a serotonin and noradrenergic reuptake inhibitor. It also weakly inhibits dopamine uptake.

Pharmacokinetics

Venlafaxine is well absorbed and achieves peak plasma concentrations in 2.5 hours. It is extensively liver metabolized and renally excreted. The elimination half-life ranges from 5–11 hours. Venlafaxine, unlike the other SSRIs, is not highly protein bound (less than 30%) (MIMS, 2002).

Effect on sleep and polysomnography

Venlafaxine reduces total sleep time (by decreasing stages 2 and 3 and increasing stage 1 sleep), and increases number of awakenings and REM latency with a reduction in total REM duration in normal and depressed subjects. Frequent periodic limb movements have been noted with venlafaxine (Luthringer *et al*, 1996; Salin-Pascual *et al*, 1997).

Side-effects

Insomnia has been reported in 4–18% of patients on venlafaxine. Cognitive function and performance in normal volunteers is not impaired and, indeed, may improve. Hyponatremia, activation of mania or hypomania and an increase in blood pressure have been reported in a small number of patients on the drug. There is insufficient information regarding the development of withdrawal symptoms, physical or psychological dependence (MIMS, 2002)

Drug interactions

Serious interactions (resembling the neuroleptic/serotonergic malignant syndrome, seizures and death) have been reported with monoamine oxidase inhibitors and, thus, concomitant use of these drugs is contraindicated (MIMS, 2002). No interaction between alcohol and venlafaxine has been documented to date. As venlafaxine is metabolized by the liver, there is the potential for an interaction between the drug and inducers or inhibitors of the cytochrome P450 system.

Mirtazapine

Mode of action

Mirtazapine acts by antagonizing central alpha-2 and specific serotonin receptors (5-HT$_2$ and 5-HT$_3$) causing increased noradrenaline and serotonin levels. These mediators are considered responsible for the drug's antidepressant activity. Mirtazapine also blocks histamine receptors resulting in its sedative properties.

Pharmacokinetics

Mirtazapine is rapidly absorbed reaching peak plasma levels within 2 hours. It is highly protein bound and has a long elimination half-life of 20–40 hours. It is metabolized by the liver, and eliminated by the kidneys and gastrointestinal tract.

Effect on sleep and polysomnography

Mirtazapine increases total sleep time, reduces sleep latency and stage 1 sleep without altering REM sleep in depressed subjects (Winokur *et al*, 2000), and increases the sleep efficiency index by increasing slow-wave sleep and reducing stage 1 sleep and decreasing the number of awakenings in normal subjects (Asian *et al*, 2002).

Side-effects

Reports are limited due to the newness of the drug. The main side-effects are transient somnolence, hyperphagia and weight gain. Unlike the SRRIs, it does not have sexual side-effects. Withdrawal is unlikely due to the drug's long elimination half-life.

Drug interactions

Mirtazapine should not be used concurrently with monoamine oxidase inhibitors. Other sedating agents such as alcohol and hypnotics should be avoided. There is a theoretical interaction between mirtazapine and inducers or inhibitors of the cytochrome P450 system (MIMS, 2002).

Anxiolytic agents (non-benzodiazepines)

Buspirone

Buspirone is a serotonergic anxiolytic and is a partial agonist at the 5-HT$_1$ receptor. It is hepatically and renally cleared.

Effect on sleep and polysomnography

There is little polysomnographic evidence on buspirone. It does not cause daytime sedation based on subjective data and MSLT studies (Seidel *et al*, 1985).

Side-effects

Dizziness, light headedness, headache, nervousness and nausea are common. Buspirone does not impair cognitive or psychomotor function (MIMS, 2002).

Drug interactions

Buspirone should not be used with monoamine oxidase inhibitors and drugs that induce or inhibit the cyotchrome P450 system.

Antipsychotics (neuroleptics)

The conventional neuroleptics include: (a) phenothiazines, eg. chlorpromazine, fluphenazine, pericyazine, thioridazine and trifluperazine; (b) butyrophenones, eg. haloperidol; (c) diphenylbuty lpiperidines, eg. pimozide and; (d) thioxanthines, eg. flupenthixol, thiothixene and zuclopenthixol. Newer agents include the atypical antipsychotics, such as clozapine, risperidone, olanzapine, sertindole, and quetiapine.

Mode of action

The antipsychotic action of the conventional agents is presumed to occur by dopaminergic inhibition of the central, especially the limbic, nervous system. The newer agents are thought to act via inhibition of serotonin receptors.

Effect on sleep and polysomnography

Antipsychotic therapy in schizophrenia may reduce slow-wave sleep, REM latency, and increase REM density (Kryger *et al*, 2000). Clozapine increases total sleep time, sleep efficiency, and increased stage 2 and 3 sleep while reducing slow-wave sleep (Lee *et al*, 2001) in patients with schizophrenia without affecting REM sleep (Hinze–Selch *et al*, 1997; Wetter *et al*, 1996). Olanzapine has been shown to increase slow-wave sleep and subjective sleep quality, in addition to reducing REM sleep and increasing REM sleep latency and density. Objective measurements of the effect of antipsychotics on daytime sleepiness are lacking.

Side-effects

Sedation, extrapyramidal symptoms, tardive dyskinesia and the neuroleptic malignant syndrome are more frequent with the older neuroleptics. While antipsychotics impair cognition in normal subjects, they either do not have any effect, or improve cognition, in schizophrenia. An important and probably under-recognized side-effect of some antipsychotics, eg. haloperidol, are circadian rhythm sleep disorders (Wirz-Justice *et al*, 1997; 2000).

Drug interactions

Antipsychotics should not be used with alcohol or other sedating medications to avoid additional central depression. They may cause hypotension when used with alpha blockers. Antipsychotics should be used cautiously with drugs that induce or inhibit the cytochrome P450 system. There may be an interaction between antipsychotics and the SSRI drugs; the latter may decrease the metabolism of the antipsychotic resulting in marked adverse effects including cognitive impairment. The conventional antipsychotics antagonise the action of levodopa and, thus, an atypical antipsychotic is recommended in this particular situation. Antipsychotics may sporadically enhance the lithium neurotoxicity and must be used cautiously as combination therapy. The newer neuroleptics should not be used with anticholinergic medication as they may potentiate anticholinergic effects (MIMS, 2002).

Lithium

Lithium carbonate is used in the treatment of bipolar disorders.

Mode of action

Lithium is thought to alter sodium transport in nerve and muscle cells (MIMS, 2002), resulting in intraneuronal metabolism of catecholamines. The specification of lithium in mania is unknown (MIMS, 2002).

Effect on sleep and polysomnography

Lithium causes sleep disturbances on polysomnography similar to depression with an increased sleep latency and number of awakenings, reduced sleep efficiency and slow-wave sleep. REM sleep is increased with a reduced latency (Kryger *et al*, 2000, Friston *et al*, 1989). Objective studies evaluating the effect of lithium on daytime sleepiness are lacking.

Pharmacokinetics

Lithium is rapidly absorbed from the gastrointestinal tract reaching peak plasma levels 2.5 to 5.5 hours after ingestion. It is cleared by the kidneys.

Side-effects

Lithium causes psychomotor and cognitive impairment and these side-effects are usually dose related. Common adverse effects include fine hand tremor, polyuria, thirst, nausea, weight gain, fatigue and mild cognitive impairment. Other more serious side-effects include the development of hypothyroidism, nephrogenic diabetes insipidus and an encephalopathic syndrome similar to neuroleptic malignant syndrome (MIMS, 2002). Sleep-walking-like behaviour has also been reported in patients on lithium, and lithium in combination with other antipsychotic medications (Landry *et al*, 1999).

Drug interactions

Drugs that should be avoided with lithium include those that alter sodium balance such as neuroleptics. There are several drugs that alter lithium concentrations. Those that increase lithium levels include metronidazole, nonsteroidal anti-inflammatory agents, diuretics and ACE inhibitors. Medications that reduce lithium concentrations include xanthines, and certain diuretics such carbonic anhydrase inhibitors. Other drugs that alter electrolyte balance, such as appetite suppressants and corticosteroids, should be used with caution. Neurotoxicity has been reported with the concurrent use of neuroleptics, antiepileptics, methyldopa, SSRIs, tricyclic antidepressants, and calcium channel blockers with lithium (MIMS, 2002).

Cardiovascular medications

Antihypertensive agents: Beta-receptor blockers

Beta-receptor blockers are commonly used antihypertensives and antianginal agents and also have a role in the treatment of heart failure. Earlier beta-blockers, such as propanolol, are lipophilic, while the later cardioselective agents tend to be hydrophilic.

Effect on sleep and polysomnography

Beta-blockers increase total wake time and number of wakenings, reduce stage 1 and REM sleep. The more lipophilic a beta-blocker is, in general, the greater the sleep disturbance due to increased central nervous system penetration (Betts *et al*, 1985; Monti, 1987).

Side-effects

The central nervous system/sleep side-effects tend to relate to the lipophilicity of the beta blocker and include fatigue, insomnia and nightmares (Koella, 1985; Dimsdale and Newton, 1992).

Angiotensin-converting enzyme (ACE) inhibitors

Angiotensin-converting enzyme (ACE) inhibitors prevent the formation of angiotensin II, a potent sympathomimetic and aldosterone agonist, and include captopril, enalapril, ramipril and cilazapril.

Effect on sleep and polysomnography

Cilazapril does not interfere with sleep, based on subjective and polysomnographic data, in normal subjects (Dietrich and Herrmann, 1989; Weichler *et al*, 1991). ACE inhibitors can be associated with increased report of nightmares when taken at bed time.

Side-effects

ACE inhibitors do not cause psychomotor or cognitive impairment (Kryger *et al*, 2000). ACE inhibitors reduce the excretion of lithium (MIMS, 2002).

Angiotensin II receptor antagonists

Angiotensin II receptor antagonists such as irbesartan, losartan and telmisartan, bind to the angiotensin II receptor and inhibit vasoconstriction, sodium reabsorption and aldosterone release (MIMS, 2002).

Effect on sleep and polysomnography

There are no polysomnographic data on the effect of angiotensin II receptor antagonists on sleep.

Side-effects and drug interactions

Side-effects are similar to those of ACE inhibitors. Insomnia has rarely been reported with losartan (Kryger *et al*, 2000).

Calcium antagonists

Calcium antagonists such as verapamil, nifedipine and amilodipine block the influx of calcium into myocardial and vascular cells thereby preventing muscle contraction.

Effect on sleep and polysomnography

There is no evidence that calcium channel blockers disturb the sleep–wake cycle (Kryger *et al*, 2000).

Side-effects and drug interactions

Fatigue is a common side-effect. As calcium antagonists are metabolized by the liver, they need to be used cautiously with drugs that are inducers or inhibitors of the cytochrome P450 system such as hypnotics and some CNS stimulants (MIMS, 2002).

Alpha-2 agonists

Alpha-2 agonists such as clonidine and methyldopa are centrally acting antihypertensives. They stimulate alpha-2 receptors of the heart and vessels and lower blood pressure by reducing sympathetic tone.

Effect on sleep and polysomnography

Alpha-2 agonists increase total sleep time, and reduce REM sleep in normal volunteers (Monti, 1987). They reduce total sleep time in patients with hypertension. Methyldopa increases REM sleep (Kryger *et al*, 2000).

Side-effects and drug interactions

Alpha-2 agonists cause sedation, nightmares, reduced concentration, headache, and fatigue (MIMS, 2002). Concurrent use of alcohol and other central nervous system depressants should be avoided.

Vasodilators, diuretics and alpha-1 antagonists

There is no information on the effect of these drugs on sleep polysomnography. Alpha-1 antagonists such as prazosin and terazosin have been associated with transient sedation (Kryger *et al*, 2000).

Antiarrhythmics agents

There is little objective or polysomographic evidence regarding the effects of antiarrhythmics on the sleep cycle. There are several subjective reports of fatigue in up to 10% of patients on a variety of antiarrhythmics (Kryger *et al*, 2000).

Lipid-lowering agents

These include the HMG-CoA reductase inhibitors, cholestyramine, fibrates such as clofibrate, gemfibrozil, probucol, colestipol, and nicotinic acid. The HMG-CoA reductase inhibitors pravastatin, simvastatin and lovostatin do not affect sleep, based on randomised double-blind placebo-controlled polysomnographic studies, except for entry and latency into stage 1 sleep (Eckernas *et al*, 1993; Kostis, *et al* 1994 Partinen *et al*, 1994). Information on the effect of other hypolipidaemic agents on sleep is lacking. There are subjective reports of fatigue and insomnia with most of the lipid-lowering drugs (Kryger *et al*, 2000; MIMS, 2002).

Antiepileptics

These include barbiturates, benzodiazepines (discussed above) and newer agents (*Figure 12.4*). The assessment of anticonvulsant medications on sleep is difficult, as comparison should be between drug-free periods versus while on treatment; and preferably on monotherapy. This is difficult to achieve in practice (Sammaritano and Shervin, 2002).

Sleep eff	% Stage 1	% Stage 2	% SWS	% REM	No full AW	RD rate	PLM rate	Total arousal rate	EDS by MSLT
?	?	?	?	?	?	+	?	?	?
+	0	0	+	+/-	?	?	?	?	-
-	+	-	-	-	+/-	-	+/-	+	-
-	?	0	-	+/-	-	?	?	?	?
+	+	0	+	-	+	0	+	+	?
?	?	?	?	+/-	?	?	?	+	+
-	-	-	0	+	+	?	?	+/-	-
-	-	-	-	+	-	?	?	-	
?	?	?	?	-	?	?	?	?	?
0	+	0	+	+/-	+/-	?	?	-	0

Figure 12.4: Chronic polysomnographic effects of major antiepileptic drugs on sleep (per consensus of available studies) (Sammaritano and Sherwin, 2002). + = improves; - = worsens; 0 = no effect; ? = insufficient data; +/- = conflicting data; AED = antiepileptic drug; TST = total sleep time; sleep eff = sleep efficency; % stages 1, 2 = percent TST in stage 1 or 2; % SWS = percent TST in stages 3 and 4; % REM = percent TST in rapid eye movement sleep; no. full AW = number of full awakenings; RD rate = respiratory disturbance events per hour of TST; EDS = excessive daytime sleepiness; MSLT = multiple sleep latency test. Note: a decrease in % stage 1 is considered a '+'.

Barbiturates

Barbiturates are older antiepileptics and include phenobarbitone, methyl phenobarbitone, and primidone.

Mode of action

Barbiturates are central nervous system depressants, through the GABA receptor (*Figure 12.1*). They exert their action by prolonging the opening time of the chloride channel and, thereby, increasing the duration of GABA inhibitory activity.

Pharmacokinetics

Barbiturates are rapidly absorbed. Most have a half-life of twelve hours or greater and are hepatically metabolized.

Effect on sleep and polysomnography

Barbiturates increase total sleep time and decrease mean sleep latency and number of wakenings in epilepsy (Kryger *et al*, 2000). They result in greater daytime sleepiness in both epileptics and normal subjects compared with other antiepileptic agents (Manni *et al*, 1993).

Side-effects and drug interactions

Barbiturates cause cognitive and psychomotor impairment on subjective and objective testing (Manni *et al*, 1993). Barbiturates should not be used with other drugs that cause CNS depression, such as alcohol, or benzodiazepines.

Other antiepileptics

These include carbamazepine, ethosuxamide, phenytoin, valproate, gabapentin, lamotrigine, tiagabine, topramate, and vigabatrin.

Carbamazepine

Carbamazepine blocks sodium channels and inhibits high-frequency, repetitive neuronal discharges. It also acts presynaptically to reduce synaptic transmission (MIMS, 2002).

Effect on sleep and polysomnography

Carbamazepine increases total sleep time and reduces sleep latency in epileptic and normal people. REM sleep is reduced in epileptic peopleon carbamazepine, but appears to be minimally altered in healthy subjects (Riemann *et al*, 1993).

Side-effects and drug interactions

Mild cognitive and psychomotor impairment has been reported with carbamazepine (Manni *et al*, 1993). Medication that is metabolized by the liver, like carbamazepine, should be avoided. Antidepressants and antipsychotics should be used with caution as they can increase the risk of generalized seizures. Concurrent use of lithium can result in neurotoxicity (MIMS, 2002).

Ethosuxamide

Ethosuxamide inhibits calcium conductance in thalamic neurons. There is a paucity of information on the effect of ethosuxamide on sleep. It has been shown to increase stage 1 sleep (Kryger *et al*, 2000). Side-effects and drug interactions are similar to carbamazepine.

Phenytoin

Phenytoin has a similar mode of action to carbamazepine. It reduces sleep latency on polysomnographic data and results in moderate cognitive and psychomotor impairment in healthy volunteers and epileptics (Kryger *et al*, 2000). Side-effects and drug interactions are similar to carbamazepine and also include gingival hypertrophy and hirsutism.

Valproate

Sodium valproate has a similar mechanism of action to carbamazepine and phenytoin. It may also prevent the degradation of gamma-aminobutryic acid (GABA) neurotransmitter. Sleep data is scanty but valproate has been shown to increase total sleep time and reduce the number of awakenings in normal people (Kryger *et al*, 2000) Valproate has improved sleep quality in patients with periodic limb movement disorder (PLMD), increasing slow-wave sleep (stages 3 and 4) without altering REM sleep (Ehrenberg *et al*, 2000). Side-effects are similar to carbamazepine and phenytoin. It causes sedation and mild cognitive and psychomotor impairment in healthy volunteers and epileptics although MSLT data does not demonstrate an adverse effect (Kryger *et al*, 2000).

Gabapentin

Gabapentin is a newer antiepileptic agent. Its mechanism of action is unclear. It is structurally related to the GABA neurotransmitter. There are no polysomnographic or MSLT data regarding its effect on sleep. Gabapentin appears to alleviate symptoms associated with restless leg syndrome (Happe *et al*, 2001). It causes sedation in 5–15% of patients (Kryger *et al*, 2000). Side-effects are similar to carbamazepine and drug interactions are few (MIMS, 2002).

Lamotrigine

Lamotrigine stabilizes presynaptic neuronal membranes by blocking sodium channels. Polysomnographic and MSLT data on the effect of lamotrigine on sleep are limited. In patients with seizures resistant to common antiepileptic agents, the addition of lamotrigine for 3months in an open study increased REM sleep and significantly reduced the number of entries into REM and stage shifts without changing other sleep variables. Daytime somnolence and neuropsychological performance with lamotrigine were unaltered compared with baseline (Placidi *et al*, 2000). Side-effects are similar to carbamazepine. Sedation has been reported in up to 13% of patients, and insomnia in up to 4 % (Kryger *et al*, 2000). Lamotrigine increases the central nervous system effects of carbamazepine and the dose of the latter needs to be reduced if used concurrently (MIMS, 2002).

Tiagabine

Tiagabine inhibits GABA uptake and thereby increases GABA neurotransmitter levels. Polysomnographic and MSLT data are scarce but there is evidence that tiagabine may improve sleep architecture in the elderly by increasing sleep efficiency and slow-wave sleep and reducing the number of wakenings (Mathias *et al*, 2001). Side-effects and drug interactions are similar to carbamazepine (MIMS, 2002).

Vigabatrin

Vigabatrin acts by irreversibly inhibiting GABA transaminase (the enzyme responsible for degrading GABA), resulting in increased GABA levels centrally. Vigabatrin does not alter sleep quality based on polysomnographic studies (Kryger *et al*, 2000). Side-effects and drug interactions are similar to carbamazepine. Sedation has been reported in 7–12% of patients, but MSLT data are lacking (Kryger *et al*, 2000).

Topiramate

Topiramate blocks sodium channels and stabilizes presynaptic neuronal membranes. It also increases the effect of GABA on post-synaptic chloride channels (MIMS, 2002). There are no objective data on the effect of topiramate on sleep. Side-effects and drug interactions are similar to carbamazepine (MIMS, 2002).

Antiparkinsonian drugs

Both Parkinson's disease and its therapeutic options cause sleep disturbances, cognitive and psychomotor impairment. Parkinson's can result in insomnia, hypersomnia, vivid dreams, nightmares, and fatigue (*Chapter 9*). Medication used in Parkinson's disease includes levodopa, ergot-derived dopamine agonists, selegiline, amantadine, apomorphine, catechol-O-methyltransferase inhibitors and anticholinergic agents. These agents will be discussed in relation to their effect on the sleep cycle.

Levodopa

Levodopa, the most commonly used antiparkinsonian drug, is a precursor of dopamine, a catecholamine that is produced in insufficient amounts by the basal ganglia in Parkinson's disease. Levodopa is converted to dopamine in the brain and is designed to replace the deficiency.

Effect on sleep and polysomnography

Sleep-related disorders have been reported in up to 75% of patients on this drug (Kryger *et al*, 2000). Levodopa tends to improve sleep in low doses and disrupt sleep at higher doses (Kryger *et al*, 2000). Levodopa reduces stage 2 sleep and REM sleep (Comella *et al*, 1993).

Side-effects and drug interactions

Sedation, insomnia, depression, hallucinations and confusion are common (MIMS, 2002). Dopamine antagonists counter the effect of levodopa. Methyldopa increases the effect of levodopa and doses need to be adjusted accordingly. Concurrent use of monoamine oxidase inhibitors can cause a hypertensive crisis and should be avoided.

Dopamine agonists

These, including bromocriptine and pergolide, stimulate dopamine receptors.

Effect on sleep and polysomnography

Bromocriptine displays similar polysomnographic sleep compared with levodopa (Kryger *et al*, 2000; Rabey *et al*, 1978). Pergolide has been shown to cause polysomnographic findings similar to narcolepsy in a patient with Parkinson's disease. 'Sleep attacks', due to dopamine agonists and levodopa, are well recognized and detailed behaviorally but not poylsomnographically (Ulivelli *et al*, 2002).

Side-effects

Common psychoneurological side-effects include hallucinations, delusions, confusion, mania and anxiety. Pergolide resulted in insomnia in 42% of patients in one study (Kryger *et al*, 2000).

Drug interactions

Alcohol should be avoided as it increases the central side-effects associated with dopamine agonists. Dopamine antagonists and vasoconstrictive sympathomimetics that may exacerbate cardiovascular effects should be avoided.

Selegiline

Selegiline (deprenyl) binds irreversibly to and inhibits monoamine oxidase B enzyme, thereby preventing the degradation of dopamine.

Effect on sleep and polysomnography

The effect of selegiline on these variables is not well studied. Insomnia has been reported in 10–32% of patients taking selegiline. Lower doses of selegiline are less likely to cause sleep disturbances compared with higher doses (Kryger *et al*, 2000). Selegiline suppresses REM sleep, increases sleep and REM latency, and reduces daytime sleepiness in narcolepsy suggesting a role for it in this disorder (Mayer *et al*, 1995; Reinish *et al*, 1995). Case reports have also implicated selegiline as a cause of REM behavior disorder in patients with Parkinson's disease (Louden *et al*, 1995).

Side-effects

Side-effects are similar to levodopa. Selegiline may worsen the side-effects of levodopa. Selegiline may interact with monamine oxidase inhibitors and SSRIs and concomitant use should be avoided (Kryger *et al*, 2000).

Anticholinergic drugs

These include benztropine, benzhexol, biperiden, orphenadrine and procyclidine. They work by blocking muscarinic receptors in the basal ganglia and reducing the excessive cholinergic activity that is thought to be part of Parkinson's disease. Objective evidence on the effects of anticholinergics on sleep is lacking. Biperiden has been shown to prolong REM latency, suppress REM sleep time and percentage in a dose-dependent manner in healthy volunteers (Gillin *et al*, 1991). Anticholinergics cause worsening of cognitive function, especially memory. This side-effect is reversible on discontinuation of the drug (Kryger *et al*, 2000).

Amantadine and apomorphine

Amantadine increases the release of dopamine presynaptically and blocks cholinergic receptors. Apomorphine stimulates dopamine receptors. There is little objective data on their effects on sleep. Amantadine, either alone or in combination, caused insomnia in 14% of patients in one study (Kryger *et al*, 2000), while apomorphine produces significant sedation and nausea.

Catechol-O-methyltransferase (COMT) inhibitor: entacapone

Entacapone inhibits COMT in the peripheral tissues preventing the breakdown of levodopa. This prolongs the clinical response to levodopa.

Effect on sleep and polysomnography

Objective studies on the effect of entacapone on sleep are lacking. A case report suggests that this drug may precipitate sleep attacks by increasing the bioavailability of levodopa (Tracik and Ebersbach, 2001).

Side-effects

Side-effects are similar to those experienced with bromocriptine.

Drug interactions

The use of non-selective monoamine oxidase inhibitors and selegiline are contraindicated as there is a risk of serotonin syndrome. Drugs metabolized by the COMT system, such as tricyclic antidepressants and venlafaxine, should be avoided as there may be an increased risk of adverse effects. Entacapone may reduce the absorption of iron and these two medications should be given 2–3 hours apart.

Histamine antagonists

These drugs are classified into histamine type 1 and histamine type 2 antagonists.

H₁ antagonists

H_1 antagonists or 'antihistamines' are used for relief of urticaria and other chronic allergic skin diseases, and seasonal and perennial allergic rhinitis. They exert their effects by binding to central and peripheral H_1 receptors.

Effect on sleep and polysomnography

Polysomnographic studies with H_1 antagonists are lacking. Diphenhydramine has been shown to reduce mean daily sleep latency and increase the percentage of inactive time using actigraphy compared with placebo (Roehrs *et al*, 2000).

Side-effects

The main side-effects with antihistamines are sedation and cognitive and psychomotor impairment. The degree of central nervous system depression is, as a rule, dependent on the extent of central binding of the drug. The older, lipophilic antihistamines, such as diphenhydramine tend to be more sedating than the newer, hydrophilic agents, eg. loratadine. Sedation and cognitive impairment have been well documented both subjectively and objectively on MSLT studies and formal psychomotor testing (Kryger *et al*, 2000). There is insufficient data to assess if tolerance to antihistamines develops with regular use (Kryger *et al*, 2000). The concomitant use of other central nervous system depressants should be avoided (MIMS, 2002)

H₂ Antagonists

These include cimetidine, ranitidine, famotidine and nizatidine, all of which are primarily used in gastroesophageal disease.These drugs bind to H_2 receptors in parietal cells and block the action of histamine and thereby gastric acid secretion.

Effect on sleep and polysomnography

A significant reduction in the sleep onset latency was noted with famotidine, in a study comparing nocturnal and daytime sleepiness using polysomnography and MSLT. All other medications had a similar effect to placebo on polysomnographic variables. There were no differences in MSLT recordings compared with placebo (Orr *et al*, 1994).

Side-effects

H$_2$ antagonists do not tend to cause sedation or cognitive and psychomotor impairment given their low lipophilicity. Headache, lethargy, drowsiness, rash, diarrhea and constipation have been reported in 1–3% of patients (MIMS, 2002).

Theophylline

Theophylline, a methylxanthine similar to caffeine, is an adenosine receptor antagonist that is used variably in airways diseases as a respiratory stimulant and bronchodilator.

Effect on sleep and polysomnography

There is subjective and objective data that theophylline disturbs sleep variably. Insomnia is a frequent complaint in up to 55% of patients. Theophylline has demonstrated significantly more arousals per hour, reduced total sleep time (Kaplan *et al*, 1993), increased sleep latency, total wake time and stage 1 sleep on polysomnography compared with placebo in healthy volunteers (Roehrs *et al*, 1995). In subjects with chronic obstructive pulmonary disease, significantly impaired sleep quality with theophylline has been demonstrated polysomnographically (Mulloy and McNicholas, 1993) while other studies of similar subjects have shown no difference in sleep quality or architecture compared with placebo (Man *et al*, 1996; Wiegand *et al*, 1999).

Theophylline appears to have variable results in the medical therapy of obstructive sleep apnea. While not as good as nasal CPAP, some studies have demonstrated that it clearly reduces obstructive events compared with placebo (Mulloy and McNicholas, 1992; Saletu *et al*, 1999). Other studies have shown no improvement in obstructive events with theophylline (Fietze *et al*, 1993).

Side-effects and drug interactions

Cognitive or behavioral impairment has not been demonstrated (Kryger *et al*, 2000). Theophylline increases the clearance of lithium.

Corticosteroids

Synthetic glucocorticoids and mineralocorticoids are used in all areas of medicine. Corticosteroids reduce REM sleep (Kryger, 2000). Prednisone, dexamethasone and hydrocortisone increase number of overnight wakings (Kryger *et al*, 2000). Hydrocortisone (a natural corticosteroid) seems to increase slow-wave sleep and dexamatezone (a synthetic steroid) to reduce it (Fehm *et al*, 1986). Aldosterone does not appear to affect sleep architecture (Kryger *et al*, 2000). Insomnia, restlesssness, cognitive, and behavioral and personality changes are thought to be common side-effects (Kryger *et al*, 2000;

Belanoff *et al*, 2001; Newcomer *et al*, 1994). Data on the effect of corticosteroids on psychomotor functioning is sparse. One study demonstrated a poorer performance on a verbal memory task in healthy volunteers given a short course of prednisone compared with placebo (Kryger *et al*, 2000).

Analgesics

The effect of analgesics on sleep has not been well studied to date. Narcotics increase wake. The administration of 50 mg or 100 mg of tramadol significantly reduced slow-wave sleep and increased stage 2 sleep in healthy volunteers and a dose of 100 mg (not 50 mg) reduced REM sleep (Walder *et al*, 2001). Well documented side-effects of narcotics include sedation, cognitive and psychomotor impairment, tolerance and dependence (MIMS, 2002).

Nonsteroidals such as aspirin disrupt sleep similarly in healthy volunteers and in those with insomnia. Aspirin and ibuprofen increase the number of polysomnographic wakenings and percentage of time spent awake, and reduce sleep efficiency compared with placebo, while ibuprofen increases sleep latency and reduces slow-wave sleep compared with placebo. Polysomnographic recordings with acetaminophen are similar to placebo (Murphy *et al*, 1994).

Anorectic agents

Evidence on the effect of slimming medications on sleep is limited. Agents that are currently available in Australia include phentermine, sibutramine and orlistat. Phentermine and sibutramine act by inhibiting noradrenaline, serotonin and dopamine reuptake. Orlistat inhibits gastrointestinal lipase. Phenteramine and sibutramine are subjectively reported to cause insomnia (Kryger *et al*, 2000). Polysomnographic data are lacking for all three medications.

References

Alderman CP, Gilbert AL, Condon JT (2000) Characteristics of tranquilizer use among Australian Vietnam War veterans. *Ann Pharmacother* **34**: 1243–7

Aldrich MS, Shipley JE, Tandon R, Kroll PD, Brower KJ (1993) Sleep-disordered breathing in alcoholics: association with age. *Alcohol Clin Exp Res* **17**(6): 1179–83

American Formulary Hospital Service (AFHS) (2002) McEvoy GK, ed. American Society of Health System Pharmacists Inc, Bethesda, Maryland

American Psychiatry Association (1995) *Diagnostic and Statistical Manual of Mental Disorders, 4th edn*. American Psychiatry Association, Washington DC

Ancoli-Israel S, Richardson GS, Mangano RM, Jenkins L, Hall P, Jones WS (2005) Long-term use of sedative hypnotics in older patients with insomnia. *Sleep Med* **6**: 107–13

Arendt J, Skene DJ, Middleton B, Lockley SW, Deacon S (1997) Efficacy of melatonin treatment in jet lag, shift work, and blindness. *J Biol Rhythms* **12**: 604–17

Asian S, Isik E, Cosar B (2002) The effects of mirtazapine on sleep: a placebo-controlled, double blind study in young volunteers. *Sleep* **25**(6): 677–9

Balderer G, Borbely AA (1985) Effect of valerian on human sleep. *Psychopharmacol* **87**: 406–9

Barratt ES, Beaver W, White R (1974) The effects of marihuana on human sleep pattern. *Biolog Psychiat* **8**(1): 47–54

Belanoff JK, Gross K, Yager A, Scatzberg AF (2001) Corticosteroids and cognition. *J Psychiat Res* **35**(3): 127–45;

Betts TA, Alford C (1985) Beta blockers and sleep: a controlled trial. *Eur J Clin Pharmacol* **28**(suppl): 65–8

Briggs GG, Samson JH, Crawford DJ (1975) Lack of abnormalities in a newborn exposed to amphetamine during gestation. *Am J Dis Child* **129**(2): 259–60

Broughton RJ, Fleming JA, George CF, Hill JD, Kryger MH, Moldofsky H *et al* (1997) Randomized, double-blind, placebo-controlled crossover trial of modafinil in the treatment of excessive daytime sleepiness in narcolepsy. *Neurology* **49**: 444–51

Broughton R, Mamelak M (1979) The treatment of narcolepsy–cataplexy with nocturnal gammahydroxybutyrate. *Can J Neurol Sci* **6**: 1–6

Brust JCM (1993) *The Neurological Aspects of Substance Abuse*. Butterworth-Heinemann, Boston

Busto U, Sellers E, Naranjo C, Cappell H, Sancehz-Craig M, Sykora K (1986) Withdrawal reaction after long term therapeutic use of benzodiazepines. *N Engl J Med* **315**: 854–9

Camí J, Farré M (2003) Drug addiction. *N Engl J Med* 349: 975–86

Cauffield JS, Forbes HJ (1999) Dietary supplements used in the treatment of depression, anxiety, and sleep disorders. *Lippincotts Prim Care Pract* **3**(3): 290–304

Centers for Disease Control and Prevention (2003) Hepatic toxicity possibly associated with kava-containing products — United States, Germany, and Switzerland, 1999–2002. *JAMA* **289**(1): 36–7

Chemelli RM, Willie JT, Sinton CM, Elmquist JK, Scammell T, Lee C *et al* (1999) Narcolepsy in orexin knockout mice: molecular genetics of sleep regulation. *Cell* **98**(4): 437–51

Clark CP, Gillin JC, Golshan S, Demodena A, Smith TL, Danowski S (1999) Polysomnographic and depressive symptoms in primary alcoholics with and without a lifetime diagnosis of secondary depression and in patients with major depression. *J Affect Disord* **52**(1–3): 177–85

Comella CL, Tanner CM, Ristanovic RK (1993) Polysomnographic sleep measures in Parkinson's disease patients with treatment induced hallucinations. *Ann Neurol* **34**: 710–4

Cnattingus S, Signorello LB, Anneren G, Clausson B, Ekbom A, Ljunger E *et al* (2000) Caffeine intake and the risk of first-trimester spontaneous abortion. *N Engl J Med* **343**(25): 1839–45

Dagan Y (2002) Circadian rhythm sleep disorders (CRSD). *Sleep Med Rev* **6**(1): 45–55

Dagan Y, Lemberg H (1999) Sleep–wake schedule disorders as a possible side effect of CNS medications. *Chronobiol Int* **16**(suppl 1): 25 [abstract]

Dagan Y, Yovel I, Hallis D, Eisenstein M, Raichik I (1998) Evaluating the role of melatonin in the long-term treatment of delayed sleep phase syndrome (DSPS). *Chronobiol Int* **15**(2): 181–90

Dahlitz M, Alvarez B, Vignau J, English J, Arendt J, Parkes JD (1991) Delayed sleep phase syndrome response to melatonin. *Lancet* **337**(8750): 1121–4

Damian MS, Gerlack A, Schmidt F, Lehmann E, Reichmann H (2001) Modafinil for excessive daytimes sleepiness in myotonic dystrophy. *Neurology* **56**(6): 794–6

Dietrich B, Herrmann WM (1989) Influence of cilazapril on memory functions and sleep behaviour in comparison with metoprolol and placebo in healthy subjects. *Br J Clin Pharmacol* **27**(suppl 2): 249S–261S

Dimsday JE, Newton PR (1992) Cognitive effects of beta blockers. *J Psychosom Res* **36**(3): 229–36

Donath F, Quispe S, Diefenback K, Maurer A, Fietze I, Roots I (2000) Critical evaluation of the effect of valerian extract on sleep structure and sleep quality. *Pharmacopsychiatry* **33**: 47–53

Drummond SP, Gillin JC, Smith TL, DeModena A (1998) The sleep of abstinent pure primary alcoholic patients: natural course and relationship to relapse. *Alcohol Clin Exp Res* **22**(8): 1796–802

Duffy A, Milin R (1996) Case study: withdrawal syndrome in adolescent chronic cannabis users. *J Am Acad Child Adolesc Psychiat* **35**(12): 1618–21

Eckernas SA, Roos BE, Kvidal P, Eriksson LO, Block GA, Neafus RP, Haigh JR (1993) The effects of simvastatin and pravastatin on objective and subjective measures of nocturnal sleep: a comparison of two structurally different HMGCo A reductase inhibitors in patients with primary moderate hypercholesterolemia. *Br J Clin Pharmacol* **35**(3): 284–9

Eddy NB, Halbach H, Isbell H, Seevers MH (1965) Drug dependence: its significance and characteristics. *Bulletin WHO* **32**: 721

Ehrenberg BL, Eisenehr I, Corbett KE, Crowley PF, Walters AS (2000) Valproate for sleep consolidation in periodic limb movement disorder. *J Clin Psychopharmacol* **20**(5): 574–8

Engber TM, Dennis SA, Jones BE, Miller MS, Contreras PC (1998) Brain regional substrates for the actions of the novel wake-promoting agent modafinil in the rat: comparison with amphetamine. *Neuroscience* **87**(4): 905–11

Eriksson, M, Larsson G, Winbladh B, Zetterstrom R (1978) The influence of amphetamine addiction on pregnancy and the newborn infant. *Acta Paediatr Scan* **67**: 95–9

Fehm HL, Benkowitech R, Kern W, Fehm-Wolfsodorf G, Paushinger P, Born J (1986) Influences of corticosteroids, dexamethazone and hydrocortisone on sleep in humans. *Neuropharmacobiology* **16**: 198–204

Feinberg I, Jones R, Walker J, Cavness C, Floyd T (1976) Effects of marijuana extract and tetrehydrocannabinol on electroencephalographic sleep patterns.*Clin Pharmacol Ther* **19**(6) 782–94

Feinberg I, Jones R, Walker J, Cavness C, March J (1975) Effects of high dosage delta 9 tetrahydrocannabinol on sleep patterns in man. *Clin Pharmacol Ther* **17**(4): 458–66

Fietze I, Warmuth R, Quispe-Bravo S, Waschke K (1993) Therapeutic consequences of obstructive sleep apnea syndrome: results of drug, mechanical and surgical treatment. *Pneumologie* **47**: 716–21

Ferraro L, Antonelli T, O'Connor WT, Tanganelli S, Rambert F, Fuxe K (1997) The antinarcoleptic drug modafinil increases glutamate release in thalamic areas and hippocampus. *Sleep* **8**(13): 2283–7

Freemon FR (1972) Effects of marihuana on sleeping states. *JAMA* **220**(10): 1364–5

Friston KJ, Sharpley AL, Solomon RA, Cowen PJ (1989) Lithium increases slow wave sleep: possible mediation by brain 5 HT2 receptors? *Psychopharmacology* (Berl) **98**: 139–40

Gentili A, Godschalk MF, Gheorgiu D, Nelson K, Julius DA, Mulligan T (1996) Effect of clonidine and yohimbine on sleep in healthy men: a double blind, randomized, controlled trial. *Eur J Clin Pharmacol* **50**(6): 463–5

Gillin JC, Rapaport M, Erman MK, Winokur A, Albala BJ (1997) A comparison of nefazodone and fluoxetine on mood and on objective, subjective, and clinician-rated measures of sleep in depressed patients: a double-blind, 8-week, clinical trial. *J Clin Psychiat* **58**: 185–92

Gillin JC, Sutton L, Golshan S, Hirsch S, Warmann C, Shiromani P (1991) Dose dependent inhibition of REM sleep in normal volunteers by biperiden, a muscarinic antagonist. *Biol Psychiat* **30**(2): 151–6

Gursky JT, Krahn LE (2000) The effects of antidepressants on sleep: a review. *Harvard Rev Psychiat* **8**(6): 298–306

Gyllenhal, C, Merritt SL, Peterson SD, Block KI, Gochenour T (2000) Efficacy and safety of herbal stimulants and sedatives in sleep disorders. *Sleep Med Rev* **4**(3): 229–51

Hagiwara M, Tsuchida A, Hyakkaku M, Nichizato K, Asai T, Nozawa Y *et al* (2000) Delayed onset of pulmonary hypertension associated with an appetite suppressant, mazindol: a case report. *Jap Circulation J* **64**(3): 218–21

Happe S, Klosch G, Saletu B, Zeitlhofer J (2001) Treatment of idiopathic restless legs syndrome (RLS) with gabapentin. *Neurology* **9**: 1717–9

Hendrickse WA, Roffwarg HP, Grannemann BD, Orsulak PJ, Armitage R, Cain JW *et al* (1994) Effects of fluoxetine on the polysomnogram of the depressed outpatients: a pilot study. *Neuropsychopharmacology* **10**: 85–91

Hinze-Selch D, Mullington J, Orth A, Lauer CJ, Pollmacher T (1997) Effects of clozapine on sleep: a longitudinal study. *Biol Psychiat* **42**(4): 260–6

Holbrook AM, Crowther R, Lotter A, Cheng C, King D (2000) Meta-analysis of benzodiazeoine use in the treatment of insomnia. *CMAJ* **162**(2): 225–33

Kaplan J, Fredrickson PA, Renaux SA, O'Brien PC (1993) Theophylline effect on sleep in normal subjects. *Chest* **103**: 93–5

Karacan I, Fernandez-Salas A, Coggins WJ, Carter WE, Williams RL, Thornby JI *et al* (1976) Sleep electroencephalographic-electrooculographic characteristics of chronic marijuana users: part I. *Ann New York Acad Sciences* **282**: 348–74

Karch SB (1996) *The Pathology of Drugs Abuse*. CRC Press, Boca Raton, Florida: 215

Kingshott RN, Vennelle M, Coleman EL, Engleman HM, Mackay TW, Douglas NJ (2001) Randomized, double-blind, placebo-controlled crossover trial of modafinil in the treatment of residual excessive daytime sleepiness in the sleep apnoea/hypopnoea syndrome. *Am J Resp Crit Care Med* **163**(4): 918–23

Koella WP (1985) CNS-related (side) effects of beta blockers with special reference to mechanisms of action. *Eur J Clin Pharmacol* **28**: 55–63

Kostis JB, Rosen RC. Wilson AC (1994) Central nervous system effects of HMGCoA reductase inhibitors: lovastatin and pravastatin on sleep and cognitive performance in patients with hypercholesterolemia. *J Clin Pharmacol* **34**(10): 989–96

Kryger MH, Roth T, Dement WC (2000) *Principles and Practice of Sleep Medicine*. 3rd edn. WB Saunders Company, London

Kuhlmann J, Berger W, Poduweit H, Schmidt U (1999) The influence of valerian treatment on 'reaction time' I volunteers. *Pharmacopsychiatry* **32**: 235–41

Lader M (1998) Withdrawal reactions after stopping hypnotics in patients with insomnia. *CNS Drugs* **10**(6): 425–40

Laffont F, Cathala HP, Kohler F (1987) Effect of modafinil on narcolepsy and idiopathic hypersomnia. *Sleep Res* **16**: 377

Lammers GJ, Arends J, Declerck AC, Ferrari MD, Schouwink G, Troost J (1993) Gammahydroxybutyrate and narcolepsy: A double-blind placebo-controlled study. *Sleep* **16**(3): 216–20

Landry P, Warnes H, Nielsen T, Montplaisir J (1999) Somnambulistic-like behaviour in patients attending a lithium clinic. *Int Clin Pharmacol* **14**: 173–5

Lee JH, Woo JI, Meltzer HY (2001) Effects of clozapine on sleep measures and sleep associated changes in growth hormone and cortisol in patients with schizophrenia. *Psychiatry Res* **103**: 157–66

Little BB, Snell LM, Gilstrap LC III (1988) Methamphetamine abuse during pregnancy: outcome and fetal effects. *Obstet Gynecol* **72**: 541–4

Louden MB, Morehead MA, Schmidt HS (1995) Activation by selegiline (Eldepryle) of REM sleep behaviour disorder in parkinsonism.*W V Med J* **91**(3): 101

Luthringer R, Toussaint M, Schaltenbrand N, Bailey P, Danjou PH, Hackett D *et al* (1996) A double blind, placebo-controlled evaluation of the effects of orally administered venlafaxine on sleep in patients with major depression. *Psychopharmacol Bull* **32**(4): 637–46

Mamelak M, Webster P (1981) Treatment of narcolepsy and sleep apnea with gammahydroxybutyrate: a clinical and polysomnographic case study. *Sleep* **4**(1): 105–11

Man GC, Champman KR, Ali SH, Darke AC (1996) Sleep quality and nocturnal respiratory function with once daily theophylline (Uniphyl) and inhaled salbutamol in patients with COPD. *Chest* **110**: 648–53

Manni R, Ratti MT, Galimberti CA, Morini R, Perucca E, Tartara A (1993) Daytime sleepiness in epileptic patients on long term monotherapy: MSLT, clinical and psychometric assessment. *Neurophysiol Clin* **23**(1): 71–6

Martin WR, Sloan JM, Sopira JD, Josinski DR (1971) Physiologic, subjective and behavioural effects of amphetamines, metamphetamine, ephedrine, phemmetrazine and methylphenidate in man. *Clin Pharmacol Ther* **12**(12 Part I): 245–57

Mathias S, Wetter TC, Steiger A, Lancel M (2001) The GABA uptake inhibitor tiagabine promotes slow-wave sleep in normal elderly subjects. *Neurobiol Aging* **22**: 247–53

Mayer G, Ewert Meier K, Hephata K (1995) Selegiline hydrochloride treatment in narcolepsy. A double blind, placebo-controlled study. *Clin Neuropharmacol* **18**(4): 306–19

Mignot E (2004) An update on the pharmacotherapy of excessive daytime sleepiness and cataplexy. *Sleep Med Rev* **8**(5): 333–8

Mitler MM, Walsleben J, Sangal RB, Hirshkowitz M (1998) Sleep latency on the maintenance of wakefulness test (MWT) for 530 patients with narcolepsy while free of psychoactive drugs. *Electroencephalogr Clin Neurophysiol* **107**(1): 33–8

Mitler MM, Dawson A, Henriksen SJ, Sobers M, Bloom FE (1988) Bedtime ethanol increases resistance of upper airways and produces sleep apneas in asymptomatic snorers. *Alcohol Clin Exp Res* **12**(6): 801–5

MIMS Annual (2002) Caswell A, Reckmann M, Sydney Wills CR, eds. MIMS. 26 edn. Bristol

Monti JM (1987) Disturbances of sleep and wakefulness associated with the use of antihypertensive agents. *Life Sci* **41**(17): 1979–88

Monti JM (1989) Effects of a reversible monoamino oxidase-a inhibitor (moclobemide) on sleep of depressed patients. *Br J Psychiat* **155**(suppl 6): 61–5

Mulloy E, McNicholas WT (1992) Theophylline in obstructive sleep apnea. A double blind evaluation. *Chest* **101**: 753–7

Mulloy E, McNicholas WT (1993) Theophylline improves gas exchange during rest, exercise and sleep in severe chronic obstructive pulmonary disease. *Am Rev Respir Dis* **148**: 1030–6

Murphy PJ, Badia P, Myers BL, Boecker MR, Wright KP Jr (1994) Non-steroidal anti-inflammatory drugs affect normal sleep in humans. *Physiol Behav* **55**: 1063–6

Newcomer JW, Craft S, Hershey T, Askins K, Bardgett ME (1994) Glucocorticoid induced impairment in declarative memory performance in adults. *J Neurosci* **14**(4): 2047–53

Nowell PD, Mazumdar S, Buysse DJ, Dew MA, Reynolds CF III, Kupfer DJ (1997) Benzodiazepine and zolpidem for chronic insomnia: a meta analysis of treatment efficacy. *JAMA* **278**(24): 2170–7

Olde Rikkert MG, Rigaud AS (2001) Melatonin in elderly patients with insomnia. A systematic review. *Gerontol Geriatr* **34**(6): 491–7

Orr WC, Duke JC, Imes NK, Mellow MK (1994) Comparative effects of H2-receptor antagonists on subjective and objective assessments of sleep. *Aliment Pharmacol Ther* **2**: 203–7

Parkes JD (1985) *Sleep and its Disorders*. WB Saunders, London

Parkes JD, Schachter M (1979) Mazindol in the treatment of narcolepsy. *Acta Neurol Scand* **60**(4): 250–4

Parrino L, Terzano MG (1996) Polysomnographic effects of hypnotic drugs. A review. *Psychopharmacology* **136**(1): 1–16

Partinen M, Pihl S, Strandberg T, Vanhanen H, Murtomaki E, Block G *et al* (1994) Comparison of effects on sleep of lovastatin and pravastatin in hypercholesterolemia. *Am J Cardiol* **73**(12): 876–80

Patrick SK, Mueller RA, Gualtieri CT *et al* (1987) Pharmacokinetics and actions of methylphenidate. In: Meltzen HY, ed. *Psycholopharmacology: The Third Generation of Progress*. Raven Press, New York: 1387–96

Pieralisi G, Ripari P, Vecchiet L (1991) Effects of a standardized ginseng extract combined with demethylaminoethanol bitartrate, vitamins, minerals and trace elements on physical performance during exercise. *Clin Ther* **13**: 373–82

Pires ML, Benedito-Silva AA, Pinto L, Souza L, Vismari L, Calil HM (2001) Acute effects of low doses of melatonin on the sleep of young healthy subjects. *J Pineal Res* **31**(4): 326–32

Piscopo JA, Goswami M, Pollak CP *et al* (1992) *A Narcolepsy Patient Role Model in Psychosocial Aspects of Narcolepsy*. The Haworth Press, New York

Placidi F, Marciani MG, Diomedi M, Scalise A, Pauri F, Giacomini P, Gigli GL (2000) Effects of lamotrigine on nocturnal sleep, daytime somnolence and cognitive functions in focal epilepsy. *Acta Neurol Scand* **102**: 81–6

Rabey J, Vardi J, Glaubman H, Streifler M (1978) EEG sleep study in parkinsonian patients under bromocriptine treatment. *Eur Neurol* **17**(6): 345–50

Reschtschaffen A, Maron L (1964) The effect of amphetamines on sleep cycle. *Electroenceph Clin Neurophysiol* **16**: 438–45

Reinish LW, MacFarlane JG, Sandor P, Shapiro CM (1995) REM changes in narcolepsy with selegiline. *Sleep* **18**(5): 362–7

Riemann D, Gann H, Hohagen F, Bahro M, Muller W, Berger M (1993) The effect of carbamazepine on endocrine and sleep EEG variables in a patient with 48-hour rapid cycling and healthy controls. *Neuropsychobiology* **27**: 163–70

Roehrs T, Merlotti L *et al* (1994) Sedative, memory, and performance of hypnotics. *Psychopharmacology* **116**(2): 130–4

Roehrs T, Merlotti L, Halpin D, Rosenthal L, Roth T (1995) Effects of theophylline on nocturnal sleep and daytime sleepiness/alertness. *Chest* **108**: 382–7

Roehrs T Merlotti L, Zorick F, Roth T (1992) Rebound insomnia in normals and patients with insomnia after abrupt and tapered discontinuation. *Psychopharmacology* **108**: 67–71

Roehrs T, Papineau K, Rosenthal L, Roth T (1999) Ethanol as a hypnotic in insomniacs: self-administration and effects on sleep and mood. *Neuropsychopharmacology* **20**(3): 279–86

Roehrs T, Turner L, Roth T (2000) Effects of sleep loss on waking actigraphy. *Sleep* **23**: 793–7

Roth T, Zorick F, Wittig R, McLenaghan A, Roehrs T (1982) The effects of Doxepin HCL on sleep and depression. *J Clin Psychiat* **43**(9): 366–8

Rugino TA, Copley TC (2001) Effects of modafinil in children with attention-deficit/hyperactivity disorder: an open-label study. *J Am Acad Child Adolesc Psychiat* **40**(2): 230–5

Rugino TA, Samsock TC (2003) Modafinil in children with attention-deficit hyperactivity disorder. *Pediatric Neurol* **29**(2): 136–42

Saletu B, Oberndorfer S, Anderer P, Gruber G, Divos H, Lachner A *et al* (1999) Efficiency of continuous positive airway pressure versus theophylline therapy in sleep apnea: comparative sleep laboratory studies on objective and subjective sleep and awakening. *Neuropsychobiology* **39**: 151–9

Salin-Pascual RJ, Galicia-Polo L, Drucker-Colin R (1997) Sleep changes after 4 consecutive days of venlafaxine administration in normal volunteers. *J Clin Psychiat* **58**(8): 348–50

Sammaritano MR, Shervin LA (2002) Effect of anticonvulsants on sleep. In: Bazil CW, Malow BA, Sammaritano MR, eds. *Sleep and Epilepsy: The Clinical Spectrum*. Elsevier Science BV, Amsterdam

Scammell TE, Estabrooke IV, McCarthy MT, Chemelli RM, Yanagisawa M, Miller M, Saper CB (2000) Hypothalamic arousal regions are activated during modafinil-induced wakefulness. *J Neurosci* **20**(22): 8620–8

Scharf MB, Lai AA, Branigan B, Stover R, Berkowitz DG (1998) Pharmacokinetics of gammahydroxybutyrate (GHB) in narcoleptic patients. *Sleep* **21**(5): 507–14

Schulz, Holtz C, Muller J (1994) The effect of valerian extract on sleep polygraphy in poor sleepers: a pilot study. *Pharmacopsychiatry* **27**: 147–51

Scrima L, Hartman PG, Johnson FH, Thomas EE, Hiller FC (1990) The effects of gamma-hydroxybutyrate on the sleep of narcolepsy patients: a double-blind study. *Sleep* **13**(6): 479–90

Seidel WF, Cohen SA, Bliwise NG, Dement WC (1985) Buspirone: an anxiolytic without sedative effect. *Psychopharmacology* **87**: 371–3

Sharpley AL, Cowen PJ (1995) Effect of pharmacological treatments on the sleep of depressed patients. *Biolog Psychiat* **37**(2): 85–98

Sharpley AL, Williamson DJ, Attenburrow ME, Pearson G, Sargent P, Cowen PJ (1996) The effects of paroxetine and nefazodone on sleep: a placebo controlled trial. *Psychopharmacology* **126**(1): 50–4

Siegel RK (1979) Ginseng abuse syndrome. Problems with the panacea. *JAMA* **241**: 1614–5

Stahl SM, Frakes DC (1995) Nefazodone and serotonin receptor modulators: a new member of a unique class of antidepressant. *Int Rev Psychiat* **7**: 29–39

Stradling JR (1993) ABC of sleep disorders. Recreational drugs and sleep. *Br Med J* **306**: 573–5

Tecce JJ, Cole IO (1974) Amphetamine effects in man: paradoxical drowsiness and lowered electrical brain activity (CNV). *Science* **185**: 451–3

Thase ME (1998) Depression, sleep and antidepressants. *J Clin Psychiat* **59**: 55–65

Tracik F, Ebersbach G (2001) Sudden daytime sleep onset in Parkinson's disease: polysomnographic recordings. *Mov Disord* **16**(3): 500–6

Trivedi MH, Rush AJ, Armitage R, Gullion CM, Grannemann MA, Orsulka PJ, Roffwarg HP (1999) Effects of fluoxetine on the polysomnogram in outpatients with major depression. *Neuropsychopharmacology* **20**: 447–59

Tunnicliff G (1997) Sites of action of gamma-hydroxybutyrate (GHB) — a neuroactive drug with abuse potential clinical toxicology. *J Toxicol Clin Toxicol* **35**(6): 581–90

Ulivelli M, Rossi S, Lombardi C, Bartalini S, Rocchi R, Giannini F *Et al* (2002) Polysomnographic characterization of pergolide induced sleep attacks in idiopathic PD. *Neurology* **58**: 341–6

US Modafinil in Narcolepsy Multicentre Study Group (1998) Randomized trial of modafinil for the treatment of pathological somnolence in narcolepsy. *Ann Neurol* **43**: 88–97

Vasar V, Appelberg B, Rimon R, Selvaratnam J (1994) The effect of fluoxetine on sleep: a longitudinal, double-blind polysomnographic study of healthy volunteers. *Int Clin Pharmacol* **9**: 203–6

Volz HP, Kieser M (1997) Kava-kava extract WS 1490 versus placebo in anxiety disorders — a randomised placebo-controlled 25-week outpatient trial. *Pharmacopsychiatry* **30**: 1–5

Walder B, Tramer MR, Blois R (2001) The effects of two single doses of tramadol on sleep: a ramdomised, cross-over trial in healthy volunteers. *Eur J Anaesthesiol* **18**: 36–42

Warot D, Corruble E, Payan C, Weil JS, Puech AJ (1993) Subjective effects of modafinil, a new central adrenergic stimulant in healthy volunteers: a comparison with amphetamine, caffeine and placebo. *Eur Psychiatry* **8**: 201–8

Weichler U, Herres-Mayer B, Mayer J, Weber K, Hoffmann R, Peter JH (1991) Influence of antihypertensive drug therapy on sleep pattern and sleep apnea activity. *Cardiology* **78**(2): 124–30

Wesensten NJ, Balkin TJ, Belenky GL (1995) Effects of daytime administration of zolpidem versus triazolam on memory. *Eur J Clin Pharmacol* **48**: 115–22

Wetter TC, Lauer CJ, Gillich G, Pollmacher T (1996) The electroencephaographic sleep pattern in scizophrenic patients treated with clozapine or classical antipsychotic drugs. *J Psychiatr Res* **30**: 411–9

Wiegand L, Mende CN, Zaidel G, Zwillich CW, Petrocella VJ, Vancey SW, Ricka KA (1999) Salmeterol vs theophylline: sleep and efficacy outcomes in patients with nocturnal asthma. *Chest* **115**(6): 1525–32

Winokur A, Sateia MJ, Hayes JB, Bayles-Dazet W, MacDonald MM, Gary KA (2000) Acute effects of mirtazapine on sleep continuity and sleep architecture in depressed patients: a pilot study. *Biol Psychiat* **48**(1): 75–8

Wirz-Justice A, Cajochen C, Nussbaum P (1997) A schizophrenic patient with an arrhythmic circadian rest–activity cycle. *Psychiatry Res* **73**: 83–90

Wirz-Justice A, Werth E, Savaskan E, Knoblanch V, Fontana Gasio P, Muller-Span F (2000) Haloperidol disrupts, clozapine reinstates the circadian rest-activity cycle in a patient with early-onset Alzheimer's disease. *Alzheimer Dis Assoc Disord* **14**(4): 212–5

Wohlgemuth WK, Krystal AD (2005) Hypnotics should be considered for the initial treatment of chronic insomnia. *J Clin Sleep Med* **1**(2): 120–4

Wong YN, Wang L, Hartman L, Simcoe D, Chen Y, Laughton W (1998) Comparison of the single-dose pharmacokinetics and tolerability of modafinil and dextroamphetamine administered alone or in combination in healthy male volunteers. *J Clin Pharmacol* **38**(10): 971–8

Wooten V (1994) Effectiveness of yohimbine in treating narcolepsy. *South Med J* **87**(11): 1065–6

Zhdanova IV, Wurtman RJ, Morabito C, Piotrovska VR, Lynch HJ (1996) Effects of low oral doses of melatonin, given 2–4 hours before habitual bedtime, on sleep in normal young humans. *Sleep* **19**: 423–31

Zhdanova IV, WurtmanRJ, Regan MM, Taylor JA, Shi JP, Leclair OU (2001) Melatonin treatment for age related insomnia. *J Clin Endocrinol Metab* **86**(10): 4727–30

Zorumski CF, Isenberg KE (1991) Insights into the structure and function of GABA–benzodiazepine receptors: ion channels and psychiatry. *Am J Psychiat* **148**(2): 162–73

CHAPTER 13

Sleep medicine and the law

Ron Grunstein and Elizabeth Ellis

Humans spend approximately one third of their existence asleep and it is important to appreciate the relevance that sleep abnormalities have to the law (Grunstein, 2000). There is increasing recognition that lack of sleep or conditions of excessive sleepiness have medicolegal ramifications. Moreover, sleep disorders are a spectrum of clinically important conditions that have generated their own medical sub-specialty of sleep medicine, methods of investigation and growing body of research literature.

This chapter addresses two major areas:

1. Violent acts arising out of sleep.
2. Medicolegal aspects of performance impaired by sleepiness.

Violence and sleep

For a public fed on a diet of television drama about the law, the topic of how violence during sleep impacts on criminality must be yet another convoluted script (Grunstein, 2000). However, it is based on the historically well-established concept of automatic behavior (automatisms). Automatisms produce acts that may result in illegal action and behaviors and, traditionally, have been the domain of the psychiatric medicolegal literature (Yeo, 2002). Automatisms may arise from wakefulness and are well described elsewhere.

The core of automatism is involuntary, comprising a complete lack of capacity to contain one's conduct. However, knowledge about sleep and its disorders accumulated over the last 30 years have shown that violent and often complicated acts arising from sleep may result in injury or death. These occur 'automatically' without conscious awareness, and the 'perpetrator' is acting without intent and, therefore, without responsibility. Defendants charged with murder or serious injury have been acquitted on the basis of automatism related to a sleep disorder. From a legal point of view, the importance is the definition of insane versus sane automatism. However, the medical expert needs to focus on the possibility of the automatisms (and, in particular, resulting violence) recurring.

Sleep-violence disorders

A range of sleep disorders may be associated with violence arising out of sleep. These sleep-violence disorders are surprisingly common and sleep-related injury from these disorders is said to affect 2% of the adult population (Ohayon *et al*, 1997). These disorders are listed in *Table 13.1*.

Table 13.1: Sleep-related violence
Sleep disorders
a. Disorders of arousal (confusional arousals, sleep drunkenness, automatic behavioral sleep-walking, sleep terrors)
b. REM sleep behavior disorder
c. Nocturnal seizures
d. Compelling hypnogogic hallucinations
e. Sleep-talking
Psychiatric disorders
1. Dissociative states (may arise exclusively from sleep)   a. Fugues   b. Multiple personality disorder   c. Psychogenic amnesia
2. Post-traumatic stress disorder
3. Malingering
4. Munchausen syndrome by proxy

Sleep-walking, night terrors and confusional arousals form parts of the spectrum of slow-wave sleep arousal disorders (SWSAD) (Mahowald and Schenck, 1996). Although common in childhood, they may persist or even develop in adulthood. These are the most common sleep disorders involved in legal proceedings related to automatism. REM sleep behaviour disorder (RSBD) (Mahowald and Schenck, 1999) also results in violence in sleep, typically punching or kicking the bed partner, but the behaviors tend to be less complex than SWSAD. Nocturnal seizures may also be associated with violent or injurious behaviors, but again are less likely to result in violence towards others. Complex behaviour may occur as part of incomplete arousal or sleep inertia in the obstructive sleep apnea syndrome (OSAS). Finally, alcohol or drugs may precipitate confusional arousal. From a medicolegal point of view this adds another layer of complexity to issue of intent (Mahowald and Schenck, 1999a).

The underlying pathophysiology and neurobiology of sleep violence is well described. Complex emotional and motor behaviors can originate from more primitive structures without involvement of the cortex (LeDoux, 1987). Animal studies provide insights into sleep-related violent behaviors in humans, and structural lesions at multiple levels of the nervous system may result in wakeful violence (Weiger and Bear, 1988).

Specific incidents reported in the medical or legal literature include somnambulistic homicide or attempted homicide, murders and other crimes with sleep drunkenness, suicide, or fear of committing suicide. These episodes may be drug induced. Inappropriate sexual behaviors have also been reported during the sleep state, presumably the results of an admixture of wakefulness and sleep.

In one case, where the confusional arousal defense was used, the defendant drove 23 km, killed his mother-in-law, and attempted to kill his father-in-law. He was acquitted with somnambulism as the legal defense (Broughton *et al*, 1994). In another case, a confusional arousal attributed to underlying, documented, severe, untreated obstructive sleep apnea was offered as a criminal defense for a man who fatally shot his wife during his usual sleeping hours. This individual was found guilty (Noffinger and Wettstein, 1995).

However, the sleep specialist should not jump to conclusions that every case of apparent sleep-related violence is genuine and has a clinical basis. Malingering must also be considered in cases of apparent sleep-related violence. In one Australian case, SWSAD was used as a defence against a murder charge. However, evidence was successfully introduced clearly showing a knife had been placed under a pillow during wakefulness in a premeditated fashion. The expert evaluation process outlined by Mahowald and Schenk provides a systematic method of minimizing the risk of malingering being confused with reality (Mahowald and Schenck, 1999a; 1999b). In addition, although not exactly a direct form of sleep violence, Munchausen syndrome by proxy has been documented as a true cause for reported sleep apnea and other unusual nocturnal spells in infants (Skau and Mouridsen, 1995). The recent Folbigg case in Australia, where a mother was found guilty of murdering her four infant children over a 6-year period, highlights the need for healthy scepticism by sleep specialists in this area.

Automatisms and the law

Fenwick has proposed the following definition of automatism (Fenwick, 1996):

> *An automatism is an involuntary piece of behavior over which an individual has no control. The behavior is usually inappropriate to the circumstances, and may be out of character for the individual. It can be complex, coordinated, and apparently purposeful and directed, though lacking in judgement. Afterwards the individual may have no recollection or only partial and confused memory for his actions. In organic automatisms there must be some disturbance of brain function sufficient to give rise to the above features.*

As discussed above, the medical view of automatism is clear, involving complex behavior in the absence of conscious awareness or intent. However, legally, there are two forms of automatism, sane and insane (Yeo, 2002). This is a complex area of law but basically a sane automatism is said to result from an external factor. In contrast, insane automatism results from an internal or endogenous cause. Mahowald and Schenk ((Mahowald and Schenck 1999a; 1999b) give examples of criminal acts resulting from altered behavior caused by hypoglycemia. If hypoglycemia is induced by injection or too much insulin, the verdict would be a sane automatism. If the same act was secondary to hypoglycemia caused by an insulinoma, that would be an insane automatism. The importance lies in the consequences of each verdict. A person in whom a sleep-walking/confusional arousal defence is successful but a verdict of insane automatism is given, may face commitment to a mental hospital for an indefinite period. On the other hand, a sane automatism decision would be followed by acquittal without any compulsory medical follow-up. The hypoglycemia analogy is complicated by the fact that insulinoma may be removed and therefore any continued imprisonment unjustified if the hypoglycemia is cured. This medicolegal conundrum implies that criminal behavior associated with epilepsy is, by definition, an insane automatism (Brown and Bird, 2001).

With regards to sleep disorders, divergent views and case law exist. In the Burgess case (Ridgway, 1996), the accused attacked his female friend who had fallen asleep watching TV. Burgess hit her over the head with a bottle and video-recorder and tried to strangle her. When she cried out, Burgess came to his senses and voluntarily called for an ambulance. A verdict of insane automatism was made favouring the expert testimony of the prosecution psychiatrist. The Court of Appeal accepted that evidence as properly leading to a conclusion that Burgess was:

> ... *suffering an abnormality or disorder, albeit transitory, due to an internal factor, whether functional or organic, which had manifested itself in violence. It was a disorder or abnormality which might recur, although the possibility of it recurring in the form of serious violence was unlikely. Therefore, since this was a legal problem to be decided on legal principles, ... on those principles, the answer was as the judge found it to be.*

In contrast, in the Parks case (Broughton *et al*, 1994) the Canadian Supreme Court upheld the verdict of not guilty on the basis of a sane automatism. The defendant was accused of having stabbed to death his mother-in-law and injuring his father-in-law in the early hours of the morning. They held that Parks was sleep-walking at the relevant time and that sleep-walking is not a neurological, psychiatric or other illness: it is a sleep disorder common in children and also found in adults. They held that there is no medical treatment apart from good health practices. It is important to note that the expert evidence in these two cases is markedly divergent.

In a recent Australian case, a confusional arousal defence was used against a charge of indecent assault. The defendant had a clear history of 'sleep-sex' with previous partners and a strong corroborated history of sleep-walking. Experts for the prosecution and defence stated that the assaults were likely to have occurred during a SWSAD episode. However, the prosecution highlighted the risks of recurrent sexual assaults and sought a verdict of insane automatism and indefinite imprisonment.

As pointed out by Mahowald and Schenk, (Mahowald and Schenck 1999b), if SWSAD is an insane automatism, then a significant percentage of the general population is legally insane. Although each case must be decided on its merits, nocturnal sleep-related violence is hardly ever a reappearing phenomenon (Guilleminault *et al*, 1995; Mahowald and Schenck, 1999). It is also reasonable to expect the defendant to undertake appropriate medical treatment and supervision. SWSAD also tends to decrease in frequency over time.

A number of medicolegal solutions have been suggested for the internal versus external, insane versus sane controversy (Mahowald and Schenck, 1999a, 1999b). These issues were highlighted by the acquittal of rock musician, Peter Buck, from a charge of assaulting flight attendants on a first-class transatlantic flight. Buck's legal team successfully used a defence of non-insane automatism, claiming that he was in a state of confusional arousal due to a use of a zolpidem tablet and some alcohol. Presumably non-insane automatism was successful as opposed to insane automatism due to the use of an exogenous agent, zolpidem. Ironically, Mr Buck is a guitarist for the band REM.

Clinical evaluation of sleep violence

Mahowald and Schenk (Mahowald and Schenck, 1999a; 1999b; 2000) have proposed a series of guidelines for the evaluation of sleep violence from a medicolegal viewpoint. These are:

- There should be reason (by history or by formal sleep laboratory evaluation) to suspect a *bona fide* sleep disorder.
- Similar episodes, with benign or morbid outcome, should have occurred previously.
- SWSAD may begin in adulthood.
- The duration of the action is usually brief (minutes).
- The behavior is usually abrupt, immediate, impulsive, and senseless — without apparent motivation.
- Although ostensibly purposeful, it is completely inappropriate to the total situation, out of (waking) character for the individual, and without evidence of premeditation.
- The victim is someone who merely happened to be present and who may have been the stimulus for the arousal.
- Immediately after return of consciousness, there is perplexity or horror, without attempt to escape, conceal, or cover up the action.
- There is evidence of lack of awareness on the part of the individual during the event.
- There is usually some degree of amnesia for the event, however, this amnesia need not be complete.
- In the case of sleep-talking or sleep-walking or sleep drunkenness, the act may: (a) occur on awakening (rarely immediately upon falling asleep) and usually at least one hour after sleep onset; (b) occur on attempts to awaken the subject; and (c) have been potentiated by alcohol ingestion, sedative or hypnotic administration or prior sleep deprivation.
- Clinical evaluation should include a complete review of sleep or wake complaints from both the victim and the bed partner (if available). This should be followed by a thorough general physical, neurological and psychiatric examination. The diagnosis may only be suspected clinically. A full polygraphic study employing an extensive scalp electroencephalogram (EEG) at a paper speed of 15 mm/s, electromyographic monitoring of all four extremities, and continuous audiovisual recording are mandatory for correct diagnosis in atypical cases.
- Establishing the diagnosis of nocturnal seizures may be particularly difficult. A normal sleep study does not exclude the possibility of SWSAD, and typical findings of abrupt confusional arousal may be lacking despite stimuli or multiple nights of monitoring. One major purpose of a sleep investigation is to determine the presence of other complicating sleep disorders.
- Given the skeptical nature of the public to the concept of crime explained by automatism due to a sleep disorder, evaluation of the defendant should take place in an expert sleep disorders center with multidisciplinary skills to maximize credibility.

Ron Grunstein and Elizabeth Ellis

Medicolegal consequences of sleepiness

Daytime sleepiness, secondary to a sleep disorder or sleep deprivation, is extremely common in modern society. Sleepiness or 'operator fatigue' is a common cause of accidents and, as such, has major implications for the legal system. Increasingly, the consequences of impaired performance caused by sleepiness are resulting in legal action. This is particularly true with fall-asleep motor vehicle accidents (MVAs) and in sleepiness-induced human error in the workplace. Such accidents may range from major disasters such as the *Exxon Valdez* attributed, in part, to human error due to sleep loss, or friendly fire accidents in the recent military action in Afghanistan.

Fatal accidents due to drivers falling asleep may have various causes but unrecognized or inadequately treated sleep disorders may be implicated (Mitler, 1996). Fall-asleep MVAs are one of the leading causes (as much as 25%) of fatal and non-fatal car crashes. Sleepiness in the workplace contributes significantly to between 30% and 90% of serious industrial accidents, including such memorable ones as Chernobyl, Three-Mile Island, *Exxon Valdez*, Bopal and the *Challenger* disaster (Leger, 1994). The total cost of accidents related to sleepiness in the United States in 1988 was estimated to be between \$43 billion and \$56 billion (Leger, 1994). Certain occupations are plagued with higher fall-asleep MVAs than others, particularly the transport industry (Stoohs *et al*, 1995).

Given the financial implications, there is increasing involvement by the legal system in determining fault and compensation. However, there are limited precedents and case law as society comes to grips with these issues. No universally accepted guidelines are available for dealing with culpability. For instance, is falling asleep at the wheel in the same category of driving under the influence of alcohol? Or, is the fall-asleep MVA of a sleep-deprived shiftworker the fault of the worker or the employer who imposed the duty hours or requested a double shift?

Because lawmakers are becoming interested in this important problem, with particular reference to limiting the driving privileges of some individuals with disorders, some of these disorders (sleep apnea and narcolepsy) are discussed further.

While there is a wide clinical spectrum of sleepiness from neurophysiological impairment to falling asleep, there are two main manifestations of sleepiness that are particularly relevant for legal issues:

❖ *Excessive daytime sleepiness:* This can result in the drowsy sufferer falling asleep while at work, driving, or elsewhere. The most common causes of excessive daytime sleepiness include sleep loss due to social or work demands, insomnia or phase disturbances associated with jet lag or shift work or disorders that cause sleep fragmentation at night such as obstructive sleep apnea (American Thoracic Society, 1994).

❖ *Sleep attacks:* The concept that patients with certain sleep disorders such as narcolepsy may have sudden, irresistible episodes of sleep that occur without warning.

There is a wide range of legal implications for an individual with sleepiness, both for the company employing that individual and for the health practitioner treating that individual. Companies face a complex series of issues related to the safety of the individual and others. These include the manufacturer's liability for products which are rendered defective by a worker's lack of vigilance (a claim made in the Firestone tyre controversy), design defects which place a worker at risk of injury, and inadequate warnings where a person is not provided with adequate information (O'Keefe, 1996). Many of these issues are beyond the scope of this book but are, in part, dealt with elsewhere (O'Keefe, 1996).

Although this analysis focuses predominantly on the Australian legal system, similarities can be found within other justice systems. Australia focuses on the specific legal obligations (duty of care) of an individual with a sleep disorder, and those healthcare practitioners associated with that individual. Although there are related implications within the criminal law and, in particular, criminal negligence, the arguments presented here are largely confined to the context of the civil law within the common law principles. Liability under tort law and within statutes will be examined for the individual with sleep disorders, the employer and the treating practitioner.

Concepts of foreseeability and proximity

When discussing duty of care, there are two important concepts: forseeability and proximity. The legal issue of proximity is more complex than just physical closeness. Proximity can involve a circumstantial relationship between, for example, employer and employee, or a causal proximity where someone may have relied on another party to take care to avoid or prevent injury. In the case of a sleepy driver or worker who causes damage to another person, a test for liability may be readily satisfied by foreseeability without either physical or causal proximity required to be argued (Ellis and Grunstein, 2001). This chapter deals only with specific issues of proximity, in the context of the relationship between the practitioner and the patient. Proximity in the context of the relationship between employers and employees is reduced as an issue when specific legislation requires employers to ensure safe working systems.

Liability for injuries when an individual falls asleep

Every driver of a motor vehicle or user of potentially hazardous machinery, whether or not they suffer from a sleep disorder, has a responsibility not to cause harm to those around them under statutory obligations and as a civil duty of care. The standard (of care) is an objective one, however, the courts have some discretion in setting this standard. The duty of care has been described by Justice Mason in *Council of the Shire of Wyong* v *Shirt* (*Council of Shire of Wyong* v *Shirt* 1980), as well as those factors that must be considered when weighing up whether negligence has occurred. In the Shirt case, the plaintif, who had suffered a cervical spine injury when diving in the shallow water of a local lake, claimed to having been misled by a sign erected by the council. The duty of care is described in two parts: that there is 'a sufficient relationship of proximity' between the parties and that a reasonable person in the defendant's position 'would foresee that carelessness on his part may be likely to cause damage to the plaintiff' (*Council of Shire of Wyong* v *Shirt* 1980).

Justice Mason (*Council of Shire of Wyong* v *Shirt* 1980) also distinguished between foreseeability and the probability of a risk of injury. Even though the probability may be very small, it may be that a reasonable person would respond to it, especially if the consequences were great. He went on to say:

> *The perception of the reasonable man's response calls for a consideration of the magnitude of the risk and the degree of the probability of its occurrence, along with the expense, difficulty and inconvenience of taking alleviating action and any other conflicting responsibilities which the defendant may have.*

In examining the test of reasonable foreseeability with sleep disorders, it is necessary to weigh up the likelihood that a driver may fall asleep at the wheel of a vehicle and have an accident and cause injury as a result of this. The courts in a number of countries have held that a driver is not liable for damages that occur as a result of a sudden unexpected event. With regard to whether falling asleep at the wheel, is an unexpected event or not for an otherwise well individual, legal opinion has been divided and the prevailing view of the High Court of Australia (*Jiminez* v *The Queen* 1992) is at odds with medical evidence (Desai *et al*, 2003).

Legal opinion has been divided as to whether falling asleep at the wheel is forseeable. In an early Canadian civil judgement, *Girling* versus *Howden* (*Girling* v *Howden* 1949), it was found that there was gross negligence in a driver falling asleep because the court assumed that a driver would know of the risks of falling asleep when driving at night and must have disregarded that risk. The judge commented that when there was every indication that the driver might fall asleep, to ignore these risks was negligent.

> *The magnitude of these plainly foreseeable dangerous risks, in my judgement, imposed a duty upon the appellant driver to take more than ordinary care to ensure that he would not fall asleep at the wheel while driving. His failure to do so is consistent only with his disregard of them as if they did not exist at all. To my mind his conduct in failing to do so, was 'a very marked departure from the standards by which responsible and competent people in charge of motor cars habitually govern themselves'.*

In this case, the judges were explicit in their condemnation of drivers who placed the public at grave risk of injury. In contrast, recent judgments have been far more qualified. In a very similar case, *Kay* versus *Mills*, Justice Milvain (*Kay* v *Mills* 1961) was prepared to accept that sleep could have come upon the defendant without any warning of drowsiness. Justice Milvain held that the judgment in *Girling* versus *Howden* did not apply because the driver claimed that sleep came upon him suddenly and without warning and that he (the driver) 'felt unconcerned at all times'. In addition, the passenger testified that there had been nothing in the driver's manner to cause concern. In 1992, in *Jiminez* versus *the Queen* (*Jiminez* v *the Queen* 1992a), the High Court of Australia appeared to agree with the approach of Justice Milvain in a criminal case with similar facts. A driver had set out at 11.00PM to drive from the Gold Coast to Sydney (a drive of approximately 1000 km) after having a nap the previous afternoon and subsequently staying awake. The driver claimed he had fallen asleep without warning after two and a half hours of driving time, at 6.00AM in the morning. When commenting on the findings of a previous case, Mason CJ stated:

> *If, in the passage which we have set out above, his Lordship was saying that falling asleep*

at the wheel is inevitably preceded by a period of drowsiness such that the driver has an opportunity to stop, then we are, with respect, unable to agree.

(Jiminez v *The Queen* 1992a)

The judges took note of the fact that the defendant had slept the afternoon before, had driven in shifts and claimed to have had no warning or concern. In finding for the driver, this judgment established that driving dangerously by falling asleep at the wheel is a strict liability offence in that the prosecution did not have to prove intent, but the defendant could plead the common law defence of an honest and reasonable mistake. In this judgment, the High Court also sought to draw the distinction between driving while sleepy and driving in a manner dangerous to the public because of that sleepiness. The implication of their findings was that a driver is not necessarily dangerous just because they have warnings that they are getting sleepy. A driver is only driving dangerously or without due care when they are so tired that their driving is dangerous. They went on to say that just because an accident is caused by a driver falling asleep, it does not mean that the driver has had sufficient warning to allow him or her to stop driving.

There has also been a technical argument as to whether or not at the point of falling asleep, driving is a voluntary act, akin to automatism (McCutcheon, 1997). If a person is unconscious or asleep, they cannot be said to have voluntary control of a vehicle or machine and, therefore, intend to perform a criminal act. The earlier judges held that drivers were responsible for allowing themselves to fall into an involuntary state. These judgements are predicated on the 'prior fault' principle (McCutcheon, 1997) that there was a period of time prior to being asleep, of voluntary conduct when a person chose to take the risk of continuing to drive. Further decisions seem to be predicated on the fact that an individual cannot be liable for damage that is caused when asleep that is, during involuntary driving (Kroon, 1990). There appears to be agreement that sleep is an involuntary state. The argument regarding liability rests on whether during the period prior to falling asleep a reasonable person could have and should have taken measures to reduce the risk.

Legal opinion is divided — the first opinion holds that falling asleep at the wheel is always foreseeable because of either symptoms or circumstances. The second opinion supports the possibility that sleep might suddenly occur without warning, such as with syncope or a seizure. The first opinion implies that, regardless of the circumstances, for the ordinary person to allow themselves to fall asleep at the wheel is negligent. In Australia, this first earlier view is encapsulated by the judgment in *Virgo* versus *Elding*, where appellant in that case had fallen asleep and his car had run off the road into a watercourse. In that case, Justice Angus Parsons stated:

It is manifest that a driver who goes to sleep at the wheel is driving without due care, and how sleep came upon him, or whether there was any premonition of its approach is an irrelevant matter.

(Virgo v *Elding* 1939)

The second opinion has been accepted because other judges are not prepared to acknowledge that there is an absolute rule that no extenuating circumstances could come to bear on a case of falling asleep behind the wheel. Although this view allows for the possibility of pathological conditions such as narcolepsy to suddenly be expressed, it is difficult to justify under ordinary circumstances and does not agree with medical evidence (Desai *et al*, 2003; Reyner and Horne 1998; Staysafe 46, 1998).

In the case of *R* versus *Hart* in the United Kingdom, there was strong support for the concept of foreseeability in a fall-asleep MVA. This accident attracted attention as the fall-asleep episode while driving a car triggered a train disaster resulting in multiple deaths and injury and, arguably, the biggest motor insurance claim in insurance history (http://www.guardian.co.uk/ selby/story/0,7369,618570,00.html). The defendant, Hart, was found guilty of causing death by dangerous driving. He admitted that he had not slept the night before the crash and had spent five hours talking on the phone. The jury rejected Hart's claims that he needed little sleep, was used to staying up all night, and was so excited that he could not have dozed off.

Recent medical evidence (Reyner and Horne, 1998) has shown that healthy people do not fall asleep without significant symptoms of sleepiness for some period of time. In this study, twenty-eight healthy drivers had their sleep restricted to five hours on the night before a driving simulation beginning at 14.30 hours. None of these subjects were on medication, none were daytime nappers and all were volunteers recruited by advertisement. The subjects were required to 'drive' an (immobile) car for two hours under realistic simulation of a dual carriage road with gentle bends, at their usual speed between lane markers. The frequency of both minor and major driving incidents increased with reports of increasing sleepiness. A minor incident was classified if one car wheel crossed the lane and a major incident was classified when all wheels ran out of the lane. Twelve subjects had major incidents that were related to their sleepiness. In each case, these incidents were preceded by periods where the subjects acknowledged that they were sleepy. Indeed, these subjects had forewarning of moderately severe sleepiness on average 45.5 minutes prior to the major incident. This would certainly amount to sufficient warning to allow a driver to stop driving and take some remedial action.

One of the authors of this study, Professor Horne, commented in correspondence with the Staysafe committee of the NSW Parliament (Staysafe 46, 1998):

> *... [the] denial of feeling sleepy before the accident is specious... I am all too aware of the Jiminez case, and in my opinion it sets a bad precedent for further cases in Australia... Here [in the UK] someone falling asleep at the wheel and having a serious accident will be prosecuted. Our legal precedents are that such a driver can be presumed to be aware of prior sleepiness, especially if they were driving in the small hours of the morning, or following long working hours.*

The consequences of the decision of the High Court in Australia have raised considerable public concern (Desai *et al*, 2003; Staysafe 46, 1998). In NSW, a significant number of driving-related offences, which may have been charged under section 52A of the Crimes Act (Crime Act 1900), have been the subject of successful application that there be no further proceedings because of sleep or black-outs (Gray, 2003).

In addition, there have been a series of unsuccessful prosecutions or successful appeals (*Jiminez* v *the Queen* 1992) based on the defence that the driver fell asleep without warning or did not remember. It appears that the prosecution now has to prove beyond reasonable doubt that the driver did not honestly believe that he was fit to drive or, if he did, that they must prove beyond reasonable doubt that it was unreasonable for him to believe so. The High Court by its decision appears to have established a precedent which is not consistent with effective public policy nor with, in some cases, effective justice. There is confusion on this issue in the legal context (Desai *et al*, 2003).

Another area of controversy is whether patients with sleep disorders, such as undiagnosed sleep apnea or narcolepsy, have the same awareness of impending sleep as those without these disorders. Although the courts seem to accept that these drivers have the propensity to fall asleep or black out without warning, until recently Australian Motor Traffic authorities have not seen fit to subject these people to medical examinations or withdraw their licenses (Desai *et al*, 2003; Staysafe 46, 1998). It cannot be effective public policy for drivers to be able to claim a condition that comes upon them without warning to avoid prosecution and still be able to continue to drive with all the attributable risks that that entails.

The question now arises as to whether an illness might increase the likelihood of falling asleep or blacking out and influence foreseeability. If a driver knew he or she was ill, but not the precise nature of the illness, and had experienced some symptoms but not the black out which caused the accident, this may be classed as an 'inevitable accident' and the driver would not be held to blame (*Smith* v *Lard* 1962).

On the other hand, an individual who is aware that they have a serious condition, even if their medical practitioner does not warn them specifically about driving, may be held liable. In *Gordon* versus *Wallace* (*Gordon* v *Wallace* 1973), the driver had been treated for ten years for high blood pressure and in a two-year period prior to the accident had had a cerebral thrombosis, angina, a heart attack and congestive heart failure. The evidence established that the driver had suffered a cardiac arrest just before hitting and injuring a pedestrian walking in a marked cross-walk. Justice Keith found:

> *I am firmly of the opinion that in driving his car at all, with his knowledge of the history of his heart disease and the repeated disabling attacks that he had suffered over a period of five years, and in the absence of specific medical advice to him that he was fit to drive, Mr Wallace was negligent in that he was doing something that a reasonably prudent man would not do in the circumstances, having regard to the duty he owed to other users of the highway.*

If a person is ill or infirm, the chance that that person may lose control of the vehicle increases. They may, however, be unaware of their diagnosis. It has been held that a person is not liable if they are not aware of their illness (Britts, 1998). On the other hand, an individual with sleep disorders may not be aware of their specific diagnosis although they may be aware of their symptoms of excessive daytime sleepiness. Mr Ian Callinan QC (now a Justice of the High Court of Australia) is quoted (Callinan, 1993) as saying:

> *A driver who suspects that he might suffer sleep apnea can hardly claim that if he is overtaken by sleep at the wheel he has been overtaken by a sudden and unpredictable event. Such a driver runs the serious risk of being charged in respect of the accident caused by his falling asleep.*

In addition, people with known illnesses that can affect their fitness to drive, would be expected to take special care not to put themselves or others at risk. Readily identifiable community-based campaigns exist in Australia for all drivers such as the 'Stop, revive, survive' slogan and 'driver reviver' stations on the roadside. Specific regulations may apply to commercial drivers such as the Motor Traffic Amendment (Driving Hours) Regulation 1998 (Motor Traffic Amendment 1998).

These regulations provide for maximum driving and work times, and minimum rest times as well as stipulating the obligations for medical examination and fatigue management training.

If an individual is made aware of their diagnosis and the risks, can society expect that they would seek treatment, or employ strategies to prevent falling asleep at the wheel or avoid driving long distances? From a public safety perspective it is easy to confirm that they should do all of the above, particularly avoid long-distance driving. When, however, an individual's livelihood is dependent on their continuing to drive long distances, personal welfare and employment security may be weighed by the driver as being of greater concern than the risks of injury to others.

In summary, everyone has a responsibility not to ignore the risks of driving when sleepy as the exact moment of falling asleep may be difficult to predict and prevent. An individual who has a condition that increases the risk of sleepiness and injury to others does have a special obligation to take effective measures to reduce that risk. The High Court in Australia in the case of *Jiminez* versus *The Queen*, by clearing the way for falling asleep at the wheel to be classed as a strict liability offence, appears to be at odds with legal opinion in other countries and medical opinion. The decision has created policy concerns in that drivers potentially have a means of avoiding responsibility for causing injury which is contrary to the public interest.

Liability of a company when an employee falls asleep

As in many countries, the Australian Federal, and all state and territory governments have legislation designed to protect employees from injury at work. In NSW, sections of the Occupational Health and Safety Act (Occupational Health and Safety Act 1983) include obligations for employers to ensure the health and safety of their employees, and employers must maintain safe systems of work to achieve this. Commonwealth of Australia provisions (Occupational Health and Safety Act) extend the obligations to prevent accidents or injury to members of the general public:

> *An employer must take all reasonably practicable steps to ensure that persons at or near a workplace under the employer's control who are not the employer's employees or contractors are not exposed to risks to their health or safety arising from the conduct of the employer's undertaking.*

These Commonwealth provisions are incorporated into the legislation of each state and territory with minor variations (Johnston, 1995). If a company's workforce is comprised of contract labour, the company may try to shift the responsibility for injuries and associated health risks to the source of the contract labour. The High Court of Australia defines an employee as someone who is engaged to work for the company as opposed to someone who is engaged for a specific job (Wallace, 1995). A significant test in determining employment is the degree of control over the working conditions of the worker (Wallace, 1995). Therefore, a company which sets up schedules which necessitate the drivers employed by its contractors to speed or work unsafe hours will still be liable for damages caused (TNT Management, 1996).

An employer is liable if an employee with a known sleep disorder causes injury to himself, fellow workers or the general public. This liability may hold because of either a failure to implement safe systems of work (Trindade and Cane, 1993) under statutory provisions or under the ordinary principles of vicarious liability in the civil courts. Mr Ian Callinan QC has stated:

> *An employer will owe a duty of care in respect of the sleep apnoea of any employee if that condition poses, and realises a threat, not only to the safety and health of other employees, but also to the employee himself suffering the condition.*

(Callinan, 1993)

The extent to which an employer will be required to accept liability will be influenced by a number of factors. These include the extent to which the implications of the condition is known and understood generally; the extent to which the condition is suspected or identified in an individual employee; the extent of a proper screening and treatment program and the way in which risk management programs have been implemented (National Road Transport Commission, 1993; Queensland Transport, 1993; Staysafe, 1994).

Guidelines established by the National Road Transport Commission (National Road Transport Commission, 1991) state that commercial transport drivers must have a medical examination to assess their fitness to drive. Within these guidelines it states that drivers must not drive with obstructive sleep apnea (OSA) unless treatment is effective (National Road and Transport Commission, 1994), a similar criterion to that of epilepsy. Conditional licenses are available with evidence that the symptoms of these illnesses are controlled. In contrast, individuals with narcolepsy are not allowed to hold a commercial vehicle license and there are no provisions for conditional licenses.

These guidelines were established for doctors giving reports at the request of authorities. The role of the medical practitioner is to decide whether the criteria are met and the authority decides what action is to be taken. The effectiveness of these medical examinations are potentially limited if they are done only at the time when a driver first receives their license. Many sleep disorders are acquired over time and may not be expressed at the early stages of a driving career. Although some transport companies do require annual screens, most use questionnaires which rely on self-reporting of symptoms. Even if specific questions on sleep disorders are included, under-reporting of snoring and sleepiness is a feature of sleep assessments (Walsleben, 1992). More objective indicators such as the body mass index (BMI) or neck size are also required to determine risk. Despite their limitations, these guidelines do encourage all practitioners to ask their patients about occupation when examining them for new illnesses or during temporary impairment, which assists in identifying people at risk at a later stage.

Under other circumstances, unless the requirement for screening for a particular disease is contained in the contract of employment, there may be no legal means of requiring an employee to undertake testing. The National Road Transport Commission Guidelines emphasize that the medical examinations are designed to protect the public and not to be used as a barrier to employment (National Road and Transport Commission, 1994). If employers have continuing concerns they may feel obliged to remove an employee from a certain position. If the employee is aggrieved by that decision, the situation would need to be resolved between the parties. It may come down to the conflicting issues of an individual's right to refuse a particular medical assessment and an employer's concern for the safety of the public, the individual and company property. The employer's rights to terminate employment under these exact conditions have not been tested in the courts. In considering this particular conflict of interests, Mr Ian Callinan QC states:

> *My opinion is, that so horrendous are the other potential consequences, so prevalent is the condition now, and so varied are the symptoms anyway, that a responsible employer would be entitled to insist upon, and an employee/driver not entitled to decline, participating in appropriate screening.*
>
> (Callinan, 1993)

Apart from the direct legal consequences, it may well be in a company's interest to monitor the health of individuals and their response to treatment for insurance purposes. Insurance companies may be able to deny liability for payment of damages if the risk of specific conditions is not disclosed or if treatment has been unsuccessful (Bennett, 1994). The statutory duty to disclose (Insurance Contracts Act 1984) obliges employers in Australia to inform the insurers of anything that they know, or might reasonably be expected to know, which might influence the insurer's decision to accept the risk of insurance. As public awareness about sleep disorders increases, it is more likely that insurance companies will contest that employers should have known about the risks of accidents in susceptible employees.

The most effective means of determining risk in sleep disorders such as sleep apnea is unclear. It would be economically unreasonable to expect a company to perform polysomnography on all its employees. Moreover, the individual patient with identifiable OSA is unlikely to have had a fall-asleep accident in the past or have one in the future, despite evidence that they are, indeed, at higher risk. This emphasizes the need both medically and legally to put in place appropriate, medicolegally reasonable risk stratification policies.

Liability of health practitioners

Most considerations of duty of care are related to the direct duty owed to the individual in the care of the practitioner. From time to time issues arise as to the duty to a third party, such as a spouse or family member, particularly if they are also in the care of the same practitioner. More recently, the duty to warn third parties who may be completely outside the (therapeutic) care of the practitioner (ie. other members of the public) has been raised. Another consideration is the duty to protect the general public by reporting specific conditions or behaviors that pose a threat to an appropriate authority. In many instances this need has been met by legislation; for example, with infectious diseases (Public Health Act 1991).

Duty to warn the patient

Health practitioners have a duty of care to their patients to provide treatment at the prevailing, acceptable standard. In Australia, health practitioners have broad guidelines on the type of information to be given to patients (Australian Professional Liability 1998). These include the likely consequences of not following the proper diagnostic procedure or treatment, or not having a procedure or treatment at all. General practitioners are not expected to recognize or manage cases of sleep-disordered breathing (American Thoracic Society, 1994). They are, however, expected to refer them to a specialist if they suspect the diagnosis. In the United Kingdom, however, clinicians are required to advise sleepy patients with OSA that they should not drive until treatment is effective (George *et al*, 2002; Taylor, 1995). In addition, the American Thoracic Society guidelines are clear (American Thoracic Society, 1994) on how specilists can reduce the risk of injury in people who have sleep-disordered breathing. These guidelines include an obligation to assess thoroughly, provide a precise diagnosis, inform the person of the risks of inadequate treatment including driving hazards, inform them of the risks of treatment and to ensure that they are adequately treated. This issue has been the subject of a recent international viewpoint manuscript (George *et al*, 2002). It is also important for the practitioner to follow up and monitoring patients with sleep disorders to ensure that treatment is effective and the individual is safe to drive.

Practitioners are also obliged to warn patients if a proposed treatment, such as a course of medication, might incidentally exacerbate sleepiness (O'Keefe, 1996). This standard of care is even higher if the practitioner is aware that an individual is at increased risk because of pre-existing sleep disorders. These obligations are clear when, for example, a physician prescribes medications such as benzodiazapines which increase the risk of accidents (Barbone *et al*, 1998). Physicians are encouraged to warn their patients not to drive when taking these drugs, particularly if they also take alcohol (O'Neil, 1998). In other areas the relationships are not as clear. A considerable amount of research is needed on the associations between the risk of accidents and behaviors such as sleep deprivation or alcohol and drug-taking in people with sleep disorders.

Practitioners who fail to provide adequate warning to a person about their own condition may also breach the duty that is owed to a third party. For example, a practitioner is aware that a patient of his is at grave risk of accident while driving and that this patient is the driver of a school bus. If the pratitioner fails to warn the patient not to drive due to the increased risk of accident, he, the practitioner, may be liable for any injuries to the third parties as it is reasonable to expect that he should have foreseen that an accident involving the bus could have occurred. This breach of duty of care to third parties is different to a breach of confidentiality to a third party, or a duty to disclose to a third party.

Duty to warn other members of the public

The duty of confidentiality is a fundamental ethical principle dating back to Hippocrates and currently expressed in the Australian Medical Association Code of Ethics (Australian Medical Association, 1996) as:

> *[I]n general, keep in confidence information derived from your patient, or from a colleague regarding your patient, and divulge it only with the patient's permission, except when a court demands.*

The logic of preserving trust between practitioner and patient during situations that do pose a risk to public safety is persuasive. If people do not feel secure in that relationship, they may not openly disclose their symptoms; they may not be treated thoroughly, and they may remain an increasing risk to themselves and to the general public.

However, the time-honoured principle of patient confidentiality has been amended to imply that it is acceptable to breach confidentiality 'where the health of others is at risk' (Australian Medical Association, 1996) which introduces a significant element of discretion. A practitioner may feel that they have an ethical duty to warn a third party, particularly if the third party is also in the care of the practitioner. If a practitioner fails to warn a third party in their care (eg. a family member of the patient with a sleep disorder), could that person sue the practitioner for breach of duty of care if that person was injured in an accident that could have been prevented had the practitioner given the warning (Intergoverment Committee, 1992)? There is currently no legislative protection in this case for either breach of confidence or the breach of duty for a failure to warn a third party. There are, however, criteria for how and when to notify partners of people with AIDS which may provide some guidance (Intergoverment Committee, 1992).

In the context of risk of accidents because of sleep disorders these criteria would be:

- the person has refused to notify those people at risk
- a real risk of injury exists
- counselling to achieve a change in behavior has failed
- advice from colleagues or an institutional ethics committee has been sought
- the person has been told that notification will occur after a reasonable time
- those notified should be obliged to keep confidential the information revealed.

It is currently debatable whether a practitioner has a duty to warn a third party who is not in the direct care of the practitioner. The Tarasoff (*Tarasoff* v *Regent* 1974) case in the USA involved a psychiatrist who was held liable for a breach of duty to a third party because the injuries were foreseeable to an individual who was identified clearly to the practitioner and, therefore, held to be in a relationship of sufficient proximity.

On 27 October 1969, Prosenjit Poddar killed Tatiana Tarasoff. The plaintiffs, Tatiana's parents, allege that two months earlier Poddar confided his intention to kill Tatiana to Dr Lawrence Moore, a psychologist employed by the Cowell Memorial Hospital at the University of California at Berkeley. They alleged that, on Moore's request, the campus police briefly detained Poddar, but released him when he appeared rational. They further claimed that Dr Harvey Powelson, Moore's superior, directed that no further action be taken to detain Poddar. No one warned the plaintiffs of Tatiana's peril. This case established that a practitioner may be liable for a person's risk-taking behaviors once injury to third parties becomes reasonably foreseeable. The precedent created by the Tarasoff case may not be as strong in some countries, such as Australia (Mendelson, 1991).

In *Duncan* versus *Medical Practitioners Disciplinary Tribunal*, Justice Jeffries described in detail the obligations to preserve confidentiality (*Duncan* v *Medical Practitioners* 1986). Duncan was a registered medical practitioner in a small rural community. Henry, one of his patients, was a bus driver by occupation and had operated a passenger service business for 30 years. In 1982, Henry suffered two heart attacks and was attended by Duncan as his general practitioner. In December 1982, Henry underwent a triple coronary artery bypass operation. After the successful operation, Henry obtained a medical certificate from the surgeon, enabling him to obtain a licence to drive passenger service vehicles.

On 27 April 1983, Henry intended to take his bus to Auckland on a charter trip. On the day before the trip, Duncan spoke to a woman who was to be a passenger on the chartered bus and told her that Henry was not fit to drive and could have a heart attack at any time. Duncan also spoke to Henry and, on discovering that he had a licence to drive a passenger service vehicle, sought assistance from the local police constable to have Henry's licence revoked. Later Duncan asked a patient at his surgery to help him organize a petition to have Henry barred from driving passenger service vehicles; the patient refused. Henry successfully complained to the Medical Practitioners Disciplinary Committee that he was being unjustly victimized by Duncan and that there had been a breach of patient confidentiality.

Justice Jefferies qualified his statements by acknowledging that there could be exceptional circumstances and if they did arise, disclosure should be limited: 'a doctor who has decided to communicate should discriminate and ensure the recipient is a responsible authority' (*Duncan* v *Medical Practitioner* 1986).

When weighing the relative merits of a particular course of action Justice Jeffries advised:

> *The doctor must then exercise his professional judgement based on the circumstances, and if he fairly and reasonably believes such a danger exists, then he must act unhesitatingly to prevent injury or loss of life even if there is to be a breach of confidence.*
>
> (*Duncan* v *Medical Practitioner* 1986)

Duty to warn statutory roads and traffic authorities

Legislators have been sufficiently concerned with the need to protect the public from undue risk that they have made statutory provisions for practitioners to report individuals without those practitioners being liable for breach of confidentiality. Statutory provisions can range from those that allow practitioners indemnity if they do report drivers (permissive) to those that state that they must report (mandatory). Within these options there can be categorical or functional reporting. Categorical reporting is required upon diagnosis of a condition and therefore allows no discretion on behalf of the practitioner except in the diagnosis itself. A well-established class of categorical reporting, for example, is that health practitioners are obliged to notify health authorities of certain infectious diseases. Functional reporting is when a person has a diagnosis and some form of functional impairment to warrant reporting. The American Thoracic Society (ATS) recommends functional reporting in their guidelines for example that OSA only be considered reportable when:

> *The patient has excessive daytime sleepiness and sleep apnea and a history of a motor vehicle accident or equivalent level of clinical concern and one of the following circumstances exists i) the patient's condition is untreatable or is not amenable to expeditious treatment (within two months of diagnosis) or ii) the patient is not willing to accept treatment or is unwilling to restrict driving until effective treatment has been instituted.*
>
> (American Thoracic Society, 1994)

Healthcare practitioners have a duty of care to their patients to provide advice and treatment at the prevailing, acceptable standard. A driver presenting with symptoms suggestive of OSA should be warned of the dangers of driving. The driver should also be warned about the early signs of drowsiness and the necessity to immediately stop driving if these occur. Finally, the driver should be referred to a sleep medicine specialist for assessment and further investigation. For medicolegal reasons, practitioners should carefully note advice about driving in patient records.

Previous national regulatory guidelines in Australia have been vague about the requirements for diagnosis of OSA and its implications for driving (Assessing Fitness to Drive, 1998; Desai *et al*, 2003; Ellis and Grunstein, 2001). A review by the Australian Sleep Association advised that the guidelines be updated to recommend that drivers proven to have OSA on polysomnography and who report or are shown to have excessive daytime sleepiness, should not drive until treatment is effective (Desai *et al*, 2003; George *et al*, 2002). The review also recommended that periodic review is required to ensure adequate treatment is maintained and that patients who do not comply with treatment while continuing to drive should be reported to licensing authorities. Although these recommendations on review and reporting are explicit, there is no clear evidence that every driver with OSA, with or without pathological sleepiness, has an increased MVA risk (George *et al*, 2002). Current national guidelines emphasize the responsibility of individuals to notify the relevant state or territory drivers' licensing authority of medical conditions that may affect their ability to drive safely, to comply with medical advice regarding satisfactory treatment, and not to pose a public risk (Assessing Fitness to Drive, 1998).

When an individual will not take responsibility for himself or herself and puts lives at risk, the Australian Medical Association Code of Ethics acknowledges that a practitioner may have an obligation to breach patient confidentiality to report the situation to the appropriate authorities (Australian Medical Association, 1996). In the case of drivers with OSA who report frequent sleepiness while driving, or MVAs caused by inattention or sleepiness, we believe a practitioner is ethically compelled to report these drivers if they do not comply with treatment or follow-up. Legislation in almost all Australian states and territories indemnifies medical practitioners in this situation (Desai *et al*, 2003; George *et al*, 2002).

There is a difference between the role and responsibilities of the general practitioner, the specialist and doctors engaged by companies for the specific purpose of screening employees. A general practitioner is not necessarily expected to be able to diagnose and assess the risks associated with complex sleep disorders. It may be difficult for them to assess the risk an individual poses to the public. They are, however, required to refer people on to specialists to have those assessments made. The standard of care expected of the specialist is greater and the obligations clearer. They must warn the individual and they may warn authorities when the risk of danger to the public outweighs the private interests of the person involved.

Conclusion

There is an increasing medicolegal workload involving issues pertinent to sleep medicine. Recent cases referred to the authors have included liability of a company for the quadriplegia sustained by a third party involved in road accident with one of its employees, a defence of extreme sleep deprivation and cognitive impairment in a young mother charged with stealing from a shop, a practitioner's failure to inform a patient about cognitive loss due to untreated sleep apnea and a defence of automatism against a charge of indecent assault where the victim was alleged to have been supplied a 'date-rape drug' beforehand. On a 'macro' scale, the legal issues in sleep research and sleep medicine are potentially enormous. Another dimension has been added, with the recognition of errors by the military due to sleep deprivation and use of ineffective countermeasures.

In the end, reasonable legal decision making and harm minimization, is only as good as the research and guidance offered by the medical field. As others have pointed out 'junk medicine' leads to 'junk justice' (Mahowald and Schenck, 2000). Finally, the escalating uncertainty and yet increasing liability in health care causes practitioners to avoid practising in certain areas of health care. This avoidance is neither in the public interest nor in the interests of the individuals needing help to improve their health and reduce their risk of injury. Health practitioners who work in sleep medicine need clearer legal guidance and adequate legislative protection when acting in the public interest.

References

American Thoracic Society (1994) Sleep apnea, sleepiness and driving risk. *Am J Respir Crit Care Med* **150**: 1463–73

Assessing Fitness to Drive (1998) Austroads Publication No AP – 56/98

Australian Medical Association (1996) *Code of Ethics*. Australian Medical Association, Sydney

Australian Professional Liability – Medical (1998) CCH Australia Ltd 40–100

Barbone F, MacMahon AD, Davey PG, Morris AD, Reid K, McDevith DG, MacDonald TM (1998) Association of road traffic accidents with benzodiazepine use. *Lancet* **352**: 1331–6

Bennett J (1994) Insuring for sleep disorders. In: *Staysafe report 1/51 Sleep Disorders, Driving Fatigue and Safe Driving*. New South Wales Parliamentary Joint Standing Committee on Road Safety, Sydney: 72–8

Britts MMG (1998) Traffic Law (New South Wales) (Sydney: LBC Information Services 7th edn, 1998) (2.2070)

Broughton R, Billings R, Cartwright R *et al* (1994) Homicidal somnambulism: A case report. *Sleep* **17**: 253

Brown S, Bird J (2001) Medicolegal aspects of epilepsy. *Seizure* **10**: 68–74

Callinan I (1993) Legal Issues: sleep apnoea and road safety. In: Lake RIE, ed. *Proceedings of a Seminar on Sleep Disorders and Road Safety*. Qld Transport Report RUB 93–1, 24—36

Council of the Shire of Wyong v *Shirt* (1980) 146 Commonwealth Law Reports 40

Crimes Act 1900 (NSW)

Desai AV, Ellis E, Wheatley JR, Grunstein RR (2003) Fatal distraction: a case series of fatal fall-asleep road accidents and their medicolegal outcomes. *Med J Aust* **178**(8): 396–9

Duncan v *Medical Practitioners Disciplinary Committee* [1986]1 NZ Law Reports 513 (NZHC)

Ellis ER, Grunstein RR (2001) Medicolegal aspects of sleep disorders: sleepiness and civil liability. *Sleep Med Rev* **5**(1): 33–46

Fenwick P (1996) Sleep and sexual offending. *Med Sci Law* **366**: 122

George CF, Findley LJ, Hack MA, McEvoy RD (2002) Across-country viewpoints on sleepiness during driving. *Am J Respir Crit Care Med* **165**(6): 746–9

Girling v *Howden* [1949] 3 Dominion Law Reports 262

Gordon v *Wallace* [1973] 42 Dominion Law Reports (3rd) 342

Grunstein R (2000) Guest editorial: Was OJ sleep-walking? *Sleep Med Rev* **4**: 319–20

Guillerninault C, Moscovitch A, Leger D (1995) Forensic sleep medicine: Nocturnal wandering and violence. *Sleep* **18**: 740

Insurance Contracts Act 1984 (Cth) s 21

Intergovernment Committee on AIDS, Legal Working Party Final Report (November 1992) 12–13 Recommendation 2.2

Jiminez v *the Queen* (1992) 173 Commonwealth Law Reports 572 FC 92/012

Jiminez v *the Queen* (1992) 173 CLR 572 FC 92/012a

Johnstone R (1995) *Occupational Health and Safety Law and Policy*. The Law Book Company, Sydney

Kay v *Mills* [1961] 28 Dominion Law Reports (2d) 554

Kroon [1990] 52 ACrimR 15

Leger D (1994) The cost of sleep-related accidents: A report for the National Commission on Sleep Disorders Research. *Sleep* **17**:84

LeDoux JE (1987) Emotion. In: Monteastle VB, Plum F, Geiger SR, eds. *Handbook of Physiology: The Nervous System: Higher Functions of the Brain, Part 1*. Williams and Wilkins, Baltimore: 419

Mahowald MW, Schenck CH (1996) NREM parasomnias. *Neurol Clin* **14**: 675

Mahowald MW, Schenck CH (1999) REM sleep behavior disorder. In: Kryger MH, Dement W, Roth T, eds. *Principles and Practice of Sleep Medicine*, edn 3. Saunders, Philadelphia

Mahowald MW, Schenck CH (1999) Sleep-related violence-forensic medicine issues. In: Chokroverty S, ed. *Sleep Disorders Medicine: Basic Science. Technical Considerations and Clinical Aspects*, edn 2. Butterworth-Heinemann, Boston: 729b

Mahowald MW, Schenk CH (2000) Parasomnias. Sleep-walking and the law. *Sleep Med Rev* 4(4): 321–39

Mahowald MW, Schenck CH (1999a) Violent parasomnias: Forensic medicine issues. In: Kryger MH, Roth T, Dement WC, eds. *Principles and Practice of Sleep Medicine*, edn 3. WB Saunders, Philadelphia

McCutcheon JP (1997) Involuntary conduct and the case of the unconscious 'driver': reflections on Jiminez. *Criminal Law J* **21**: 71–9

Mendelson D (1991) Could Tarasoff happen in Australia. *J Psychiatry Law* **19**: 38–59

Mitler MM (1996) Sleepiness and human behavior. *Curr Opin Pulm Med* **2**: 488

Motor Traffic Amendment (Driving Hours) Regulation 1998 (NSW)

National Road Transport Commission (1993) *Sleep Disorder, Driving Fatigue and Safe Driving*. National Road Transport Commission, Melbourne: April

National Road Transport Commission Act 1991 (Cth)

National Roads and Transport Commission Medical Examinations of Commercial Vehicle Drivers Nov 1994

Noffinger EA, Wettstein RM (1995) Homicidal behavior and sleep apnea; a case report and medicolegal discussion. *Sleep* **18**: 776

Occupational Health and Safety Act 1983 (NSW) s9–11

Occupational Health and Safety (CE) Act (Cth)

Ohayon MM, Caulet M, Priest RG (1997) Violent behavior during sleep. *J Clin Psychiatry* **58**: 369

O'Keefe R (1996) Sleep disorders in the law of torts. *J Law Med* **3**: 283–95

O'Neil D (1998) Benzodiazepine and driver safety. *Lancet* **352**: 1324–5

Public Health Act 1991 (NSW) s14

Queensland Transport November, 1993

Reyner LA, Horne JA (1998) Falling asleep whilst driving: are drivers aware of prior sleepiness? *Int J Legal Med* **111**(3): 120–3

Ridgway P (1996) Sleep-walking — Insanity or Automatism. Murdoch University Electronic Journal of Law. Vol 3 (www.murdoch.edu.au/elaw/issues/v3n1/ridgeway.html)

Skau K, Mouridsen SE (1995) Munchausen syndrome by proxy: A review. *Acta Paediatr* **84**(9): 977–82

Smith v *Lard* [1962] South Australian S Report 88

Staysafe 28 Seminar (1994) Parliament House, Sydney

Staysafe 46 Falling asleep at the wheel — legal and licensing implications of driver fatigue (1998) Report 19/51. Parliament House, Sydney

Stoohs RA, Bingham L, Itol A *et al* (1995) Sleep and sleep-disordered breathing in commercial long-haul truck drivers. *Chest* **107**: 1275

Tarasoff v *Regent (Board of the University of California)* 1 [1974] 118 Californian Reports 129; 529 P2d 553

Taylor JF (1995) *Medical Aspects of Fitness to Drive: a Guide for Medical Practitioners.* HMSO, London

TNT Management Pty Ltd v *Brown* (1996) 23 MVR 240

Trindade F, Cane P (1993) *Law of Torts in Australia*, 2nd edn. Oxford University Press, Melbourne

Virgo v *Elding South Australian* Supreme Court Reports 294, 1939

Wallace M (1995) *Health Care and the Law*. The Law Book Company, Sydney

Walsleben JA (1992) The measurement of daytime wakefulness. *Chest* **101**(4): 890–1

Weiger WA, Bear DR (1988) An approach to the neurology of aggression. *J Psychiatr Res* **22**: 85

Yeo S (2002) Clarifying automatism. *Int J Law Pyschiatry* **25**: 445–58

CHAPTER 14

Assisting ventilation during sleep

David Hillman and Amanda Piper

Non-invasive ventilation (NIV)

Hypoventilation results when respiratory muscles are weak or excessively loaded. If the imbalance between load and capacity to cope is severe enough, the patient is ventilator dependent and continuous ventilatory assistance is required until the underlying causes have successfully been addressed. Under such circumstances, assistance is most commonly applied in the form of intermittent positive pressure ventilation (IPPV) delivered invasively, via an endotracheal tube or tracheostomy, and the patient is nursed in an intensive care unit.

In more subtle forms of imbalance, the need for ventilatory assistance may be intermittent, often being restricted to sleep where, because of sleep-associated decreased ventilatory drive, increased diaphragm dependence and decreased upper airway patency, vulnerability to hypoventilation is greatest. In such cases, or when the requirement for continuous ventilatory assistance is likely to be short-term, non-invasive ventilatory assistance (NIV) may be used with IPPV delivered via a nose or face mask. Older forms of NIV using intermittent negative pressure applied to the chest wall by cuirass, poncho wrap or tank ventilators have been supplanted by this method.

This chapter discusses the indications and contraindications for NIV, the types of ventilator available for application of this therapy and how they are adjusted, commonly used mask interfaces, and other adjuncts to treatment commonly used in combination with it.

Use of NIV

The boundaries for use of NIV continue to expand in the treatment of both acute and chronic respiratory failure.

Acute respiratory failure

In acute respiratory failure, invasive ventilatory assistance (tracheal intubation and IPPV) remains the gold standard, although the need for it is often obviated by NIV. In such circumstances, NIV may be used as (British Thoracic Society [BTS] Guidelines, 2002):

- a holding measure to assist ventilation earlier than invasive ventilation would be considered
- a therapeutic trial with a view to intubation if it fails.
- a ceiling of treatment in patients who are not candidates for tracheal intubation by choice and/or severity of underlying disease or disability.

The most common clinical setting in which NIV is used acutely is acute exacerbations of chronic obstructive pulmonary disease (COPD). Several randomized controlled trials have demonstrated a decrease in hospital mortality, intubation rate and length of stay with this treatment (Bott *et al*, 1993; Brochard *et al*, 1995; Kramer *et al*, 1995; Plant *et al*, 2000b). Evidence for its efficacy in other acute settings is accumulating with the recent publication of controlled trials demonstrating its efficacy in a variety of conditions (Antonelli *et al*, 1998; Keenan and Brake, 1998). Indications include various causes of type 2 respiratory failure (primary ventilatory failure) including:

- acute neuromuscular disease (eg. Guillain Barre syndrome) (Vianello *et al*, 2000)
- infective exacerbations of cystic fibrosis or bronchiectasis
- decompensated obstructive sleep apnea/obesity hypoventilation
- chest trauma (Gregoretti *et al*, 1998)
- post-operative respiratory failure (Pennock *et al*, 1999)
- asthma (Fernandez *et al*, 2001).

It has also been used in cases of type 1 respiratory failure (primary hypoxaemic failure) including:

- pneumonia (Confaloneri *et al*, 1999)
- mucous plugging
- acute respiratory distress syndrome (Rocker *et al*, 1999)
- cardiogenic pulmonary edema (Masip *et al*, 2000)
- post-transplant and in immunocompromised patients (Antonelli *et al*, 2000; Hilbert *et al*, 2001).

In these acute settings, NIV is initially applied semi-continuously (see below) to support ventilation allowing time for treatment of the underlying condition to be implemented and take effect.

Chronic respiratory failure

NIV is generally considered in chronic respiratory failure where the underlying disorder is relatively stable, with sufficient wakeful ventilatory capacity not to be fully ventilator dependent, but associated with significant sleep-related hypoventilation. In such cases, ventilatory support is provided continuously during sleep and either intermittently or not at all during wakefulness, depending on the ability of the patient to maintain gas exchange unassisted.

Sleep is always a more vulnerable time for ventilation than wakefulness as the ventilatory drive is diminished, breathing is more diaphragm dependent, the upper airway is vulnerable to narrowing and collapse and arousal responses are depressed. These changes are more profound during REM than non-REM sleep. Sleep-related hypoxemia and hypercapnia, if severe, can cause a secondary disorder of ventilatory drive as the ventilatory control system becomes desensitized to these stimuli. If unrecognized and untreated, daytime respiratory failure supervenes and persists until the nocturnal hypoventilation is controlled using NIV (Piper and Sullivan, 1994).

The most common conditions treated in this way are the restrictive chest wall disorders:

- neuromuscular diseases associated with respiratory muscle weakness, such as the muscular dystrophies, myotonic dystrophy, and tetraplegia
- kyphoscoliosis
- old thoracoplasty
- obesity hypoventilation.

While there have been no randomized controlled studies of its use in these conditions, numerous uncontrolled studies have shown such consistent benefit that it is unlikely that a more formal study could now be ethically undertaken (Shneerson and Simonds, 2002).

The use of NIV in the ongoing management of chronic respiratory failure in COPD (beyond an acute exacerbation) is controversial, although a controlled trial appears to demonstrate longstanding improvement in dyspnoea and daytime gas exchange (unassisted) when the therapy is applied during sleep (Clini *et al*, 2002).

Contraindications to NIV

There are a number of contraindications to NIV (BTS Guideline, 2002) some of which could be considered absolute, including:

- respiratory arrest, pauses or gasping respiration which indicate (if assisted ventilation is to be used at all) the need for immediate intubation
- cardiac or haemodynamic instability
- the need for prolonged (>24–36 hours) continuous ventilatory support
- the requirement for a very high fractional inspired O_2 concentration (FiO_2), which is difficult to deliver via the inherently leaky high flow non-invasive systems
- respiratory diseases associated with a high impedance and therefore use of consistently high (>20–25 cm H_2O) inflation pressures which are associated with greater discomfort, propensity for leaks around the mask interface and aerophagia
- aspiration risk, either because of a mechanical gastrointestinal problem or neurological derangement, such as bulbar weakness or altered conscious state not solely attributable to CO2 narcosis, in which case the airway protection of invasive methods is required. In the case of CO2 narcosis, individual judgment is required but the therapy is frequently successfully used in such settings, although published experience is limited (Adnet *et al*, 2001)
- conditions associated with copious secretions where tracheal intubation allows direct access to the lower airway for suctioning
- recent facial upper airway or gastrointestinal surgery or trauma, again requiring the airway protection of tracheal intubation
- an uncooperative, confused and/or agitated patient
- an undrained pneumothorax, which will require drainage before positive pressure ventilation can be safely applied
- end-stage terminal illness, in which case this intervention is unjustifiably intrusive.

Timing intervention with NIV

Timing intervention varies according to whether NIV is to be used in the setting of acute (including acute on chronic) or chronic failure.

Acute respiratory failure

In the case of acute respiratory failure, timing of intervention is dictated by the immediate clinical situation both in terms of bedside observation and, importantly, arterial blood gases when the patient is established on appropriate O_2 therapy.

Intervention should be considered in the presence of a combination (Kramer *et al*, 1995; Brochard *et al*, 1995) of any of the following:

- severe dyspnoea with use of accessory muscles
- respiratory rate >25–30 breaths per minute
- pH <7.3 and partial pressure of carbon dioxide in arterial blood (PaCO2) >55 mm Hg
- partial pressure of oxygen (PaO_2)/FiO_2 <200 (which is equivalent to a PaO_2 <45 mm Hg (= arterial O_2 saturation (SaO_2) <80%) on air).

If these criteria are fulfilled but there is a rapid clinical improvement with initial treatment before instigation of NIV, arterial blood gases should be repeated.

Chronic respiratory failure

In the setting of chronic respiratory failure, knowledge of ventilation during sleep is highly desirable as ventilation is more vulnerable then than during wakefulness. With progressive neuromuscular disorders, sleep-related hypoventilation may precede established daytime respiratory failure by months or even years. Where to intervene along this evolutionary pathway requires careful judgment. In these cases, and in the other conditions that culminate in chronic respiratory failure, NIV should be considered in the presence of:

- symptoms suggesting disrupted sleep, such as repeated awakenings which may or may not be associated with dyspnea, morning headaches, and somnolence
- severely impaired daytime ventilatory capacity (in general with an FEV_1 of <40% predicted normal) (Hukins and Hillman, 2000)
- wakeful respiratory failure
- significant sleep-related hypoventilation, indicated by more than 1–2% of sleep spent at an SaO_2 <80%, an increase in transcutaneous PCO_2 of >6–8 mmHg, or a markedly elevated $PaCO_2$ on waking arterial blood gas measurement.

The rate of evolution of these changes is an important indicator. Progression on repeated measurement increases the case for intervention.

Other clinical indicators suggesting significant sleep hypoventilation which requires investigation and, perhaps, intervention with NIV include:

- persistent respiratory failure not readily explained by daytime ventilatory capacity which appears adequate (FEV_1 >40% predicted normal)
- difficulty weaning from ventilatory support
- repeated episodes of acute respiratory failure not readily explained
- right heart failure or polycythemia not explicable on daytime PO_2
- persistent base excess on arterial blood gases, indicating buffering of overnight CO_2 retention (Hukins and Hillman, 2000).

NIV for acute respiratory failure is delivered in the hospital setting, optimally in a high dependency area where there are adequate nursing resources to offer the patient close attention, particularly during the initial phases of therapy (Elliot *et al*, 2002). When used for chronic failure, while therapy is often initiated in hospital, it is either self-administered at home or administered with the aid of a carer. In such cases, patients and/or their carers need to be carefully instructed in its use.

Applying NIV

Types of ventilators

Ventilators used to deliver non-invasive ventilatory assistance fit into two broad categories: devices designed to deliver a preset pressure during inspiration and devices designed to deliver a preset volume (Meecham Jones and Wedzicha, 1993). Pressure-preset devices are the most prevalent and have two inherent advantages over volume-preset devices for NIV. Firstly, delivery of a preset pressure means that a larger volume will be delivered in the presence of leak, compensating for its presence. Such leaks are commonplace with NIV, either around the mask or through the mouth where a nasal mask is used. In addition to this inherent leak compensation, a number of commonly used NIV ventilators incorporate specific leak compensation methods which allow them to function adequately even in the presence of substantial leak (up to 30 L/min).

Secondly, pressure-preset devices limit peak airway pressure delivered to the patient. This is an advantage for NIV as discomfort, excessive mask leaks and aerophagia may result if excessive pressures (in general inspiratory pressures >20 cm H_2O) are applied. With volume-preset devices, inspiratory pressure may become excessive if the preset volume is delivered against increased impedance to ventilation because of greater upper airway, lung or chest wall resistance or elastance.

The remaining discussion will refer primarily to pressure-preset devices because they are in common use for NIV.

Modes of operation, respiratory rate, within breath timing

Three basic modes of operation are available:

❖ **Timed.** Where the respiratory rate is set by a ventilator control. This rate is set to one of comfort for the patient, which is often close to his/her resting respiratory rate when unassisted. The percentage of each breath spent in inspiration is independently set, usually to 40% (providing an inspiratory to expiratory ratio of 1:2.5). This percentage can be increased (usually to no more than 50%) where gas exchange is disordered and increased alveolar recruitment is desired. It may be decreased (usually to no less than 30%) where a longer expiratory time is desired (eg. in airflow obstruction). Note that inspiratory and expiratory times are determined by respiratory rate (which determines the length of each breath) and inspiratory to expiratory ratio. The timed mode can work well in patients with neuromuscular disease, but is less successful in respiratory conditions associated with elevated impedance to ventilation (eg. obstructive disorders), and/or erratic breathing patterns. In such cases, synchrony between patient inspiratory effort and ventilator assistance may be lost with loss of efficiency of ventilatory assistance. As a result, timed mode is not now commonly used.

❖ **Spontaneous.** Where onset and offset of inspiratory assistance by the ventilator are determined by patient effort, the ventilator inspiratory cycle is triggered by a small increase in inspiratory flow generated at the onset of inspiratory effort. It is terminated when inspiratory flow reduces to a similar threshold at the end of spontaneous inspiratory effort. This mode ensures patient–ventilator synchrony; provided that the patient makes sufficient effort to trigger the device and that this effort is detected reliably by the ventilator. Such detection is dependent on effective management of and compensation for leaks (so that the ventilator does not misinterpret flow associated with leak as either a signal that inspiratory effort has started or that it has not ceased). While their leak compensation is very good, some devices also allow the operator to set a minimum and maximum inspiratory time to ensure that the device does not deliver its inspiratory pressure indefinitely in the presence of a large inadequately compensated leak. Spontaneous mode is a useful mode of ventilatory assistance where the patient has adequate respiratory drive to trigger reliably the ventilator, including during REM sleep when drive is at its nadir.

❖ **Spontaneous/timed (S/T).** This operates in the same way as spontaneous mode except that where the ventilator fails to detect an inspiratory effort after a preset time it delivers a 'mandatory breath'. The preset time is determined by the respiratory rate setting on the ventilator. In S/T mode rate is usually set to about 20% below the patient's own spontaneous rate on the ventilator, so that it is only activated by an inordinate pause between spontaneously initiated breaths. If the rate is set at ten breaths a minute, the ventilator will allow six seconds between spontaneous breaths before imposing a mandatory breath. If set at twelve breaths a minute, it will allow five seconds, and so on. This mode is a useful development on spontaneous mode for those cases where the ventilator is not reliably triggered, as it ensures a mandatory minimum level of ventilatory assistance. For example, it is commonly the case in patients with advanced respiratory muscle weakness that respiratory effort is particularly weak in REM sleep, and substantial hypoventilation can occur if 'spontaneous' mode is used because of failure to trigger assistance at an appropriate rate.

In addition to the settings referred to above, a number of devices also allow the rate of rise of inspiratory pressure (rise time) to be controlled. This can be as little as 100 msec and as great as 900 msec. Short rise times are effective, but can be uncomfortable as inspiratory pressure is suddenly delivered at its maximum level. Longer rise times can improve comfort but, if excessively long relative to the length of inspiration, can compromise inspiratory assistance by truncating the length of time over which the preset maximum inspiratory pressure is delivered. In practice, the range of rise times commonly used is 100–300 msec.

Setting inspiratory and expiratory pressures

The end-expiratory and end-inspiratory pressures delivered by these devices are independently adjustable. Depending on individual clinical circumstances, the end-expiratory pressure is adjusted to:

- overcome upper airway obstruction, in the case of obstructive sleep apnea
- recruit alveoli, in the case of disordered gas exchange
- treat pulmonary edema, in the case of left ventricular failure
- counteract intrinsic PEEP (Appendini *et al*, 1994) in the case of airflow obstruction with dynamic hyperinflation.

The usual working range is 5–10 cm H_2O, with adjustment made against clinical response. Most devices deliver a minimum level of EPAP of approximately 2.5 cmH_2O as they maintain airflow to the mask interface during expiration to eliminate CO_2 from the deadspace of the mask.

Inspiratory pressure is set above the expiratory level, the difference between the inspiratory and expiratory pressures determining the amount of pressure assistance delivered with each breath. Low levels of pressure assistance are unlikely to be efficacious and excessive levels are uncomfortable, can cause excessive mask and mouth leaks, and are often associated with aerophagia. Therefore, the usual working range of inspiratory pressures used is between 10 and 20 cmH_2O. The precise level is determined by tolerance of therapy and clinical response, including gas exchange on therapy (judged by indirect and direct measures of arterial blood gas tensions).

Choosing the mask interface

There are a wide variety of mask interfaces available for delivery of NIV. They fit into two broad categories:

- face masks, which cover the nose and mouth
- nasal masks.

There is a great deal of choice within each of these broad categories. Choosing the correct interface is vital for comfort and acceptability and, therefore, success of treatment. General considerations when choosing the specific interface include:

- the nature of the presentation (acute versus chronic, see below)
- a comfortable, leak-free fit
- nasal patency
- ability to maintain mouth closure
- dentition and dental occlusion (relationship of upper and lower dental arches)
- patient's dexterity — both for mask assembly and placement
- patient's preference
- anticipated length of therapy
- local expertise and experience.

In considering the choice between face and nose masks, face masks should always be fitted with an anti-asphyxia valve which opens if the ventilator becomes disconnected or fails (as with a power black-out). These interfaces are useful in:

- acute disease, as they offer better control of ventilation than nasal masks, which allow variable mouth leak particularly where high airway pressures are used
- where the patient is naive to NIV therapy and more disconcerted by mouth leak and less able to coordinate palatal muscle activity to control it
- where there is facial muscle weakness, causing excessive mouth leaks
- where there is high impedance to ventilation, so that high inspiratory pressures have to be used (increasing propensity to mouth leak)
- where the nose is blocked.

Nasal masks are less intrusive and claustrophobic than face masks, but offer less direct control of the delivery of positive pressure. They are commonly used where NIV is commenced electively and often used in the acute setting. Where face masks are used to commence therapy acutely, it is often possible to change to a nasal mask after a day or so, once the patient is used to NIV. If efficacious, nasal masks are generally preferred for long-term use. A chin strap may be needed to help control mouth leaks during sleep with these masks.

Daily application of NIV

Acute respiratory failure

Providing it is adequately tolerated, NIV is initially applied continuously or semi-continuously in acute respiratory failure. Respites from therapy are dictated by ability to comply with therapy and rate of rise of PCO_2 and/or capacity to maintain oxygenation off therapy. During this phase of therapy, invasive therapy is kept under consideration.

As acute respiratory failure resolves, time off therapy during wakefulness is gradually increased. Support during sleep is maintained until daytime (wakeful) support is no longer needed. Ongoing improvement sees support during sleep discontinued if there is no reason to suspect persistent sleep-related hypoventilation, as may occur in acute or chronic respiratory failure.

Chronic respiratory failure

In chronic respiratory failure, NIV is often only needed during sleep because of the vulnerability of ventilation during this state. In advanced cases, periodic daytime respite may be needed to supplement nocturnal support, particularly during daytime naps if these are taken.

Additional therapies

Oxygen therapy

Oxygen therapy is added to treatment where there is adequate CO_2 control but persistent hypoxemia that is not eliminated by adjusting the ventilatory parameters (Plant *et al*, 2000a). It is generally delivered to the mask at flow rates of $1-2L/min$ or more, titrated against arterial O_2 saturation ($\approx 90\%$) and $PaCO_2$. The BiPAP 'Vision' ventilator and other critical care ventilators allow O_2 therapy to be more accurately titrated as they are fitted with an O_2 blender and connected to a high flow O_2 source so that they can deliver up to 100% O_2 if required.

Humidification

Humidification is often needed to prevent mouth and nasal drying with consequent rhinitis. In such cases, the humidifier is placed in series with the ventilator and the chamber temperature is set to humidify the gas passing through it to the required degree. In the acute setting, heated humidifiers should be used rather than heat moisture exchangers, as the latter have been shown to increase work of breathing (Lellouche *et al*, 2002).

Posture

Elevating the upper body can be extremely useful in the presence of obesity and diaphragm weakness, which compromise ventilation, particularly in the dependent regions of the lungs. The lateral posture can be useful in improving ventilation in the presence of obstructive sleep apnea, scoliosis or old thoracoplasty.

Monitoring therapy

In judging adequacy of therapy it is important to determine whether its aims are being met and, if so, at what cost. The general aims of therapy are to relieve symptoms, reduce disability, increase longevity and improve quality of life.

The specific aims of therapy are to control or correct the derangement in arterial blood gases, at a minimum achieving adequate oxygenation without excessive CO_2 retention. This consideration applies to blood gases both on and off NIV. In the chronic setting, benefits of correcting the sleep-related hypoventilation should include restoration of more normal sleep architecture, control of

respiratory failure, and resolution of right-heart failure and polycythemia where present.
In judging adequacy, the following should be monitored:

- patient comfort and mental state
- heart rate and respiratory rate
- synchrony of patient inspiratory effort with ventilator mediated breaths
- use of accessory muscles of inspiration
- amplitude of chest wall displacement
- abolition of paradoxical chest wall motion, where present
- arterial blood gases
  - indirectly, by continuous monitoring of SaO_2 and, if available, transcutaneous PCO_2
  - directly, measuring these 1–2 hours after commencement of therapy in the acute setting and repeating at 4–6 hours if little improvement (BTS Guidelines, 2002)
- measuring ventilation during sleep in the chronic setting, paying particular attention to oxygenation and transcutaneous PCO_2 (or waking $PaCO_2$ where this is not available).

Treatment failure

Treatment failure is indicated by:

- worsening breathlessness, tremor, headache
- increasing heart rate, respiratory rate
- deterioration in conscious state
- arterial blood gases that fail to improve or deteriorate
- development of new complications, such as nasal bridge ulceration (with prolonged application of the mask interface), pneumothorax (a rare complication with pressure-preset devices), and sputum retention
- intolerance of, or asynchrony with, the ventilator (these are often related) which fails to respond to troubleshooting, such as resolving leaks
- patient's wish to discontinue therapy despite encouragement.

Illustrative cases: practical applications of the technique

The following case descriptions are intended to illustrate how this therapy may be applied in clinical practice.

Case study 1: Acute exacerbation of chronic obstructive pulmonary disease (COPD)

Mrs Adele Stewart is a 66-year old female with known COPD who is brought into the Emergency Department after a family member found her unconscious in bed at home. She has complained of increased shortness of breath over the last four days but refused to go to hospital or have the local doctor visit. She has used continuous home O_2 for the past eighteen months, with three admissions for acute exacerbations in 7 months. There is no known history of cardiac or neurological disease. Her medications include inhaled bronchodilators and steroids as well as spironolactone for peripheral edema.

On arrival she is receiving 6 L/min of oxygen through a mask, with an arterial saturation of 97% and a respiratory rate of 40 breaths per minute. Her Glasgow Coma Score (GCS) is 6. On auscultation, she has basal inspiratory crepitations with reduced air entry bilaterally. The chest X-ray shows hyperexpanded lung fields but no pneumothorax or consolidation. Arterial blood gases taken shortly after arrival are as follows: pH 7.01, $PaCO_2$ 186 mmHg, PaO_2 126 mmHg, bicarbonate 44, base excess (BE) 5 and SaO_2 98%.

Issues regarding the appropriateness of intubation and resuscitation are discussed with Mrs Stewart's son and daughter. They report that their mother had previously expressed her wish not to be intubated. Therefore, bi-level ventilatory support is commenced. The spontaneous mode is used with an inspiratory positive airway pressure (IPAP) of 20 cmH$_2$O and expiratory positive airway pressure (EPAP) of 5 cmH$_2$O, while rise time is set at 100 ms. Initially, 4 L/min of supplemental oxygen is used to maintain a SaO_2 between 85% and 92%. A face mask is also employed. With this set up, good patient–machine synchrony is achieved.

After 1 hour of bi-level support, pH has risen to 7.13 with a $PaCO_2$ 13 mmHg. The patient has become more responsive, though disorientated. After further discussion with the family, the patient is documented for full active therapy short of intubation. Bi-level support is continued and the patient is transferred to the respiratory ward. Three hours later, the GSC has improved to 13, although the patient remains agitated. The mask is removed and Mrs Stewart is placed on 3 L/min of nasal prong oxygen. However, within minutes, the SaO_2 falls to 67% and her level of consciousness deteriorates. Bi-level mask support is recommenced. Once again, as her level of consciousness improves, Mrs Stewart exhibits signs of agitation and confusion. Physical restraints are used to maintain the mask in place and after 20 minutes the patient settles.

Ventilatory support is continued overnight. Next morning, the respiratory rate has fallen to 20 breaths per minute and blood gases have significantly improved with a pH 7.34, $PaCO_2$ 72 mmHg and PaO_2 74 mmHg. The restraints are removed and Mrs Stewart is placed back on nasal prong oxygen. She is alert and orientated and the do not resuscitate (DNR) orders are discussed with her and she agrees with the management plan. She continues using mask support, removing it for meals.

By late afternoon, her pH is 7.4 and $PaCO_2$ 55 mmHg. The mask is removed and Mrs Stewart is placed on 2 L/min nasal prong oxygen. She continues on bi-level support at night only for another four days with the IPAP reduced from 20 to 17 cmH$_2$O. At this stage, Mrs Stewart expresses the wish to be discharged home without further intervention, refusing recommendations to attend pulmonary rehabilitation.

Is NIV indicated?

In appropriately selected patients, particularly those with hypercapnic respiratory failure, NIV has emerged as an effective method for avoiding intubation (Brochard *et al*, 1995; Phua *et al*, 2005; Ram *et al*, 2004), reducing complications associated with mechanical ventilation (Girou *et al*, 2000), and improving survival (Plant *et al*, 2000b). However, those with a lower baseline pH level are less likely to respond positively to NIV therapy (Ambrosino *et al*, 1995), especially in the ward situation (Plant *et al*, 2000a). Although treatment of patients with such severely abnormal baseline clinical parameters does not preclude the use of NIV, a low threshold for more definitive intervention in a more highly monitored environment would have to be considered. As the family believed the patient would not have wanted invasive intervention, it was appropriate for a trial of NIV to be undertaken, recognizing the realistic likelihood of therapy failure.

Which device?

Both volume- and pressure-preset devices have been used with equal success in the management of acute exacerbations of COPD. However, pressure-preset modes of ventilatory support are more commonly used, often in the form of portable bi-level devices. The aim of NIV therapy is to improve gas exchange while reducing respiratory effort. A number of studies have shown that a similar degree of blood gas improvement can be achieved with either volume- or pressure-preset devices. Volume-preset machines appear to reduce the work of breathing to a greater extent than pressure-preset devices, while the latter are generally perceived by the patient to be more comfortable (Girault *et al*, 1997). The type of device chosen to deliver NIV is probably not as important as the skill and experience of the staff in setting up the equipment and altering settings to match best the ventilatory needs of the individual patient.

What interface?

The choice of interface in the acute setting is guided largely by the ability of the patient to maintain mouth closure and their tolerance of NIV. As a significant number of patients with acute decompensated COPD are dyspneic and unable to consciously or comfortably maintain a mouth seal, a full face mask is frequently the mask of initial choice. Once the patient has settled and their respiratory condition improved, changing to a nasal mask may be possible. Such decisions need to be based on both patient comfort and their physiologic response to the equipment used. It has been shown that facial masks and nasal prong masks are more effective in decreasing PaCO$_2$, but that nasal masks are better tolerated (Navalesi *et al*, 2000)

Monitoring and ongoing management

Not infrequently, worsening of hypercapnia and acidosis will occur if inappropriately high levels of oxygen are used. A recent investigation has demonstrated that around 20% of hypercapnic COPD patients were able to correct their pH once the FiO$_2$ was reduced (Plant *et al*, 2000b). Therefore, the initial step in management is to maintain a SaO$_2$ level within the range of 85–92%.

In the acute setting, NIV is usually used continuously for the first 6–24 hours, depending on the patient's response to therapy. Oximetry, respiratory rate and mental state are useful parameters to monitor progress during this time. Close observation of the patient's respiratory pattern and their interaction with the ventilator is mandatory during the initial stages of therapy to identify any problems and correct them rapidly. This may involve altering pressures, changing interfaces, or instituting treatments to aid secretion removal. Once the patient appears less distressed and gas exchange is improved, a short period off the ventilator is attempted. During this time fluids may be given and oral care attended to. Periods of ventilator use are then interspersed with ventilator-free time based on patient tolerance and level of respiratory distress. Daytime use is reduced and then withdrawn, although nocturnal use may continue for longer if tolerated by the patient. In some instances, long-term nocturnal ventilation may be indicated. This should be discussed with the patient and follow-up investigation arranged once the patient is discharged and again medically stable.

Case study 2: Myotonic dystrophy with established respiratory failure

Mrs Lucy Stiefel, a 53-year-old woman with myotonic dystrophy is referred for assessment of possible sleep-disordered breathing. She was first diagnosed with myotonic dystrophy in her mid-20s and has experienced progressive muscle weakness since that time. She feels her deterioration has accelerated in the last 6 months, with increased breathlessness, worsening daytime sleepiness and occasional morning headaches. Lung function studies show an overall restrictive pattern with a FEV$_1$ of 1 L (34% predicted), an FVC of 1.12 L (32% predicted), and TLC of 43% predicted. Her maximum inspiratory mouth pressures are –60 cmH$_2$O (83% predicted) and expiratory pressure 30 cmH$_2$O (32% predicted).

A diagnostic sleep study is performed. Her baseline N-REM saturation is low at 85–88%, with the occasional hypopneic event noted. However, during REM episodes, significant falls in SaO$_2$ occurred to a minimum value of 36%. Concurrently, transcutaneous carbon dioxide (PtcCO$_2$) rose by a maximum of 14 mmHg, mirroring the rise in arterial PaCO$_2$ from an evening value of 52 mmHg to an awakening value of 65 mmHg.

She is started on bi-level support, commencing with daytime practice sessions. She takes to the therapy readily, and sleeps around 4 hours the first day. She returns with her husband the second day for further monitoring and equipment training. The couple are sent home for a week to use therapy on settings on IPAP 14 cmH$_2$O and EPAP 6 cmH$_2$O in the spontaneous mode.

Mrs Stiefel returns for a formal bi-level titration study, which shows that IPAP of 15 cmH$_2$O and EPAP of 5 cmH$_2$O best maintained nocturnal gas exchange. When reviewed 2 months later in clinic, clock time on the device indicates a mean nightly use of 5.3 hour per night. Her awake CO$_2$ has fallen to 47 mmHg and she reports feeling less sleepy during the day.

Is NIV indicated in this patient?

Even without the results of the sleep study to confirm severe sleep-disordered breathing, there should have been a high index of suspicion of a problem in this patient. She had symptoms that could be consistent with nocturnal hypoventilation (morning headaches and sleepiness) along with breathlessness. Her awake CO_2 levels were raised and she had a significant restrictive pattern on lung function testing. Sleep-disordered breathing is common in patients with myotonic dystrophy, and should be investigated as part of an overall management program, especially if the patient's clinical condition is deteriorating. Unlike other neuromuscular disorders, the degree of respiratory muscle weakness alone does not fully explain the abnormalities in sleep breathing and gas exchange seen in myotonic dystrophy. It appears that these patients may also have brainstem abnormalities that could account for changes in respiratory drive and daytime somnolence, that are independent of sleep-disordered breathing (Gilmartin *et al*, 1991; Ono *et al*, 1998).

Which machine?

The diagnostic sleep study demonstrated that the nature of the breathing disorder was hypoventilation due to reduced inspiratory effort, primarily in REM sleep. Frank apneas were not seen at any time. Therefore, a bi-level device set in the spontaneous mode was the initial choice of machine for this patient.

Determining settings

This patient needed sufficient inspiratory positive airway pressure (IPAP) to support each spontaneously initiated breath and enough end positive expiratory pressure (EPAP) to ensure upper airway stability. In commencing therapy, daytime practice sessions were undertaken using starting pressures of IPAP $10 \, cmH_2O$ and EPAP $4 \, cmH_2O$ in the spontaneous mode. IPAP was increased in $1 \, cmH_2O$ increments as tolerated by the patient to the maximum level the patient comfortably tolerated, being guided by both SaO_2 and leak.

Choice of interface

Prior to fitting a mask, the patient's nasal patency was checked to ensure an adequate nasal airflow could be achieved. It was also established that the patient was able to maintain relaxed lip closure when awake. From a practical point of view in this patient, a nasal mask was going to be easier to position and care for, given her poor eyesight and lack of manual dexterity. However, mouth leaks could be a problem, reducing the effectiveness of ventilatory support. The patient was started with a nasal mask, but it was discussed with her the likely need for a chinstrap or a change to a face mask at a later stage if leaks with the nasal mask were experienced.

Monitoring and management

NIV was commenced using daytime practice periods to acclimatize the patient to the mask and pressures, while monitoring the patient's response to therapy. An oximeter was used to gauge how altering pressures affected gas exchange. The patient accepted therapy readily, falling asleep within minutes of the mask being placed on her face. This provided an opportunity to observe the interaction between the patient and machine during sleep. It became apparent almost immediately that mouth leaks were a significant problem, with values of 18–24 L/min being recorded while SaO_2, which had initially improved from 87–93%, fell again to 86–87% during these leak episodes. A chinstrap was added which lead to improvements in both leak and SaO_2.

The patient slept for around four hours without problems. Training in fitting the mask and chinstrap was commenced, though it became quickly obvious that she would have difficulties managing the mask and chinstrap unaided. She and her husband were asked to return the following day for further instruction. Acclimatization to therapy can be commenced on either an inpatient or an outpatient basis, depending on the skills and confidence of patient and/or carers, the level of acuity of the patient, and local resources. Our usual approach is to commence therapy on an inpatient basis to identify and correct early on any problems or side-effects that could affect the patient's willingness to benefit from, or continue on, therapy. In this case, the patient was not keen to stay in hospital. Her husband rapidly became proficient in fitting and adjusting the mask and chinstrap and the couple lived close to the hospital. Given these circumstances, management of acclimatization as an outpatient seemed appropriate.

Follow-up and compliance

Once the patient was sleeping on the device for at least 4 hours a night, an overnight bi-level titration study was arranged. This provided the opportunity to ensure that settings chosen were appropriately controlling all aspects of the sleep disordered breathing and to identify any factors that could limit either the use of therapy or its effectiveness. In particular, poor synchrony between the patient and the machine from mouth leak, failure to trigger consistently or persisting upper airway instability were all potential problems that may have affected gas exchange or sleep quality in this patient.

Once established on therapy, ongoing review of the patient and their progress is important. Our routine approach is to review the patient two to three months after initiating therapy to compare baseline objective and subjective parameters with their current state. Compliance with therapy is also documented using the clock hours that are recorded by the machine. Any problems or questions that have arisen with therapy are discussed. Adjustments to settings or equipment are not uncommon as the patient's clinical condition can change considerably after the institution of therapy. Continued review then occurs at regular intervals, usually every 6 months. A regular review program is important, particularly in patients with a progressive underlying disorder, not only to fine tune therapy, but also to discuss issues related to progressive disability, medical directives about end-stage care and other management options.

Case study 3: Duchenne muscular dystrophy and evolving respiratory failure

Liam Passlow is a 14-year-old boy with Duchenne muscular dystrophy who presents to clinic with symptoms of daytime sleepiness. He denies any morning headaches or problems maintaining sleep at night. Spirometry shows an FEV_1 of 0.5 L and a FVC of 0.6 L. He is able to generate -25 cm H_2O of inspiratory pressure and 20 cmH_2O of expiratory pressure measured at the mouth. An arterial blood gas taken during the afternoon shows a pH of 7.37, a $PaCO_2$ of 42 mmHg, a PaO2 of 87 mmHg with a BE of 0. A sleep study is performed which shows SaO_2 maintained at 94–95% in N-REM sleep, with falls to a minimum of 76% during REM sleep. During these REM episodes, $PtcCO_2$ rose by a maximum of 11 mmHg.

Liam is offered a trial of NIV but declines. The signs and symptoms of worsening respiratory failure are discussed with him and his family, and treatment options in the case of an acute respiratory deterioration outlined.

Three months later he presents with worsening dyspnea. His $PaCO_2$ awake is 44 mmHg with a PaO_2 of 77 mmHg. He is commenced on NIV (bi-level support in S/T mode) and sleeps during an afternoon practice session, as well as overnight, without difficulty. On settings of IPAP 12cm, EPAP 4 cm and a backup rate of 16 breaths per minute, SaO_2 is maintained at or above 94% with no discernible rise in $PtcCO_2$ during REM. The following day, he practises with a volume-preset ventilator and that night a further sleep study is performed to check the effectiveness of settings. With a tidal volume of 400 mls, rate of 16 beats per minute and inspiratory time of 1.75 secs, ventilation is similarly effective. However, after around 4 hours on the device overnight, he wakes complaining of abdominal bloating and refuses to use the machine again. After 2 more days acclimatizing to the bi-level device, he returns home. After 10 days use he reports his dyspnea has improved and declines further therapy at this time.

He is followed at 12-week intervals to monitor his lung function and symptoms. Over the next twelve months a gradual rise in awake CO_2 and bicarbonate are noted. A sleep study performed just prior to recommencing NIV demonstrated falls in SaO_2 during REM to 60% with $PtcCO_2$ rises of 16 mmHg. His awake $PaCO_2$ is 52 mmHg. Shortly after, he presents with headache and difficulty breathing. He is commenced on nasal mask therapy and accepts therapy without incident. After a short period of stabilization in hospital he is discharged home on nocturnal therapy. He continues to be followed up regularly and remains compliant with therapy after 6 years.

When should NIV be commenced?

The decision to commence therapy is not a difficult one when the patient presents with severe symptoms and unstable respiratory failure. However, intentionally leaving intervention to such a late stage in the disease process puts the patient at risk of deteriorating acutely and rapidly, to the point where intubation and ventilation may become the only option to sustain life. Ideally, NIV should be commenced much earlier to prevent such a situation. At the other end of the spectrum, early initiation of NIV, before the onset of symptoms or hypoventilation, has been advocated as a means of slowing the deterioration in lung function and breathing. A randomized controlled trial designed to test this approach found no benefit in the 'prophylactic' use of NIV in normocapnic, symptom-free Duchenne muscular dystrophy patients (Raphael *et al*, 1994). In addition, such early intervention may discourage the patient from pursuing therapy longer term if they feel it is inconvenient, uncomfortable or of no benefit.

In practice, NIV is usually commenced when patients report symptoms consistent with sleep disruption or nocturnal hypoventilation, or, when there is evidence of isolated abnormal nocturnal or diurnal blood gas tensions. Therefore, the first task of the clinician is to identify those at risk of developing nocturnal hypoventilation and investigating those individuals appropriately. Clinicians should not rely on patients reporting symptoms to initiate investigation into sleep-disordered breathing. A sedentary lifestyle coupled with a gradual adaptation to their respiratory limitation means that patients may not be aware of symptoms. For this reason, a number of investigators have sought to develop daytime predictors of nocturnal breathing problems based on wakeful blood gases and lung function as well as symptoms (Hukins and Hillman, 2000). In our practice, once the patient has been identified as vulnerable to sleep-related hypoventilation, baseline polysomnography is performed to document the degree and nature of any abnormality present.

If the patient denies symptoms, daytime CO_2 is normal, and breathing during sleep is only mildly deranged, then NIV may be postponed for a time. Much will depend on the patient's willingness to trial therapy. In this clinical case, the patient and family were not ready to accept the need for respiratory support until a respiratory crisis was reached, despite well-documented deteriorations in both awake blood gases and nocturnal gas exchange.

Clinically, our preference would have been to introduce therapy when nocturnal desaturation was first identified. Unable to achieve this, we endeavored to provide sufficient information to the patient and his family about NIV and invasive ventilation, so that informed decisions could be made should an emergency situation arise. By maintaining close contact and ongoing monitoring, we were able to ensure that appropriate intervention was instituted as soon as the patient was willing to undertake it.

Which device?

In this patient, either a volume- or a pressure-preset device was considered to be suitable. The pressure-preset (bi-level device) was likely to have been more comfortable, easier to use and less expensive. On the other hand, the internal battery and alarm features of the volume preset device available would have been more suitable for someone with a progressive disorder, where eventual ventilator dependence and daytime ventilation through a mouth piece may have been considered. The patient was trialed on both devices and though both were equally effective in terms of gas exchange, the side-effect profile and patient comfort were better with the bi-level device.

What settings?

As described previously, daytime practice sessions were used to acclimatize the patient to the sensations of the mask and airflow delivery. This patient was young and anxious so in the initial stages a low IPAP of 9 cmH$_2$O and an EPAP of 4 cmH$_2$O were used. However, once the patient felt comfortable on these settings, the IPAP was raised to 11 cmH$_2$O. The S/T mode of support was used because the patient failed to trigger the ventilator adequately during sleep, particularly REM. In this circumstance, his breathing rate was determined by the back-up rate set on the ventilator. The overnight sleep study used to confirm settings were effective, leak was minimized and sleep architecture was not adversely affected.

What interface?

For comfort, a nasal mask, which the patient found comfortable and the family found easy to apply, was chosen as the initial interface. As is normal practice in our unit, a chinstrap was not used during the initial trial periods but the possibility that one might be needed if significant mouth leaks occurred during sleep was discussed and later used.

Ongoing management

Although the patient declined pursuing therapy on several occasions, close monitoring and follow-up continued in an attempt to avoid a crisis situation. Each follow-up visit was used as an opportunity to educate the patient and his parents about his condition, the natural evolution of breathing problems that occur in neuromuscular disorders and therapy options. In particular, signs and symptoms that indicated the urgent need for intervention were emphasized. A management plan was provided to try and increase the likelihood that any deterioration was recognized and treated appropriately. It took some time for this patient and family to acknowledge the presence of a significant breathing problem that required ongoing intervention. However, once this barrier was overcome, the patient readily accepted therapy and benefited from it.

Regular reviews were arranged to monitor his nocturnal ventilation needs, as well as plan and manage other aspects of his care such as swallowing status, nutritional needs and family support. A percutaneous endoscopic gastrostomy (PEG) feeding tube was inserted several years later when weight maintenance became an issue. As his respiratory muscle weakness increased, ventilation increased into daytime use. He was trained to use a mouthpiece and provided with a volume-preset ventilator for daytime use.

Case study 4: Chronic respiratory failure due to COPD

Mrs Delia MacLean is a 52-year-old woman with severe COPD. She has an FEV_1 of 0.5 L, a FVC of 1.5 L and a residual volume of 185% predicted. Her daytime CO_2, which had been 42 mmHg, rose to 51 mmHg over an 18-month period, while her PaO_2 fell from 71 mmHg to 65 mmHg. A sleep study was requested to identify any sleep-disordered breathing and to monitor her response to low flow oxygen therapy.

The diagnostic study showed a low baseline SaO_2 between 85–88% during N-REM sleep. During periods of REM sleep, there were episodes of reduced nasal airflow and chest wall movement resulting in falls in SaO_2 to minimum levels of 45–50%, while $PtcCO_2$ rose by a maximum of 13 mmHg (*Figure 14.1*, top panel). The following night 1 litre/minute of supplemental oxygen was used during sleep. This maintained SaO_2 above 93% in both NREM and REM sleep, while rises in $PtcCO_2$ during REM remained in the 12–15 mmHg range. Comparison of evening and morning arterial blood gases showed that $PaCO_2$ had risen from 51 mmHg in the evening to 55 mmHg.

For the next 2 years Mrs MacLean was regularly monitored by her respiratory physician. She was again referred for investigation when she began to complain of morning headaches and her wakeful arterial blood gases showed a pH of 7.37 and $PaCO_2$ of 60 mmHg. A sleep study on NIV showed that an IPAP of 13 cmH_2O and EPAP of 4 cmH_2O with 1 litre/min supplemental oxygen was effective in maintaining SaO_2 >92% in all sleep stages. Morning blood gases show the $PaCO_2$ had fallen to 55 mmHg. She was tolerating the therapy well andhappy to continue using it at home.

At review 3 months later, Mrs MacLean's $PaCO_2$ had fallen to 48 mmHg and the overnight sleep study shows SaO_2 is maintained >92% on the previous settings. The rise in $PtcCO_2$ during

REM sleep is 4mmHg (*Figure 14.1*, bottom panel). She continues using nocturnal mask bi-level support at home.

Is NIV indicated in this patient?

In patients with COPD, ventilation during sleep is decreased, particularly during episodes of rapid eye movement sleep and can result in significant sleep-related hypoxemia and hypercapnia. This nocturnal oxygen desaturation appears to be related to a fall in tidal volume associated with reduced respiratory effort, as evidenced by a reduction in the mean inspiratory pleural pressure generated (Fletcher *et al*, 1983). This is partly due to a reduction in respiratory drive along with increases in upper airway resistance (Ballard *et al*, 1995). At the same time, the responsiveness to increases in CO_2 is reduced. Although the use of supplemental oxygen therapy can prevent or limit desaturation and has been shown to improve survival (MRC Working Party, 1981; NOTT group, 1980), in some patients it can also worsen hypercapnia.

Theoretically, NIV should be of value in maintaining ventilation during sleep, thereby improving daytime blood gases and other functional parameters. However, discordant results from a number

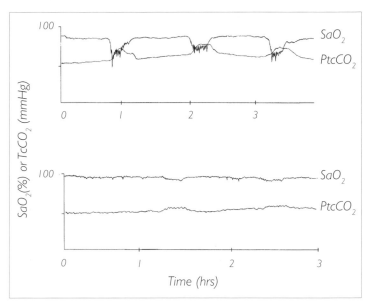

Figure 14.1: Overnight oxyhaemoglobin saturation (SaO_2) and transcutaneous carbon dioxide ($PtcCO_2$) from Case 4, a patient with chronic respiratory failure due to COPD. Top panel: Representative portion of the tracing from the diagnostic sleep study night. Marked nocturnal desaturation occurred during episodes of REM sleep, accompanied by increases in $PtcCO_2$ — REM hypoventilation. Bottom panel: Representative portion of the $SaO_2/PtcCO_2$ tracing from the review night on bi-level support. With the use of NIV, SaO_2 was maintained within an acceptable range with low-level supplemental oxygen. Importantly, rises in $PtcCO_2$ were minimal during REM sleep, suggesting that the therapy was set in such a way that effective control of nocturnal hypoventilation was achieved.

of trials addressing this question have only served to muddy the waters, rather than clarify this issue (Wijkstra *et al*, 2002; Wijkstra, 2003). Of the six randomized trials to date addressing this question, two have reported beneficial effects (Clini, 2002; Meecham Jones *et al*, 1995) while the other four have found no clear-cut advantage of NIV to standard oxygen therapy (Casanova *et al*, 2000; Gay *et al*, 1996; Lin, 1996; Strumpf *et al*, 1991).

There are several reasons that could explain these conflicting results, primarily related to the types of patients studied and the approach to monitoring and titrating of settings that many investigators have taken. In a number of studies, patients have been selected on the basis of a diagnosis of stable COPD only, and not on the presence of hypercapnia or nocturnal oxygen desaturation (Casanova *et al*, 2000; Clini *et al* 2002; Strumpf *et al*, 1991). Given the rationale for using NIV is to prevent nocturnal hypoventilation, it could be reasonably argued that improvements in gas exchange, sleep quality and daytime function are unlikely if the patient is not presenting with these problems. While there is no evidence to support the routine use of NIV in patients with COPD, there are subgroups of patients who will respond positively to this therapy. In our practice, patients are assessed and trialed on therapy if they are hypercapnic with symptoms (disrupted sleep and morning headaches), if they have demonstrated worsening hypercapnia with use of nocturnal oxygen therapy, or are shown to have significant sleep-related hypoventilation, especially during REM sleep.

Which machine?

In this patient a spontaneous mode of bi-level support was used. The diagnostic sleep had demonstrated that during REM sleep the fall in SaO_2 was related to reduced chest wall movement, and not due to apnea or a slowing of respiratory rate. Therefore, the goal was to provide sufficient inspiratory support to each inspiratory effort made by the patient to increase tidal volume. Overall, the choice of the type of machine to be used in the home will depend on local experience, patient comfort and the efficacy of the device in improving gas exchange during sleep. The cost and simplicity of bi-level devices makes them an attractive choice for NIV therapy in this setting.

What settings?

The EPAP was kept low ($4\,cmH_2O$) and the IPAP increased to the maximum tolerated comfortably by the patient. A spontaneous mode with low EPAP and sufficient IPAP to improve chest wall movement and improve gas exchange was the goal of intervention, in particular, during periods of REM sleep.

Which mask?

This choice was based both on effectiveness and patient comfort. The patient was offered the opportunity to experience both nasal and face masks and found she preferred using a face mask. This choice may have, in part, been influenced by the need to use a chinstrap with the nasal mask to minimize mouth leak. During the daytime practice sessions, it became quickly apparent that with the onset of sleep, significant mouth leak occurred associated with a fall in SaO_2, and frequent arousal. This problem was corrected when a chinstrap was added. Having experienced both set-ups, the patient found the face mask easier to apply and less cumbersome than a nasal mask and chinstrap.

Monitoring and management

This patient was managed as an inpatient. After acclimatizing to the mask and bi-level machine on the ward for two days and nights, a nocturnal sleep study was performed. The purpose of the study was to determine the effectiveness of settings and the impact of ventilatory support on sleep quality. It appears that success with therapy depends greatly on how effectively nocturnal CO_2 can be controlled with NIV (Meecham Jones *et al*, 1995). This requires careful titration of ventilator settings and attention to mask leaks to ensure adequate ventilatory assistance, including assurance of ventilator–patient synchrony.

Accessories

Although not required by all patients, if rhinitis or significant mouth dryness are a problem, humidification may be used. The majority of patients also require supplemental oxygen through the machine. Oxygen flows need to be carefully titrated to ensure that improvements in SaO_2 have been achieved as much as possible by the settings on the ventilator. If SaO_2 levels remain below 90% after pressure titration, oxygen should be added.

Follow-up

The variable findings of randomized studies of NIV in COPD emphasize the need to evaluate the efficacy of therapy, and compliance to it, on a regular basis. Some investigators have reported a significantly poorer compliance to this therapy long-term compared to patients with restrictive disorders (Criner *et al*, 1999). Poor patient selection may account for some of this problem. In addition, clinicians may fail to recognize that mouth leak could be contributing to a poor clinical response and, therefore, not take appropriate steps to correct this. If a patient fails to respond to therapy it is important to establish why. Although there is controversy as to the role of routine polysomnography in adjusting the settings for NIV, there is no doubt that oximetry alone is insufficient to monitor the effectiveness of therapy, especially where supplemental O_2 is being used. Although leaks may cause reduced chest wall excursion or poor synchrony between the patient and machine that could be picked up with simplified respiratory monitoring, arousals from sleep causing sleep fragmentation and failure to achieve REM sleep could still be overlooked. Even if review polysomnography is not part of the routine follow-up of patients, it should be undertaken in those who fail to respond appropriately to therapy or who report problems coping with it.

Case study 5: Duchenne muscular dystrophy presenting in established respiratory failure

Lucas Merchant is 22-year-old man referred for assessment and management of significant daytime respiratory failure with a background of Duchenne muscular dystrophy. His daytime arterial blood gases confirmed that he was in acute or chronic respiratory failure, with a pH of 7.29, a $PaCO_2$ of 81 mmHg and PaO_2 of 45 mmHg, while the BE was 10. His spirometry showed an FEV_1 of 0.5 L and a FVC of 0.55 L. His initial sleep study demonstrated severe sleep disordered breathing (*Figure 14.2*, top panel). The use of supplemental oxygen at 1 L/min improved SaO_2 to 88–89%, but at the expense of further CO_2 retention, with $PtcCO_2$ rising 26 mmHg above previous sleep levels.

The following night he was studied on NIV delivered via a volume-preset ventilator. This was only partially successful. Significant mouth leaks persisted that could not be effectively controlled with a chinstrap, resulting in low airway pressure and loss of effective ventilation. The patient was changed to a full-face mask, with maintenance of airway pressure and significant improvements in sleep SaO_2. He was discharged home after acclimatization to therapy and training of his family on how to manage NIV.

Over the next few weeks his clinical status and blood gases continued to improve, with his CO_2 falling to 48 mmHg and his PaO_2 increasing to 77 mmHg during spontaneous breathing. He was followed up 6-monthly, then yearly, to check blood gases, sleep parameters and overall functional capacity.

For the next 4 years he remained stable and well. However, at a routine review a blood gas taken during spontaneous wakeful breathing in the afternoon showed a rise in $PaCO_2$ to 63 mmHg and a pH of 7.34. On questioning, he reported feeling less well than previously, with daytime tiredness. The overnight sleep study demonstrated good gas exchange in NREM sleep with SaO_2 values 95% or greater. However, during REM sleep, repetitive episodes of upper airway obstruction occurred, with airway pressures of > 35 cmH$_2$O being generated by his volume-preset ventilator, while SaO_2 fell to a minimum of 70% (*Figure 14.2*, top panel). It was felt that the problem was upper airway obstruction due to his large tongue blocking his airway during mouth breathing through the face mask.

A nasal mask was again trialled, in conjunction with a chinstrap. This combination now allowed delivery of effective ventilatory support with SaO_2 maintained $> 94\%$ through the night with an early morning $PaCO_2$ of 41 mmHg from an evening value of 61 mmHg (*Figure 14.2*, bottom panel).

He continued relatively unchanged for another 2 years, when he was changed to a pressure-preset device in S/T mode in place of volume preset therapy. He found this mode of support increased comfort during sleep, although he continued to use his volume-preset ventilator for short periods during the day via a mouthpiece. Over the succeeding years this regimen continued with a gradual increase in his dependence on daytime ventilatory support.

A sleep study review after 13 years of non-invasive ventilatory support demonstrated excellent nocturnal ventilation through a nasal mask with chinstrap, with SaO_2 levels $> 95\%$ and no rise in PtcCO$_2$. However he was, by then, using mouthpiece ventilation

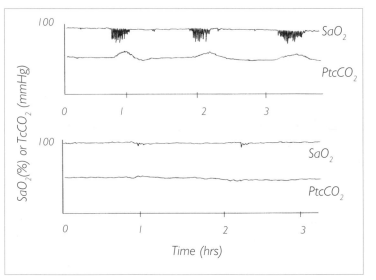

Figure 14.2: SaO$_2$ and PtcCO$_2$ tracings from the treatment nights of a patient with Duchenne Muscular dystrophy managed with nocturnal mask ventilation. Top panel: During a follow-up review where the patient was using a full face mask and volume preset ventilator, significant falls in SaO$_2$ during REM sleep occurred along with rises in PtcCO$_2$. During these episodes, although high airway pressures were generated, there was little or no chest wall movement, suggestive of upper airway obstruction. Bottom panel: illustrates the improvement in gas exchange on a subsequent night when the face mask was replaced with a nasal mask and chinstrap. The patient had a large tongue and during the night of nasal mask ventilation, movement of the tongue forward during the inspiratory phase of ventilatory support could be observed. This forward displacement aided in creating a seal during inspiration. In all patients, but particularly those with progressive disorders, it is important to distinguish between disease progression and technical problems in order to appropriately manage any deterioration in the patient's condition.

via the volume-preset device for the majority of the day. He was satisfied with his lifestyle, and despite almost total dependence on ventilatory support had wheelchair mobility and continued to participate well in his family and community groups.

Is NIV indicated?

As illustrated in this case, oxygen therapy in any patient with a nocturnal hypoventilation syndrome will improve nocturnal saturation; however, it frequently does so at the expense of a higher apnea/hypopnea index, worsening sleep quality and increased CO_2. Severe hypercapnia and changes in pH may occur even when low flow oxygen is given, especially when hypercapnia is already present (Masa *et al*, 1997; Plant *et al*, 2000a). Where nocturnal hypoventilation is present or suspected, NIV must be considered as first line therapy. Should the patient reject this approach, appropriate nocturnal and daytime monitoring needs to be employed to ensure that the use of oxygen therapy does not simply hasten further hypercapnia.

Which device?

This case illustrates how both volume and pressure preset ventilators can be used at various times both during the evolution of the disease and across 24 hours to provide adequate ventilatory support to meet the patient's clinical needs and lifestyle demands. Where a patient fails to respond as expected to mask ventilation, a sleep study can be valuable in determining if the problem is a technical one (insufficient volumes or pressures, overventilation, leak), or if there has been a change in the patient's underlying condition.

Although the various types of machines differ in terms of built-in features and bench-top performance, there is no evidence that these differences have a significant impact on the clinical outcomes. However, where a patient does not respond to therapy satisfactorily using one type of device, it is worth trialing another type to see if a better outcome can be achieved (Schonhofer *et al*, 1997; Smith and Schneerson, 1997). Where both types of device are equally effective, patients tend to find pressure-preset devices more comfortable (Schonhofer *et al*, 1997). In addition, an advantage of pressure-preset devices over their volume-preset counterparts is their ability to compensate for leak. They do this by varying flow to maintain airway pressure. Clinicians should not become complacent in thinking that maintaining airway pressure is the same as maintaining effective ventilation. If a significant leak is present (usually through the mouth), sleep disruption and deterioration in gas exchange will occur (Meyer *et al*, 1997).

Which interface?

For patients using NIV on a long-term basis, the therapy must be well tolerated and used regularly if an effective outcome is to be achieved. Compliance with therapy can only be expected if the patient is satisfied and comfortable with the interface. Although most patients in the home setting are likely to use a nasal mask, there are a range of interface types and mask designs that can be considered to provide the most comfortable and appropriate delivery of therapy.

When choosing an interface for therapy, clinicians will be guided by a number of factors including mask availability and sizing, experience with fitting, nasal patency, the patient's dentition and facial anatomy. In most cases, a nasal mask will be the first choice when initiating therapy.

These come in a wide range of sizes and styles. If the patient is unable to maintain lip closure and minimize leak when awake, it is not likely that they will do so when asleep. This can be seen in patients with myotonic dystrophy or facial muscle weakness due to other neuromuscular disorders such as motor neuron disease. Likewise, patients with a prominent overbite or retrognathia can find it difficult to keep their lips together even with the use of a chinstrap. In these situations, a face mask should be trialed.

Other patients may do well during wakefulness with a nasal mask but with sleep onset, or during REM sleep, the mouth will open, resulting in clinically significant mouth leaks. In some patients an appropriately fashioned chinstrap can be enough to aid lip closure effectively. If this fails, and mouth leaks during sleep are large enough to disturb sleep or cause effective ventilation to be lost, a face mask needs to be considered. Nasal prongs or plugs are useful where there is a problem with pressure areas on the nasal bridge or in some cases of claustrophobia. They are also helpful as an alternate interface for patients requiring more than 12 hours ventilatory support a day.

Mouthpieces also have a role here. By alternating between masks, nasal plugs and mouthpieces many patients are able to maintain, comfortably and effectively, ventilatory support across a 24-hour period for months, even years, without problems of skin breakdown or ulceration. Since it is the patient who must ultimately wear the mask, their preference once a number of different masks are trialed is important. Other considerations such as cleaning of the mask, simplicity of mask assembly and ease with which the mask can be placed or removed can all influence the type and style of mask the patient will use.

Monitoring therapy

Once NIV is commenced, polysomnography is performed during nocturnal ventilation and at regular ongoing intervals to ensure that the therapy is as effective as it possibly can be, with particular emphasis on the presence and clinical impact of any mouth leaks. Follow up is especially important for those individuals with progressive disorders to determine if deterioration in nocturnal ventilation, or a change in their primary disorder, is responsible for a decline in awake blood gases or change in symptoms.

The first step is to check the equipment the patient is using to ensure that the device and accessories have been set up as prescribed. Compliance with therapy is also an important factor that will influence the patient's response to therapy, and should be recorded regularly. Failure to achieve improvements in symptoms and/or blood gases may simply reflect insufficient use. Timer devices are now built into most devices providing useful information about average nightly use. If the patient is compliant with therapy, and the equipment is set up and operating as it should, then a repeat sleep study on therapy can be useful in establishing problems in the interaction between the patient and the machine, or inadequate/inappropriate settings.

In this clinical case, the polysomnogram allowed us to identify an unexpected but significant technical problem with therapy that had resulted in worsening of nocturnal and daytime blood gases. Failure to recognize and correct this problem would have resulted in the patient unnecessarily increasing his daytime use of therapy to improve blood gases. In progressive disorders, as further respiratory muscle weakness becomes apparent, deterioration in blood gases despite NIV has to be expected. Although some patients respond initially to changes in pressures or rate, eventually the duration of ventilatory assistance will need to be increased. The patient and their carers need to be informed of this eventuality to ensure that this is the way they wish to proceed when the need arises. Alternative management approaches, such as tracheostomy and palliation, as well as advanced medical directives, are other crucial issues that need to be discussed. However, prior to setting off on this path it is critical to identify any reversible causes of a decline in the patient's condition to ensure that the patient does not prematurely extend the use of NIV from overnight to daytime.

Case study 6: Motor neuron disease and increasing ventilator dependence

Kim Choy is a 65-year-old man who presented with worsening daytime dyspnea and inability to lie flat. He was troubled by disturbed sleep, waking unrefreshed and occasional morning headaches. These symptoms had been apparent for at least the last 4 months. He had a significant fall in vital capacity erect to supine (1.9 L erect to 0.7 L supine). Although a formal diagnosis of motor neurone disease had not been made, this was considered the most likely cause of his respiratory muscle dysfunction. His muscle weakness appeared to be confined primarily to the diaphragm and some left hand weakness. He was otherwise ambulatory and independent.

A sleep study was performed. This demonstrated fragmented sleep, with frequent hypopneas. Only stages I and II sleep were seen. His awake blood gases showed a $PaCO_2$ of 61 mmHg and PaO_2 of 50 mmHg. He was commenced on NIV as an inpatient and accepted it immediately, falling to sleep within minutes of therapy commencing. He remained in hospital for 4 days while he and his wife were trained in the use of the equipment. He used a nasal mask and chinstrap and a pressure-preset machine set in the S/T mode.

During the admission motor neuron disease was confirmed and long-term management options and issues were raised with him. A repeat sleep study on NIV was performed prior to discharge and demonstrated good control of nocturnal gas exchange with the reappearance of REM sleep. By discharge his wakeful spontaneous $PaCO_2$ had fallen to 51 mmHg.

According to normal clinical practice, Kim Choy was reviewed two months later to check the effectiveness of settings and to determine how he and his wife were coping with therapy. The patient reported feeling well, sleeping through the entire night on the device. A check of the machine time clock confirmed a mean usage of 8–9 hours/day. However, his wakeful $PaCO_2$ had increased again to 62 mmHg. On questioning, it was found that the patient had not used a chinstrap after the first week at home as 'he had trained himself to keep his mouth closed during sleep'. A sleep study was undertaken which quickly demonstrated large mouth leaks (*Figure 14.3a*). A chinstrap was added, with a significant improvement in both sleep quality and nocturnal gas exchange (*Figures 14.3b* and *14.3c*). The importance of minimizing leak was discussed with the patient who agreed to use the chinstrap.

Further follow-up 6 and 12 months later showed maintenance of daytime CO_2 in the range of 48–49 mmHg. He continued using ventilatory support for 26 months, initially at night only, but over time this increased to daytime use as well. He became increasingly short of breath off the machine and could no longer ambulate. When use of ventilatory support had extended to around

20–22 hours a day, he elected palliative care services to manage his dyspnea and reduced his time on ventilatory support. Mr Choy died around 8 days later.

Is NIV indicated?

Early in the history of its use, NIV was often considered inappropriate in patients with MND and other rapidly progressive neuromuscular disorders, as clinicians feared it might simply prolong the dying process. It is now offered to patients with MND with the aim of palliating symptoms and is used primarily at night and for short daytime periods. However, with disease progression, bulbar function will deteriorate, compromising upper airway protection and increasing the risk of aspiration. These issues and limitations of NIV should be discussed with the patient at the outset of initiating therapy. However, many patients are willing to trial and use this form of therapy if it improves their quality of life in the time that they have left.

Monitoring and follow-up

In the clinical case described here, follow-up early on was crucial to ensure the patient received the maximum benefit from therapy. Excessive air leaks through the mouth during sleep had caused a failure of effective ventilatory support. This problem is common in patients with facial muscle weakness using a nasal mask. Once the cause was identified, and the patient convinced of the need

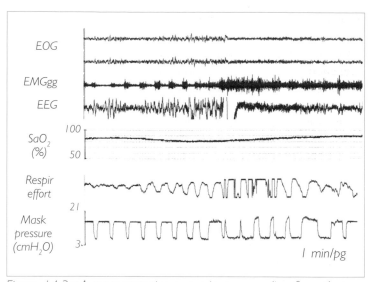

Figure 14.3a: A representative one minute recording from the polysomnogram performed in Case 6 during his routine 2-month review. The initial part of the study was performed without a chinstrap. Sleep was severely disrupted with prolonged inspiratory times and poor chest wall movement. Gas exchange was not well maintained. It appeared that large mouth leaks were the cause. Note also the continued high inspiratory activity apparent in the submental EMG (EOG = electrooculogram; EMGgg = submental electromyogram; EEG = electroencephalogram; respir effort = respiratory effort).

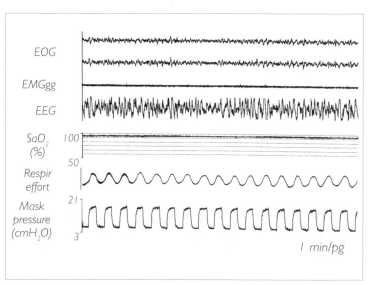

Figure 14.3b: An example from the polysomnogram showing NREM sleep once a chinstrap had been added, correcting the leak. Note the improvement in both sleep quality and oxygenation. Abbreviations as for Figure 14.3a.

to adopt the solution, improved nocturnal ventilation resulted in better daytime function and gas exchange.

A crucial element of patient management in this situation is to discuss with the patient issues related to disease progression, particularly their wishes regarding life-support measures. Patients need to be fully informed about the progressive nature of the disorder and the loss of function that will ensue, including increasing ventilatory dependence and loss of bulbar function. To date, in our experience, patients commenced on non-invasive support have not opted to be transferred to invasive support via tracheostomy. This type of decision is an individual one that will be influenced by a number of factors, including the patient's attitude towards loss of independence, feelings of being a burden on their family and cost.

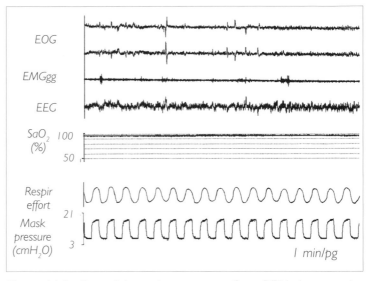

Figure 14.3c: Part of the polysomnogram from REM sleep on the same night with the chinstrap still in place. Leak was effectively controlled with a normal I:E ratio seen in the mask pressure channel. With improved nocturnal gas exchange, daytime blood gases also improved. Understanding the potential technical problems that can arise with mask ventilation is important in order to maximise the effectiveness of therapy longer term. Abbreviations as for Figure 14.3a.

Specific advanced directions about management, especially in an acute situation, need to be discussed and emphasized. Patients need to be informed that the purpose of NIV is to relieve symptoms, especially those related to sleep-disordered breathing. It is not primarily intended to prolong life, and its use may not be feasible especially in the presence of severe bulbar dysfunction. It needs to be made clear to the patient that respiratory deterioration will continue with eventual ventilator dependence which, together with bulbar dysfunction, is not manageable using NIV.

If the patient is suitable for and wishes to extend NIV to a more continuous basis, some number of management challenges will arise. The patient needs to have access to a number of different types of interfaces, including mouthpieces. Equipment may need to be upgraded or modified to allow it to be attached to and run off an electric wheelchair battery in order for the patient to maintain mobility. Additional alarms such as 'disconnect' or 'power off' should be added to ensure patient safety. A back-up device is advisable for the severely ventilator-dependent patient. With the advent of bulbar dysfunction, gastrostomy feeding tubes may be required to augment or replace oral intake, while tracheostomy is an option when the patient is no longer able to adequately protect the upper airway. Pharmacological and physical means of reducing oral secretions may also need to be employed.

The benefits of extending survival with ventilation will need to be balanced against the extra demands of treatment on the carers, the patient's level of discomfort and the patient's perception of their quality of life. After weighing up these factors some patients will decide to limit the period of time they will allow themselves to use ventilatory support daily or to cease it altogether. Once such a decision is made, it is important to have palliative care services involved to ensure that the patient remains comfortable and that any respiratory symptoms are alleviated promptly.

Accessories

As muscle weakness progresses the risk of aspiration increases, while the ability to mobilize and expectorate secretions is reduced. Techniques for assisting cough will need to be taught. These are of particular importance during episodes of chest infection. Manually assisted coughing can aid the force of expiration, and is usually more effective when combined with techniques to augment inspiration (Sivasothy *et al*, 2001). This can be achieved by using the volume-preset ventilator to provide a larger tidal volume or breath stacking. The insufflator–exsufflator is a commercially available device that is used to deliver high inspiratory pressures and then can be switched to negative pressure to generate a high expiratory flow to mobilize secretions. Caregivers need to be trained in applying these techniques.

Conclusion

NIV is effective in improving gas exchange in many causes of acute and chronic respiratory failure, and its role in the treatment of these conditions continues to grow. In the acute setting it can often be used at an earlier stage than one where intubation and invasive ventilation would be considered, often obviating the need for this. With acute exacerbations of COPD it has been shown to decrease in-hospital mortality and length of stay and has become a standard treatment for this common problem. It has a major role in the management of chronic respiratory failure due to restrictive chest wall disorders, such as those caused by respiratory muscle weakness, skeletal deformity and morbid obesity. Its role in the ongoing management of chronic respiratory failure in COPD remains to be defined, although some trials appear to demonstrate benefits for sleep quality and daytime gas exchange. Although the clinical circumstances will differ from patient to patient, the basic principles for establishing effective therapy are similar. Success of the treatment depends on the appropriateness of patient selection, the ability of the patient to tolerate therapy, and the skill of the clinician in choosing a device and interface that best meets the ventilatory need of the patient. Appropriate monitoring and follow-up are essential to ensure that changes in settings or interfaces are promptly identified so that ventilatory support is optimized and side-effects minimized.

Suggested reading

British Thoracic Society Guideline (2002) Non-invasive ventilation in acute respiratory failure. *Thorax* **57**: 192–211

Mehta S, Hill NS (2001) Non-invasive ventilation. *Am J Respir Crit Care Med* **163**: 540–77

References

Adnet F, Racine SX, Lapostolle F, Cohen Y, Cupa M, Minadeo J (2001) Full reversal of hypercapnic coma by noninvasive positive pressure ventilation. *Am J Emerg Med* **19**: 244–6

Ambrosino N, Foglio K, Rubini F, Clini E, Nava S, Vitacca M (1995) Non-invasive mechanical ventilation in acute respiratory failure due to chronic obstructive pulmonary disease: correlates for success. *Thorax* **50**: 755–7

Antonelli M, Conti G, Bufi M *et al* (2000) Non-invasive ventilation for the treatment of acute respiratory failure in patients undergoing solid organ transplantation. *JAMA* **283**: 235–41

Antonelli M, Conti G, Rocco M *et al* (1998) A comparison of non-invasive positive pressure ventilation and conventional mechanical ventilation in patients with acute respiratory failure. *N Engl J Med* **339**: 429–35

Appendini L, Patessio A, Zanaboni S *et al* (1994) Physiologic effects of positive end-expiratory pressure and mask pressure support during exacerbations of chronic obstructive pulmonary disease. *Am J Respir Crit Care Med* **149**: 1069–76

Ballard RD, Clover CW, Suh BY (1995) Influence of sleep on respiratory function in emphysema. *Am J Respir Crit Care Med* **151**(4): 945–51

Bott J, Carroll MP, Conway JH *et al* (1993) Randomised controlled trial of nasal ventilation in acute respiratory failure due to chronic obstructive airways disease. *Lancet* **341**: 1555–7

British Thoracic Society Guidelines (2002) Non-invasive ventilation in acute respiratory failure. *Thorax* **57**: 192–211

Brochard L, Mancebo J, Wysocki M *et al* (1995) Non-invasive ventilation for acute exacerbations of chronic obstructive pulmonary disease. *N Engl J Med* **333**: 817–22

Casanova C, Celli BR, Tost L, Soriano E, Abreu J, Velasco V, Santolaria F (2000) Long-term controlled trial of nocturnal nasal positive pressure ventilation in patients with severe COPD. *Chest* **118**: 1582–90

Clini E, Sturani C, Rossi A, Viaggi S, Corrado A, Donner CF, Ambronsio N (2002) The Italian multicentre study on non-invasive ventilation in chronic obstructive pulmonary disease patients. *Eur Respir J* **20**: 529–38

Confaloneri M, Potena A, Carbone G, Della Porta R, Tolley EA, Meduri GU (1999) Acute respiratory failure in patients with severe community-acquired pneumonia. A prospective randomized evaluation of noninvasive ventilation. *Am J Respir Crit Care Med* **160**: 1585–91

Criner GJ, Brennan K, Travaline JM, Kreimer D (1999) Efficacy and compliance with noninvasive positive pressure ventilation in patients with chronic respiratory failure. *Chest* **116**: 667–75

Elliot MW, Confalonieri M, Nava S (2002) Where to perform noninvasive ventilation? *Eur Respir J* **19**: 1159–66

Fernandez MM, Villagra A, Blanch L, Fernandez R (2001) Non-invasive mechanical ventilation in status asthmaticus. *Intensive Care Med* **27**: 486–92

Fletcher EC, Gray BA, Levin DC (1983) Nonapneic mechanisms of arterial oxygen desaturation during rapid eye movement sleep. *J Appl Physiol* **54**: 632–9

Gay PC, Hubmayr RD, Stroetz RW (1996) Efficacy of nocturnal nasal ventilation in stable, severe chronic obstructive pulmonary disease during a 3-month controlled trial. *Mayo Clin Proc* **71**: 533–42

Gilmartin JJ, Cooper BG, Griffiths GJ *et al* (1991) Breathing during sleep in patients with myotonic dystrophy and nonmyotonic respiratory muscle weakness. *Q J Med* **78**: 21–31

Girault C, Richard J-C, Chevron V, Tamion F, Pasquis P, Leroy J, Bonmarchand G (1997) Comparative physiologic effects of noninvasive assist-control and pressure support ventilation in acute hypercapnic respiratory failure. *Chest* **111**: 1639–48

Girou E, Schortgen F, Delclaux C, *et al* (2000) Association of noninvasive ventilation with nosocomial infections and survival in critically ill patients. *JAMA* **284**: 2361–7

Gregoretti C, Beltrame F, Lucangelo V, Burbi L, Conti G, Turello M, Gregori D (1998) Physiologic evaluation of non-invasive pressure support ventilation in trauma patients with acute respiratory failure. *Intens Care Med* **24**: 785–90

Hilbert G, Gruson D, Vargas F *et al* (2001) Non-invasive ventilation in immunosuppressed patients with pulmonary infiltrates, fever, and acute respiratory failure. *N Engl J Med* **344**: 481–7

Hukins CA, Hillman DR (2000) Daytime predictors of sleep hypoventilation in Duchenne muscular dystrophy. *Am J Respir Crit Care Med* **161**: 166–70

Keenan SP, Brake D (1998) An evidence-based approach to noninvasive ventilation in acute respiratory failure. *Crit Care Clin* **14**: 359–72

Kramer N, Meyer TJ, Meharg J, Cece RD, Hill NS (1995) Randomised, prospective trial of noninvasive positive pressure ventilation in acute respiratory failure. *Am J Respir Crit Care Med* **151**: 1799–806

Lellouche F, Maggiore SM, Deye N, Taille S, Pigeot J, Harf A, Brochard L (2002) Effect of the humidification device on the work of breathing during noninvasive ventilation. *Intensive Care Med* **28**: 1582–9

Lin CC (1996) Comparison between nocturnal nasal positive pressure ventilation combined with oxygen therapy and oxygen monotherapy in patients with severe COPD. *Am J Respir Crit Care Med* **154**: 353–8

Masa JF, Celli BR, Riesco JA, Sanchez de Cos J, Disdier C, Sojo A (1997) Non-invasive positive pressure ventilation and not oxygen may prevent overt ventilatory failure in patients with chest wall disease. *Chest* **112**: 207–13

Masip J, Betbes AJ, Vecilla F *et al* (2000) Non-invasive pressure support ventilation versus conventional oxygen therapy in acute cardiogenic pulmonary oedema: a randomized trial. *Lancet* **356**: 2126–32

Medical Research Council Working Party (1981) Long-term domiciliary oxygen in chronic hypoxic cor pulmonale complicating chronic bronchitis and emphysema. *Lancet* **1**: 681–6

Meecham Jones DJ, Paul EA, Jones PW, Wedzicha JA (1995) Nasal pressure support ventilation plus oxygen compared with oxygen therapy alone in hypercapnic COPD. *Am J Respir Crit Care Med* **152**: 538–44

Meecham Jones DJ, Wedzicha JA (1993) Comparison of pressure and volume preset nasal ventilator systems in stable chronic respiratory failure. *Eur Respir J* **6**: 1060–4

Meyer TJ, Pressman MR, Benditt J *et al* (1997) Air leaking through the mouth during nocturnal nasal ventilation: effect on sleep quality. *Sleep* **20**: 561–9

Navalesi P, Fanfulla F, Frigerio P, Gregoretti C, Nava S (2000) Physiologic evaluationof noninvasive mechanical ventilation delivered with three types of masks in patients with chronic hypercapnic respiratory failure. *Crit Care Med* **28**: 1785–90

Nocturnal Oxygen Therapy Trial Group (1980) Continuous or nocturnal oxygen therapy in hypoxemic chronic obstructive lung disease. *Ann Intern Med* **93**: 391–8

Ono S, Takahashi K, Jinnai K *et al* (1998) Loss of catecholaminergic neurons in the medullary reticular formation in myotonic dystrophy. *Neurology* **51**: 1121–4

Pennock BE, Crawshaw L, Kaplan PD (1994) Non-invasive nasal mask ventilation for acute respiratory failure. Institution of a new therapeutic technology for routine use. *Chest* **105**: 441–4

Phua J, Kong K, Hoe Lee K, Shen L, Lim TK (2005) Non-invasive ventilation in hypercapnic acute respiratory failure due to chronic obstructive airway pulmonary disease vs other conditions: effectiveness and predictors of failure. *Intensive Care Med* **31**: 533–9

Piper AJ, Sullivan CE (1994) Sleep-disordered breathing in neuromuscular disease. In: Saunders NA, Sullivan CE, eds. *Sleep and Breathing*. 2nd edn. Marcel Dekker, New York

Plant PK, Owen JL, Elliott MW (2000a) One year prevalence study of respiratory acidosis in acute exacerbations of COPD: implications for the provision of non-invasive ventilation and oxygen administration. *Thorax* **55**: 550–4

Plant PK, Owen JL, Elliott MW (2000b) Early use of non-invasive ventilation for acute exacerbations of chronic obstructive pulmonary disease on general respiratory wards: a multicentre randomized controlled trial. *Lancet* **355**: 1931–5

Ram FS, Picot J, Lightowler J, Wedzicha JA (2004) Non-invasive positive pressure ventilation for treatment of respiratory failure due to exacerbations of chronic obstructive pulmonary disease. Cochrane Database of Systematic Reviews (3): CD004104

Raphael JC, Chevret S, Chastang C, Bouvet F (1994) Randomised trial of preventative nasal ventilation in Duchenne muscular dystrophy. *Lancet* **343**: 1600–4

Rocker GM, Mackenzie MG, Williams B, Logan PM (1999) Non-invasive positive pressure ventilation. Successful outcome in patients with acute lung injury/ARDS. *Chest* **115**: 173–7

Schonhofer B, Sonneborn M, Haidl P, Bohrer H, Kohler D (1997) Comparison of two different modes of noninvasive mechanical ventilation in chronic respiratory failure; volume versus pressure controlled device. *Eur Respir J* **10**: 184–91

Shneerson JM, Simonds AK (2002) Non-invasive ventilation for chest wall and neuromuscular disorders. *Eur Respir J* **20**: 480–7

Sivasothy P, Brown L, Smith IE, Shneerson JM (2001) Effect of manually assisted cough and mechanical insufflation on cough flow of normal subjects, patients with chronic obstructive pulmonary disease (COPD), and patients with respiratory muscle weakness. *Thorax* **56**: 438–44

Smith IE, Shneerson JM (1997) Secondary failure of nasal intermittent positive pressure ventilation using the Monnal D: effects of changing the ventilator. *Thorax* **52**: 89–91

Strumpf DA, Millman RP, Carlisle CC, Grattan LM, Ryan SM, Erickson AD, Hill NS (1991) Nocturnal positive-pressure ventilation via nasal mask in patients with severe chronic obstructive pulmonary disease. *Am Rev Respir Dis* **144**(6): 1234–9

Vianello A, Bevilacqua M, Arcaro G, Gallan F, Serra E (2000) Non-invasive ventilatory approach to treatment of acute respiratory failure in neuromuscular disorders. A comparison with endotracheal intubation. *Intens Care Med* **26**(4): 384–90

Wijkstra PJ (2003) Non-invasive positive pressure ventilation (NIPPV) in stable patients with chronic obstructive pulmonary disease (COPD). *Respiratory Med* **97**(10): 1086–93

Wijkstra PJ, Lacasse Y, Guyatt GH, Goldstein RS (2002) Nocturnal non-invasive positive pressure ventilation for stable chronic obstructive pulmonary disease. Cochrane Database of Systematic Reviews (3): CD002878

Index